Clinical Phonetics

Third Edition

Clinical Phonetics

Lawrence D. Shriberg
University of Wisconsin–Madison

Raymond D. Kent
University of Wisconsin–Madison

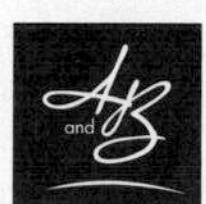

Boston New York San Francisco
Mexico City Montreal Toronto London Madrid Munich Paris
Hong Kong Singapore Tokyo Cape Town Sydney

Executive Editor and Publisher: Stephen D. Dragin
Editorial Assistant: Barbara Strickland
Editorial-Production Coordinator: Joe Sweeney
Editorial-Production Service: Heckman & Pinette
Composition and Prepress Buyer: Linda Cox
Manufacturing Manager: Megan Cochran
Cover Administrator: Linda Knowles
Electronic Composition: Publishers' Design and Production Services, Inc.

For related titles and support materials, visit our online catalog at www.ablongman.com

Library of Congress Cataloging-in-Publication Data
Shriberg, Lawrence D.
Clinical phonetics / Lawrence D. Shriberg, Raymond D. Kent.—3rd. ed.
p. cm.
Includes bibliographical references and index.
ISBN 0-205-36833-6 (alk. paper)
1. Speech therapy. 2. Phonetics. 3. English language—Phonetics. I. Kent, Raymond D. II. Title.

RC423 .S515 2003
616.85'5—dc21 2002028027

Printed in the United States of America

10 10 09

To our families:
Linda, Elizabeth, Kathryn, and Janet
Jane, Laurel, and Jason

Contents

Foreword

I feel a little like a godparent to *Clinical Phonetics.* I witnessed its birth in the first edition, followed its development in the second edition, and now am looking at its extraordinary maturity in this third edition. Its parents, Shriberg and Kent, have done a masterful job over the years in expanding, modernizing, and making the book user friendly to instructors and students. Both authors are steeped in research and its translation to clinical endeavors. This shows in every nook and cranny of the text. This is an important book, and it demonstrates a special brand of passion for its topic. As a teacher, I feel palpable excitement in examining the galley proofs for the book. The next generation of students has something very special here, and Shriberg and Kent are to be admired for the teaching skills they demonstrate in the assembly of this exciting third edition of the book. This is *the* text on the topic. It stands head and shoulders and more above other contenders, and its solid base and quality make it a model for those who would aspire to blend basic science and practical application.

Those who have used earlier editions of this book will find this new edition to preserve the best of the traditions of earlier versions and to add to them some very attractive new features. The authors lay these out in detail in their Preface to this edition, where they discuss how they have expanded teaching examples and made them more readily accessible. These are not cosmetic changes to the second edition of *Clinical Phonetics.* They are full-blown substantive additions. Some of the many include new information on languages other than American English, new information on acoustic phonetics, new information on speech sampling and audio recording, new information on dialect and language variation across cultures, new information on contemporary analysis of infant vocalizations, new CD-ROMs, and a new Web site with supplementary materials.

This third edition of *Clinical Phonetics* is a new one-of-a-kind and raises the standard even further for the discipline. I can't imagine teaching a course in clinical phonetics without using this new text. Having had the opportunity to see all three editions of this text, it is safe to say that this third time really is the charm. Applause to Shriberg and Kent once again.

Thomas J. Hixon
University of Arizona

Preface

Welcome to the third edition of *Clinical Phonetics.* Like the peripatetic pink bunny, *CP* seems to have kept on trucking into the next millennium. A special thanks to those instructors who have been with us since the second or perhaps even the first edition! Thanks too, for your continued positive comments and specific suggestions for this revision.

The most frequent request during the past few years was to try to expand the teaching examples and to make them readily accessible. We have tried to do both. Although the fundamentals of phonetic transcription have not changed since the first edition, media options for skills acquisition have increased significantly. We hope the features described below enhance both the teaching and the learning experience for students and instructors as you complete a course of study in clinical phonetics.

WHAT'S NEW

This third edition of *Clinical Phonetics* retains the ten chapters designed for a semester-length course. We have also kept the appendixes that provide reference materials and other information for additional reading and applied needs in the clinic and laboratory. The "What's Old" section of the Preface to the Second Edition includes useful information on the transcription system taught in this textbook. Instructors using this book for the first time should also read Notes to Instructors, which includes class-tested suggestions for alternative ways to use the book and the audio examples. We have also updated references wherever possible throughout the text. Clearly, however, many of the classic papers in phonetics stand as the best and, for many topics, as the only available sources of information or data. The following are the major text and media enhancements in *Clinical Phonetics,* 2003:

- Chapter 4, Vowels and Diphthongs, has additional information on vowels in languages other than American English, including a section on the difficulties in learning vowels in a second language.
- Chapter 5, Consonants, has new information on consonants that occur in other languages, with a section on trills, clicks, ejectives, and voiced implosives.
- Chapter 6, Diacritics and Sounds in Context, includes an expanded discussion of coarticulation.
- Chapter 10, Acoustic Phonetics, provides a discussion of formant frequencies for vowels in different languages (with implications for second-language learning) and expanded coverage of the suprasegmental features of loudness, vocal effort, and boundary effects.
- Appendix E, Procedures for Speech Sampling and Audio Recording, has been expanded to include technical information on the selection and use of alternative microphones and recorders for analog and digital recording.
- A new appendix, Appendix F, Dialect: Language Variations across Cultures, written by Linda Carpenter (University of Wisconsin–Eau Claire), focuses on concepts and skills needed for phonetic transcription of regional, social, and foreign dialects; it also includes new audio examples.
- A new appendix, Appendix G, Infant Vocalizations, describes contemporary systems for the transcription of babbling and other vocalizations produced by infants.
- A new appendix, Appendix H, Anatomic Bases of Developmental Phonetics, provides basic summaries of the anatomic development of the respiratory, laryngeal, and articulatory systems of speech production.
- A new set of four CDs has been made available for the transcription skills modules, including the new Appendix F audio samples. Both the CDs and a comparable set of audiocassette tape recordings may be obtained by contacting a bookstore, your local Allyn & Bacon sales representative, or the Allyn & Bacon order department, (800) 852-8024, for instructors, or (800) 278-3525 for student purchases.
- A *Clinical Phonetics* Web site (http://www.ablongman.com/shriberg) provides a number of instructional resources for instructors and students. The Web site includes instructions on how to download the PEPPER font, which is available at no cost at http://www.waisman.wisc.edu/phonology/. The PEPPER font includes all of the main character and diacritic symbols used in *Clinical Phonetics.* Instructors and students should find this font useful for quizzes and for other manuscript needs requiring electronic entry of phonetic symbols. The *Clinical Phonetics* Web site also includes additional transcription practice samples from persons with a variety of speech disorders, sample quizzes for

each of the ten chapters and eight appendixes, technical support information for the PEPPER font, and links to other sites that have interesting audio examples and other information on phonetics transcription.

ACKNOWLEDGMENTS

In addition to the dozens of people whom we have thanked for their significant contributions to the prior editions of *Clinical Phonetics,* we are very grateful to the following colleagues for their expert assistance and guidance with this revision. Our sincere thanks to:

Katherina Hauner, Waisman Center, University of Wisconsin–Madison, for her thorough, thoughtful, and cheerful editorial assistance with every aspect of this revision.

Linda Carpenter, University of Wisconsin–Eau Claire, for her well-articulated discussion of dialects and the unique challenges they pose in contemporary clinical phonetics.

Jane McSweeny, Waisman Center, University of Wisconsin–Madison, for her assistance with a variety of tasks reflecting her expertise in phonetic transcription of child speech-sound disorders, including selection and authorship of supplementary audio examples for the *Clinical Phonetics* Web site.

Peter Flipsen, Jr., University of Tennessee, Knoxville, for his significant contributions to the CD samples and authorship of supplementary practice material for the *Clinic Phonetics* Web site.

Martin Ball, John Esling, Ben Maassen, and Thomas Powell for their gracious assistance in providing phonetics materials and resources for the appendixes.

Connie Nadler and Steve Pittelko, Waisman Center, University of Wisconsin–Madison, and Ron Holder, University of Tennessee, Knoxville, for their expert mastering of the CDs and supplementary audiocassette samples.

We would also like to thank the following reviewers: Anna Marie Schmidt of Kent State University and Alice T. Dyson of the University of Florida.

Steve Dragin, Executive Editor and Publisher, Allyn & Bacon, for his consistent support of *Clinical Phonetics* over the years and his congenial guidance with all aspects of the current revision.

Barbara Strickland, Editorial Assistant, Allyn & Bacon, for her valued editorial assistance and contributions at every step of the publication process.

Larry Shriberg
Ray Kent

Preface to the Second Edition

It has been over a decade since the first edition of *Clinical Phonetics.* Many words of encouragement from colleagues who have used this text over the years suggested that it was time for a revision. We have it on good authority that the most important need was to "get a new binding—one that doesn't self destruct!" Sorry about that. Many thanks to all instructors who developed ingenious ways to keep intact their well-annotated, but ever disintegrating, desk copies.

WHAT'S NEW?

Content

Revisions in the content of this second edition focus primarily on updating and expansion. Because each section of the book is used in one phonetics course or another, we have not deleted any of the original chapters. Thus, instructors will find everything pretty much in the same place. The only deletion is the former Appendix F, which provided references for phonological analysis—these procedures are now taught routinely in courses in developmental phonological disorders.

We hope we have added some nice treats throughout the text. We have updated references throughout the book. Students should know that many older references in phonetics remain the classic or perhaps only source of information on some topics. Expansions in the text include information on the assessment of prosody and an overview of microcomputer systems for acoustic analysis. Expanded and new appendixes include the following:

Appendix D: research findings on the reliability of phonetic transcription.

Appendix E: guidelines for speech sampling and audiotape recording.

Appendix F: multicultural and multilingual considerations in phonetic transcription.

Appendix G: systems to transcribe infant vocalizations.

Format

Revisions in the format of the text (e.g., two-column text) should enhance readability and ease of use and reference. The graphics and subheadings now include color for emphasis. Frequently used tables have been placed in the inside cover pages for ready reference. The index has been redone too.

Audiotapes and Clinical Phonetics Font

The audiotapes that accompany the text may be obtained by contacting your local sales representative or bookstore.

A font that produces all of the symbols and diacritics in *Clinical Phonetics* is available for several platforms. Instructors and researchers should find the font, termed the PEPPER Font, useful to insert phonetic symbols in quizzes and manuscripts requiring broad and narrow phonetic transcription characters. Students and clinicians should find it useful for papers and clinical reports.

WHAT'S OLD?

A Note on the *Clinical Phonetics* Transcription System

Our primary motivation when we wrote the first edition of *Clinical Phonetics* was to offer students in communicative disorders a phonetics book that was directly relevant to clinical application. This is not to say that traditional courses in phonetics are not worthwhile to students in communicative disorders, but simply to reflect our experience that students who took traditional phonetics instruction were often at a loss when faced with clients who had speech disorders. Surely not everyone believes as we do. However, our opinion is shared by many; so many, in fact, that the International Phonetic Alphabet (IPA) was revised in 1989 to include symbols for the transcription of disordered speech. These additions were termed the "Extensions to the International Phonetic Alphabet" and were sanctioned by the International Phonetic Association. In describing the rationale for these additions, Duckworth, Allen, Hardcastle, and Ball wrote, "People working with individuals who have speech which is not the same as that of the adult community in which they live, have long recognized the limitations of the International Phonetic Alphabet (IPA) for transcribing such speech" (*Clinical Linguistics and Phonetics,* Volume 4, p. 273). We believe that the limitations are significant and therefore welcome the Extensions to the IPA, which are included in Appendix A, Table A-6 of this edition.

Some readers may wonder why we did not simply accept the Extensions to the IPA as a solution to the transcription of disordered speech. There were two reasons. The first was a practical one—it was easier to retain the special symbols introduced in the first edition. These symbols were used in the text and in the answer keys for the transcription exercises. The second—and major—reason was that we preferred the simplicity of the original system to the IPA Extensions. The original system established conventions for the placement of the special "diacritic" symbols. In our teaching experience, the arbitrary placement of diacritic symbols was a stumbling point for students who not only had to remember the symbol for a particular sound modification but also where to place that special symbol in the transcription. We believed, and continue to believe, that life could be easier. Therefore, we continue to use the original system with only minor modification. The modification is designed to make things even easier by enhancing the consistency of symbol location.

Another innovation in the first edition was a system of stress marking based on numbers rather than on the stress symbols used in the IPA. We have retained the number system because it has served us well in clinical transcription and because it overcomes some difficulties with the stress-marking conventions of the IPA. One of these difficulties is that, in complex transcriptions, the stress marks of the IPA tend to be hard to distinguish from other phonetic symbols. The IPA stress marks are easily lost in the symbol-rich world of clinical transcription. The number-based system we favor separates stress marks from the other symbols used in phonetic transcription. This physical separation makes it much easier to scan a transcription for information on stress because the stress marks are always located in the top line of the transcription. Of course, we teach our own students both the IPA system and our number-based system. Ultimately, the students can select the system they prefer. And that is our advice to all readers of this book: Use the system that is most convenient and most useful to you.

ACKNOWLEDGMENTS

The Preface to the First Edition included a hefty list of persons whose efforts and talents made possible the first edition of *Clinical Phonetics.* To each of you—these many years later—thanks once again. *Thanks also to:*

The many friends and colleagues who have taken the time to express kind words about the value of *Clinical Phonetics* in their training programs. In the blur of professional activities within one's discipline, this positive feedback has really meant a lot to us.

Mary Anne Reeves, a former student and later phonetics instructor at the University of Wisconsin–Madison, who provided a detailed list of typographic errors in the first edition and thoughtful suggestions for changes in form and content.

Karen Carlson, a clinical instructor at the University of Wisconsin–Madison. Drawing on her broad experience with nonnative-English-speaking persons, Karen has authored a unique set of transcription guidelines for clinical transcription in multicultural and multilingual environments.

Jamie Murray-Branch, a clinical instructor at the University of Wisconsin–Madison, and her lovely daughter Charmaine, for illustrating the process of speech sampling, transcription, and analysis.

Shirley Hunsaker, photographer at the Waisman Center for Mental Retardation and Human Development, for the excellent photographs.

Darlene Davies, San Diego State University; Michael Moran, Auburn University; Susan Moss-Logan, University of Central Arkansas; and Roberta Wacker-Mundy, SUNY-Plattsburgh, whose thoughtful reviews of the first edition of *Clinical Phonetics* helped us formulate our approach to this edition.

David Wilson, Senior Systems Programmer at the University of Wisconsin–Madison, for creative collaboration in the design, coding, and documentation of the PEPPER Font.

Jane McSweeney, Program Assistant at the University of Wisconsin–Madison, for competent editorial assistance at many phases of this project.

Diane Austin, Research Specialist at the University of Wisconsin–Madison, for remarkable excellence in coauthoring the PEPPER Font and associated graphics, and for thorough and congenial copyediting of this busy manuscript.

Thomas Hixon, University of Arizona, a long-time friend and colleague whose gracious and supportive Forewords have launched both editions of *Clinical Phonetics.*

Larry Shriberg
Ray Kent

Preface to the First Edition

A preface allows authors an "up front" opportunity to express their hopes, regrets, and thanks. Here are ours.

We hope that this book does the job it was intended to do. Several years ago we recognized that something was missing in phonetics textbooks. The existing textbooks lacked materials that taught the specific information and perceptual skills needed by speech-language clinicians. This book and the companion audiotapes are our attempt to meet this need. Our goal has been to assemble information and teach the discrimination skills that are relevant for the use of phonetics in the practice of clinical speech-language pathology. We won't retrace here our lengthy journey toward that end. Moreover, we will spare the reader a list of the features that we believe make our effort unique among available phonetics texts. We hope that instructors will find these materials to be as effective with their students as we have found them to be with ours. And for students, clinicians, and others who will progress through this series, we hope you will find it to be an efficient and enjoyable learning experience.

Regrets about what couldn't be included in the scope of this book would require another lengthy list—a list we also will not present here. Instructors will quickly discern for themselves what could not be accommodated within our goals for this text. Phonetics is taught in a variety of course structures within programs that cover communication disorders. We believe that this textbook has the flexibility to be used successfully, with supplementary readings and assignments provided as needed by course instructors.

One list we very much do want to present includes the names of the many persons who assisted us in developing both the text and the audio materials.

Our deepest thanks to:

Wayne Swisher, for co-authoring a 1972 paper on an articulation scoring system that was to become the prototype for the audiotape modules used in this text.

Kathleen Gruenewald and Joan Kwiatkowski, who are the excellent clinician-examiners on several of the lengthier tape segments.

Carol Caldwell, Catherine Jackson, Julie Baran Peterson, and Linda Wurzman, who each provided effective and efficient research assistance in culling, dubbing, and transcribing tape segments for possible inclusion in the series.

Shelly Bezack, Jill Brooks, Denise Dinan, Michele Goodman, Constance Kemper, and Sylvia Thompson, who each volunteered to participate in several pilot studies of phonetic transcription in audio versus video modes.

The several classes of undergraduate students who provided detailed feedback and suggestions for discrimination training.

Frederick Baecker, Stanley Ewanowski, Robert Nellis, and Francesca Spinelli, who each lent time and expertise to provide audio and visual materials used throughout the text.

William Horne, for his tireless, thorough guidance in preparation of the audiotapes.

Helen Goodluck, who provided expert counsel on source materials for Appendix F.

Anne J. Smith, whose scholarly research assistance is reflected throughout the text, particularly in the appendix materials dealing with phonetics systems and statistical summaries.

Thomas Klee and Christine Dollaghan for their thorough and efficient assistance with final stages of manuscript preparation, including the Index.

Mary Louise Edwards, Mary Elbert, and Elaine Paden, our expert listeners, who provided phonetic transcriptions of all audio materials and extremely useful suggestions on program content.

John Bernthal, Raphael Haller, and David Kuehn, for their productive editorial reviews of the manuscript.

Thomas Hixon, for his usual insightful review of the manuscript and his assistance with other phases of the project.

Carole Dugan, for a remarkable effort and performance in typing the manuscript.

The administrative and secretarial staffs at the Department of Communicative Disorders, University of Wisconsin–Madison, and at the Boys Town Institute for Communication Disorders in Children for their consistent support.

L. D. Shriberg
R. D. Kent

Notes to Instructors

We are mindful of the problems instructors face in becoming familiar with a new textbook. These notes bring together facts, impressions, and suggestions collected during field tests of this book with undergraduate students. Many of these observations concern the audiotaped discrimination modules. We hope both new and experienced instructors will find these comments relevant to their teaching task.

TECHNICAL NOTES

The audio materials were selected from a library of over 350 tapes originally made in public schools and speech-language clinics. Approximately 1500 individual sound and word segments were isolated for reproduction. These tape segments were fed by a Sony TC-27 audiotape recorder to a Crown Series 800 audiotape recorder, which was biased and equalized for Ampex 470 mastering tape. The master tapes, in turn, were fed from an Ampex Model 351 audiotape recorder through a 150 Hz high-pass filter to the Crown Series 800 recorder. The intensity of the most intense sound on each tape segment was balanced on the Crown recorder to peak within ± 1 dB of the calibration tone setting. The four audiocassette tapes and compact discs that accompany the text were reproduced from these master tapes and supplementary samples.

Field tests have been conducted with first-generation cassette dubs to ensure that they contain sufficient signal information for discrimination purposes. Their quality and fidelity have been endorsed by consultants and by the panel of five expert judges who contributed to the keys that accompany the tapes. We strongly discourage dubbing copies of the audio examples. Aside from violating copyright, important signal components might be lost from second-generation dubs.

CONTENT NOTES

Four particular content areas of this book warrant brief comment here.

We have found that intuition and verbal descriptions do not always help students to understand how sounds are produced. In writing this book, we have relied almost exclusively on tracings from X-ray films to illustrate the articulatory configurations of English sounds. Accordingly, the student can learn how sounds are produced from factual illustrations rather than contrived drawings. Only a few simplifications have been made in adapting the original X-ray tracings to published illustrations. We intentionally have oriented the X-ray tracings to face both left and right, because we believe it is important that the student be able to imagine vocal tract shapes no matter which way a speaker is facing. In our experience, students benefit from drawing vocal tract shapes for different sounds, and we recommend this exercise as a useful part of phonetics education.

The diacritic system presented in Chapter 6 and used in the transcription modules departs in some ways from other diacritic systems we have seen. The primary innovation in the system used in this book is the spatial orientation or location of the diacritic marks: all marks denoting a general class of sound modification, such as tongue articulation, laryngeal function, or velopharyngeal function, are placed in the same position relative to the phonetic symbol that is being modified. Thus, the various modifications of tongue articulation—such as dentalization, lateralization, palatalization, and rhotacization (a term we favor over retroflexion)—are all marked by placing the appropriate diacritic mark *below* the phonetic symbol that represents the sound segment. We have tried as much as possible to use the conventional characters for the diacritic marks, but we have changed their transcription positions. One benefit of this innovation is that it becomes easier for the student to remember the diacritic marks—because all marks of a particular class go in the same place. Another benefit is that the spatial position of a diacritic can carry some clinical meaning. For example, because the diacritics pertaining to velopharyngeal function are placed above the phonetic symbol being modified, the clinician can determine from a quick scan of a transcription the number and variety of modifications in velopharyngeal function.

A chapter entitled "Acoustic Phonetics" appears as the last chapter in the book. For those instructors who wish to include content in this area, we have provided a fairly detailed treatment of this topic. However, the remainder of the text has been written to be essentially independent of the information on acoustics. Thus, the student does not need to understand the acoustic information to read or apply the other information given in the text. Because the acoustics chapter has a relatively dense information content compared to the other chapters, students may require more time and guidance with it.

A fourth content area that instructors should consider is the material in the appendixes. Appendix B, in particular, is a consolidation of data that is useful for many types of class assignments, including preclinical exercises in the rationale for assembling stimulus materials. Beginning students are especially motivated to learn statistical information about English linguistic forms if this information is made "relevant" for their upcoming clinical practice. The materials in each of the other appendixes are also designed for use in clinical transcription in communicative disorders.

The final content note concerns the material and audio examples in Appendix F, Dialects. We have retained this new text and audio materials in an appendix so that instructors can decide where to position this topic in their course syllabus. Our experience indicates that some phonetics classes will want to schedule this information early in the semester, whereas other instructors may find it convenient to schedule consideration of speech differences after speech disorders. Alternatively, these materials may be included in a class focusing specifically on diversity issues in communicative disorders. Whichever the instructional approach, the appendix was written to provide undergraduates who are new to communicative disorders with a reasonably compact introduction to the history, issues, and procedural considerations associated with the transcription of dialects. The audio samples are provided only to demonstrate the latter needs across regional, social, and foreign dialects. As with different types of speech disorders, instructors will want to supplement the audio examples with examples relevant to their locale and relevant cultural communities. For instructors and students interested in pursuing specific issues in transcription of dialects, the transcriptions provided on the Web site should provide a good basis for instructor–student and student–student dialogue on alternative approaches using the clinical phonetics transcription system and other systems.

TRAINING NOTES

The key to the acquisition of discrimination skills is clearly *practice*. Questionnaire-discussion sessions with our students have yielded the following comments and suggestions about discrimination practice.

Time

Students should not be asked to do "too much, too soon." Of all comments about the program, this one was made most often by students. In the press of other coursework, students need to schedule time each day and each week to practice on the audio modules. Many students like to go over each module several times, returning later to certain modules as needed. Quizzes must be scheduled carefully to allow for adequately spaced practice throughout the semester.

Assistance

Some form of assistance should be available on a regular basis throughout the program, particularly for beginning students. Such help may be provided by the instructor, a teaching assistant, another student, or some other way to students when they simply "don't get it." Some approaches to group and individually guided assistance are listed as follows (see also Chapter 7).

- Classroom demonstrations using acoustic displays can be helpful in contrasting visually the target sound or sound errors with other sounds in question.
- Students can accomplish production-perception practice in pairs or in small groups. One person can produce (simulate) predetermined errors from a laboratory workshop, for example, while others transcribe what they hear on paper or at the blackboard. Differences in production and perception should then be discussed, with corrective feedback provided by the instructor and other students as necessary.
- The instructor can make recordings in which the same word is used in contrast drills; for example, "see" [s i], [s̪ i], [s̯ i], [s̢ i]. Students practice saying the same word with the different speech errors, gradually increasing their rate of production. Word forms can proceed from simple ("see") to more complex ("Mississippi").
- Students can generate their own lists of helpful comments, in addition to those provided in the text, describing how they have learned to make a particular sound change. As the text stresses, students must become able to produce each sound change readily before learning to discriminate it from other sound changes.
- Students can make their own recordings of particular sound changes. Students can trade recordings, score them, and discuss differences in conjunction with the instructor or within their own student sessions.

Grading

Instructors have several alternatives in grading the skills development portion of any academic coursework. In the ideal situation, instructors would use criterion-referenced grading of phonetics skill acquisition, assigning each student a grade based on the level of skill demonstrated at the conclusion of a period of training. This approach seems most ethical from the perspective of the consumer; that is, it will provide information about students' skill levels as they enter clinical practicum. However, a number of other grading practices are also defensible. Such matters are ultimately left to instructors to arrange within the context of their curricula in communication disorders. However, three issues related to any grading system are important to note here.

First, instructors will need to provide audio materials for quizzes. We have found it useful to use a combination of instructor stimuli (normal speech and error simulations) and audio samples from children (normal speech and errored speech) to test students' acquisition of discrimination skills. Such materials are initially challenging to construct. Over time, the instructor will accumulate a large pool of reliable recorded items, much like the accumulation of a set of useful objective test questions.

Second, the instructor needs to establish clearly the criteria used for determining grades based on the percentage of agreement between students' responses and the keys for quizzes. Appendix D describes three bases for calculating agreement—exact agreement, functional equivalence, and near functional equivalence. We have used each of these criteria, our choice depending on the difficulty level of the discrimination task. What is important is that students know exactly which criteria will be used to convert their quiz performance into grades. When considering grading criteria, the instructor should keep in mind that published studies involving speech errors (for example, / r /, / s / distortions) routinely report interjudge agreement percentages no higher than 75 to 80 percent (see also Chapter 7).

Especially in the early stages of a phonetics course, we have found it beneficial to use a rather lax criterion in grading transcription quizzes. One particular device that we have used is to give students a second-choice selection in transcription. That is, students are allowed to enter a second-choice symbol above their first-choice symbol. For example, in transcribing the word *dog,* a student who is unsure whether the vowel is / ɔ / or / ɑ / can write

ɑ
/ d ɔ g /

Although this option runs a certain risk of abuse (such as second-choice symbols for every element in a transcription), we never encounter such overuse. In fact, few students use the option as often as we might expect. However, students appreciate having a second choice, particularly for more subtle auditory discriminations. Some phonetic decisions are difficult to make, and not all errors in transcription are equal. As experiments have shown, not even the experts agree exactly in their phonetic transcriptions of the same utterance.

Third, as noted previously, it is important to gauge carefully the frequency and timing of quizzes throughout a period of training. We have found frequent quizzes covering small amounts of material to work well. Students need time to assimilate and consolidate their developing phonetics skills. If they feel rushed, fears and frustrations develop. Ideally, students should be allowed to schedule each quiz as they are ready, rather than scheduling the perceptual quizzes in large groups. Students especially appreciate efforts to allow for individual differences in level of entrance skills and in rates of learning throughout the training period.

PROGRAM NOTES

Students have indicated that there are benefits from the experience of progressing through the text and the audio modules beyond the informational content and skills acquisition. Instructors may wish to include lecture or discussion materials to augment the following observations made by students.

- They enjoy the opportunity to hear examples of children talking, an experience that for most beginning students is both educational and entertaining.
- They appreciate the opportunity to hear clinicians talking to children with speech errors, particularly to learn how competent clinicians talk to children who have severe intelligibility deficits.
- They profit from the exposure to several procedures for obtaining speech samples from children, including standard articulation tests and continuous speech sampling procedures.
- They learn to respect the variety of spoken forms of languages and individual differences across cultures and among speakers.
- They develop the discipline needed for learning independently, including learning to arrange their own listening schedule and study group sessions with other students.
- They experience the pride of accomplishment—with reference to the clinical phonetics component of speech pathology, they feel prepared to meet the challenge of their first clinical practicum assignment.

L. D. S.
R. D. K.

Contents of the Audio Samples

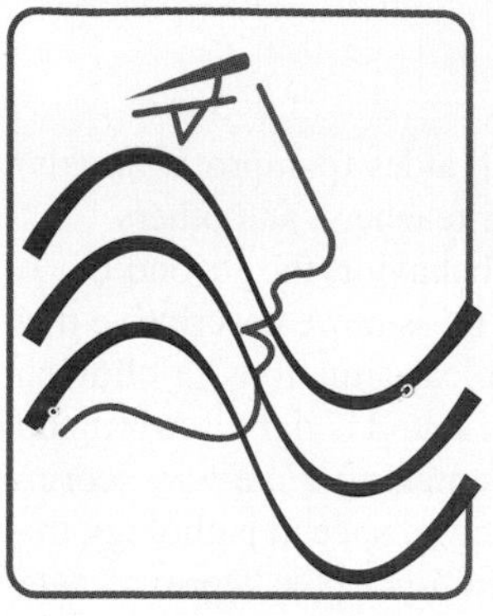

Overview of Clinical Phonetics

1

WELCOME

Beginning a new course of study is exciting. If this is one of your first courses in a program leading to a degree in communication disorders, we welcome you to a dynamic and challenging field. We hope that your interests and needs in phonetics will be met by this text. This opening overview is intended to help you get the "big picture" before you begin a chapter-by-chapter progression through this series.

What is **clinical phonetics,** and what role does it play in the training of a speech-language clinician?

CLINICAL PHONETICS

Phonetics is the study of the perception and production of speech sounds. Although subdisciplines within phonetics, such as articulatory phonetics and acoustic phonetics, are well established, formal accounts of phonetics as it applies to clinical areas are limited. In coining the term *clinical phonetics,* we acknowledge that application of phonetics in the clinical arena is a legitimate area of study in its own right. Beyond the basic concepts of phonetics, which are covered in Chapters 2 to 5 of this text, there is a need for a discipline that deals with phonetics as it applies to disorders; hence, clinical phonetics. For our purposes in this book, clinical phonetics includes two major domains: informational and perceptual.

The Informational Domain of Clinical Phonetics

Clinical phonetics includes a wealth of descriptive information about speech sounds. Students often have difficulty understanding how such information is relevant to clinical practice. We hope you will perceive in this text the importance of phonetic knowledge to your skills in assessing and managing people with communication disorders. A personal anecdote might illustrate this point.

A student once asked one of the authors for an opinion on therapy materials she was preparing. Although this student was *not* a major in communication disorders, she was called upon in her student teaching practicum to help a child who had trouble "pronouncing his *s*'s." She had constructed a word list for working on the *s* sound in the word-final position; here are some of the items on her list:

base

face

hose

What's wrong here? Without the benefit of the most basic information in phonetics, this well-meaning student was going to ask the child to say the *z* sound, not the *s* sound, in the word *hose.*

The point of this example is that knowledge about speech sounds is basic to efficient and effective clinical practice. Clinicians who are well grounded in phonetics will possess the tools to assess and manage people with communication disorders. Knowledge of facts such as how often speech sounds occur in running speech is essential when dealing with a child or adult who is not making sounds correctly, for whatever reason.

We have presented descriptive information about sound production verbally and pictorially. Because it is difficult to understand how sounds are produced from verbal descriptions alone, many illustrations accompany the text. Virtually all of the illustrations of speech sound formation are based on X-ray materials collected by author Raymond D. Kent. We believe that many phonetics texts rely on impressionistic drawings that often mislead the reader about how sounds really are formed. Therefore, we decided at the outset to use, as much as possible, illustrations that relate directly to anatomical reality. Careful study of these illustrations should give the student the ability to visualize the positions and motions of the speech structures. This ability is invaluable to the specialist in communication disorders.

The Perceptual Domain of Clinical Phonetics

In addition to acquiring knowledge in the informational domain of clinical phonetics, a person who wishes to become competent in clinical phonetics must also acquire adequate skill in making perceptual discriminations. Figure 1-1 depicts 24 situations in which discrimination skill is needed in clinical speech pathology. The 24 blocks in this figure embrace levels of increasing skill, from those that can be learned fairly rapidly to those that require considerable training to acquire. That is, each sequentially numbered block requires more skill than the numbered blocks that precede it. The validity of this hierarchical arrangement has been tested and supported (Shriberg and Swisher, 1972). This conceptual representation has served as the basis for revisions of several programs to teach clinical phonetics; the present text is the final outcome of these efforts. You will have the opportunity to acquire discrimination skill in each of the 24 clinical situations depicted in Figure 1-1. Here we describe each of the axes on this three-dimensional representation of the perceptual domain of clinical phonetics.

System Complexity. The vertical axis in Figure 1-1 includes the three systems used in clinical phonetics. Each of these systems is appropriate in certain situations in assessing and managing people with communication disorders.

In the lowest row, blocks 1 to 8, **two-way scoring** refers to dichotomous decision making about speech behavior. A clinician must decide if a target behavior is "correct" or "incorrect," "right" or "wrong," "socially acceptable" or "socially unacceptable," or some other binary decision. In Chapter 7 more will be said about such decisions. The points to be made here are that a dichotomous decision about behavior, termed two-way scoring, is the easiest of the three systems in terms of complexity; and, of the three systems, it is most often used. Two-way scoring is done not only by clinicians but also by people who may be assisting with a child's management program, such as speech aides (paraprofessionals); the child's parents, caregivers, or teachers; and others.

Five-way scoring of speech behavior, the second tier of blocks in Figure 1-1 (cells 9 to 16), is more descriptive than two-way scoring. For some clinical situations, a clinician needs to know not only whether a sound is right or wrong but also what type of error a child is making. Five-way scoring is the traditional system of scoring in speech pathology that provides such information. In addition to the "correct" category, four "wrong" categories specify the type of error. A sound can be deleted altogether (**deletion** or **omission**), replaced by another sound (**substitution**), not said quite correctly (**distortion**), or said correctly but preceded or followed by an intrusive sound (**addition**). These five categories—"correct," "deletion," "substitution," "distortion," and "addition"—constitute the five-way system of scoring. Again, practical information on matters pertaining to five-way scoring will be presented in Chapter 7.

Finally, at the highest level of the model presented in Figure 1-1 is **phonetic transcription.** There is a fundamental distinction between the two scoring systems (two-way scoring and five-way scoring) and phonetic transcription. Whereas each of the scoring systems involves judgments about speech—they require the clinician to "score" a behavior—phonetic transcription is concerned only with *description* of behavior. The task in phonetic transcription is to represent what the child says rather than to score or judge it by some arbitrary standard. The degree of precision required in transcription depends on the clinician's purpose, as discussed in detail in Chapter 7. Depending on the number and

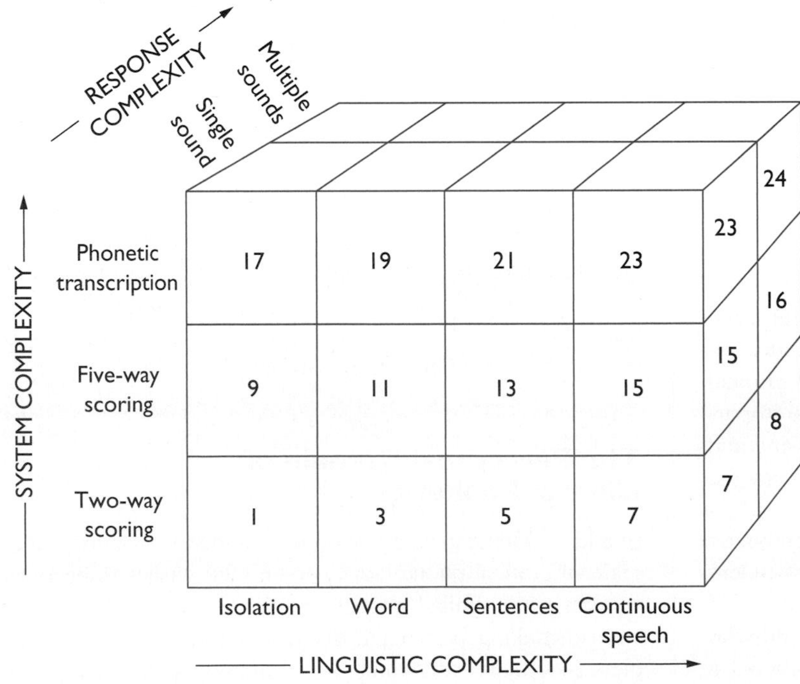

FIGURE 1-1
The perceptual domain of clinical phonetics. A person who wishes to become competent in clinical phonetics must acquire adequate discrimination skills for each of the clinical situations depicted in this representation.

type of symbols used, clinicians can do a **broad transcription** or a **narrow (close) transcription** of behavior. As depicted in Figure 1-1, phonetic transcription requires the highest level of skill from a clinician. Whereas speech aides, parents, caregivers, teachers, and so forth may be trained for two-way and even five-way scoring, phonetic transcription typically is done only by clinicians.

Linguistic Complexity. The horizontal axis in Figure 1-1 divides speech into four linguistic contexts of increasing **linguistic complexity,** as indicated by higher numbers. The far left blocks require the clinician to score or transcribe speech sounds in *isolation.* For example, a child is asked to say a sound, *s,* or a series of sounds, *s, f, z,* which the clinician scores or transcribes. When a sound is embedded in a *word, sentence,* or *continuous speech,* the task of discriminating one or more sounds is more difficult. This left-to-right hierarchy also generally parallels a child's progress in a management program. Clinicians and others who work to help a child carry over skills to new situations must be competent in making perceptual discriminations within all four linguistic contexts.

Response Complexity. The third dimension in the model, **response complexity,** captures an important situational difference between scoring and transcribing. For some clinical tasks, represented in Figure 1-1 by the odd-numbered blocks, the clinician need only score or transcribe one **target sound** per linguistic unit. For other tasks, represented by the even-numbered blocks, the clinician is required to score or transcribe two or more sounds per word. For example, some tests of a child's articulation proficiency are designed to test only one target sound or target cluster per word (for example, "*p*ig," "cu*p*," "cu*ps*"). Other articulation tests, however, require the clinician to score two or as many as four targets per word (for example, "*p*i*g*," "*c*u*ps*," "*s*i*ts*," "*sq*ui*rr*e*l*," "*b*u*s-f*i*sh*"). Obviously, because of memory constraints and other speech processing variables, the multiple-target tests are more difficult to score or transcribe than the single-sound articulation tests.

SUMMARY

The perceptual domain of clinical phonetics as portrayed in Figure 1-1 includes 24 discrimination situations. In one situation, a clinician may need to make only correct/incorrect decisions about one isolated target sound (Block #1). In another situation, a clinician may need to transcribe phonetically continuous speech (Block #24). This text will provide you with discrimination training in each of the 24 situations depicted in Figure 1-1. Trends in clinical practice support the need for clinicians to be comfortable transcribing samples of continuous conversational speech.

As you begin your study of clinical phonetics, we hope you will keep in mind two objectives—to acquire a firm knowledge of descriptive information about the phonetics of American English and to acquire discrimination skills for the clinical situations represented in Figure 1-1. In our view, demonstrated competence in each of these areas of clinical phonetics is the ethical responsibility of anyone who tests or attempts to change the articulatory behavior of another person.

GLOSSARY

Addition a speech production error in which a sound is incorrectly added (before or after) to another sound.

Broad transcription includes symbols to represent the consonants, vowels, and diphthongs produced in a speech sample.

Clinical phonetics applications of phonetics in the clinic, including information about speech sounds and the perceptual skills used in phonetic transcription.

Deletion a speech production error in which a sound is omitted (also termed an *omission*).

Distortion a speech production error in which a speech sound is recognizable as the correct sound but is not produced exactly correctly.

Five-way scoring a perceptual system in which speech sounds are classified as typical versus one of four error types: an addition, a deletion (or omission), a substitution, or a distortion.

Linguistic complexity the context in which a sound to be transcribed is embedded, which may range from a sound in isolation to a sound occurring in conversational speech.

Narrow (close) transcription includes symbols to represent both the target sounds (consonants, vowels, and diphthongs) and symbols that describe slight variations in the production of the target sounds.

Phonetics study of the perception and production of speech sounds.

Phonetic transcription use of symbols to represent the production of speech sounds.

Response complexity the number of target sounds to be transcribed, which may vary from only one sound to all sounds occurring in a section of speech.

Substitution a speech production error in which a speech sound is replaced by another speech sound.

Target sound the sound to be transcribed, as it occurs in isolation or together with other speech sounds.

Two-way scoring a perceptual system in which speech sound productions are dichotomized into two classes representing typical versus atypical behavior (e.g., correct vs. incorrect, right vs. wrong, etc.).

EXERCISES

Fill in the information that describes each clinical situation depicted in Figure 1-1. Answers for the first situation are provided. (See "Answers to Exercises" at the back of the book.)

	Linguistic Complexity	*System Complexity*	*Response Complexity*
1. A clinician asks a child to say some words, each of which contains one *r* sound (e.g., *r*ug, *r*abbit, ca*r*). After each word, the clinician records whether or not the child said the *r* sound correctly.	(word)	(two-way scoring)	(single sound)
2. A clinician is interested in knowing whether an adult client is saying *s* and *sh* correctly at work. The client obtains a 10-minute recording of her speech at the office. The clinician scores all occurring *s* and *sh* sounds as correct or incorrect.			
3. As part of his management program, a boy reads 20 sentences, each of which is composed of several words containing one or more *l* sounds. After each sentence, the clinician scores each *l* sound as correct, distorted, substituted for, added to, or deleted.			
4. An audio recording is made of a 5-year-old girl with extremely delayed speech who is talking about her favorite television program. The clinician later transcribes the entire speech sample.			
5. A speech-language pathologist administers a word-level articulation test with multiple targets per word (e.g., *t*e*l*e*v*i*s*ion, u*mbr*e*ll*a, *s*ci*ss*o*rs*). Each target sound is scored as correct, distorted, substituted for, added to, or deleted.			

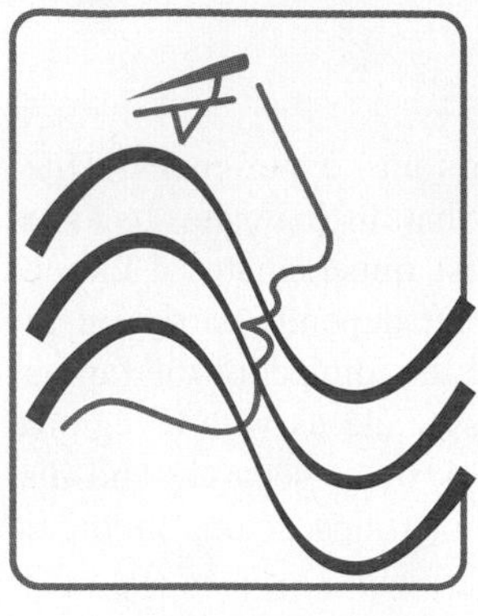

Linguistic Phonetics

2

Now the world had one language and a common speech.

—(Genesis 11:1; NIV)

In the biblical story of the tower of Babel, people tried to build on the plain in Shinar a city, with a tower that would reach to the heavens. Upon seeing the city and the tower under construction, God said, "If as one people speaking the same language they have begun to do this, then nothing they plan to do will be impossible for them. Come let us go down and confuse their language so they will not understand each other" (Genesis 11:6; NIV). In so doing, God confused the language of the entire world.

LANGUAGE, SPEECH, AND DIALECT

Estimates of the number of languages in the world vary, but we may say conservatively that there are over 3000. In this book we are concerned with spoken language, that is, a symbolic system in which meanings are communicated by speech. Physically, **speech** is both a pattern of the movements of the speech organs and a pattern of acoustic vibrations. Speech is most conveniently studied in physical terms by observing the movements of the speech structures (tongue, lips, jaw, and so on) and by recording the acoustic signal that the speech structures generate. Therefore, the study of sounds in a spoken language generally includes a description of how individual sounds are formed and information on the acoustic or auditory properties of a sound. For example, we might try to describe the sound represented by the first letter in the word *see* by examining the action of the tongue and by talking about the "noise" that we hear when this sound is uttered.

Spoken language is rooted deeply in human cultures and in the human race itself. Sapir comments on the antiquity of language as follows:

The universality and the diversity of speech leads to a significant inference. We are forced to believe that language is an immensely ancient heritage of the human race, whether or not all forms of speech are the outgrowth of a single pristine form. It is doubtful if any other cultural asset of man, be it the art of drilling for fire or of chipping stone, may lay claim to a greater age. I am inclined to believe that it antedated even the lowliest developments of material cultures, that these developments, in fact, were not strictly possible until language, the tool of significant expression, had itself taken shape. (Sapir, 1921, pp. 22–23)

All of us, except for people with severe vocal or hearing impairment, learn speech as the primary and first modality of language. The parent gauges a child's progress in learning language by the child's utterance of sounds that resemble words in the adult's spoken language. Parents eagerly await their child's first crude attempts at saying "mama" or "dada." As the child matures in linguistic ability, the parents may marvel as the child utters sentence-length expressions, sometimes containing words that the parents had not heard the child say before. Gradually, the child learns to name objects, to express needs and desires, and to remark on attitudes and emotions. Speech becomes a unique and powerful bond by which one person communicates ideas to another. An American visitor in a foreign land who needs directions or advice anxiously asks the persons he or she encounters, "Do you speak English?" in expectation of the simple "Yes" that will open the door to spoken language.

Nations or cultures often are identified by their language. People speaking the same language share not only a communication system but also usually a cultural heritage. Naturally, people who live close together in the same geographic area and who need to communicate with one another will use a common language. These people constitute a **speech community** (a group of people who live within the same geographical boundaries and use the same language). The United States may be called an American-English speech community because most of its citizens speak the same language, American English. However, we can identify smaller speech communities within the United States. For example, the city of Los Angeles has a Mexican-American speech community composed of people who share the Spanish language.

Within a country such as the United States, we encounter speakers who use American English but differ from other speakers of that language in pronunciation, vocabulary, or grammatical construction. These different usage patterns within a language are called **dialects.** Many dialects are

regional dialects because they are characteristic of people who live in a certain region.

"Appendix F: Dialects" provides a detailed examination of regional, social, and foreign dialects and includes procedural suggestions for phonetic transcription. The following are some introductory perspectives.

For most purposes in this book, we will assume the dialect of General American English (GAE). But do not be concerned if your pronunciation departs on occasion from that described in this text. We do not use GAE because it is "better" than any other dialect but simply because it is the most commonly used in the United States. We think of dialects as descriptive, not prescriptive. Prescriptive comments are evaluative judgments and state, implicitly or explicitly, preferences for one dialect over another. Descriptive comments simply describe dialectal variations without evaluative judgments.

Because a speaker of New England dialect uses the same language as a speaker of Southern American dialect, they communicate with little difficulty, aside from relatively minor differences in pronunciation and vocabulary. The distinction between language and dialect is one of degree. If two dialects of the same language diverge more and more in pronunciation, vocabulary, and grammatical structure, they may become recognized as different languages as communicative interaction diminishes.

Each of us belongs to a speech community and uses a certain dialect. The authors of this book share American English as a language but differ in dialect, one being a native of the Boston area and the other being a native of Montana. Thus, the authors share a language but not a dialect. Because the written form of language usually does not vary appreciably across dialects, our dialectal differences did not interfere with the writing of this book. However, in preparing the audio samples that accompany the book, dialectal differences were immediately apparent. The author from Boston "dropped" his *r*'s (*car* became *caw* or *cah* to the other author's ears), and the author from Montana used the same vowel for the words *cot* and *caught.* The authors also differ in other aspects of pronunciation because of dialectal differences. For example, the author from Montana occasionally pronounces words like *palm* and *calm* with an *l* because his parents pronounce them that way. The author from Boston pronounces them without an *l.* Despite the many differences in pronunciation, the two authors wrote a book in the same language (although our writing styles may differ somewhat). In written language many dialectal differences disappear. The two authors spell *car, caught,* and *palm* the same way, despite their differences in pronouncing each of these words.

In addition to a dialect, each person has a unique form of spoken language that is called an **idiolect** (*idio-* meaning personal or distinct; *-lect* apparently borrowed from *dialect*). The idiolect is determined by our membership in a speech community, by our regional background, by our social class, and by various individual factors and experiences. Thus, the idiolect is the speech pattern that distinguishes us as individuals. When the impressionist impersonates a famous personality, the success of the act depends partly on the impressionist's ability to recreate the idiolect of the famous person. Whereas dialects may associate us with a regional or social class, our idiolects mark us as separate and distinct speakers within the broader groups of our linguistic association.

The remainder of this chapter introduces concepts and terms useful in the study of written and spoken language. Keep in mind as you read that speaking and writing are modes of language expression. That is, the spoken word and the printed word are not language per se but expressions of language. The **sign language,** or manual communication, used by the deaf is another mode of language expression. We know of a young man born deaf and blind who communicates by still another mode—he uses a tactile coding device that allows him to "feel" language through his fingers and to type his message on a keyboard.

Speech can be understood even though it may not be heard. Expert speech readers (also called lipreaders, though they "read" more than lips) can understand much of what a speaker says by observing the visible movements that accompany speech. Finally, the user of a special method called Tadoma "feels" speech by placing a hand against a speaker's face. All this is simply to underscore the point that speech is a popular, but not a necessary, mode of language.

Now let us consider some basic units of linguistic analysis, beginning with the morpheme and the phoneme. Our examination will include both written and spoken language.

THE MORPHEME

The **morpheme** is the minimal unit of meaning, or, more formally, the morpheme is the smallest unit of language that carries a semantic interpretation. The list of morphemes in a language is called the **lexicon** of that language. Individual morphemes may be stems, endings for plurals and verb tenses, and other suffixes and prefixes. Thus, the word *cat* is a single morpheme, whereas the words *cats* and *catlike* each consist of two morphemes.

cats = cat + s (the plural ending or suffix is a morpheme)

catlike = cat + like

Each word in a language is made up of one or more morphemes, but an individual morpheme is not necessarily a word. As shown above, the plural ending *s* in the word *cats* is a morpheme even though *s* is not a word in the English language. Any word in the **dictionary** of our language is composed of stems, suffixes, prefixes, and endings for tense, possession, and pluralization, and these constituent parts of words are the morphemes of the language. *Words make up the dictionary of the language, and morphemes make up the lexicon of the language.*

Sometimes a morpheme of the English language does not look familiar when it is taken out of a word and placed in isolation. Consider the words *desist, consist, resist, insist,* and *persist.* Notice that each of these words is composed of a stem (*sist*) and a prefix (*de, con, re, in,* or *per*). Now, the stem *sist* probably does not look like an English word to you. And, in fact, it is not a word but rather a morpheme that is derived from the Latin word *sistere,* meaning "to stand (set)" or "to cause to stand." The Latin word survives in our language as a part of some of our words even though the morpheme *sist* does not occur by itself as a word in our dictionary. The derivation of English words like *desist* is revealed by morphemic analysis, as illustrated below.

desist = de (from) + sist = "to stand from" or "to stop"

consist = con (together) + sist = "to stand together" or "to be formed of"

resist = re (back) + sist = "to stand back" or "to oppose"

insist = in (in, on) + sist = "to stand on" or "to demand"

persist = per (through) + sist = "to stand through" or "to persevere"

Here are some additional examples of morphemic decomposition.

relentless = re + lent + less

morpheme = morph + eme

subnormal = sub + norm + al

feather = feather

cupboards = cup + board + s

transmittal = trans + mit + al

permitting = per + mit + ing

teeth = tooth + plural

The study of morphemes is called **morphemics** or **morphology,** and it embraces issues even more complicated than those hinted at in the examples given above. Languages differ greatly in their morphology, and these differences contribute to part of the complexity in this area of linguistic study. For the purposes of this text, a **morphemic transcription** is a written record of the morphemic content of an utterance. Such a transcription might be made if a clinician wants to analyze a language sample from a child. It should be emphasized that such a transcription has as its goal the recognition of meaningful elements rather than individual speech sounds.

THE PHONEME

Just as a word has one or more constituent morphemes, a morpheme has one or more constituent phonemes. A **phoneme** is a basic sound segment that has the linguistic function of distinguishing morphemes. For example, consider the words in the following list:

cat mat fat rat bat pat vat hat

First, notice that each of these words is a single morpheme because each is a meaningful unit that cannot be broken down further into two or more meaningful units.[1] Notice further that any two of these words differ only in the initial sound. In other words, the morphemes are distinguished by the sound segments denoted in these words by the alphabet letters (or **graphemes**) *c, m, f, r, b, p, v, h.* The sounds represented by these letters are phonemes of the English language, and they are identified by their role in morphemic contrasts. In fact, the linguist discovers the phonemes in a language by examining **minimal contrasts,** or contrasts between two morphemes that differ in only one sound segment. The linguist knows that *p* and *b* are distinct phonemes in English because of their roles in contrasting pairs like *pay–bay* and *cup–cub.*

It is important to recognize that phonemic contrasts are linguistic contrasts and therefore have the potential to produce entirely different morphemes and words. Changing, say, the *p* in *mop* to a *b* yields a new word that has no semantic similarity to *mop* (that is, there is no similarity in meaning). Is there ever sound change that does not result in a linguistic change? Yes. Consider the initial consonant sound in *key* and the initial consonant sound in *coo.* Despite the difference in spelling (*k* versus *c*), you probably will agree that both words *key* and *coo* begin with the same sound (call it a *k* sound). Yet, as you can verify yourself by touching your finger to your tongue as you say each word, the initial *k* sounds are not made in exactly the same way. Actually, the sound in *coo* is produced farther back in the mouth than the *k* sound in *key.* To most speakers of English, these two *k* sounds sound alike, in fact, identical. But to a speaker of Arabic, they sound quite different. In Arabic, the frontal *k* sound is a different phoneme than the back *k* sound, so to the Arabic speaker, these two sounds seem as different as a *p* and *b* seem to us. This difference, which to an English speaker is barely detectable because it is a nonphonemic difference, is very obvious to the speaker of Arabic (in which the difference is phonemic). Children learn to produce these two different kinds of *k* sounds in English; but, because the difference is nonphonemic, they grow up with little appreciation of the difference between them. Another example of a nonphonemic sound change can be demonstrated with the second *n* in *nine* and *ninth.* If you hold your finger just behind your upper front teeth so that your fingertip touches the gum line, you should notice that as you say the two words, your tongue comes farther forward for the *n* in *ninth* than for the *n* in *nine.*

To sum up, a phonemic difference between two sound segments means not only that they sound different but that the difference can be linguistically significant insofar as it

[1]Although *at* is a morpheme, the isolated consonants *c, m, f,* etc., are not morphemes. Therefore, *at* is not a base form in these words.

yields two different morphemes or words. Of course, not every sound change in a given word will produce another word in our language. If we substitute a *w* for the *v* in *vat,* we do not get a new English word. But we know that *w* and *v* are different phonemes because some pairs of contrasting morphemes (like *vine–wine*) do exist. The study of such differences is called phonemics.

The symbols that are used to represent phonemes of a language are placed between virgules, or slashes (/ /), to distinguish them from graphemes and other kinds of symbols. The phonemic symbols are included in a universal symbol system called the International Phonetic Alphabet (IPA).[2] Some of the symbols in this system are like those in the alphabet of written (or printed) English. The phonemic symbols /p/, /b/, /f/, /v/, /t/, /d/, /k/, /g/, /s/, /z/, /m/, /n/, /l/, /r/, and /h/ represent the same sound segments that ordinarily are conveyed by these letters in printed words. However, the student who studies phonemes also has to learn some symbols that may not be familiar at all, such as /ŋ/, /ʒ/, /ð/, and /ɝ/. The phonemes of English number about 42 to 44, depending on which phonetician does the counting. This number is only a fraction of the total number of phonemes used in the 3000 or so languages of the world; but, even at that, the number of phonemes used in all the different languages (about 100 phonemes) is very small compared to the total number of morphemes in these languages.

The relationships between morphemic and phonemic composition are shown for the word *cats* in Figure 2-1. As indicated previously, the word *cats* is composed of two morphemes, *cat* + *s.* The morpheme *cat,* in turn, is composed of the three phonemes /k/ + /æ/ + /t/, or initial consonant + vowel + final consonant. Note that /s/ is only one phonemic realization of the plural morpheme: In a word like *dogs,* /z/ is the phonemic realization.

PHONOLOGY AND PHONETICS

Phonology is the study of sound systems of language, that is, the structure and function of sounds in languages. Phonetics is the study of how speech sounds are produced and what their acoustic properties are. Thus, two major areas of study in phonetics are **articulatory phonetics** (concerned with how sounds are formed) and **acoustic phonetics** (concerned with the acoustic properties of sounds). Phonetics is closely related to phonology but differs in the sense that two languages could have the same inventory of phonetic units, with exactly the same articulatory and acoustic descriptions, but use this inventory differently to convey meaning. That is, the two languages could have a different phonology. We entitled this chapter "Linguistic Phonetics" to draw attention to its linguistic focus and to show how the study of phonetics is related to the general study of language structure and function. This book is entitled *Clinical Phonetics* because we are concerned ultimately with the study of speech sounds that depart from the phonetic system of the speech community. Whereas phonetics is generally concerned with the study of sounds in normal adult speech, the branch of **clinical phonetics** focuses on the sounds that become the professional concern of the speech-language pathologist. Several years of teaching phonetics to aspiring speech-language clinicians have convinced us that the standard course in phonetics, dealing primarily, if not entirely, with the correct sound productions of adult speakers, does not satisfy the needs of clinical application. We have seen many students trained this way throw up their hands in frustration when they first encounter a child with multiple misarticulations, many of which defy description by the methods that work so well with the normal adult talker.

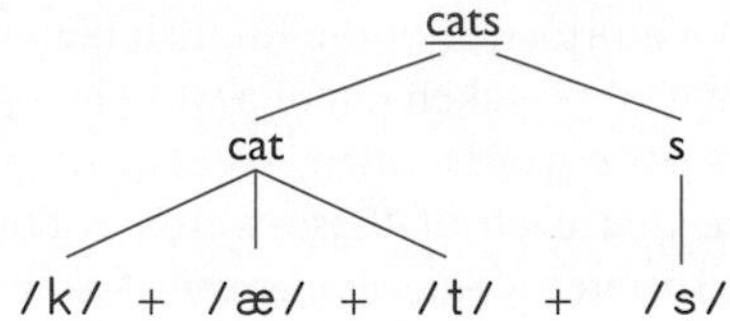

FIGURE 2-1
Morphemic and phonemic analyses of the word *cats.*

THE ALLOPHONE

Although each phoneme in a language is identified by what the linguist calls minimal pairs of contrasting morphemes (*pill* versus *bill,* for example) and is represented by a single symbol from the IPA (/p/ or /b/, for example), the phoneme is not a single, invariant sound. In fact, a phoneme is really a class or family of sounds, and the members of the family are called **allophones.** An allophone may be defined as a phonetic variant of a phoneme, that is, as one of the members of the phoneme family. Two allophones of the same phoneme never contrast to produce two different morphemes; only phonemes have this linguistic function. We already have discussed two examples of allophonic variation in connection with the word pairs *key–coo,* and *nine–ninth.* Recall that in the words *key* and *coo* the initial consonant is produced differently even though we hear the two versions (or allophones) as being the same phoneme. Such phonetic differences between allophones do not produce different morphemes or words, but they are important nonetheless. The allophonic variations in speech are significant in the sound patterns of a language, and failure to use them correctly can sometimes result in striking deviations, as we will discuss later in this book.

The conditions under which a given allophone occurs are described as being either **free variation** or **complementary**

[2]A copy of the IPA table of symbols is included in Appendix A of this text.

distribution. Allophones are said to be in free variation when they can be exchanged for one another in a given phonetic context (or neighborhood of other sounds). For example, the final sound in the word *pop* has two primary allophones: a released allophone for which a burst of air can be heard when the lips abruptly open and an unreleased allophone for which the lips do not open with an audible burst. As you can demonstrate for yourself, either the released or unreleased allophone can be used in producing the final sound of the word *pop.* Therefore, the two allophones are said to be in free variation for this phonetic context.

Allophones are said to be in complementary distribution when they are not normally exchanged for one another in a certain phonetic context. For example, we described earlier two major allophones of the *k* sound, one produced with a relatively fronted tongue position (as in the word *key*) and one with a relatively backed tongue position (as in the word *coo*). The fronted allophone occurs in the context of vowel sounds that have a tongue position near the front of the mouth, and the backed allophone occurs in the context of vowel sounds that have a tongue position near the back of the mouth. Hence, the fronted allophone occurs in the words *key, kit, cape, ken,* and *cat* but not in the words *coo, cook, coat,* or *cot.* Because the fronted and backed allophones do not occur in the same context, they are said to be in complementary distribution. This term indicates that the conditions of occurrence of one allophone complement the conditions of occurrence of another allophone.

Phonemic symbols are placed within virgules, for example /k/. **Phonetic symbols,** that is, symbols used to represent allophones or phonetic variants of phonemes, are placed within brackets, for example [k]. Because a given phoneme may have a large number of allophonic variants, phonetic symbols may be modified by special marks called **diacritic marks.** For instance, if we wish to transcribe phonetically the initial consonant in *key,* we could write [k̟], where the diacritic mark under the *k* denotes a tongue position toward the front of the mouth. Similarly, we can characterize the difference between the second *n* in *nine* and in *ninth* by transcribing the latter as [n̪], where the diacritic mark symbolizes a dental (toward the teeth) modification of the tongue position during the consonant production. Such small changes in sound production will be considered in detail in the course of this text.

The relationships among morphemic, phonemic, and allophonic analyses of the word *cats* are illustrated in Figure 2-2. This illustration is like that in Figure 2-1 except that the appropriate allophonic variants have been added to indicate the phonetic realization of the phonemes /k/, /æ/, /t/, and /s/. Hence, this illustration demonstrates three levels of analysis: morphemic, phonemic, and allophonic. Similarly, we can speak of three kinds of transcription:

morphemic transcription, or the identification of meaningful units;

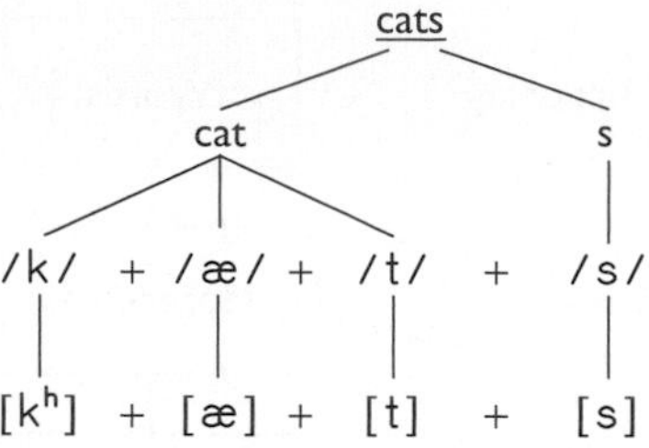

FIGURE 2-2
Morphemic, phonemic, and allophonic (phonetic) analyses of the word *cats.*

phonemic transcription, or the identification of sound segments that have linguistic significance in the speaker's language; and

phonetic transcription, or the identification of the allophonic variants in a speaker's pattern of sounds.

A pictorial summary of the terms introduced in this chapter is given in Figure 2-3.

THE MORPH AND THE PHONE

A few more fundamental terms are needed to complete this brief introduction to linguistic phonetics. Individual morphemelike shapes encountered in a language sample are called **morphs.** Most morphs indeed turn out to be morphemes, but some may not. The *o* in *drunkometer* is a morph but not a morpheme, because it is not a minimal unit of meaning. Some linguists refer to the *o* as a meaningless morph. Hence, the individual morphs discovered in a linguistic analysis are shapes that may or may not be morphemes. Of course, the vast majority of morphs in any natural language are morphemes. Until a given unit has been confidently established as being a morpheme, it may be called a morph.

Any particular occurrence of a sound segment of speech is a **phone.** Thus, phonemes and allophones are identified by examining phones. Just as morphs are the raw material for morphemic analysis, so are phones the raw material for phonemic and phonetic analysis.

Neologisms, or newly coined words, sometimes introduce some strange twists in word derivations. For example, a word of recent coinage is *workaholic,* which is used to describe someone who works to excess. Thus, the legendary hard-driving executive who neglects his or her family might be called a workaholic. This word was formed as a parallel to alcoholic, or someone who drinks to excess. However, if we attempt to break *workaholic* into its morphemic subparts, we discover that we have the three apparent units *work + ahol + ic.* Both *work* and *ic* are in fact legitimate morphemes of the English language, but *ahol* does not have morphemic status, being rather like the meaningless morph *o* in *drunkometer.* No doubt some etymologists (those who study word deriva-

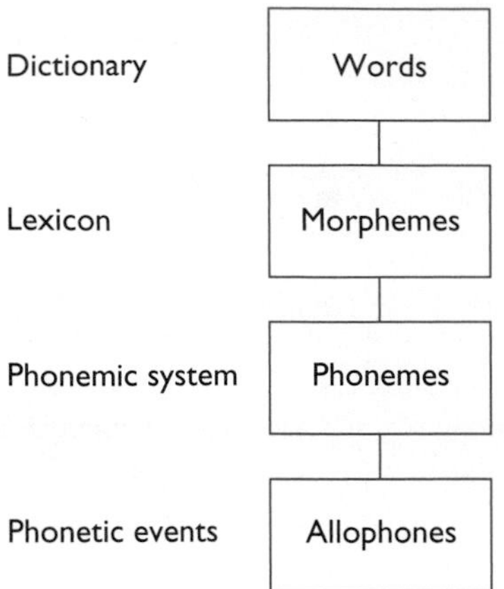

FIGURE 2-3
Some units of linguistic analysis pertinent to the study of phonetics. Higher-level units, such as phrases and sentences, are not shown in this drawing, but they also figure in the study of phonetics.

tions) deplore such coinages as *workaholic,* but if this principle is extended to other forms, such as jogaholic, sexaholic, and footballaholic, it may become a fixture of the English language.

THE ALPHABET AND THE ALLOGRAPH

An **alphabet** (from the Greek *alpha* + *beta*) is a set of letters or other characters used for the writing of a language. The elements of an alphabet are not always directly related to the way the language is pronounced. The same letter in English may be associated with several different sounds. For example, the alphabet letter *g* represents very different sounds in the words *go, gist,* and *weigh.* Similarly, the same sound can be represented by many different alphabet letters (singly or in combination). For example, the sound that is most commonly represented by the letter combination *sh,* as in *ship,* also is represented by *s* as in *sugar, ss* as in *tissue, ch* as in *machine, ti* as in *creation, ci* as in *precious,* and *x* as in *anxious.* Such sound–letter confusions are a source of difficulty to children (or non-English-speaking persons) learning to read the English language.

Different letters or combinations of letters that represent the same phoneme are called **allographs.** Thus, for the *sh* sound, as in *ship,* a partial listing of allographs is: *sh, s, ss, ch, ti, ci, x.* Note that any one of these allographs may itself represent different phonemes. The combination *ch* also represents the sounds in the words *chasm* and *chair.* In this book, the allographs for the vowels and consonants of English are listed at the ends of the chapters for these two major sound classes.

Some letters are occasionally silent. Examples are the *e* in *came,* the second *b* in *bomb, h* as in *honor, gh* as in *weigh, n* as in *damn,* and *g* as in *paradigm.* Interestingly, the phonetic significance of these "silent" letters sometimes is revealed through affixing (adding prefixes or suffixes). Consider the following pairs: *bomb–bombastic; damn–damnation; paradigm–paradigmatic.* Thus, silent letters are not always useless accidents in the development of a written language. Some letters can be either pronounced or silent in the same position in a word: Compare *hour, honest,* and *honor* with *humble, hat,* and *hospital.* Moreover, a letter in a word may be either silent or not depending on who says it. Some people pronounce the words *human, humor,* and *humid* with the same initial sound as that in *happy,* but other people drop the *h.* This ambiguity with *h* may reflect the influence of spelling. As Kerek (1976) observed, words like *hospital, heritage,* and *humble* were not produced with an *h* sound as late as the eighteenth century, but the fact that these words are spelled with *h* has reestablished their pronunciation with an *h* sound. Perhaps the same fate will come to *hour, honor,* and *honest,* which are now pronounced without an *h* sound.

POSITIONAL AND CONTEXTUAL TERMINOLOGY FOR PHONETIC DESCRIPTIONS

Certain terms are widely used to describe the position of a sound with respect to a linguistic unit or to describe the context within which a sound occurs. The terms **initial, medial,** and **final** are used to denote sound locations at the beginning, middle, or end of a word, respectively. For example, the *t* sound is both word-initial and syllable-initial in the word *turn* but only syllable-initial in the word *return.* Syllable-initial and syllable-final sounds also are called **releasing** and **arresting** sounds, respectively. That is, a sound at the beginning of a syllable is said to release the syllable, whereas a sound at the end of a syllable is said to arrest the syllable. Medial sounds occur somewhere within a word or syllable, not at the beginning or end of it. However, the medial position can occur in quite different phonetic contexts in different words; consider the sound *b* in the words ru*bb*er, tooth*b*rush, and a*b*ove.

With some exceptions to be discussed later, all syllables contain a vowel. Therefore, it is often convenient and useful to describe consonant positions relative to the location of a vowel. The term **prevocalic** notes that a sound (usually a consonant) occurs before a given vowel, and the term **postvocalic** denotes that a sound occurs after a given vowel. In the word *tub,* the *t* sound is prevocalic and the *b* sound is postvocalic.

Geminate (from the Latin *geminus,* meaning "twin") sounds occur together as a pair, that is, two adjacent sounds are the same. For example, the two *k* sounds are geminates in the word *bookkeeper* (the double letters *oo* and *ee* are not truly phonetic geminates because these pairs each represent a single sound). Geminate sounds occur word-medially (as in *bookkeeper*) or across word boundaries (as in *sad day*).

The two major types of syllables are **open** and **closed.** An open syllable is one that does not end in a consonant, whereas a closed syllable does end in a consonant. *Law, see, throw,* and *spry* are open syllables (note that the *w* in *throw* is not pronounced as a consonant). *Lot, seep, throat,* and *sprite* are closed syllables. What then is a syllable? Actually the syllable is difficult to define. We prefer to think of syllables as highly adaptive units for the articulatory organization of speech. A syllable is a grouping of speech movements, usually linked together with other syllables in a rhythmic pattern.

The difficulty of giving a physical definition of syllable can be demonstrated in a simple tape-editing experiment. If you record on magnetic tape certain two-syllable words like *wrestling, tussling,* or *nestling* and then cut off the segment of the tape recording that contains the *-ing* portion of the word, you will now hear the words as *wrestle, tussle,* and *nestle.* Notice that the vowel of the second syllable of the original two-syllable word has been discarded, yet we still hear two-syllable words. This experiment shows us that syllables are relational units, that is, units that are defined with respect to their function in an utterance. Furthermore, it is not always easy to break up a word into syllables. Where does the first syllable end and the final syllable begin in the word *cupboard?*

Some phonetics books mention syllables without ever defining what a syllable is. Of the definitions we have seen, none is satisfactory. It is instructive to look at a couple of examples. Calvert (1980) defines a syllable as "a cluster of coarticulated sounds with a single vowel or diphthong[3] nucleus, with or without surrounding consonants" (p. 179). Aside from the inherent contradiction of allowing some "clusters" to consist of one element (like the first syllable *o-* of *obey*), this definition is not totally satisfactory because it does not allow for syllabic consonants. These consonants, to be discussed in more detail later, are like vowels in serving as the nucleus of a syllable. For example, the word *button* typically is pronounced with only one vowel (represented by the alphabet letter *u*), yet it seems to contain two syllables. The second syllable is formed by the syllabic consonant *n,* that is, a consonant that acts like a vowel. In addition the term *coarticulated* doesn't help much. This term (which also will be discussed in more detail later) means that the movements for adjacent sounds overlap one another. Such overlapping of movements or articulations has been thought to be a useful way of defining syllables because the overlapping indicates a cohesiveness or "belonging together." However, studies of speech production have made it clear that overlapping commonly occurs across word boundaries and across what almost anybody would call a syllable boundary. Certain kinds of overlapping occur even between adjacent vowels (which can be in different words). In short, coarticulation, or overlapping of movements, is not restricted to any one kind of unit.

Kantner and West (1941) define a syllable as a "unit of speech containing a peak of sonority [loudness or carrying power] and divided from other such peaks by a hiatus or a weakening of sonority" (p. 62). But the sonority criterion is difficult to apply consistently. In words such as *piano, chaos,* and *trio,* the syllable divisions marked by / in the syllabifications pi/an/o, cha/os, and tri/o are not necessarily associated with a change in sonority so much as with a change in vowel quality. In fact, if we look at the actual physical power in these words, it is not always easy to identify distinct peaks that correspond to the number of syllables we hear.

The difficulty in defining the syllable does not mean that it is an unimportant unit in the study of phonetics. The syllable is a useful construct and plays a role in the explanation of many phonetic phenomena. It is well to study Malmberg's comments on the syllable:

> *It [the syllable] is one of the fundamental notions of phonetics. If phoneticians are not always in agreement about defining a syllable, it is partly because different points of view have been chosen for its definition (acoustics, articulatory, functional), partly because the apparatus which has been used up to now has not enabled phoneticians to locate the boundaries of syllables on the graphs or tracings obtained. But it would be an error to conclude that the syllable as a phonetic phenomenon does not exist and that the grouping of phonemes in syllables is a mere convention without any objective reality. . . . Even a person without any linguistic training usually has a very clear idea of the number of syllables in a spoken chain. (Malmberg, 1963, p. 65)*

A formal definition of *syllable* will be postponed until Chapter 6.

GLOSSARY

Acoustic phonetics the branch of phonetics that deals with the acoustic properties of sounds; acoustics is a subfield of physics that deals with the generation and transmission of sound.

Allograph any one alphabet letter or combination of letters that represents a particular phoneme. One phoneme may be represented (spelled) by several different allographs.

Allophone one of the sound variants within a phoneme class, often used in a specified phonetic context.

Alphabet a system of written symbols used to express a language.

Arresting another name for syllable-final sounds; they arrest (stop) the syllable.

[3] A diphthong is a sequence of vowel sounds that behaves phonemically as a single vowel.

Articulatory phonetics the branch of phonetics that deals with how sounds are formed; also called *physiological phonetics.*

Clinical phonetics the branch of phonetics that deals with errors or abnormalities in the production of sounds.

Closed a syllable that ends in a consonant.

Complementary distribution a term used to describe two or more allophones of a particular phoneme that occur in mutually exclusive phonetic contexts.

Diacritic mark a special symbol used to modify a phonetic symbol to indicate a particular modification of sound production.

Dialect different usage patterns within a language; speakers of one dialect may or may not easily understand speakers of another dialect of the same language.

Dictionary an inventory of the words in a language, usually together with their meaning.

Final the final position or segment in a word, e.g., the *t* in the word *bat* is a final consonant.

Free variation a term used to describe allophones that may be exchanged for one another in a particular phonetic context.

Geminate sounds that occur together as a pair, such as the two *k* sounds in *bookkeeper* or the two *s* sounds in *gas supply.*

Grapheme a unit in the writing system of a language.

Idiolect an individual or personal pattern of language usage. Each user of a language has an idiolect.

Initial the first position or segment in a word, e.g., the *b* in the word *bat* is an initial consonant.

Lexicon an inventory of the morphemes in a language.

Medial a middle position or segment in a word (i.e., not initial or final); the *b* is medial in the words *rubber, rebut,* and *toothbrush.*

Minimal contrast a sound segment distinction by which two morphemes or words differ in pronunciation. Minimal contrasts are basic to the discovery of phonemes in a language.

Morph an individual morphemelike shape in a language sample.

Morpheme the smallest unit of language that carries a semantic interpretation (meaning).

Morphemic transcription a written account of the morphemic content of a language sample.

Morphemics the study of morphemes; a subfield of linguistics.

Morphology that part of linguistics concerned with the study of morphemes, the meaning-bearing elements of a language.

Open a syllable that does not end in a consonant.

Phone a particular occurrence of a speech sound segment.

Phoneme a basic speech segment that has the linguistic function of distinguishing morphemes (the minimal units of meaning in a language).

Phonetic symbol a written character that represents a particular speech segment.

Phonetic transcription a written account of the sound segments in a spoken language sample.

Phonology the study of the structure and function of sounds in language.

Postvocalic occurring after a vowel, e.g., the *t* in *eat* is a postvocalic consonant.

Prevocalic occurring before a vowel, e.g., the *b* in *bee* is a prevocalic consonant.

Regional dialect a pattern of language usage that is shared by people living in a particular geographic region. A language may have several regional dialects.

Releasing another name for syllable-initial sounds; they release (begin) the syllable.

Sign language a system of communication that uses manual symbols, such as hand positions, postures, and movements to express language.

Speech a mode of language expression based on sounds emitted through the mouth and nose.

Speech community a group of people who live within the same geographic boundaries and use the same language.

EXERCISES

1. Morphemic analysis. Count the number of morphemes contained in each of the following words.

   Example: The word *stairways* contains three morphemes (*stair* + *way* + *s*)

Word	*Number of Morphemes*
(a) lightened	________
(b) table	________
(c) morphemic	________
(d) recruitment	________
(e) dismissed	________
(f) television	________
(g) finger	________
(h) singers	________
(i) revealing	________
(j) imposition	________

2. By adding prefixes and suffixes to the stem *pose,* create as many words as you can. For example, the word *imposition* (no. 1-j above) is formed by adding the prefix *im* and the suffixes *it* and *ion* to the stem *pose.*

3. Phonemic analysis. Count the number of phonemes contained in each of the following words.

Example: The word *chair* contains three phonemes: the initial consonant, the vowel, and the final consonant.

Word	*Number of Phonemes*
(a) daughter	______________
(b) laughter	______________
(c) phone	______________
(d) cupboard	______________
(e) cellophane	______________
(f) knead	______________
(g) Chicago	______________
(h) finger	______________
(i) singer	______________
(j) six	______________

4. Sequential phonemic constraints. In this list of twelve "words," only half of them are really words in the English language. The other six are words that have been made up for this exercise. Separate this list of words into two groups—one group for words that you think could be found in an English dictionary, and the other group for words that you would not expect to find in an English dictionary. The "real" words are sufficiently rare that you probably have never heard of them. After you have made up the two lists of words, explain the factors that you used in making your decisions.

(a) fsew	(g) skeg
(b) grith	(h) dlut
(c) srin	(i) shlar
(d) scute	(j) gvise
(e) trave	(k) spile
(f) ktun	(1) knar

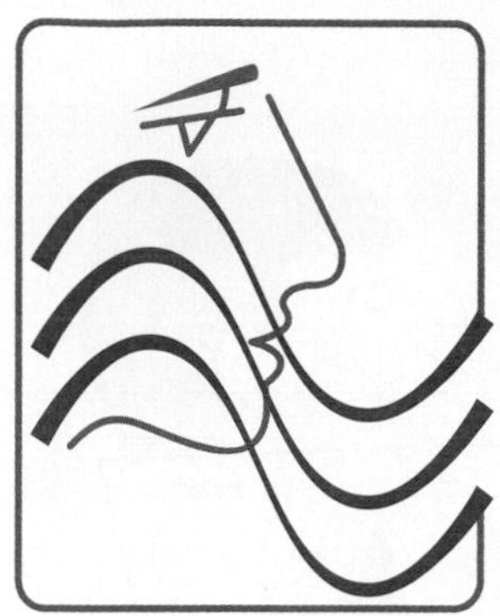

The Three Systems of Speech Production 3

The human vocal tract may be described as an apparatus for the conversion of muscular energy into acoustic energy.

—(J. C. Catford, 1968, p. 310)

Speech is produced by the carefully controlled action of over 100 muscles in the chest, abdomen, neck, and head. We can simplify the description of speech production by considering three major functional systems—**respiratory, laryngeal,** and **supralaryngeal** (or pharyngeal-oral-nasal). These three systems are illustrated in Figure 3-1.

THE RESPIRATORY SYSTEM

The respiratory system, consisting primarily of the lungs, rib cage, abdomen, and associated muscles, acts like a pump to provide the movement of air needed for speech production. All sounds in the English language normally are **egressive,** meaning that they are produced with a flow of air that moves outward from the lungs. Kantner and West (1941) wrote, "All English sounds normally produced have one factor in common: they are based upon the utilization of the moving column of air furnished by the expiratory phase of the process of respiration" (p. 39). Some languages include **ingressive** sounds, or sounds produced with an inward flow of air. The respiratory system supplies the forces of air that are used to generate most sounds. For egressive sounds, air that has been drawn into the lungs during inspiration is then forced outward through the mouth or nose. As one speech scientist,

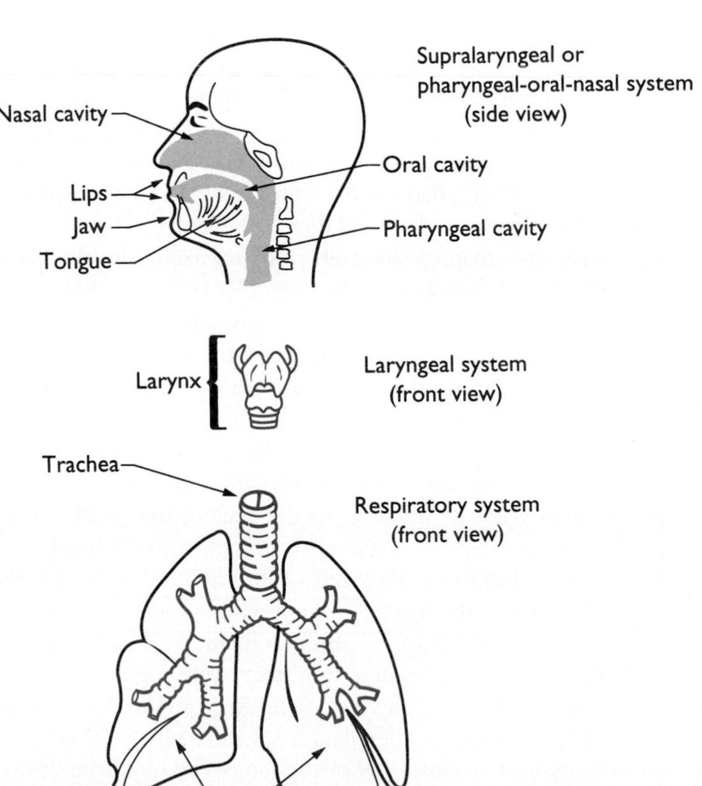

FIGURE 3-1
The three systems of speech production: respiratory, laryngeal, and supralaryngeal. Some parts of the respiratory system are not shown in the drawing, for example, the rib cage.

Thomas Hixon, puts it, speaking is a process of making oneself gradually smaller. That is, after we make ourselves larger by taking in air through inspiration, the air is driven out in small pulses that are formed into sounds.

The role of the respiratory system in speech can be summarized as follows:

1. During inspiration, air is drawn into the lungs as the result of muscle contractions that increase the volume of the **thoracic,** or chest, **cavity.**
2. The muscles of the respiratory system release air into the larynx and supralaryngeal system for the purpose of generating speech.
3. In situations when an unusually strong burst of air is required—as when special emphasis or loudness is desired—the respiratory muscles can act to provide this additional pulse of energy by a forceful squeezing of the thoracic cavity.

Speech that is continued for more than a few seconds necessarily takes on the rhythm of respiration—cycles of inspiration and expiration. This pattern gives rise to a unit called the **breath group,** which is simply the sequence of words or syllables produced on a single expiration. The breath group is distinctive of speech and is not necessarily well defined in other types of communication, such as manual signing or typing. That is, a person who uses manual signs, such as in American Sign Language, does not need to pause the flow of signs to take in a breath. In ordinary conversation, we typically speak for no more than 10 seconds on a single breath. Normally, we interrupt for inspiration at syntactically appropriate places, such as phrase or clause boundaries. Therefore, breath groups often coincide with syntactic units.

THE LARYNGEAL SYSTEM

The air from the lungs travels up through the laryngeal system, where voice is produced. The **larynx,** or "voice box," is made up largely of cartilage and muscles and is situated on top of the **trachea,** the air pipe that connects the lungs with the larynx (Figure 3-1). Inside the larynx are the **vocal folds,** small cushions of muscle (Figure 3-2). The vocal folds are about three-quarters of an inch (or 17 millimeters) long in an adult male. Their length is shorter in women and in children. At the front, they attach close to the "Adam's apple." If you put your finger on your throat, you should be able to feel a small notch at the top of your larynx. The vocal folds attach just below this notch and have their other place of attachment on tiny cartilages located at the back of the larynx. A physician or speech pathologist can examine the vocal folds by using a special mirror, as shown in Figure 3-2.

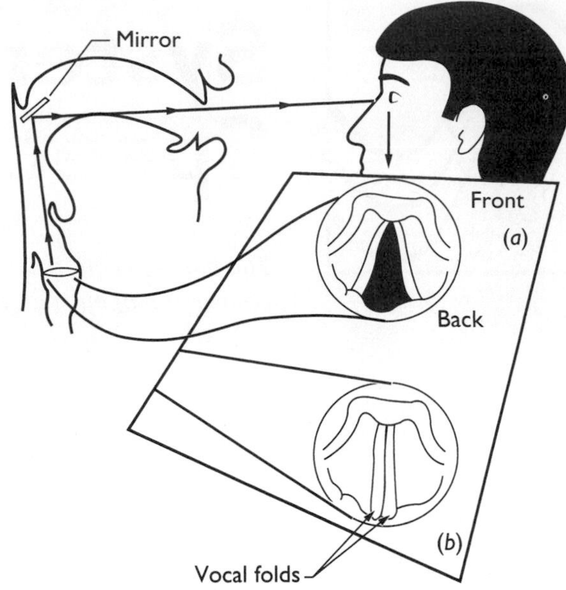

FIGURE 3-2
Viewing the vocal folds with a laryngeal mirror. In *(a)* the vocal folds are shown in their abducted (open) state. In *(b)* the vocal folds are in their adducted (drawn together) state.

During breathing, the vocal folds are kept apart so that air can move freely into and out of the lungs. When voice is required, the vocal folds are brought together so that air escaping from the lungs can set them into vibration. This process is like the production of a sound that results when a person suddenly releases an inflated balloon. The vocal folds vibrate in a similar way. The muscles of the larynx bring the folds together just tightly enough so that the force of air developed in the lungs can blow them apart. But each time they are blown apart, they come together again because of restoring forces. The successive pulses of air from the vibrating vocal folds generate the sound of voice. The neck of the rapidly deflating balloon does the same thing, first opening as a burst of air escapes and then closing again. Curious as it seems, the escaping air itself is one reason why the vocal folds (and the balloon mouthpiece) can close again. The rapidly moving air momentarily creates a lower pressure between the vocal folds (or the lips of the balloon mouthpiece), and this force helps to restore closure.

The deflating balloon is a crude analogy of the respiratory-laryngeal action in voice production (Figure 3-3). Inflation of the balloon is similar to the inspiration of air that precedes voice production. As the neck of the balloon is released, air escapes—just as air is driven from the lungs once the vocal folds are separated. Then, as just explained, the vocal folds, or the lips of the balloon mouthpiece, are forced to vibrate as the air rushes through them. And, of course, the balloon, like a person's thoracic cavity, gradually gets smaller as the air flows out of it. As you can demonstrate very easily yourself, the vocal folds can be set into vibration both by air that flows *out* of the lungs and by air that flows *into* the lungs. That is, we can phonate, or produce voice, during either expiration (the usual way) or inspiration, so

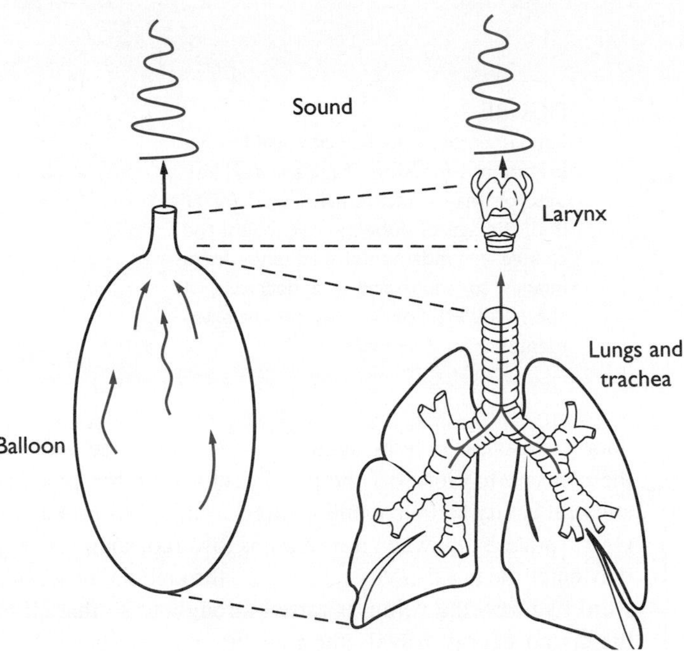

FIGURE 3-3
Balloon analogy of respiratory-laryngeal action in voice production. Air escaping from the deflating balloon causes neck of balloon to vibrate with a fluttering sound. Similarly, the air driven outward from lungs causes vocal folds to vibrate.

long as the vocal folds are positioned properly. If the folds are not closed sufficiently, voice will not be produced because the air will move through them like air through a straw.

As a consequence of the alternating opening and closing motions of the vocal folds, small pulses of air enter the chambers of the mouth and nose. Figure 3-4 shows the sequence of events in vocal fold vibration. In the words of Denes and Pinson (1963), "The vibrating vocal cords [folds] rhythmically open and close the air passage between the lungs and mouth." The rate of vocal fold vibration, or the number of opening–closing cycles in a unit of time, is about 125 per second for an adult male. In an adult female, the rate is higher, averaging about 250 per second. Higher rates of vibration occur for young children; for example, the cry of a newborn baby has an average rate of vocal fold vibration of about 500 per second. The developmental variation in rate of vibration is graphed in Figure 3-5. It is because of these differences in the rate of vibration that voices have different pitches. A man's voice sounds lower in pitch than a woman's or a child's because his vocal folds vibrate at a slower average rate. When we change the pitch of our voices during speaking or singing, the vocal folds vibrate at different rates. For example, we sing up a musical scale by making our vocal folds thinner and more tense so they vibrate at higher rates. The rate of vocal fold vibration is commonly called the **fundamental frequency of the voice,** symbolized as f_0. A high fundamental frequency is associated with a high pitch and a low fundamental frequency with a low pitch. Fundamental frequency is expressed in units called Hertz (abbreviated Hz). One **Hertz** is defined as one complete cycle of vibration per second. Hence, 20 Hz would mean 20 complete vibrations per second, which is approximately the lower limit of the frequency range of the human ear. If an adult male has an average rate of vocal fold vibration of 125 per second, then we can say that his f_0 is 125 Hz. During ordinary conversational speech, a talker's f_0 changes almost

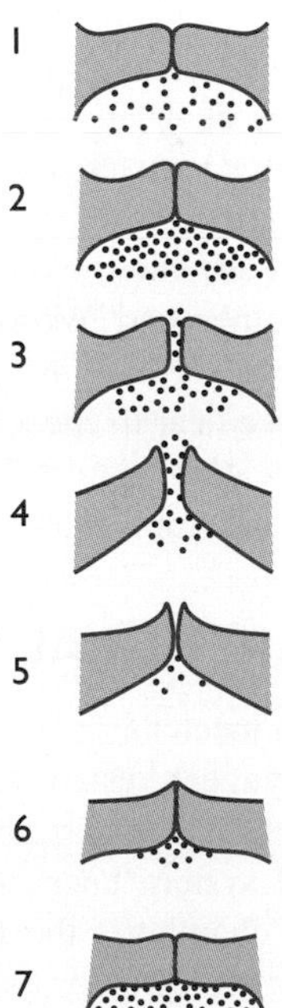

FIGURE 3-4
Series of events in vocal fold vibration. (1) Folds are closed and air pressure builds up beneath them. (2) Folds just before they burst apart in response to air pressure. (3) Folds burst apart, and air flows through them. (4) Folds are maximally open. (5) Folds begin to close. (6) Folds are closed. (7) Cycle begins again.

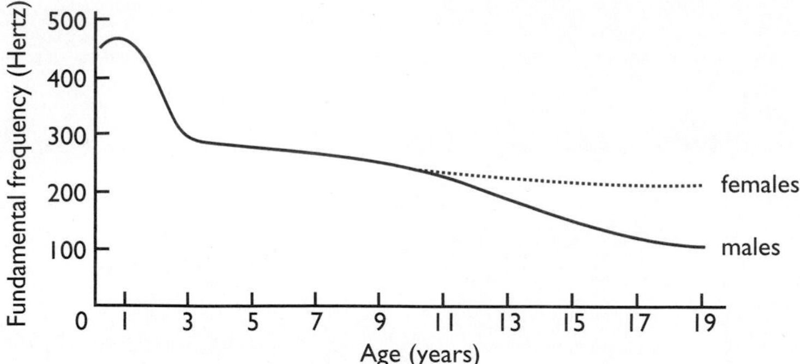

FIGURE 3-5
Fundamental frequency of vocal fold vibration as a function of age and sex. Values for males and females are similar until the age of puberty. For males, the change in fundamental frequency from infancy to adulthood is a decrease of about 400 Hz. For females, the developmental change is smaller.

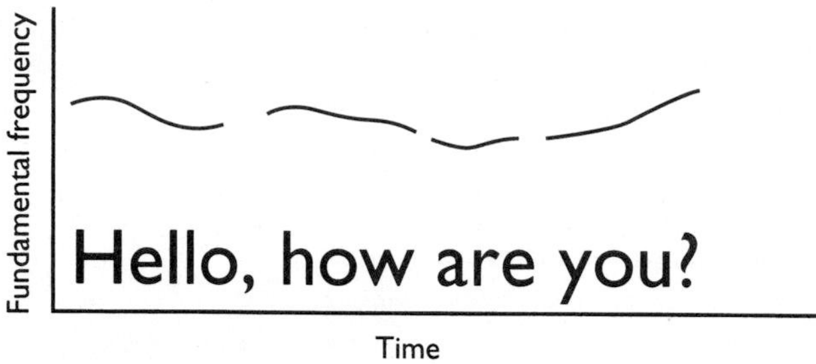

FIGURE 3-6
Variation in fundamental frequency of the voice during the utterance "Hello, how are you?"

continuously, as shown in the graph of Figure 3-6. These changes underlie much of what is called the **intonation** of speech. Intonation is used to mark sentences as declarative or interrogative, to place emphasis or stress on certain words, or to signal emotions and attitudes.

But, to quote Kantner and West (1941), "The sound waves produced at the vocal folds are still far from being the finished product that we hear in speech" (p. 45). The finishing is done by the resonating chambers of the pharynx, nose, and mouth and by the structures that valve the breath stream.

THE SUPRALARYNGEAL SYSTEM

The part of the speech mechanism that lies above the larynx is called the supralaryngeal system (*supra* is a morpheme that means "above"). This system also may be called the pharyngeal-oral-nasal system because it consists of three major air cavities or chambers, the pharyngeal, oral, and nasal (Figure 3-7). Lying directly above the larynx is the pharynx, or pharyngeal cavity, which is essentially a muscular tube. The pharynx divides into two other cavities, the oral (or mouth) and the nasal (or nose). Sound energy from the larynx travels up through the pharynx and then enters the oral cavity, the nasal cavity, or both. The direction of sound travel is determined by the position of the **velum,** or **soft palate.** The velum is rather like a hanging door. When the door is raised, it presses against the back and side walls of the pharynx to close off the nasal cavity from the pharynx and oral cavity so that sound is directed into the oral cavity. On the other hand, when the velum is lowered, sound energy may enter the nasal cavity and escape through the nose. In a word like *fast,* the velum is raised throughout so that all of the sound energy travels through the oral cavity. This is called **oral radiation of sound** energy. For a word like *man,* the sound energy travels through the nose for the nasal consonants *m* and *n* and through *both* mouth and nose for the intervening vowel. You can demonstrate the importance of the nasal cavity for these nasal consonants by pinching your nose tightly as you say the word *man.* The speech of a person with a severe cold gives a similar lesson: Because of the stopped-up nasal passages, *man* may sound like *bad.* An even more effective demonstration is to attempt to produce a sustained *m* sound with your nostrils closed. How long can you make the sound?

Most of the sounds in English are formed by modifying the **pharyngeal, oral,** and **nasal cavities**. These modifications are accomplished by activation of the muscles of the head and neck, which work to move the velum, jaw, tongue, lips, and pharyngeal walls. The process of articulation is one of movement, and the moving structures are called **articulators.** For example, the tongue is an articulator. A tracing of an X-ray view of the articulators is shown in Figure 3-8. Some articulators, like the tongue, change in both shape and position, whereas others, like the jaw, change only in position. Let us examine the role of the major articulators in speech production, remembering as we do so these words of Raymond H. Stetson (1951), ". . . speech is a series of movements made audible."

Velopharynx: Velum and Pharyngeal Walls

The velum, or soft palate, operates as a valve to open or close the entrance to the nasal cavity, thus permitting **nasal radiation of sound** energy. As just discussed, during respiration and during the production of nasal sounds, the velum is lowered. During oral (nonnasal) sounds or during such activities as sucking or blowing, it is raised. Articulation of the velum is illustrated in Figure 3-9, which was derived from X-ray

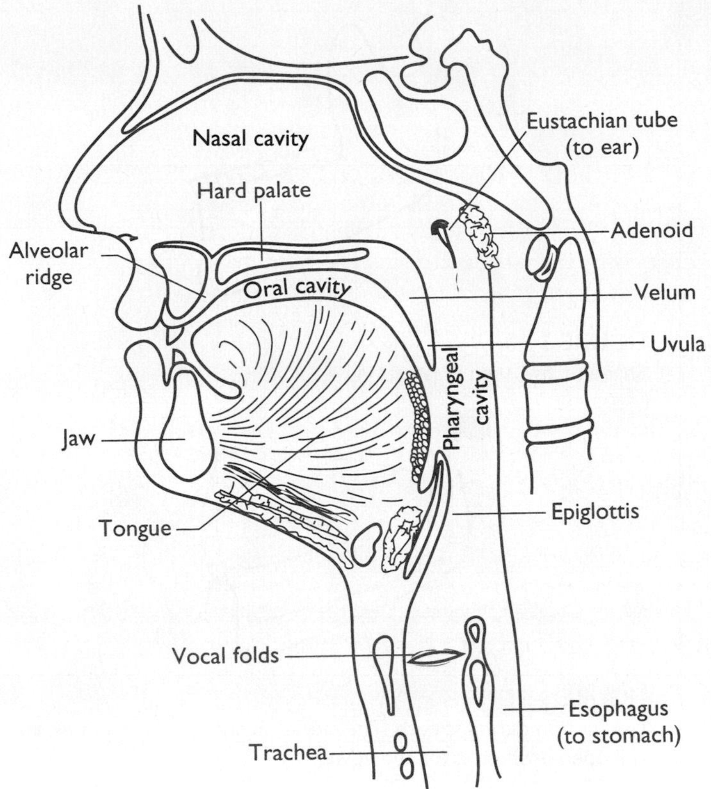

FIGURE 3-7
Structures of the supralaryngeal (pharyngeal-oral-nasal) system. The larynx also is shown.

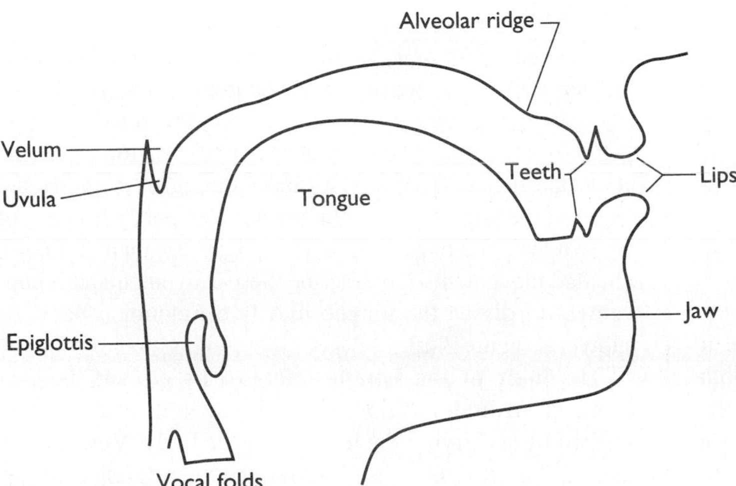

FIGURE 3-8
Tracing of an X-ray photograph of the articulators.

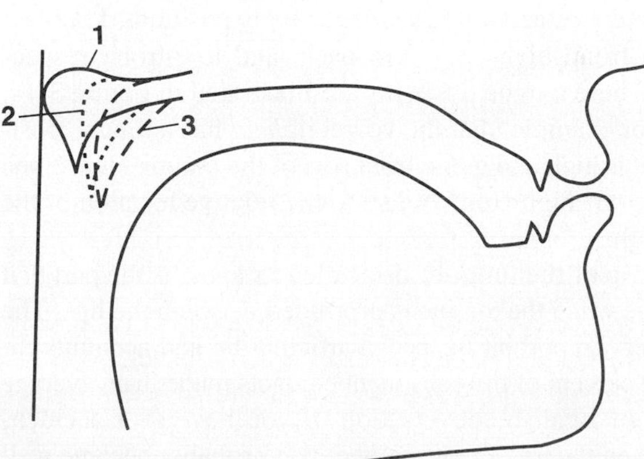

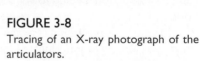

FIGURE 3-9
Articulation of velum, represented by positions for (1) *s* sound in *soon,* (2) *n* sound in *soon,* and (3) normal rest breathing. Velopharyngeal port is open for positions (2) and (3).

pictures of a person talking. Velar positions are shown for three events: (1) an elevated position during the oral sound *s* in the word *soon,* (2) a lowered position during the nasal sound *n* in *soon,* and (3) the normal resting position of the velum during quiet rest breathing through the nose.

Although articulation of the velum is a primary factor in closure of the **velopharyngeal port** (the opening between the oral-pharyngeal and nasal cavities), inward movements of the lateral walls of the pharynx also can assist in closing the port. The combined action of the elevating velum and the constricting pharyngeal walls often produces a purse-string effect, in which the velopharyngeal port is closed by movements on at least three sides. Opening of the velopharyngeal port is accomplished by the reverse actions, that is, lowering of the velum and outward movements of the lateral walls of the pharynx. Not all speakers rely on the purse-string type of closure—some appear to depend more on elevating and lowering movements of the velum to control the degree of opening at the velopharyngeal port. Still another pattern of velopharyngeal closure involves a bulging of the back wall of the pharynx, so that the back wall appears to move forward to meet with the elevating velum. This type of velopharyngeal closure is most common in individuals who have an abnormality of the velum, such as a cleft palate or a short palate. The student of communicative disorders should take note of the fact that speakers vary widely in the pattern of velopharyngeal valving.

The velum might be regarded as a muscle-and-flesh extension of the bony hard palate that forms the roof of the mouth. The pendulous tip of the velum, which you probably can see if you open your mouth widely as you look in a mirror, is called the uvula. The anatomy of the velopharyngeal region is illustrated in Figure 3-7.

Jaw

The jaw, or **mandible,** is important primarily because it contributes to movements of the tongue and lower lip, both of which are supported by the jaw. As the jaw moves, the tongue and the lower lip tend to move with it. The jaw has a hingelike motion made possible by a joint located close to the ear on either side of the head. The hinge is formed at a place called the **temporomandibular joint,** where the jaw (mandible) inserts into the temporal bone of the skull. Because of this hinge joint, the jaw rotates along an arc of opening and closing. However, the joint is constructed so that the jaw can move slightly forward and backward as well, so that some degree of mandibular protrusion and retrusion is possible. The shape of the jaw is illustrated in Figure 3-10. Jaw motion during speech is shown in Figure 3-11. The jaw positions shown here were obtained from X-ray pictures of the word *saw.* For the *s* sound, the jaw assumes a relatively closed (or elevated) position, whereas for the following vowel, it assumes a relatively open (or lowered) position.

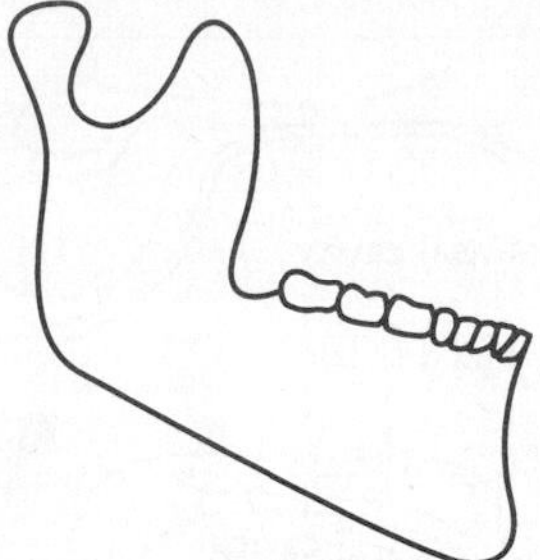

FIGURE 3-10
Shape of jaw, seen in lateral view.

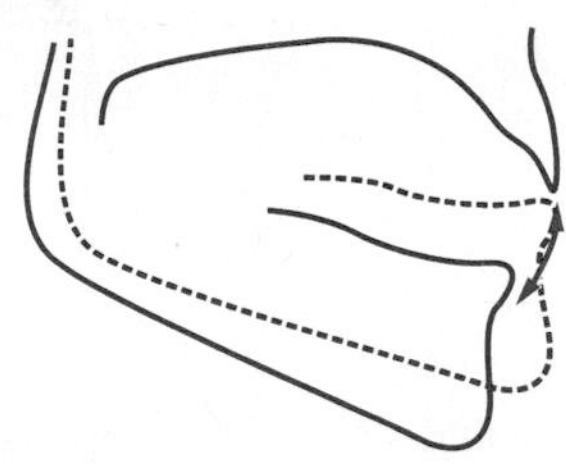

FIGURE 3-11
Jaw motion during speech. The closed position is for *s* in *saw,* and the open position is for the vowel.

Tongue

The tongue is a muscular organ that has no internal skeleton but derives skeletal support from the jaw and the hyoid bone (these bony structures and the tongue are illustrated in Figure 3-12). In addition, various muscles attach the tongue to the skull, the palate, the pharynx, and the epiglottis. Partly because of the variety of its attachments and partly because of its own versatile musculature, the tongue is capable of complicated movements. To describe these movements, it is convenient to divide the tongue into five functional parts, as shown in Figure 3-13.

The **body of the tongue** refers to its primary bulk or mass. The overall position of the tongue in the mouth is described by specifying the location of the body. Vowel articulation, in particular, is described with reference to the tongue body. For example, the four vowels in the words *heat, hoot, hot,* and *hat* have tongue body positions described as high-front, high-back, low-back, and low-front, respectively. These tongue positions are illustrated in Figure 3-14. Note, for example, that the vowel in *heat* has a tongue position that is high and in the front part of the mouth. Hence, the description "high-front" refers to the relative location of the bulk of the tongue.

The **tip of the tongue,** also called its apex, is the part that is visible when the tongue is protruded between the lips. The tip is very important in speech articulation and accounts for over 50 percent of the consonant contacts made in an average sample of English conversation. If you have ever accidentally bitten the tip of your tongue, you probably became well

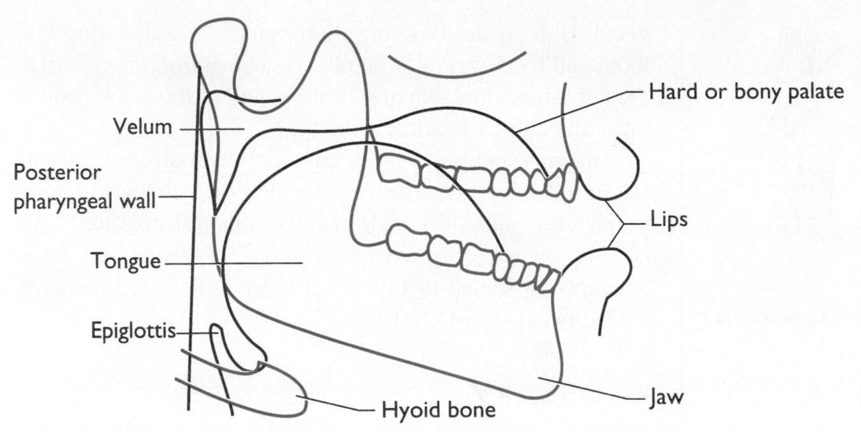

FIGURE 3-12
Skeletal or bony structures of the articulatory system shown by red lines. Tongue and lips are also shown (compare with X-ray tracing in Figure 3-9).

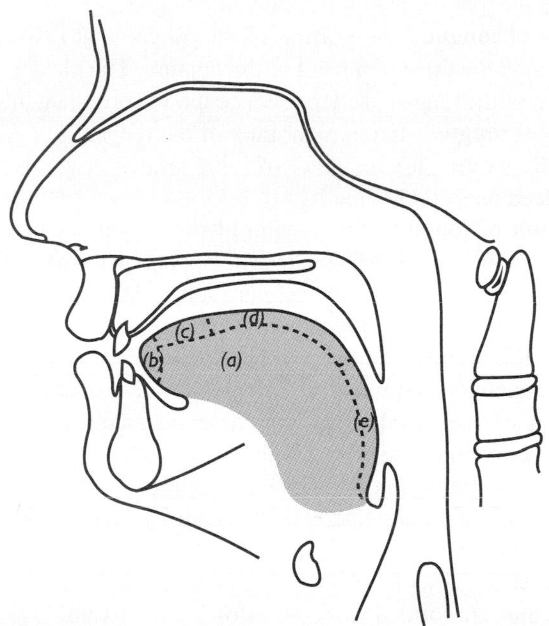

FIGURE 3-13
Functional divisions of tongue: *(a)* body, *(b)* tip or apex, *(c)* blade, *(d)* dorsum, and *(e)* root.

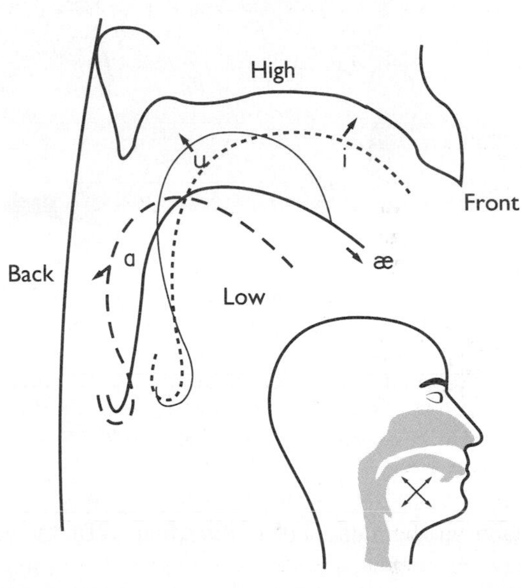

FIGURE 3-14
Tongue positions for the vowels in the words *heat* (high-front tongue position), *hoot* (high-back position), *hot* (low-back position), and *hat* (low-front position).

aware of how often it is used in making English speech sounds. The underlined letters in this sentence are produced with the tip of the tongue making contact somewhere in the mouth. Obviously, the tip is kept very busy in the task of speaking.

The **blade of the tongue,** located just behind the tip, is the part that makes the constriction for the *sh* sound in *sheep.* The blade is used in making constrictions for only a small number of sounds, but it also plays a role in shaping the tongue for other speech sounds.

The **dorsum of the tongue** (also known as the back) is the portion used in making the first sounds in the words *key* and *go* and the last sound in *thing*. This rather large segment contacts the roof of the mouth. As you might be able to determine from saying the three words given, the actual point of closure varies along the ceiling of the oral cavity. Indeed, the dorsum makes its articulations with both the hard palate and the soft palate.

The **root of the tongue** is the long segment that forms the front wall of the pharynx. The root does not actually make contacts or closures for English consonants, but it is important in shaping the vocal tract for vowel and consonant sounds.

Lips

The upper and lower lips contribute to speech articulation primarily by opening and closing, as in production of the

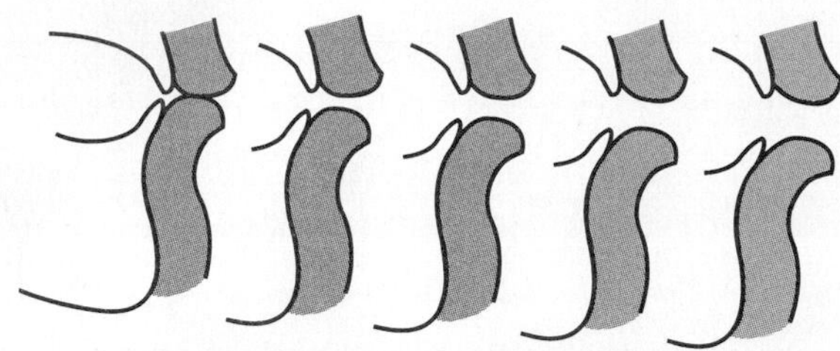

FIGURE 3-15
Lip opening for *p* sound as in *pa*. Lip and jaw positions are shown at intervals of 6.7 milliseconds (0.0067 second).

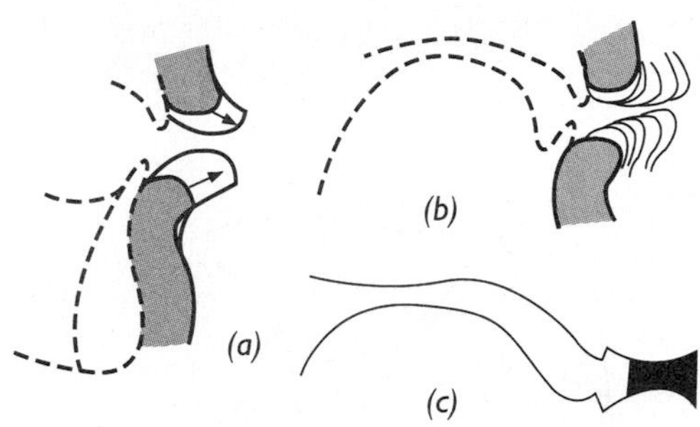

FIGURE 3-16
Articulation of lip rounding or protrusion. Drawing *(a)* shows unrounded and rounded lips. Drawing *(b)* shows successive lip positions as seen in intervals of 20 milliseconds (0.02 second) in an X-ray motion picture. Drawing *(c)* shows lengthening of vocal tract (shaded portion) caused by lip rounding.

word *pop,* and by rounding, or protruding, as for the vowel in *you.* Like the tongue, the lower lip is supported by the jaw, so that jaw movement usually moves the lower lip as well. In most people, the lower lip moves more than the upper lip. The two basic lip articulations are shown in Figures 3-15 and 3-16. Figure 3-15 illustrates the opening of the lips for a release of a *p* sound. Successive positions of lips and jaw are shown at intervals of 6.7 ms (*ms* is an abbreviation for milliseconds, or divisions of 1/1000 of a second). The separation of the lips is accomplished in about 35 ms or one-thirtieth of a second. Figure 3-16 depicts progressive lip positions during an articulation of protrusion. The positions are shown at intervals of 20 ms, in part *(b)* of the figure. The lengthening of the vocal tract caused by lip protrusion is illustrated by the blackened segment in part *(c)* of the figure.

CONCLUSION

It should be emphasized that the three systems described in this chapter interact strongly with each other in the production of speech and that each system is complicated enough to require a book for a reasonably complete description. We have simplified matters greatly by comparing the respiratory system to an air pump or balloon, by likening the vibrating vocal folds to the flapping mouthpiece of a deflating balloon, and by describing the pharyngeal-oral-nasal system as a set of articulators that are a critical part of the conversion of muscular energy to sound energy.

Anatomy and physiology have not been discussed in detail in this book because it is assumed that students of communicative disorders will receive this information from courses on anatomy and physiology. However, the basic concepts presented in this chapter are sufficient for the introductory study of phonetics.

GLOSSARY

Articulator an anatomic structure capable of movements that form the sounds of speech. The primary articulators are the tongue, jaw, lips, and velopharynx.

Blade of tongue the portion of the tongue that is located behind the tip and in front of the dorsum. The blade is the part of the tongue used to produce the *sh* consonant in *she.*

Body of tongue the mass or bulk of the tongue.

Breath group the sequence of syllables and/or words produced on a single breath.

Dorsum of tongue the portion of the tongue located between the root and the blade. The dorsum is the part of the tongue used to produce the *g* consonant in *go.*

Egressive associated with outflowing air; egressive sounds are formed from an outflowing airstream.

Fundamental frequency of voice the basic rate of vibration of the vocal folds; fundamental frequency is the physical correlate of vocal pitch.

Hertz the term that denotes one complete cycle of vibration; Hertz, abbreviated Hz, is the unit of frequency measurement.

Ingressive associated with inflowing air; ingressive sounds are formed from an inflowing airstream.

Intonation the pattern of fundamental frequency and sound duration in speech.

Laryngeal system the system of speech production identified anatomically with the larynx and functionally with control of phonation and voicing.

Larynx the "voice box" of speech; a structure made up of cartilage, muscles, and other tissues located within the neck. The larynx is located on top of the trachea and below the pharynx and serves to valve the airstream from the lungs.

Mandible the lower jaw, the bony structure that provides skeletal support for the tongue and lower lip.

Nasal cavity the space between the nares (nostrils) and the entrance into the pharynx.

Nasal radiation of sound transmission of sound through the nasal cavity (rather than through the oral cavity).

Oral cavity the space between the lips and the entrance to the pharynx.

Oral radiation of sound transmission of sound through the oral cavity (rather than through the nasal cavity).

Pharyngeal cavity the space between the division of the oral and pharyngeal cavities and the entrance to the larynx; its anterior boundary is the root of the tongue, and its posterior boundary is the pharyngeal wall.
Respiratory system the part of the speech production mechanism consisting of the lungs, rib cage, abdomen, and associated muscles. The respiratory system provides the major airstream of speech.
Root of tongue the part of the tongue that reaches downward from the dorsum of the tongue to the epiglottis and larynx.
Soft palate the soft-tissue structure that articulates to open or close the velopharynx.
Supralaryngeal system the system of speech production consisting of the pharyngeal, oral, and nasal structures.
Temporomandibular joint the hinge joint by which the jaw, or mandible, attaches to the temporal bone of the skull.
Thoracic cavity the chest cavity, containing the lungs, heart, and other organs.
Tip of tongue the forwardmost portion of the tongue, visible upon protrusion of the tongue from the mouth. The tip of the tongue is used to produce a large number of sounds, including the *th* consonant in *though* and the *t* consonant in *two.*
Trachea the "windpipe" that connects the lungs with the larynx, or "voice box."
Velopharyngeal port the opening between the oropharynx and the nasal cavity, which can be closed to prevent the nasal transmission of sound.
Velum the soft palate, especially its muscular portion; the velum articulates to open or close the velopharynx.
Vocal folds the paired cushions of muscle and other tissue that vibrate within the larynx to produce the sound of voicing.

EXERCISES

1. Draw an outline of the vocal tract and label the following: tongue body, root, dorsum, blade, and tip; lips, velum, jaw, alveolar ridge, velopharyngeal port, and pharynx.
2. Discuss the following and check your answers with the material in the text.
   (a) The difference between nasal and oral (nonnasal) consonants.
   (b) The meaning of the term *articulator.*
   (c) The function of the respiratory system in speech.
   (d) The interaction between tongue and jaw and lip and jaw in speech production.
   (e) The time pattern of vocal fold vibration.
3. Say the following words and name the oral articulators used for the sounds represented by the italicized letters.

   *Example: sh*oe—blade of tongue

   (a) *p*ay ____________________
   (b) *g*ee*s*e ____________________
   (c) *f*ir*m* ____________________
   (d) *l*i*k*e ____________________
   (e) *th*i*ng* ____________________
   (f) *ch*air*s* ____________________
   (g) *c*i*p*her ____________________
   (h) *b*a*th*e ____________________
4. Read aloud the following passage and, as you do so, circle the italicized letters that represent sounds made with the lips and place a check (✔) over the italicized letters that represent sounds made with the tongue.

   Al*th*ough the to*ng*ue is *v*ery i*mp*orta*nt* in spee*ch* ar*t*iculatio*n*, *th*ere are *s*everal re*p*orts of *p*erso*ns* who produ*c*e intelligible *s*peech e*v*en a*f*ter *m*o*s*t of *the* to*ng*ue has *b*een sur*g*ically remo*v*ed (often because of *c*ancer). I*nd*i*v*iduals so*m*etimes co*mpens*ate *s*urprisi*ng*ly well for da*m*age to the arti*cul*ators.

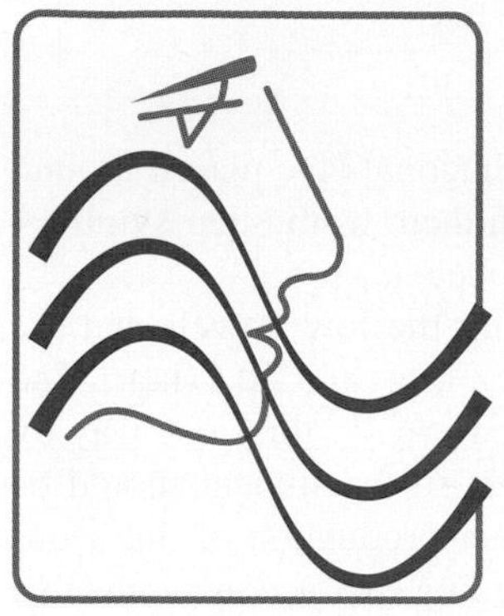

Vowels and Diphthongs 4

What is a **vowel**? This seemingly innocent question creates more difficulties than the beginning student of phonetics might imagine. The famous phonetician, Kenneth L. Pike, wrote about vowels and consonants as follows:

> *The most basic, characteristic, and universal division made in phonetic classification is that of consonant and vowel. Its delineation is one of the least satisfactory. . . . Frequently for descriptions of single languages the division is assumed, with no attempt to define it. The distinction is often presented as if it were clearcut, with every sound belonging to one or the other of the groups. Jones [another famous phonetician], for example, says, "Every speech-sound belongs to one or the other of the two main classes known as Vowels and Consonants." Later, however, various sounds are mentioned by him which have to be discussed separately under different rules, or with various kinds of reservation, because they do not neatly catalog themselves. Occasionally, in contrast to this, a writer frankly admits that his definition either of vowels or of consonants is unsatisfactory.* (Pike, 1943, p. 66)

Wise, in his book *Applied Phonetics,* also was highly cautious in defining consonant and vowel.

> *For consonant and vowel, at least, the student has had serviceable, if unformulated, definitions already in mind from ordinary school experience, which have been sufficient for the time. Actually, the formulation of exact definitions, even of consonant and vowel, is a difficult matter, and a very controversial one. The student must understand that the definitions in this book will not necessarily be approved by critics and other writers of phonetics texts.* (Wise, 1957, pp. 65–66)

Given this introduction, the reader may appreciate the rather involved definition: *A vowel is a speech sound that is formed without a significant constriction of the oral and pharyngeal cavities and that serves as a syllable nucleus.* By "significant constriction" we mean that the cavities are never narrowed to the degree observed for consonants, such as the underlined sounds in yes, keep, rope. Thus, the vowels are associated with a relatively open tract from the larynx through the lips. By "syllable nucleus" we mean that only one vowel sound can occur within the boundaries of a syllable unit and that, therefore, individual vowels can be identified with individual syllables. When the doctor asks you to open your mouth and say "ah," he or she is asking you to produce a vowel. This sound is convenient for the physician's purposes because it keeps the tongue low in the mouth (hence out of the way) and because the patient can sustain this sound for a long time if necessary (hence affording considerable time for observation). Vowels usually are voiced (produced with vibrating vocal folds), but not always. Whispered speech contains vowels that are not associated with vibrating vocal folds. The definition given here (to which occasional reservations might be added as we progress through the phonetic swamp) stresses three aspects of vowel production: (1) a spatial one—the articulators are positioned so as not to constrict the oral and pharyngeal cavities; (2) a temporal one—the sound of interest can be sustained indefinitely; and (3) a functional one—a syllable (with some exceptions) must include a vowel as its nucleus.

A pure vowel, that is, a vowel having a single, unchanging sound quality, is sometimes called a **monophthong** (from the Greek *mono,* meaning "one" and *phthongos,* meaning "voice" or "sound"). The IPA represents these sounds with single symbols, such as /u/ (who), /ɪ/ (hid), or /æ/ (had). But sometimes vowel-like sounds are produced with a gradually changing articulation and hence with a complex, dynamic sound quality. For example, consider the vowel-like sounds in the words *how, eye,* and *hoy.* If you place your finger or a pencil on the top of your tongue as you say these words, you should be able to detect a slow motion. This movement may be very small in the case of *how,* but much larger for *eye* and *hoy.* In addition, for both *how* and *hoy,* you should be able to see (or feel) a change in the shape of the lips. The vowel-like sounds in these words are called **diphthongs** (*di* meaning "two" and *phthongos* meaning "sound"). In the IPA, diphthongs are represented by a digraph, or pair of symbols such as /aɪ/ for the sound of *eye.* That is, the sound is presumed to begin with an /a/-like vowel and to end with an /ɪ/-like vowel. The tongue gradually changes its position from /a/ to /ɪ/, and the slowness of the articulatory motion helps to distinguish the diphthongs from certain "gliding" consonants, such as the *y* in *you* and the *w* in *we*.

VOWEL ARTICULATION

The position of the tongue distinguishes among almost all of the vowels in the English language. Tongue position can be described according to two dimensions: a dimension of high–low (superior–inferior) and a dimension of front–back (anterior–posterior).

Tongue Height (the High–Low Dimension of Tongue Position)

The term **tongue height** is used here to refer to the relative vertical position of the tongue body. In some cases, tongue height can be determined as the position of the highest point on the tongue, but this procedure has shortcomings. Difficulties with existing phonetic feature systems for vowels are reviewed later in this chapter, and the reader is forewarned that the features used here are not exact descriptions of vowel articulation. The features conform to general articulatory properties of vowels and are motivated largely by the requirements of simplicity and convenience.

In English and most other languages, the tongue has a range of vowel positions in the high–low (or superior–inferior) dimension. Vowels produced in the highest position, in which the tongue is close to the roof of the mouth, are called **high vowels.** Vowels produced in the lowest position, with the tongue depressed in the mouth, are the **low vowels.** Intermediate tongue positions along the high–low dimension are specified with such descriptors as mid-high, mid, or mid-low. Say the following pairs of words to yourself as you try to describe the height of the tongue for each vowel as either *high* or *low*.

heat–hat	hoot–hot
Pete–Pat	soup–sop
meat–mat	mood–mod
leak–lack	Luke–lock
ease–as	you–yaw

In each pair, the first word contains a high vowel, and the second word contains a low vowel. You can verify the difference in tongue height by touching your finger or a pencil to your tongue as you say the vowel sounds in the words *heat–hat–hoot–hop*. The vowels in *heat* (and in *he* and *ease*) and in *hoot* (and *who* and *you*) are the high vowels. We must emphasize that *high* is a relative term and does not necessarily mean that /i/ (he) and /u/ (who)[1] can be measured to have exactly the same elevation of the tongue. For some speakers, the tongue position for /u/ (who) is lower than that for /i/ (he), but the /u/ is the highest of the vowels produced in the back of the oral cavity. Similarly, /i/ is the highest of the vowels produced in the front of the oral cavity.

Remember that the virgules or diagonals are placed around phonemic symbols to distinguish them from other symbols, such as letters of the ordinary alphabet.

The vowels in *hat* and *hop* are the low vowels and are given the phonemic symbols /æ/ (hat) and /ɑ/ (hop). The latter key word is not pronounced exactly the same way by all speakers of American English, so the student should be very careful to compare his or her production of this word with the words on the tape recording that accompanies this text. Other frequently used key words for vowel /ɑ/ are *father, pot, calm, ah,* and *psalm.* This vowel often is confused with other vowels to be discussed later, so we want to give the student advance warning that /ɑ/ (hop) is another hazard of the phonetic swamp. Special attention to the recorded sample vowels is highly recommended.

X-ray pictures of the vocal tract are helpful in visualizing the differences between the high and low vowels. The line drawings in Figure 4-1 were derived from X-ray films of vowel production. Composite drawings of two vowels are shown to illustrate the differences between /i/ (he) and /u/ (who) and between /æ/ (hat) and /ɑ/ (hop). Note that for both /i/ (he) and /u/ (who), the tongue is high in the mouth and the jaw is in a nearly closed (or elevated) position, whereas for /æ/ (hat) and /ɑ/ (hop), the tongue is low in the mouth and the jaw is relatively open (or lowered). Because the tongue is supported by the jaw, it is natural to produce the low vowels /æ/ (hat) and /ɑ/ (hop) by dropping the jaw, which causes the tongue to assume a low position.

It should be recognized that although tongue and jaw tend to work together in vowel articulation (for example, vowels with a high tongue position are also produced with a closed jaw position), the tongue can move independently of the jaw. Figure 4-2 shows how the high tongue position for vowel /i/ can be accomplished with jaw positions ranging from closed to open (over an inch of opening, in fact). Of course, in order for the tongue to reach a high position when the jaw is open, the tongue must push up very high relative to the jaw, as shown at the bottom of Figure 4-2.

Other vowels assume intermediate positions along the high–low continuum of tongue positions. These sounds will be described in detail after the front–back dimension of tongue positioning has been discussed. But, in the meantime, the reader can get some idea of the variations in tongue height by saying the words (or even better, just the vowel sounds) in this list: *meat, mit, mate, met, mat.* These words are arranged roughly in descending order of tongue height for the vowel, so you should be able to feel the tongue assuming progressively lower positions as you read through

[1]Note: In the first part of this book, we will always follow a phonetic symbol with a parenthesized key word to help you remember the sound that is represented. For example, the phonemic symbols and key words for the high vowels mentioned above are

/i/ (he)
/u/ (who)

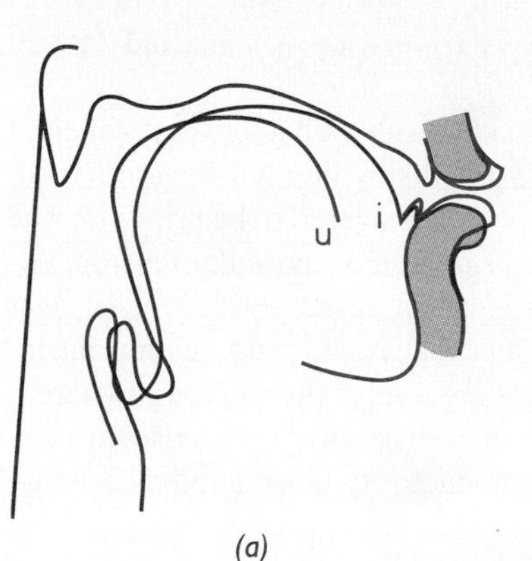

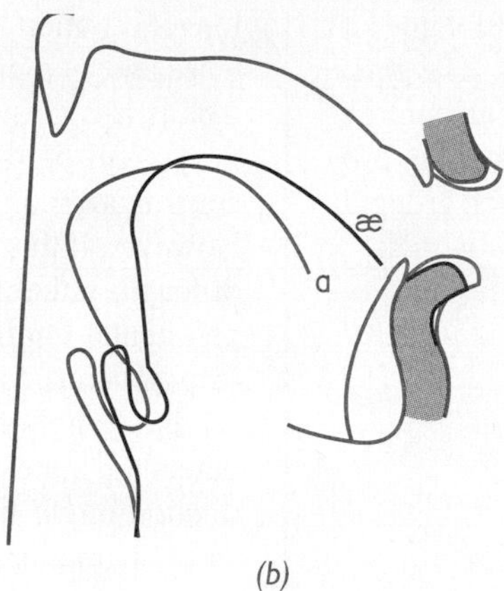

FIGURE 4-1
X-ray tracings of the corner or point vowels. *(a)* Black line shows high-back /u/ *(who)*, and red line shows high-front /i/ *(he)*; *(b)* black line shows low-back /ɑ/ *(hop)*, and red line shows low-front /æ/ *(hat)*.

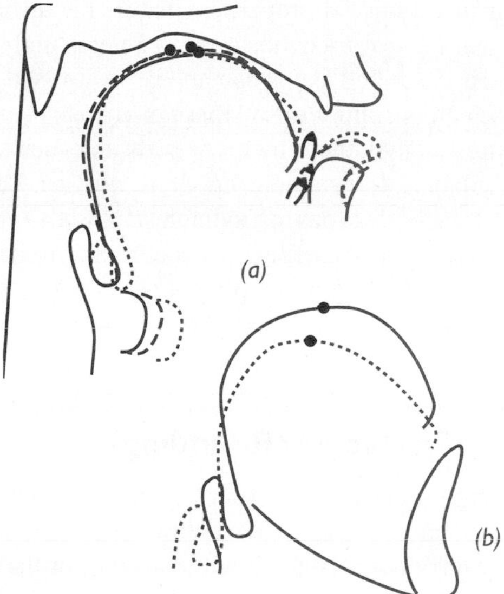

FIGURE 4-2
X-ray tracings showing high-front vowel /i/ produced with various degrees of jaw opening. The filled circle on the dorsum of the tongue is the location of a small marker attached to the tongue surface. *(a)* Articulatory configurations of /i/ with normal closed jaw position (dotted line), large jaw opening (dashed line), and very large jaw opening (solid line); *(b)* the stretching of tongue relative to jaw is shown by this composite of tongue shapes for normal (dotted line) and very large (solid line) jaw openings.

the list. We say "roughly" because individual speakers vary somewhat in the tongue height feature of vowel articulation. Read the list forwards and backwards to get a feeling of changes in tongue height.

Tongue Advancement (the Front–Back Dimension of Tongue Position)

In any given language, the vowels may vary along a dimension of front–back (anterior–posterior). We will refer to this dimension as **tongue advancement,** although it might just as well be called tongue retraction. Ladefoged (1971) uses the term "backness" to label a similar dimension of tongue position. For the vowels of English, we will use three descriptors of tongue advancement: front, central, and back. Thus, there are fewer variations for tongue advancement than for tongue height. As you say the pairs of words in Table 4-1, try to describe the position of the tongue for each vowel, using the choices of front, central, and back.

In Column 1, the first word in each pair contains a front vowel, and the second word contains a back vowel. In Column 2, the first word contains a front vowel, and the second word a central vowel. Finally, in Column 3, the first word has a central vowel, and the second word a back vowel.

Examples of vowels for each of the three places of front–back tongue position are given in Table 4-2. Say the words in each list and try to verify the descriptions of front, central, and back. It may help if you say only the vowel in each word.

TABLE 4-1

Column 1	Column 2	Column 3
heat–hoot	heat–hurt	hurt–hoot
hat–hot	hat–hut	hut–hot
pit–put	pit–putt	putt–put

TABLE 4-2

Front Vowels	Central Vowels	Back Vowels
seat	but	call
that	bird	tune
wet	luck	load
guess	supper (both vowels)	log
did	once	push
late	firm	took

One more exercise that helps to give the feel of tongue advancement is to say the following word triads. The three words in each row are arranged in order of front–central–back, so you should be able to feel the tongue assuming progressively backward positions for the words in each group. It may help if you say only the vowel in each of the words.

heat	hurt	hoot
hat	hut	hot
Sam	sum	psalm
deed	dud	dude
lick	lurk	look
weigh	were	woe

We can fix endpoints or extremes on the front–back dimension by using the vowels /i/ (heat), /u/ (hoot), /æ/ (hat), and /ɑ/ (hop or ah). That is, for a high tongue position, the extremes in tongue advancement are given by the vowels /i/ (high-front) and /u/ (high-back). For a low tongue position, the extremes in advancement are the vowels /æ/ (low-front) and /ɑ/ (low-back). Figure 4-3 shows how these four vowels compare in terms of tongue positions. Notice that the overall tongue positions, often even the positions of a given point on the tongue, are arranged in the form of a **vowel quadrilateral,** having the vowel corners /i/, /u/, /æ/, and /ɑ/ and the corresponding articulatory descriptions of high-front, high-back, low-front, and low-back. We will return to this quadrilateral description of vowels in a moment, but first we must consider two other features of vowel production.

Tenseness or Length

The terms **tense** and **lax,** representing extremes along a continuum of tenseness, are occasionally used in phonetic descriptions of vowels. Although these terms are very difficult to define, they are used to represent aspects of vowel articulation not covered by the other features. Basically, the feature or dimension of tenseness refers to the degree of muscle activity involved in the vowel articulation and to the duration of the vowel. Tense vowels have greater muscle activity and longer duration than lax vowels. For example, /i/ in *heat* is tense and /ɪ/ in *hit* is lax; /u/ in *Luke* is tense and /ʊ/ in *look* is lax.

As will be discussed later in this chapter, experimental confirmation of the tense–lax distinction has been difficult. However, if this distinction is considered to be primarily one of length rather than one of degree of muscular tension, experimental confirmation is much easier. In fact, it is clear from several acoustic studies that vowels vary in their intrinsic duration. Some vowels are almost always long, whereas others are almost always short. Therefore, the tense–lax distinction might be more satisfactorily considered as a long–short distinction.

To a degree, the vowels traditionally described as tense can be distinguished from those described as lax by examining their distributional properties, that is, the different phonetic conditions of their occurrence. Interestingly, none of the vowels described as lax can appear in stressed open syllables, which is simply to say that lax vowels cannot terminate a stressed syllable. The lax vowels do occur in stressed closed syllables, for example, *hit, book, nut, get.* Tense vowels occur in both types of syllables: closed—*heat, boot, caught;* open—*he, blue, law.* Hence, tense and lax vowels are treated differently in the phonology of English, and this fact alone is sufficient reason to divide vowels into tense and lax groups for phonetic purposes.

Lip Configuration (Rounding)

Lip configuration can be described by a variety of terms (such as rounding, protrusion, retraction, spreading, eversion, and narrowing), but we will consider for the most part only two states of the lips—rounded or unrounded. **Rounded vowels** are produced with the lips in a pursed and protruded state, so that they form a letter O when viewed from the front. **Unrounded vowels** are formed without such pursing or protrusion. See the examples in Figures 4-4 and 4-5. Occasional reference to these figures will be made as individual vowels are described in this chapter.

The best example of a rounded English vowel is the vowel /u/ (who), but even with this vowel we must be

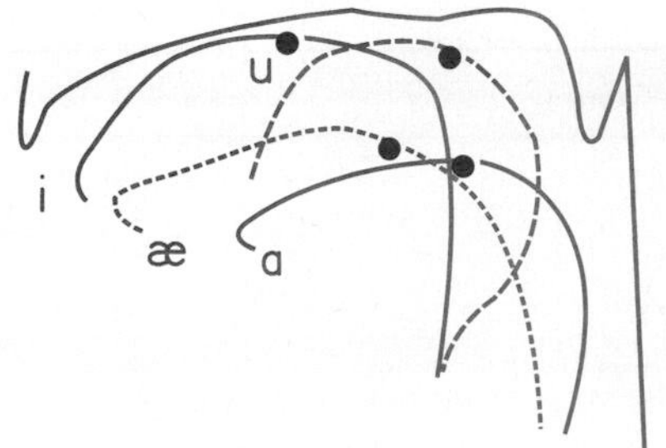

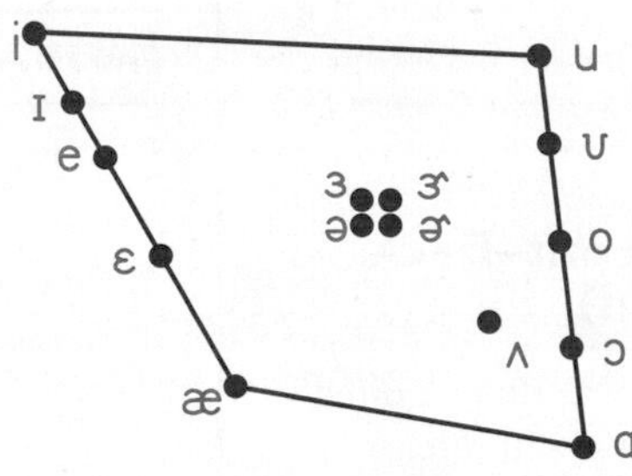

FIGURE 4-3
Vowel quadrilateral formed with vowels /i/, /u/, /ɑ/, and /æ/ as its corners. Tongue positions for vowels are specified as points falling on the sides of, or within, the quadrilateral diagram.

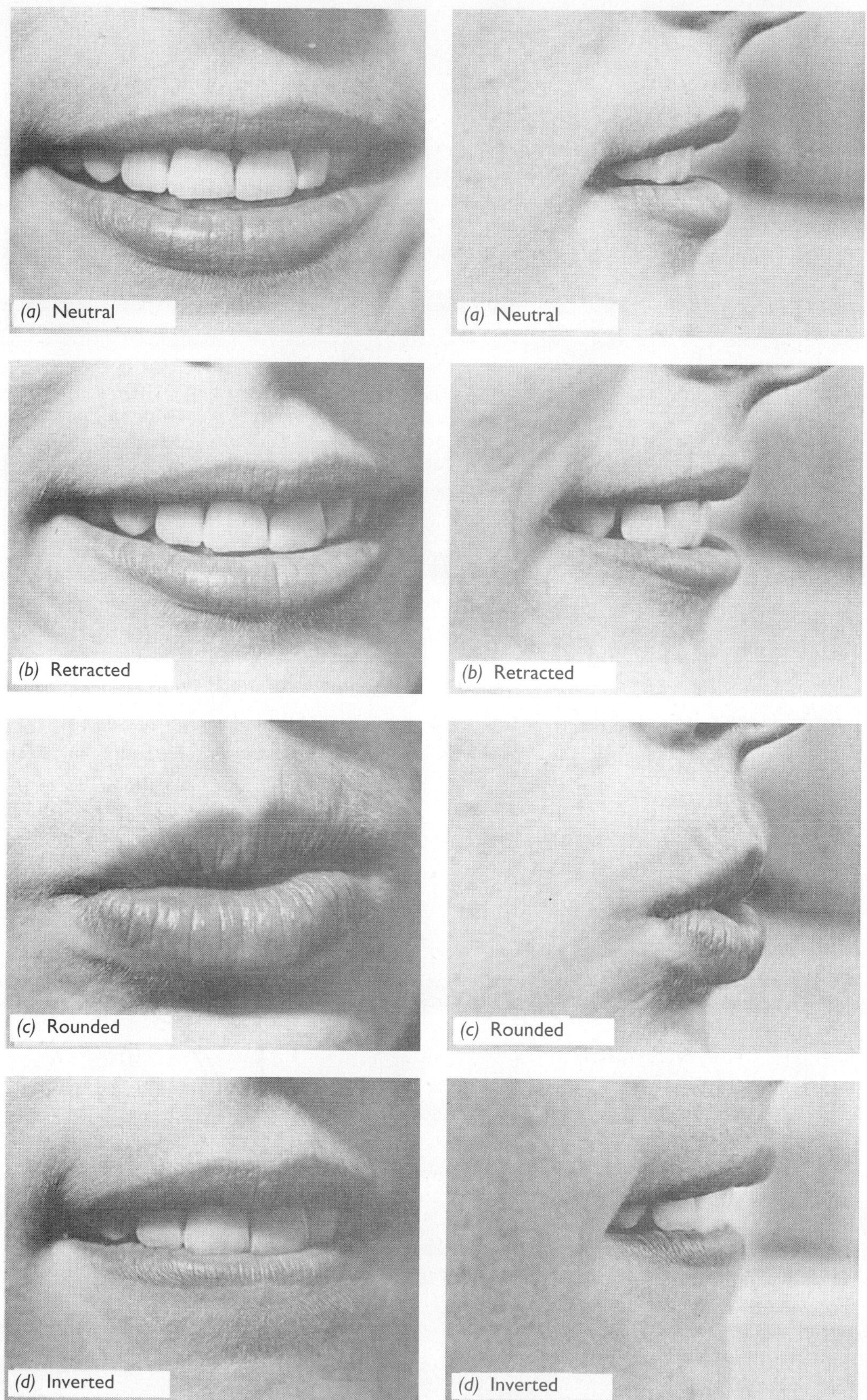

FIGURE 4-4
Major shapes of mouth opening or lip configuration, shown in side and front views: *(a)* neutral, *(b)* retracted, *(c)* rounded, and *(d)* inverted.

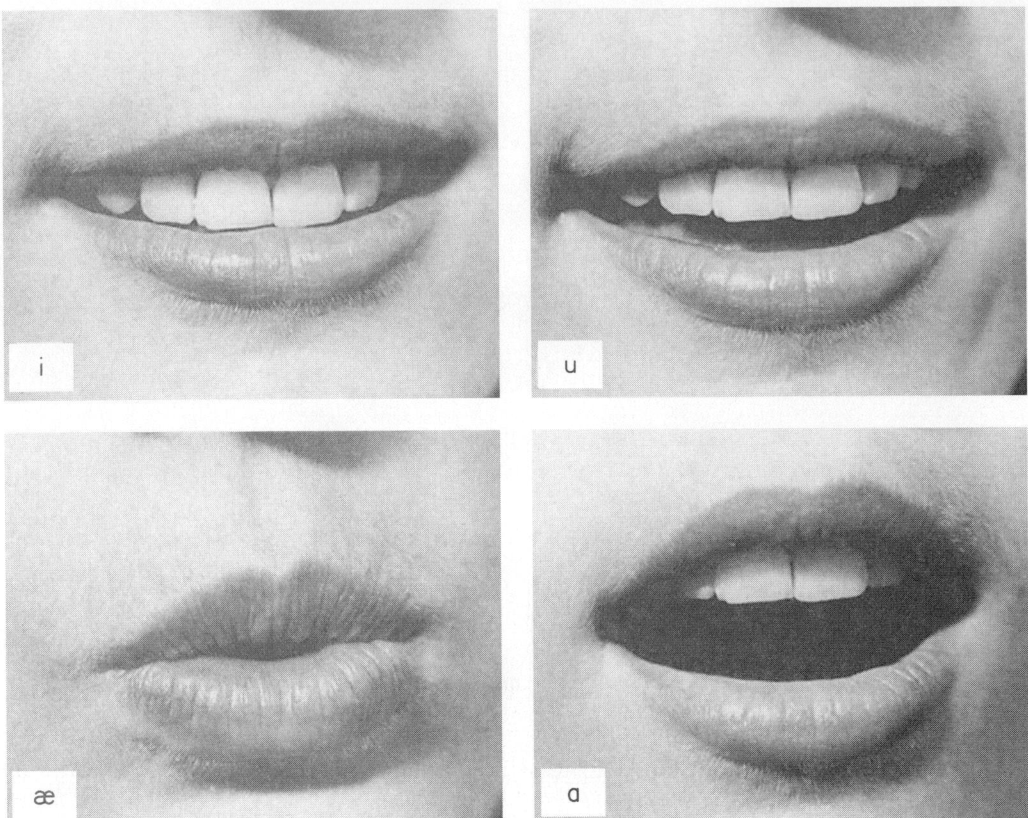

FIGURE 4-5
Photographs of the mouth opening for the vowels in the words *he, who, had,* and *palm.* The phonemic symbols for these vowels are /i/, /u/, /æ/ and /ɑ/, respectively.

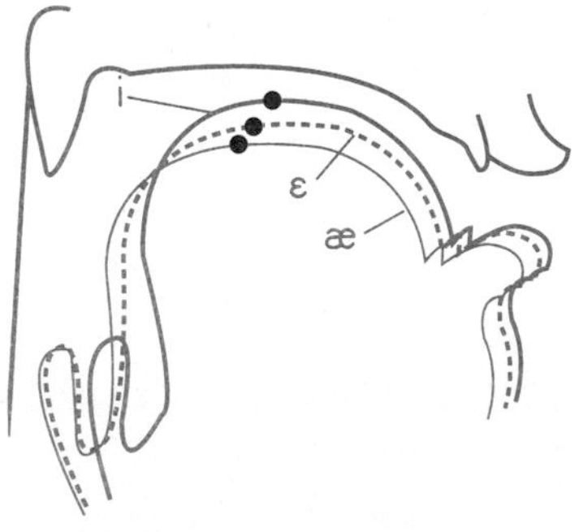

FIGURE 4-6
Composite of X-ray tracings for the front vowels /i/ *(heed)*, /ɛ/ *(head)*, and /æ/ *(had)*. For all three vowels, the tongue is positioned near the front of the oral cavity. The vowels are distinguished primarily by the feature of tongue height. Note that mouth opening varies but lips are unrounded.

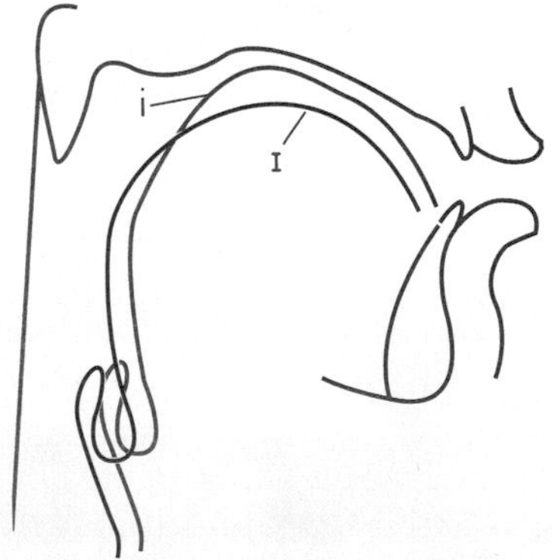

FIGURE 4-7
Comparison X-ray tracings for high-front /i/ *(heed)* and high-mid-front /ɪ/ *(hid)*. Vowel /i/ is shown by black line, /ɪ/ by red line.

cautious because not all speakers produce a rounded /u/. Vowels /i/ (he) and /æ/ (had) are examples of unrounded vowels. As mentioned earlier, lip rounding lengthens the vocal tract, and such lengthening can produce a significant acoustic change in the vowel sound. In English, only some of the back and central vowels are typically rounded. Included among the rounded back vowels are /u/ (pool), /ʊ/ (pull), /o/ (pole), and /ɔ/ (pawl). The best example of a rounded central vowel is /ɝ/ (bird). No front vowel in English is rounded, although many other languages contain rounded front vowels, as you may know if you have studied French, German, or Swedish.

Vowel Description: Tongue Height, Tongue Advancement, Tenseness, and Lip Rounding

English vowels can be described by considering three series or groupings: the **front series,** the **central series,** and the **back series.** The front and back series correspond to two sides of the vowel quadrilateral, as discussed previously. The vowels in each series are differentiated on the basis of tongue height, tenseness, and rounding. Thus, the three series are divisions according to tongue advancement, and the vowels within a series are distinguished by the other three features. Some cautions in the use of these terms are given at the end of the chapter.

THE FRONT SERIES

The front series includes the following vowels: /i ɪ e ɛ æ/, all of which are unrounded. The articulatory configurations for selected front vowels, as determined from X-ray studies, are shown in Figure 4-6. Note that the tongue is carried near the *front* of the mouth and that the lips are in an *unrounded* state. According to Dewey (1923), who determined the relative frequencies of occurrence of phonemes in standard English prose, the front vowels as a group made up about 20 percent of all sounds recorded. Within the class of vowels and diphthongs, the front vowels accounted for about half of the tokens. Thus, the front vowels have a rather high frequency of occurrence in the English language. Other data on frequency of occurrence are given in Appendix B.

Vowel /i/ (He)

Articulatory Description: High-Front, Tense, and Unrounded Vowel (Figures 4-7 and 4-5). This vowel is produced with the tongue in the extreme front and high position and therefore qualifies as a **point,** or **corner, vowel** on the vowel quadrilateral. The articulation is described as tense because the tongue musculature has a relatively tensed state and the duration is long (compared to /ɪ/, for example). You might be able to verify the difference in tension or overall muscle activity by placing your fingers under the fleshy part of your chin as you say the vowels /i/ (heed) and /ɪ/ (hid). Many speakers feel a greater tension for /i/ than for /ɪ/. Because /i/ is a high vowel, the jaw usually is held in a closed position, to assist the tongue in arching to its high position in the mouth. The velopharynx normally is closed for /i/, but it may be open if the vowel is in a nasal context (for example in the words *me* or *mean*). When the velopharynx is closed, the velum tends to be held in a high position because velar elevation usually is higher for high vowels than for mid or low vowels. For all English vowels, the possibility of nasalization exists for production in nasal contexts. Although we will not repeat this fact in each description that follows, this possibility should be kept in mind. Lip rounding is not tolerated well for /i/, as it causes a marked change in phonetic quality.

Articulatory Summary

Lips:	Unrounded, possibly everted or retracted.
Jaw:	Closed or elevated position.
Tongue:	Tongue body held in high-front position, so that maximal constriction occurs in the palatal region; pharynx is widely opened, with advancement of tongue root.
Velopharynx:	Normally closed unless sound is in nasal context; velum tends to be quite high.

Special Considerations and Allophonic Variations. Although the IPA treats /i/ as a monophthong, some linguists regard it as being diphthongized (/i y/). Vowel /i/ rarely is used before *r* within the same syllable. Vowel /ɪ/ (described next) is used in this position. Other allophonic variations of /i/ are described in the discussion of nasalized vowels in this chapter.

Words for Vowel Recognition or Transcription Practice. Until the student has had some transcription experience with consonants, it is recommended that he or she simply pronounce each word carefully and identify the vowel under consideration. After the student has studied consonants, these words may be used for practice in phonetic transcription.

s*ee*d	C*ae*sar	Ph*oe*nix
rel*ea*se	p*eo*ple	l*ea*p
r*ee*ling	mach*i*ne	est*ee*m
kn*ea*d	bel*ie*ve	c*ei*ling
l*ea*se	pr*e*vious	ben*ea*th
pl*ea*se	an*e*mic	tr*ea*tise

Vowel /ɪ/ (Hid) (Also Transcribed /ɩ/ in a Previous Version of the IPA)

Articulatory Description: High-Mid, Front, Lax, and Unrounded Vowel (Figure 4-7). This vowel differs from /i/ in that /ɪ/ is slightly lower (hence, high-mid), relatively lax, and shorter in overall duration. The following word pairs give contrasts of /i/ and /ɪ/: *lead–lid, weak–wick, sheep–ship, team–Tim, seen–sin, heed–hid.* As you say each pair, you should be able to tell that the second vowel, compared to the first, is lower, lax, and shorter. Because /ɪ/ is produced with a relatively high tongue position, the jaw usually is held in a closed position, but on occasion rather open positions can be tolerated. Lip rounding is tolerated better for /ɪ/ than for /i/, especially with reduced vowel duration, but rounding is unusual for either vowel. In word-final position in words like cit*y*, mudd*y*, pett*y*, and pit*y*, the choice between /i/ and /ɪ/ can be difficult. However, most phoneticians prefer /ɪ/ in these situations. One practical reason for this preference is the distinction between words such as *warranty–warantee,* for which /ɪ/ is suited for the former and /i/ to the latter.

Articulatory Summary

Lips:	Unrounded, sometimes slightly rounded or retracted.
Jaw:	Closed position, ranging to mid-open.
Tongue:	Tongue body in a high-mid and front posture, so that maximal constriction is developed in palatal region; pharynx not as widely opened as in the case of / i /.
Velopharynx:	Normally closed unless sound is in nasal context.

Allophonic Variations. See nasalized vowels and centralized vowels.

Transcription Words

l*i*mp	d*i*d	c*i*ty
l*i*st	w*o*men	r*i*ch
c*y*st	tr*i*ck	m*i*ddle
b*i*d	w*i*ck	qu*i*ver
sl*i*d	shr*i*mp	M*i*ck*ey*
t*i*ll	r*i*p	s*i*mple
sw*i*m	W*i*ll*y*	pick*i*ng

Vowel /e/ (Chaos—First Syllable)

Articulatory Description: Mid-Front, Tense, and Unrounded Vowel (Figure 4-8). The vowel /e/ is a monophthongal variant of the sound that more commonly occurs as the diphthongized form /e͡ɪ/, which is described in detail later in this chapter. The monophthong is shorter than the diphthong and does not have the tongue raising that is characteristic of the diphthong. The jaw usually assumes a mid position but may be as closed as that for the vowel /ɪ/. The lips are unrounded.

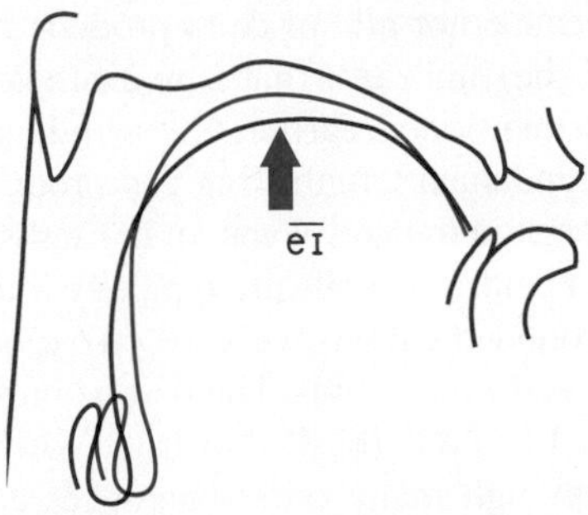

FIGURE 4-8
X-ray tracings for the monophthong /e/ *(vacation)* and the diphthong /e͡ɪ/ *(day)*. Black line shows tongue position for /e/, and red line shows the final position assumed after articulation of the diphthong /e͡ɪ/. Hence, the diphthong is produced with a gradual movement in the direction of the arrow.

Articulatory Summary

Lips:	Unrounded.
Jaw:	Mid position.
Tongue:	Tongue body in a mid and front position, creating a maximal constriction of the vocal tract in the palatal region; the constriction is less than that for /ɪ/.
Velopharynx:	Normally closed unless sound is in nasal context.

Allophonic Variations. See nasalized vowels and diphthong /e͡ɪ/.

Transcription Words. Note: The monophthong often occurs in these examples.

ob*e*yance	loc*a*te	incorpor*a*te
oper*a*te	holid*a*y	*e*ighteenth
ball*e*t	alter*a*tion	c*a*pon
ch*a*otic	s*e*ance	st*a*ying

Vowel /ɛ/ (Head)

Articulatory Description: Low-Mid, Front, Lax, and Unrounded Vowel (Figure 4-9). Vowel /ɛ/ is somewhat lower than /e/ (v*a*cation) and therefore has the articulatory description of low-mid-front (in the lower part of the mid range). This vowel is rather short, and in fact its short duration often distinguishes it from vowel /æ/ (had) more than does any other difference. The musculature is in a lax state, as is usually the case for short vowels. The jaw typically is in a mid position, tending to be somewhat more open (lower) than it is for /e/ (ch*a*os). The lips are unrounded.

Articulatory Summary

Lips:	Unrounded.
Jaw:	Mid position.
Tongue:	The tongue body is in a low-mid and front position, so that the constriction of the vocal tract tends to be uniform along its length (that is, there is no region of marked constriction).
Velopharynx:	Normally closed unless sound is in nasal context.

Allophonic Variations. See nasalized vowels. Both /æ/ (described next) and /ɛ/ are used before *r* in words like *chair, care, carry,* and *rare,* but /ɛ/ is more common in general American usage.

Transcription Words

b*e*t	f*e*rry	b*e*rry
ag*ai*n	att*e*mpt	m*e*rry
fr*ie*nd	regr*e*t	*e*xpect
*a*ny	sp*e*ll	rep*e*nt
s*e*nd	t*ea*r	m*e*ssage

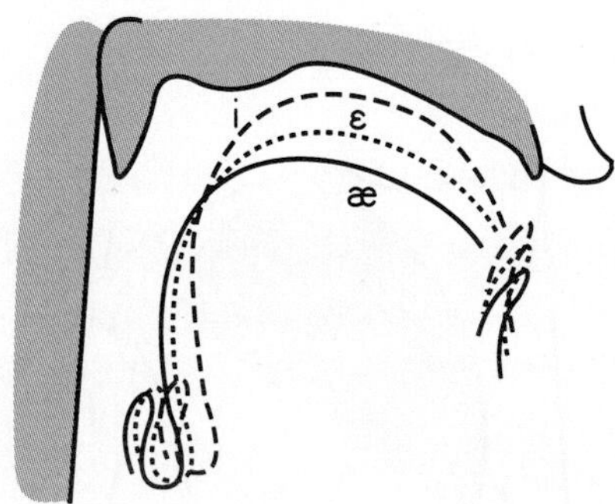

FIGURE 4-9
Composite of X-ray tracings for the vowels /i/ *(heed)*, /ɛ/ *(head)*, and /æ/ *(had)*.

Vowel /æ/ (Had)

Articulatory Description: Low-Front, Lax, and Unrounded Vowel (Figure 4-9). (Note: The IPA describes this sound as high-low-front, to indicate that it has a slightly higher tongue position than the non-English /a/.)

For speakers of General American English, the vowel /æ/ is the lowest front vowel; but for speakers with /a/ in their dialect, /æ/ is slightly higher than /a/. Vowel /æ/ tends to be long in duration but is sometimes described as lax because relatively little muscular tension can be felt under the chin during its articulation (compare /i/ to /æ/). Frequently, however, the major distinction between /æ/ and /ɛ/ is one of duration, and for this reason /æ/ is called long (and sometimes tense). Because /æ/ is quite low, the jaw assumes a low or open position. The lips are unrounded, often even retracted, as shown in Figures 4-4 and 4-5.

Articulatory Summary

Lips:	Unrounded, frequently retracted.
Jaw:	Open position.
Tongue:	Low-front in mouth, nearly the lowest front vowel in the IPA and in fact the lowest front vowel in General American speech.
Velopharynx:	Normally closed unless sound is in a nasal context; velar position during velopharyngeal closure tends to be low compared to other front vowels.

Allophonic Variations. See nasalized vowels. Also, /æ/ often is diphthongized in some dialects and idiolects, for example, /k æ t/ (cat) → /k æ ɪ t/ or /k æ ə t/.

Transcription Words

b*a*d	*a*lab*a*ster	h*a*mmer
s*a*ss	h*a*ng	*A*lab*a*ma
h*a*nd	h*a*ndsome	S*a*n Diego
*a*nswer	pl*a*ster	pi*a*no
cr*a*ss	*a*n*a*logous	st*a*ndard
gl*a*ss	*a*lcohol	bl*a*nd

Vowel /a/

(Eastern *path* or the initial segment of the diphthongs in *high* and *how;* see diphthong section later in this chapter.)

Articulatory Description: Low-Front, Lax, and Unrounded Vowel (Figure 4-10). This vowel was omitted from the vowel quadrilateral in Figure 4-3 because it rarely appears in isolated production in English. Sometimes it is used to denote the onglide, or first segment, of the diphthongs in *high* (or *buy, sign, aisle*) and *how* (or *round, house, town*). However, our own observations of vocal tract X-rays indicate that for Midwesterners, these diphthongs often begin with a segment that is very nearly like low-back /ɑ/. Vowel /a/ can be heard in the Eastern speech in words such as *path, park,* or *barn.* Although the IPA lists /a/ as the low-front vowel, many phonetics texts assign this description to /æ/. Because of the infrequent appearance of /a/, we prefer to regard it as an allophone or dialectal variation. For further discussion, see the section on diphthongs later in this chapter.

THE CENTRAL SERIES

The central vowels are /ɝ ɜ ɚ ə ʌ /, which are produced with a tongue body position roughly in the center of the mouth. Tongue height varies little among these vowels except that /ʌ/ is both lower and farther back than the other central vowels. The two vowels /ɝ ɜ/ often are rounded, but the degree of rounding varies considerably with speaker and dialect. The vowels /ə ʌ/ usually are not rounded. The weak or unstressed /ɚ/ is variable in rounding. Some speakers round it most of the time, whereas other speakers do not round it at all. Estimates of the relative frequencies of these vowels are uncertain because of problems in phonetic transcription and dialectal variation, but Dewey (1923) gives the relative frequency of occurrence of /ʌ/ and /ə/ as 2.33 and 4.63 percent, respectively. Within the group of vowels and diphthongs in Dewey's study, these two vowels make up almost one-fifth of the total usage.

The central vowels cannot be described without reference to stress. Whether good or bad, it is a characteristic of the IPA that both segmental and suprasegmental properties can influence phonemic transcription. That is, sometimes one symbol is selected over another because of a perceived difference in stress (the emphasis or prominence given to a syllable). For example, each of the two vowels in the word *further* has *r* coloring, but the vowels differ in stress. The first vowel receives more stress than the second. This difference is represented phonetically by transcribing the first vowel as /ɝ/ and the second vowel as /ɚ/. Therefore, the phonemic transcription of *further* is /f ɝ ð ɚ/. The vowels /ə/ and /ʌ/ also are described as having different stress, with /ʌ/ being more stressed than /ə/. For example, in the words *amuck* and *abut,* the first vowel is produced with less stress than the second. Therefore, the words are transcribed /ə m ʌ k/ and /ə b ʌ t/. The importance of stress in transcribing the central vowels often is underestimated by the beginner, and we have found that many students stumble in this area.

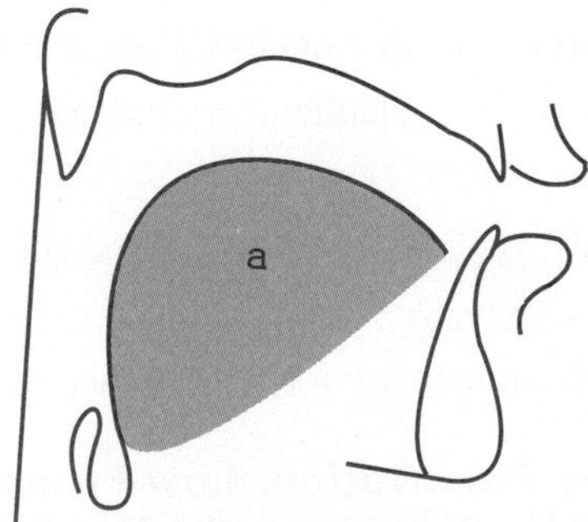

FIGURE 4-10
X-ray tracing of articulatory configuration for vowel /a/ (Eastern *path*).

Vowel /ɝ/ (Her)

Articulatory Description: Mid-Central, Tense, and Rounded Vowel (Figure 4-11). Vowel /ɝ/ has a mid-central position and usually is produced with some degree of rounding. The degree of rounding varies across speakers. As noted in the introductory comments on central vowels, /ɝ/ may be regarded as the stressed counterpart to /ɚ/ (which is unstressed). Vowel /ɝ/ is sometimes described as **r-colored, retroflex,** or **rhotacized.** Some vowels followed by consonantal /r/ occasionally are confused with /ɝ/ (see the description of /r/ in the chapter on consonants). Note the distinction between /ɝ/ in *burr* and the vowel + /r/ combination in *bar, bore, bear,* and *beer.*

Articulatory Summary

Lips:	Usually rounded.
Jaw:	Mid-open position.
Tongue:	Tongue body in mid-central position, often bunched in the palatal region.
Velopharynx:	Normally closed except for nasal contexts.

Allophonic Variations. See nasalized vowels, vowels /ɜ / and /ɚ/, and consonant /r/.

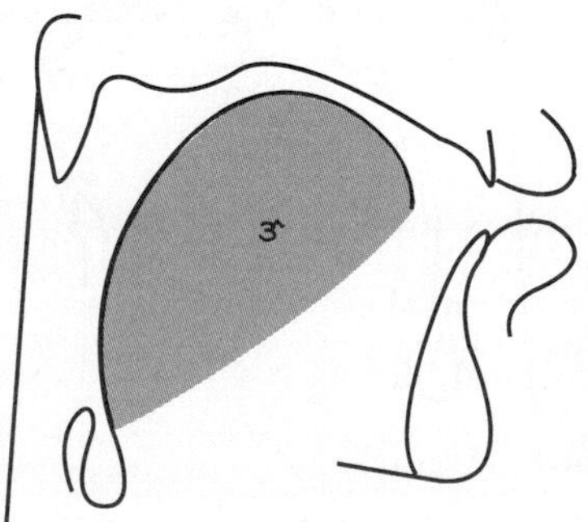

FIGURE 4-11
X-ray tracing of articulatory configuration for vowel /ɝ/ (*her*).

Transcription Words

sir	ret*ur*n	perv*er*se
le*ar*n	b*ur*ner	t*ur*pentine
ch*ur*ch	ass*er*t	s*er*pent
*ir*k	w*or*ker	st*irr*up
w*or*thy	p*ur*ged	k*er*nel
w*or*k	div*er*t	in*er*t

Vowel /ɜ/ (British or Southern Her)

Articulatory Description: Mid-Central, Tense, and Rounded Vowel. Vowel /ɜ/ is similar to /ɝ/ and replaces it as a dialectal variant in British, Southern, and occasionally Eastern speech. Perhaps the best description of /ɜ/ is "/ɝ/ without the *r* coloring." /ɜ/ does not normally occur in General American speech, but it does occur in some dialects and in developing speech. Some children who have difficulty with /ɝ/ will substitute /ɜ/ for it.

Vowel /ɚ/ (Further, Sometimes Called Schwar)

Articulatory Description: Mid-Central, Lax, and Rounded Vowel (Figure 4-12). Vowel /ɚ/ is the unstressed counterpart to /ɝ/ and shares with /ɝ/ a mid-central tongue position and *r* coloring. Generally, we will restrict /ɚ/ to unstressed (low-level stress) conditions. Thus, /ɚ/ does not occur in isolated single-syllables. For such words, /ɝ/ is the preferred symbol, for example, *word* /wɝd/. Although /ɚ/ generally is described as rounded, it may be produced as unrounded by some speakers. That is, lip rounding is not an invariant characteristic.

Articulatory Summary

Lips:	Rounded, but not necessarily so.
Jaw:	Usually closed to mid position.
Tongue:	Mid-central tongue body, with a bunching toward the palatal area (Figure 4-12).
Velopharynx:	Normally closed except in nasal contexts.

Allophonic Variations. See nasalized vowels and vowel /ɝ/. In some dialects (particularly Eastern) and some individual usage, /ɚ/ may be produced as /ə/, for example, the final /ɚ/ in *brother, sister, butter.*

Transcription Words

north*er*n	stup*or*	murd*erer*
upp*er*	laqu*er*	murm*ur*ing
rul*er*	surg*er*y	earn*er*
stirr*er*	loit*er*ing	high*er*
merg*er*	work*er*	barb*er*

Vowel /ʌ/ (Hub)

Articulatory Description: Low-Mid, Back-Central, Lax, and Unrounded Vowel (Figure 4-13). This vowel is produced with a tongue body position that is shifted somewhat toward /ɑ/ from the mid-

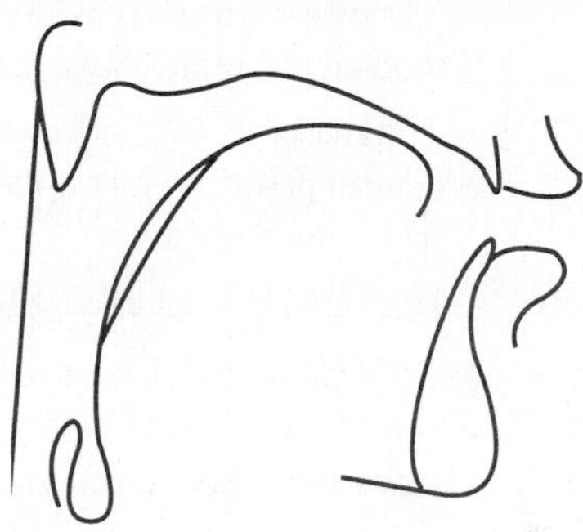

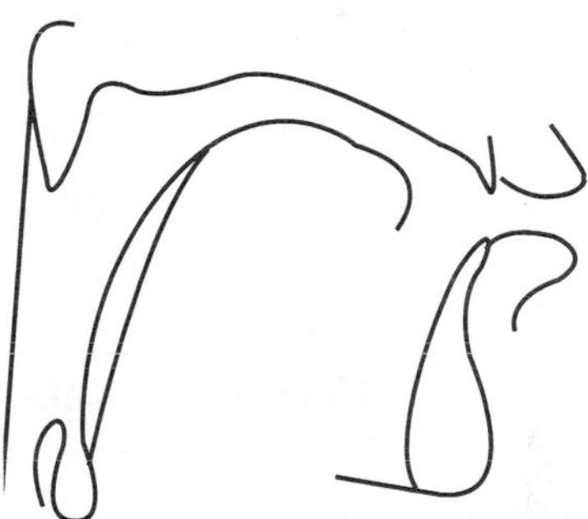

FIGURE 4-12
X-ray tracings of articulatory configurations for vowel /ɚ/ (*further*). The red line is the lingual midline, which is indented because of grooving of the tongue. Because the two tracings are from different words (*honor* and *polar*), the configurations vary slightly.

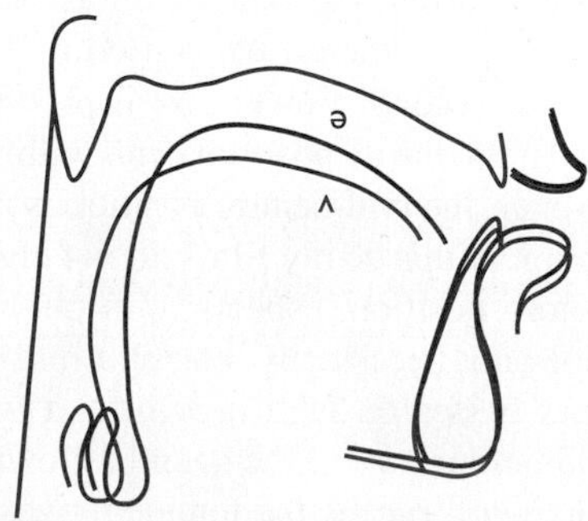

FIGURE 4-13
X-ray tracings of articulatory configurations for vowels /ʌ/ (black line) and /ə/ (red line). The vowels occur together in the word *abut* /ə b ʌ t/, which is a useful key word for their contrast.

central position. It may be regarded as lying about midway along an axis between the central position and the position for /ɑ/ (to be described). In addition, /ʌ/ is shorter in duration than /ɑ/. The lips are not rounded, and the jaw usually is quite open but ranges from relatively open to relatively closed, depending upon phonetic context, stress, and other factors.

Articulatory Summary

Lips:	Unrounded.
Jaw:	Varies over a fairly wide range but tends to be relatively open.
Tongue:	Tongue body is in a low-mid, back-central position, just up and forward from that for /ɑ/.
Velopharynx:	Normally closed except for nasal contexts.

Allophonic Variations. See nasalized vowels and vowel /ə/.

Transcription Words

r*ou*gh	cl*u*tter	s*u*pper
n*u*t	t*u*mble	n*u*mber
ab*u*t	s*o*me*o*ne	*u*pset
en*ou*gh	r*u*ckus	p*u*ppet
s*u*n	l*u*strous	*o*nce
tr*u*st	c*u*stomer	b*u*cket

Vowel /ə/ (Above, Sometimes Called Schwa)

Articulatory Description: Mid-Central, Lax, and Unrounded Vowel (Figure 4-13). Vowel /ə/, also known as the **schwa** vowel, is the unstressed counterpart to /ʌ/. As noted earlier, the stress contrast appears in the words *above* and *abut,* where /ə/ is used in the first syllable and /ʌ/ in the second. Vowel /ə/ is produced with the tongue in the mid-central position and with the lips unrounded. However, the mid-central position is rather an idealized description in that X-ray films do not always reveal a stable articulatory position, especially in phonetic context. The tongue does not necessarily stop at a mid-central position but instead passes through it or near it while moving from the sound before /ə/ to the sound following /ə/. For example, in the word *ruckus* the tongue moves almost continuously from the *k* to the *s*. Often, what we hear as the vowel /ə/ is a short duration vocalic segment brought about by continuous tongue movement. The jaw ranges between closed to mid-open position.

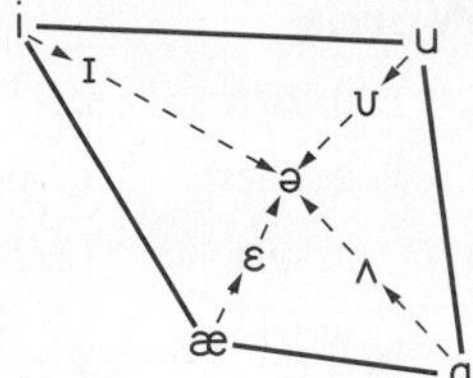

FIGURE 4-14
Diagram of vowel reduction. Reduction occurs along the red lines; for example, /i/ reduces to /ɪ/, and /ɪ/ reduces to /ə/. Schwa /ə/ is the maximally central, maximally reduced vowel.

Generally speaking, /ə/ does not receive more than tertiary (third-level) stress, although some phoneticians occasionally use it with higher stress levels. One reason to restrict it to the weakest stress level is that its use can be taken as evidence of unstressing, or **reduction.** In normal adult speech, some vowels are reduced greatly in duration compared to others. When the reduction is great enough, almost any vowel can approach /ə/, although this reduction is especially likely for the vowel /ʌ/. A diagram of vowel reduction is shown in Figure 4-14. The arrows indicate the direction of vowel changes as a result of reduction. Normally, the duration of /ə/ is quite short. For example, when adult speakers say the sentence "We saw you hit the cat," the vowel /æ/ in *cat* is five times as long as the vowel in *the.*

Articulatory Summary

Lips:	Unrounded.
Jaw:	Closed to mid-open position.
Tongue:	Ideally mid-central in isolated production, but tongue position is often not stable in connected speech.
Velopharynx:	Normally closed except when in nasal context.

Allophonic Variations. See nasalized vowels and previous discussion. Vowel /ə/, or schwa, is the ultimately unstressed vowel in that it has the shortest duration and the most nearly central tongue position.

Transcription Words. Note: Because we will try in this book to restrict the use of /ə/ to conditions of weak stress, it will not be used in single syllables produced in isolation. Such words necessarily carry first-level or primary stress.

*e*nough	lustr*ou*s	im*i*tate
*a*gain	cust*o*mer	radi*u*m
*a*but	pupp*e*t	purp*o*se
ruck*u*s	*a*wait	relig*io*n
tel*e*phone	*a*mount	rust*e*d

THE BACK SERIES

This series includes the vowels / u ʊ o ɔ ɑ /, all of which except / ɑ / tend to be rounded. Figure 4-15 is a composite illustration of the articulatory configurations for some of these vowels. Notice that the tongue is positioned near the back of the mouth for these vowels, but there is some variation in their position along a front–back dimension. The drawings also show lip rounding for three of the vowels. Because the tongue is in the back of the mouth, the region of greatest constriction is in the pharynx or near the velum. In Dewey's (1923) study of frequency of occurrence, these vowels constituted 12 percent of the vowels and diphthongs and about 4 percent of all sounds recorded. However, these figures do not include the diphthongs, three of which involve a back vowel.

Vowel /u/ (Who)

Articulatory Description: High-Back, Tense, and Rounded Vowel (Figures 4-5 and 4-15). The tongue is in the extreme high-back position, so that /u/ is one of the point vowels. The articulation constricts the oral cavity in the velar region. The tenseness of the articulation can be sensed by comparison of /u/ with the lax /ʊ/ (book). The tense–lax (or long–short) contrast of /u/–/ʊ/ is analogous with that of /i/–/ɪ/. Like /i/, /u/ usually is produced with a closed jaw position to aid the tongue in reaching its high articulation. Although most speakers produce /u/ with rounding and protrusion of the lips (Figures 4-4 and 4-5), some persons make this sound with a narrowed opening but little protrusion. The acoustic consequences of narrowing and protrusion of the lips are highly similar.

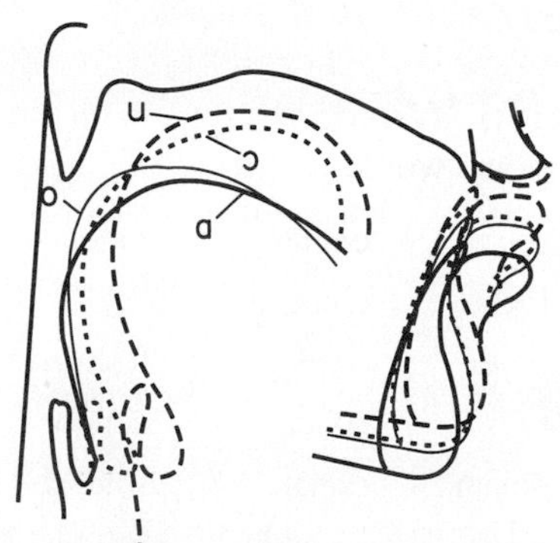

FIGURE 4-15
Composite of X-ray tracings for the back vowels /u/ (dashed line) /ɔ r/ (dotted line), /o/ (thin solid line), and /ɑ/ (thick solid line). The tongue is carried toward the back of the oral cavity for all these vowels, but tongue height and mouth opening vary among them. All except /ɑ/ are rounded. The configuration for /ɔ r/ represents a rhotacized modification (to be discussed later) and should not be taken as a typical example of /ɔ/.

Articulatory Summary

Lips:	Rounded and/or narrowed.
Jaw:	Closed position.
Tongue:	Tongue body in high-back position; tongue root is advanced so that lower pharynx is wide; maximal constriction in velar region.
Velopharynx:	Normally closed except when sound is in nasal context; velum tends to be high.

Special Considerations and Allophonic Variations. Some phoneticians regard the /ju/ combination, as in the words *use, you,* and *excuse,* to be a diphthong. Frequently, tongue movements from a consonant to /u/ are gradual, almost glidelike in character. As shown in Figure 4-16, /u/ sometimes has an allophonic variant of a front, rounded vowel in words like *commune.*

Transcription Words

s*ue*	n*oo*dle	st*u*dent
*oo*ze	dil*u*te	ball*oo*n
dr*ew*	poll*u*te	all*u*de
can*oe*	ast*u*te	st*u*pid
cr*ui*se	cr*ue*l	*u*seful
n*ew*	r*u*dely	*u*niverse

Vowel /ʊ/ (Book, also Transcribed /ɷ/ in a Previous Version of the IPA)

Articulatory Description: High-Mid, Back, Lax, and Rounded Vowel (Figure 4-17). Compared to /u/, /ʊ/ is lax, slightly lower, and shorter in duration. Note the contrast of /u/ and /ʊ/ in these word pairs: *Luke–*

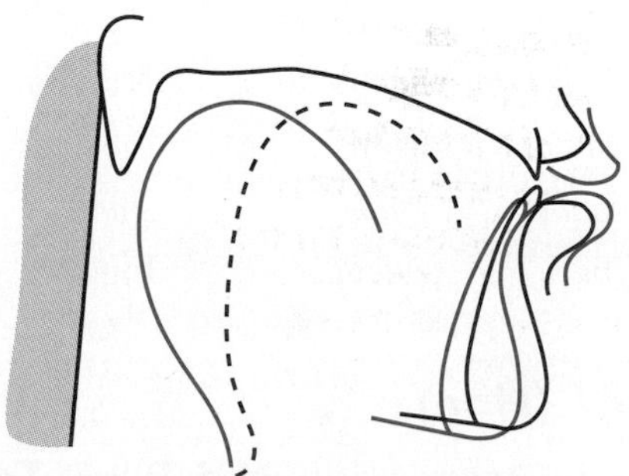

FIGURE 4-16
X-ray tracing for the second vowel in the word *commune* (dashed line) compared to tracing for vowel /u/ (solid line). Note that configuration shown by dashed line resembles a rounded front vowel.

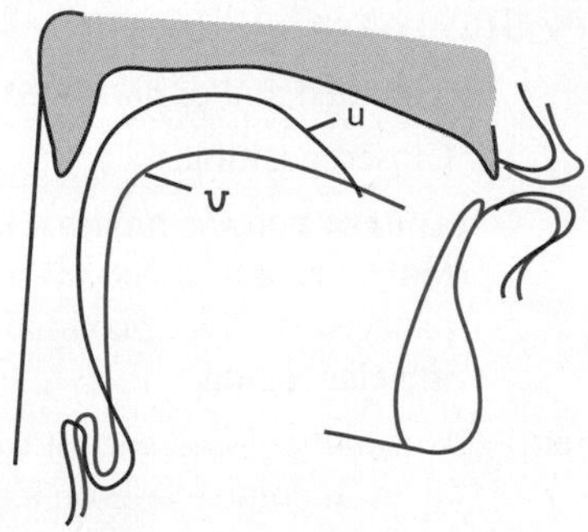

FIGURE 4-17
X-ray tracings of articulatory configurations of vowels /u/ (black line) and /ʊ/ (red line). Vowel /ʊ/ is essentially a reduced version of /u/, being shorter in duration, more central in tongue position, and less rounded.

look, cooed–could, fool–full, wooed–would, and *stewed–stood.* Jaw position usually is closed for /ʊ/. Lip rounding frequently is not as pronounced as with /u/ and may be neglected altogether.

Articulatory Summary

Lips:	Rounded in most cases.
Jaw:	Closed position, but ranging to mid-open.
Tongue:	Tongue body in high-mid and back position, with width of pharynx less than for /u/.
Velopharynx:	Open only for nasal contexts.

Allophonic Variations. See nasalized vowels. See /ʌ/, described in the central series. Note that some words can be pronounced with either /ʊ/ or /u/: *hoof, roof, root, broom.*

Transcription Words

w*oo*d	underst*oo*d	br*oo*k
h*oo*f	g*oo*d	f*u*llness
sh*ou*ld	c*oo*k	r*oo*k
n*oo*k	p*u*ll	sh*oo*k
b*u*ll	s*u*gar	f*oo*t

Vowel /o/ (Hoe)

Articulatory Description: Mid, Back, Tense, and Rounded Vowel (Figure 4-18). The pure or monophthong /o/ usually occurs in syllables of no more than secondary stress, such as the first syllable in *notation*. In syllables receiving primary stress, the diphthong /o͡ʊ/ is more likely to occur than the monophthong /o/. Tongue position for /o/ is slightly lower than for /ʊ/, and a distinct rounding of the lips usually can be seen. For diphthong /o͡ʊ/, the tongue makes a raising gesture from /o/ roughly to /ʊ/. Jaw position varies from closed to mid, depending upon phonetic context, stress, and other prosodic variables.

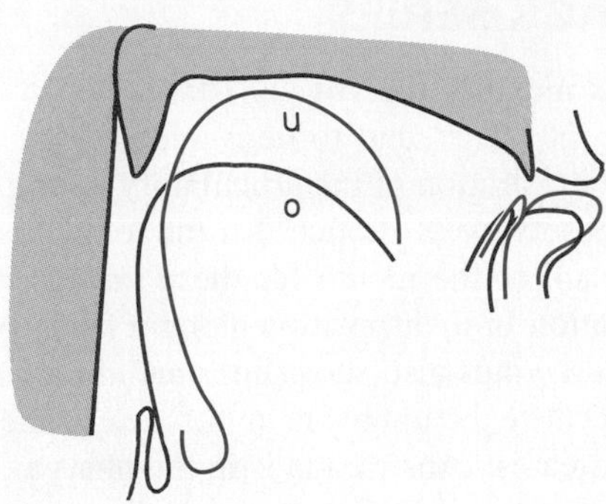

FIGURE 4-18
X-ray tracing of articulatory configuration of vowel /o/ (black line) compared with that of vowel /u/ (red line).

Articulatory Summary

Lips:	Rounded.
Jaw:	Closed to mid position.
Tongue:	Tongue body is in a back position, not quite as high as for /ʊ/, resulting in a constricted region in the pharynx.
Velopharynx:	Normally closed, except when sound is in nasal context.

Allophonic Variations. See nasalized vowels and diphthong /o͡ʊ/.

Transcription Words. Note: both /o/ and /o͡ʊ/ may occur in some words.

r*o*tate	c*o*llate	r*o*de*o*
l*o*cate	em*o*tion	s*o*l*o*
m*o*de	r*oa*d	R*oa*n*o*ke
t*oe*s	r*o*llcall	den*o*te
*o*cean	d*o*nate	s*o*ldier
*o*de	sh*ou*lder	foll*ow*

Vowel /ɔ/ (Awl)

Articulatory Description: Low-Mid, Back, Tense, and Rounded Vowel (Figure 4-19). Tongue position is similar to that for /o/ but is slightly lower. The lips are rounded. The jaw usually is in a mid position. Speakers

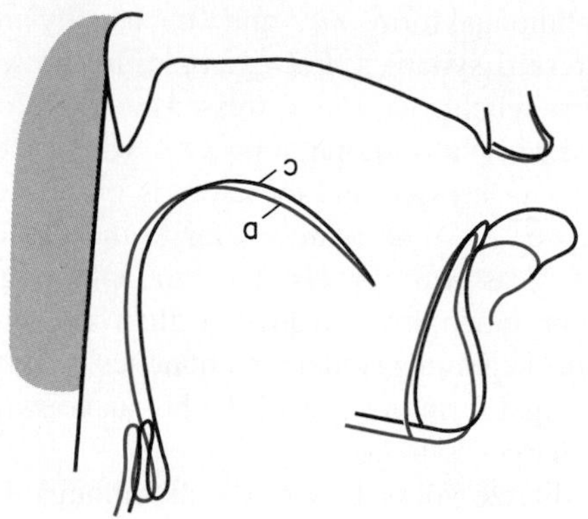

FIGURE 4-19
Comparison X-ray tracings of the articulatory configurations of vowels /ɔ/ (black line) and /ɑ/ (red line). Vowel /ɔ/ *(awl)* is higher than /ɑ/ and is rounded.

vary considerably in the use of /ɔ/, with dialectal alternation of /ɔ/ and /ɑ/ (described next) being quite common. Words typically pronounced with /ɔ/ are *taut, brought, all,* and *wash.*

Articulatory Summary

Lips:	Rounded, though often not as much as for /u/ or /o/.
Jaw:	Mid position.
Tongue:	Tongue body is in a low-mid and back position, so that the most constricted region of the vocal tract is in the mid-pharyngeal segment.
Velopharynx:	Normally closed except for nasal contexts.

Allophonic Variations. See nasalized vowels. Either /ɔ/ or /o/ can be used before *r* in words like *tore, port, more,* and *sport.* Vowel /ɔ/ is similar to the British vowel /ɒ/ (Br. *hot*) but tends to be longer. See description of /ɑ/.

Transcription Words

*aw*l	d*o*g	qu*a*rrel
*ou*ght	c*ou*gh	h*au*nt
c*au*ght	*o*ffice	f*o*reign
*o*range	c*o*rd	l*au*rel
l*aw*	*o*rigin	m*o*ral

Vowel /ɑ/ (Hop)

Articulatory Description: Low, Back, Tense, and Unrounded Vowel (Figures 4-5, 4-15, and 4-19). The vowel /ɑ/ with its low-back tongue position, completes the vowel quadrilateral. The lips are unrounded and widely open (Figure 4-5). The jaw is in an open position; in fact, for most speakers, this vowel is the most open vowel. The region of greatest constriction of the vocal tract is between the root of the tongue and the mid to lower pharynx. Because the use of this vowel varies widely with dialect, selection of a key word is troublesome. Generally useful key words include *father, calm, hot, barn,* and *ah.* In attempting to say /ɑ/, the speaker should be careful to place the tongue in the extreme low-back position, avoid rounding, and allow ample duration.

Articulatory Summary

Lips:	Unrounded and widely open.
Jaw:	Open.
Tongue:	Tongue body is in the extreme low and back position, so that the pharynx is constricted. The front cavity is larger than for any other vowel.
Velopharynx:	Open only for nasal contexts, but the velum can be lower than for other vowels.

Special Considerations and Allophonic Variations. See nasalized vowels. Depending on dialect, the vowel /ɑ/ may be replaced by /ɒ/ or /ɔ/ or /a/.

Transcription Words

p*o*t	sl*o*t	imp*o*ster
cl*o*d	c*o*mmon	h*o*ller
b*a*lm	c*o*llege	h*o*nor
f*o*lly	d*o*ll	s*o*cket
*o*pera	h*o*lly	adm*o*nish

DIPHTHONG ARTICULATION

As mentioned in the introduction to this chapter, diphthongs are vowel-like sounds produced with a gradually changing articulation. These sounds are represented in phonetic transcription by digraph (two-element) symbols that are meant to describe the onglide, or initial segment, and the offglide, or final segment. Thus, the digraph symbol represents in articulatory terms a position of origin and a position of destination.

Actually, the choice of a digraph symbol for the English diphthongs is not easy, and an examination of this problem takes us into another part of the phonetic swamp. Appendix A lists the various symbols that have been proposed for the diphthongs of American English. The reader should be aware of this diversity and not necessarily expect any two

TABLE 4-3
Diphthongs of American English

	Symbol	Key Words
Phonemic	/a͡ɪ/	bye, eye, aisle
	/ɔ͡ɪ/	boy, toy, oil
	/a͡ʊ/	bough, how, owl
Nonphonemic	/e͡ɪ/	bay, hay, pail
	/o͡ʊ/	bow, hoe, pole

phoneticians to use the same diphthong symbols. In this text, with some exceptions, we will use the symbols of the IPA. The two symbol elements are connected with an overhead bar to indicate their phonemic unity.

The phonetic symbols and selected key words for the diphthongs of American English are given in Table 4-3. Notice that three of the diphthongs /a͡ɪ/ (bye), /ɔ͡ɪ/ (boy), and /a͡ʊ/ (bough) are called *phonemic,* whereas the diphthongs /e͡ɪ/ (bay) and /o͡ʊ/ (bow) are *nonphonemic.* The phonemic diphthongs cannot be reduced to monophthongs, but the nonphonemic diphthongs can. This difference can be illustrated with the words in the following columns.

bind	/ba͡ɪnd/	bond	/band/
loin	/lɔ͡ɪn/	lawn	/lɔn/
down	/da͡ʊn/	Don	/dan/

In the column at the left, the phonemic diphthongs occur in common English words. Imagine saying each of these words by producing only the first element in each diphthong and omitting the second element, that is, reducing the diphthong to a monophthong. If you do this, *bind* should sound something like *bond, loin* should sound something like *lawn,* and *down* should sound something like *Don.* In short, reducing the diphthong to a monophthong results in a new morpheme. As was explained in Chapter 2, morphemes are distinguished by phonemic contrasts. Hence, the diphthong in *loin* is phonemically distinct from the monophthong in *lawn.* The phonemic diphthongs /a͡ɪ/ (bye), /ɔ͡ɪ/ (boy), and /a͡ʊ/ (bough) cannot be reduced or simplified to monophthongs.

The nonphonemic diphthongs /e͡ɪ/ (bay) and /o͡ʊ/ (bow) can be, and often are, reduced to monophthongs without producing different phonemes. The words *bait, state,* and *nape* commonly are produced with the diphthong /e͡ɪ/, but they can be produced with the monophthong /e/ without any change in their morphemic status. Similarly, the words *boat, soap,* and *tote* commonly are produced with the diphthong /o͡ʊ/, but they can be produced with the monophthong /o/. Thus, for these two diphthongs, the diphthongal and monophthongal forms are allophonic variations, not distinct phonemes. The diphthongal forms /e͡ɪ/ and /o͡ʊ/ occur most commonly in heavily stressed syllables, whereas the monophthongal forms /e/ and /o/ usually are found in weakly stressed syllables. For example, in the word *vacation,* the first syllable *va-* is not stressed and therefore usually is produced with the monophthong /e/, whereas the second syllable *-ca-* is stressed and therefore is produced with the diphthong /e͡ɪ/. Some writers refer to the monophthongs /e/ and /o/ as *pure* vowels. The monophthongal or pure forms occur much less frequently than the diphthongal forms, so the beginning student in phonetics is advised to use the diphthongal form in cases of doubt—at least until his or her ear is sharpened to hear the difference.

To familiarize yourself with the diphthongs, look at the words below and write in the blanks the diphthongs that are used.

life ____________
Troy ____________
Dane ____________
bone ____________
coy ____________
side ____________
sewed ____________
weighed ____________
bound ____________
cry ____________
cloud ____________
home ____________
toys ____________
cow ____________
braid ____________
known ____________
pout ____________
pray ____________
Roy ____________
Ray ____________
town ____________
blow ____________

As Appendix A shows, there is little agreement among phoneticians as to which vowels should be used to symbolize the English diphthongs. Most phoneticians do agree that two symbols are required, one to represent the **onglide,** or beginning position, and another to represent the **offglide,** or ending position. However, different phoneticians often hear different vowels for both the onglide and offglide segments, so that the diphthong in *bye* is variously transcribed as /aɪ/, /ay/, /ai/, /ɑɪ/, /ɑy/, /ɑi/, /ae/, and so on. Actually, it is not surprising that different sounds are heard because X-ray and acoustic studies have shown that a given diphthong is not always produced with exactly the same onglide and offglide segments. In fact, even an individual speaker may use different onglide and offglide segments from one occasion to another, depending on phonetic context (that is, the influence of surrounding sounds), his or her rate of speaking, and the degree of stress. Figure 4-20 illustrates the variation in onglide and offglide positions for diphthong /a͡ɪ/ uttered at different speaking rates. Notice that different degrees of tongue movement are used. Hence, one production might sound as though it ends with /i/, and another might sound as though it ends with /ɪ/. The student of phonetics should keep this variability in mind and recognize that the phonetic symbols are partly a matter of convenience and best guess. When we produce a diphthong symbolized as /a͡ɪ/, we do not always move the tongue exactly from a position for /a/ to one for /ɪ/. Rather, these vowels serve as the approximate targets for the diphthong's onglide and offglide segments.

We have examined diphthong articulation in several speakers of General American speech, Midwestern dialect, using both acoustic analysis (spectrograms) and X-ray motion pictures. Onglide and offglide segments obtained from X-ray analyses are illustrated for the five English diphthongs in Figures 4-21, 4-22, 4-23, 4-24, and 4-25. We recommend that the student study these illustrations while making these sounds, attempting to feel the changes in lip, tongue, and jaw positions.

Diphthong /a͡ɪ/ (Bye; Figure 4-21)

The IPA symbol /a͡ɪ/ is somewhat misleading as an articulatory description of this sound because, at least in Midwestern speech, the onglide is highly similar to the low-back /a/ (Kent, 1970). The offglide is highly variable and depends on stress, speaking rate, and phonetic context. The variation in the tongue movement for /a͡ɪ/ is illustrated in Figure 4-20. This drawing was obtained from X-ray films of diphthong /a͡ɪ/ uttered at two different speaking rates, slow and fast. For the slow production shown in *(a)*, the tongue movement is much greater than for the fast production shown in *(b)*. Indeed, both acoustic and X-ray studies have shown that diphthongs produced at increasingly faster rates of speech have progressively smaller movements, up to some limiting movement needed for recognition of the sound. Figure 4-20 shows that a diphthong does not have a stable and invariant offglide. In fact, the onglide also varies somewhat with phonetic context and speaking rate (Kent, 1970).

Thus, the diphthong cannot be defined as a movement from one invariant vocal tract configuration to another invariant vocal tract configuration. Neither the configuration of the onglide or offglide nor the amount of articulator movement is constant from one condition to another. The phonetic symbols used to represent diphthongs are thus best approximations and should not be taken literally as accurate descriptions of the movements that a speaker makes. A given

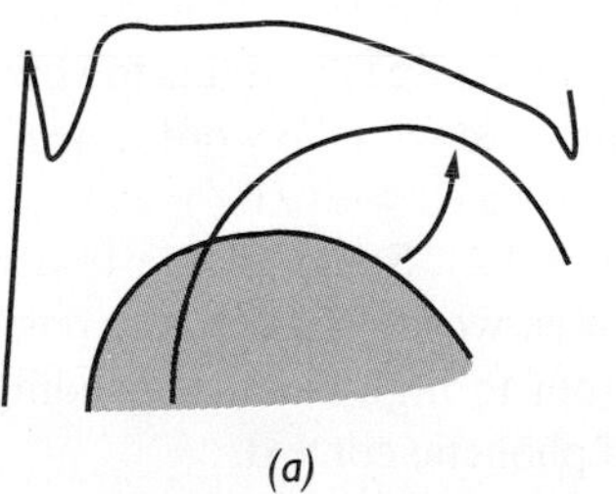

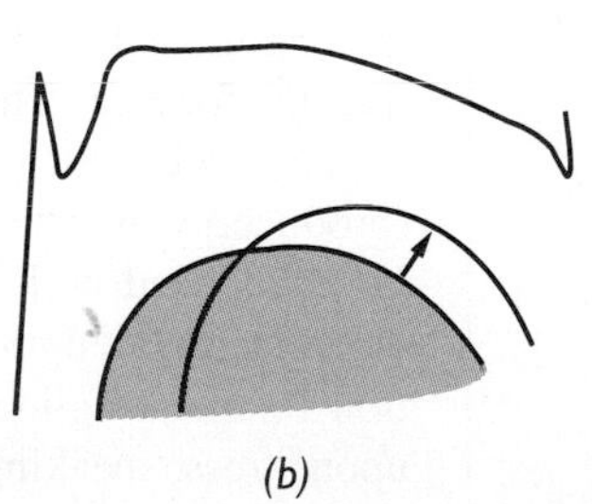

FIGURE 4-20
Articulations of diphthong /a͡ɪ/ *(bye)* at a slow speaking rate *(a)* and a rapid speaking rate *(b)*. Onglide position is shown by shaded region and offglide position by the heavy outline. At the more rapid rate, tongue movement is reduced.

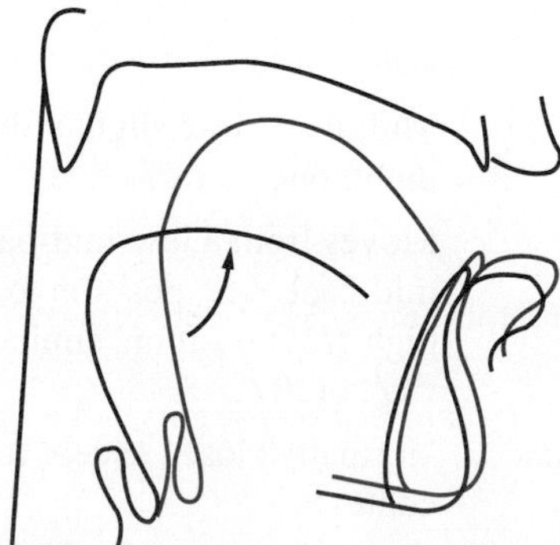

FIGURE 4-21
Articulation of diphthong /a͡ɪ/ *(bye)* shown as onglide (black line) and offglide (red line) configurations.

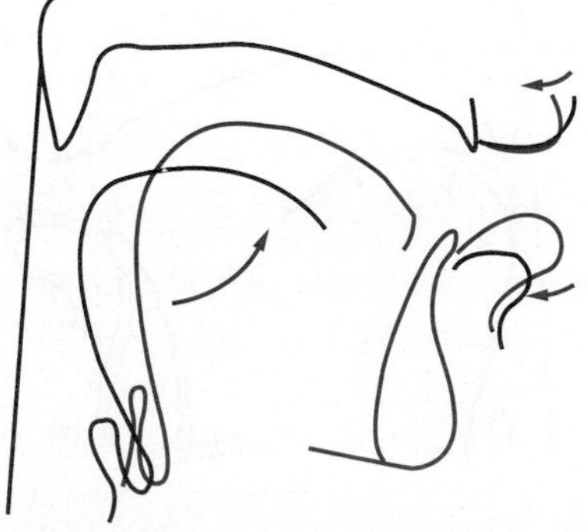

FIGURE 4-22
Articulation of diphthong /ɔ͡ɪ/ *(boy)* shown as onglide (black line) and offglide (red line) configurations.

diphthong actually has a range of onglide and offglide configurations.

Articulatory Summary

Lips:	Unrounded; usually make a slight to moderate closing motion during the diphthong.
Jaw:	Mid-open to open for the onglide, then closes somewhat for the offglide.
Tongue:	Moves from a low-back onglide to a mid-front or high-front offglide. The onglide is similar to /a/ or /ɑ/ and the offglide may be like /e/, /ɪ/, or /i/.
Velopharynx:	Normally closed, except for nasal contexts.

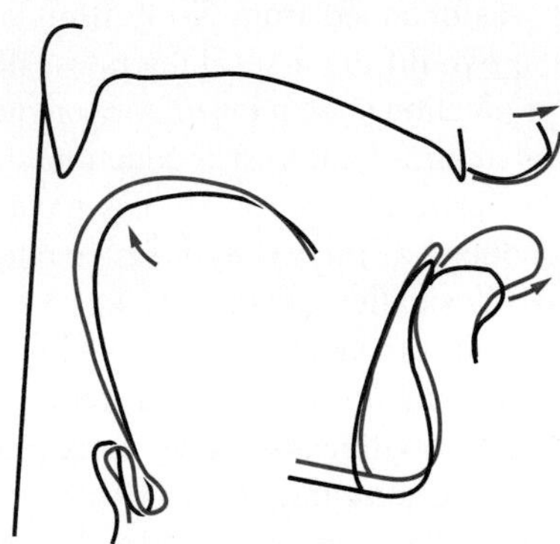

FIGURE 4-23
Articulation of diphthong /ɑ͡ʊ/ *(bough)* shown as onglide (black line) and offglide (red line) configurations.

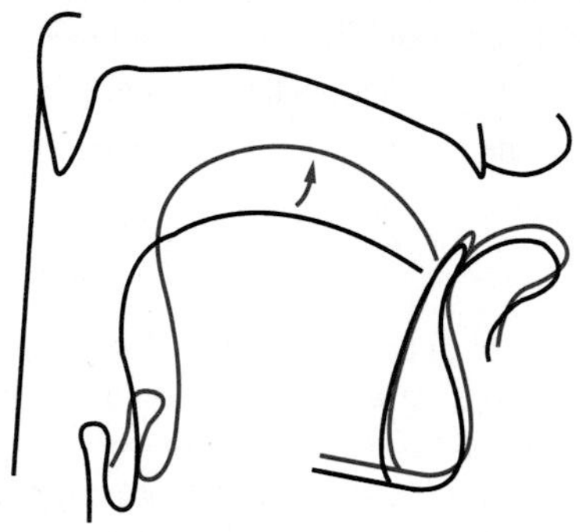

FIGURE 4-24
Articulation of diphthong /e͡ɪ/ *(bay)* shown as onglide (black line) and offglide (red line) configurations.

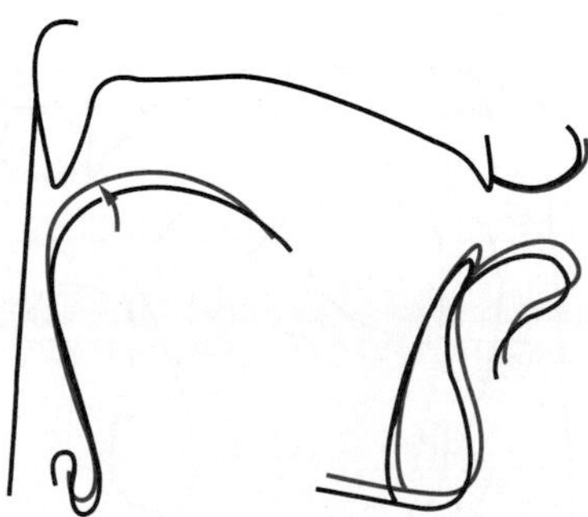

FIGURE 4-25
Articulation of diphthong /o͡ʊ/ *(bow)* shown as onglide (black line) and offglide (red line) configurations.

Allophonic Variations. See nasalized vowels and monophthongization.

Transcription Words

s*igh*	style	n*igh*ttime
*ai*sle	m*igh*t	Fr*i*day
m*i*ne	s*i*lo	W*y*oming
t*y*ke	r*i*ot	rh*y*me
l*i*ke	tr*i*al	*i*ce
br*i*ne	l*igh*tning	b*i*cycle

Diphthong /ɔ͡ɪ/ (Boy; Figure 4-22)

This diphthong is produced with coordinated movements of the lips and tongue. The lips move from a rounded or protruded state to an unrounded state. The tongue position for the onglide is low-mid-back, like that for /ɔ/, or mid-back, like that for /o/. The similarity of the /ɔ͡ɪ/ onglide to vowels /ɔ/ and /o/ can be demonstrated with the words *tawing* (produced with /ɔ/), *toeing* (produced with /o/), and *toying* (produced with diphthong /ɔ͡ɪ/). Some people find it difficult to distinguish these three words. The tongue position for the offglide is mid-front to high-front, depending upon stress, speaking rate, and phonetic context.

Articulatory Summary

Lips:	Move from a rounded to an unrounded state.
Jaw:	Mid; may close slightly during the diphthong.
Tongue:	Moves from a low-mid-back /ɔ/ or mid-back /o/ position to a mid-to-high-front position, similar to /e/, /ɪ/, or /i/.
Velopharynx:	Normally closed except for nasal contexts.

Allophonic Variations. See nasalized vowels and monophthongization.

Transcription Words

pl*oy*	sirl*oi*n	dec*oy*
t*oy*	typh*oi*d	ann*oi*nt
R*oy*	cl*oi*ster	f*oy*er
sp*oi*l	all*oy*	destr*oy*
b*oi*l	r*oy*al	ann*oy*
*oi*l	p*oi*nt	turqu*oi*se

Diphthong /a͡ʊ/ (Bough; Figure 4-23)

The lips and tongue have coordinated movements of rounding and raising, respectively. As was the case for /a͡ɪ/, the onglide of /a͡ʊ/ in Midwestern speech is highly similar to vowel /ɑ/ and may be described as low-back or low-mid-back. As shown in the illustration, the tongue makes a raising motion of small extent, toward the position for /ʊ/. The lips are unrounded and usually relatively open for the onglide, then they gradually move to a rounded state for the offglide. The IPA symbol /a͡ʊ/ is misleading in that, strictly speaking, it indicates a tongue movement from low-front to high-mid-back. But, as shown in Figure 4-23, the movement is almost entirely one of raising from a low-back or low-mid-back position.

Articulatory Summary

Lips:	Move from a relatively open, unrounded state to a rounded state.
Jaw:	Mid-open to open for the onglide; often closes somewhat for the offglide.
Tongue:	Moves from an onglide position of low-back (similar to /ɑ/) or low-mid-back (similar to /ɔ/) to an offglide position of mid-back (similar to /o/) or high-mid-back (similar to /ʊ/).
Velopharynx:	Normally closed except in nasal contexts.

Allophonic Variations. See nasalized vowels and monophthongization.

Transcription Words

c*ow*	*ou*ster	h*ou*sewife
r*ou*nd	d*ow*nt*ow*n	*ou*tcast
fl*ou*t	t*ow*er	d*ou*btful
cl*ow*n	al*ou*d	d*ow*nsp*ou*t
st*ou*t	ast*ou*nd	tr*au*ma
c*ou*ch	ch*ow*der	*ou*rselves

Diphthong /e͡ɪ/ (Bay; Figure 4-24)

Diphthong /e͡ɪ/ is essentially an allophone, alternating with the monophthong /e/. The diphthong is more likely to occur when the syllable is strongly stressed or the speaking rate is slow. The articulatory positions for the onglide are those for vowel /e/, and the positions for the offglide are roughly those for /ɪ/. However, the actual extent of tongue and jaw movement varies with stress, speaking rate, and phonetic context.

Articulatory Summary

Lips:	Mid-open and unrounded.
Jaw:	Mid; may close somewhat during the diphthong.
Tongue:	Moves from a mid-front /e/ to a high-mid-front /ɪ/.
Velopharynx:	Normally closed except in nasal contexts.

Allophonic Variations. See nasalized vowels, monophthongization, and vowel /e/.

Transcription Words

w*ay*	m*ay*be	l*ay*man
p*ai*d	n*eigh*bor	str*aigh*t
tr*a*de	fianc*ee*	dissu*a*de
*eigh*t	tod*ay*	s*ai*lor
st*ea*k	w*ay*side	h*a*lo
wh*ey*	par*a*de	d*ay*time

Diphthong /o͡ʊ/ (Bow; Figure 4-25)

Diphthong /o͡ʊ/ alternates allophonically with /o/. The diphthong is more likely to occur when the syllable is strongly stressed or the speaking rate is slow. The onglide is vowel /o/: mid-back tongue position and rounded lips. The offglide is essentially vowel /ʊ/: high-mid-back tongue position and rounded lips. The diphthong gesture can be characterized as a raising tongue movement and a slight narrowing of the lips.

Articulatory Summary

Lips:	Rounded with progressive narrowing.
Jaw:	Mid-open; often closes slightly during the diphthong.
Tongue:	Moves from a mid-back /o/ position to a high-mid-back /ʊ/.
Velopharynx:	Normally closed except in nasal contexts.

Allophonic Variations. See nasalized vowels, monophthongization, and vowel /o/.

Transcription Words

m*o*de	br*oo*ch	sh*ou*lder
n*o*	ye*o*man	b*o*lder
sl*ow*	m*ou*lded	t*oa*ster
b*eau*	sn*ow*man	ab*o*de
h*oe*	*ow*ner	r*oa*ming
s*ew*	l*oa*ned	r*o*lling

SPECIAL NOTES ON THE PHONETIC PROPERTIES OF VOWELS

Some Cautions about Vowel Features

The terms used in this book to describe vowel articulation were chosen for their simplicity and general relevance to observed patterns of vowel articulation. However, these terms are not entirely accurate for all speakers. For example, it is not exactly true that the vowels within the front, central, or back series are always satisfactorily distinguished by descriptions of tongue height. Ladefoged (1971) commented that the tongue shapes for the back vowels "can be considered as differing simply in terms of the single parameter called tongue height only [by] neglecting large and varied differences in the front–back dimension" (p. 69). Differences in the front–back dimension (advancement) are evident in Figure 4-15. For example, the tongue position for /u/ and /o/ is more fronted than the position for /ɑ/. In view of these difficulties in the description of tongue height, phoneticians have sought other descriptions of vowel articulation. Ladefoged writes as follows on one possibility:

> *The only way of regarding the articulatory positions of the back vowel as being approximately equidistant is by reference to the position of the point of maximum constriction of the vocal tract. This point, which was suggested as a reference point by Stevens and House (1955), gets progressively farther away from the glottis by roughly equal steps on a logarithmic scale as one goes from* a *to* u. . . . *But specification of tongue shape in terms of the position of the point of maximum constriction is very misleading when applied to front vowels. There is, for instance, no articulatory or acoustic discontinuity corresponding to the discontinuity in this form of specification which occurs when one goes from* ɛ *(in which the maximum constriction is near the hard palate) to* æ *(in which it is nearer the pharynx . . .).* (Ladefoged, 1971, p. 69)

Ladefoged concluded that there is no one simple set of parameters that is equally accurate for describing the tongue shapes of different vowels. Similarly, Nearey (1978) remarked in his evaluation of phonetic feature systems for vowels that "It would appear that neither the traditional features nor recent modifications of them stand up to empirical tests. . . . Indeed, empirical research since the thirties has produced evidence that weighs heavily against the notion of invariant articulatory specification in anything like that implied by traditional phonetic theory" (p. 69).

Even the description of tongue height for the front vowels is not without contradictions. Russell (1928); Ladefoged, DeClerk, Lindau, and Papcun (1972); and Nearey (1978) reported that actual measurements of tongue height show that /e/ and /æ/ can be higher than /ɪ/, in disagreement with traditional phonetic theory.

Matters are even worse for the tense–lax distinction, especially when articulatory correlates for this dimension are sought in studies of tongue shape. Although Perkell (1971) proposed that vowels usually called "tense" have an advanced tongue root and that vowels usually called "lax" have a constricted pharynx, Ladefoged et al. (1972) and Nearey (1978) did not confirm these observations. One study of the electrical activity in contracting muscles (electromyography) provided only modest support for the idea that tense vowels involve greater muscle activity. Raphael and Bell-Berti (1975) reported that, of twelve muscles studied with this method, only two showed consistently greater activity for the tense vowels than for the lax vowels. Generally, the durational difference between tense and lax vowels has fared better than other correlates when tests are made. Tense vowels are longer in duration than lax vowels.

Obviously, systems of articulatory description for vowels are not perfect. Accordingly, the system used in this book should be used with that recognition. It should suffice for general articulatory description and most clinical purposes, but its details should not be accepted uncritically. It is partly because of the inadequacies of phonetic feature systems for vowels that we include many drawings based on X-ray pictures of vowel articulation. Where verbal descriptions fail, these drawings should help to fill the gap. It is recommended that the illustrations be studied closely and compared against the vowel features used in verbal description.

Tongue and Jaw Interaction

It has been proposed that when the tongue positions for different vowels are compared relative to the jaw, the tongue shapes fall into a small number of groups or families (Lindblom and Sundberg, 1969). An illustration of this idea is shown in Figure 4-26 for vowels produced by author Kent. Note that the front vowels /i/, /ɛ/, and /æ/ have fairly similar shapes and might be grouped together as one family. Vowels /o/, /ɑ/, and /ʌ/ might be grouped in another family. Vowel /u/ has a tongue shape unlike that for any other vowel but quite similar to that for the velar consonants (the final sounds in the words *back, dog,* and *ring*). These results may indicate that a talker does not have to make as

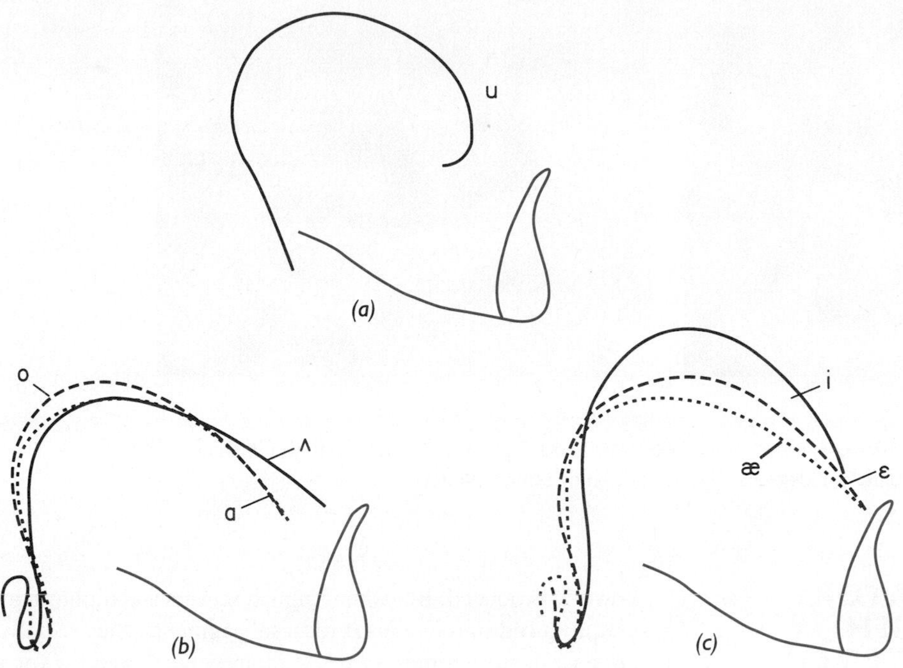

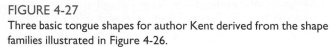

FIGURE 4-26
Tongue shapes for selected vowels of author Kent, shown relative to the jaw. The shapes fall into three families: *(a)* high-back, *(b)* low-back, and *(c)* front vowels.

many adjustments of the tongue as there are vowels in the language. A small number of tongue shapes, combined with various positions of the jaw (and lips) can suffice to produce several different vowels. The three basic tongue shapes for author Kent are shown in Figure 4-27. The shape drawn with a solid line represents the front vowels fairly well; the shape drawn with a dotted line satisfactorily represents low-back to mid-back vowels; and the shape drawn with a dashed line represents the high-back vowel /u/.

Of course, one should bear in mind that a speaker can produce all of the English vowels while clenching a pencil between the teeth or with the jaw propped open (Figure 4-2). Hence, we know that the tongue, without the aid of jaw movement, can make adequate adjustments for the vowels of English. What results like those in Figure 4-26 may tell us is that, when both tongue and jaw are free to vary, the tongue tends to assume a small number of preferred shapes relative to the jaw.

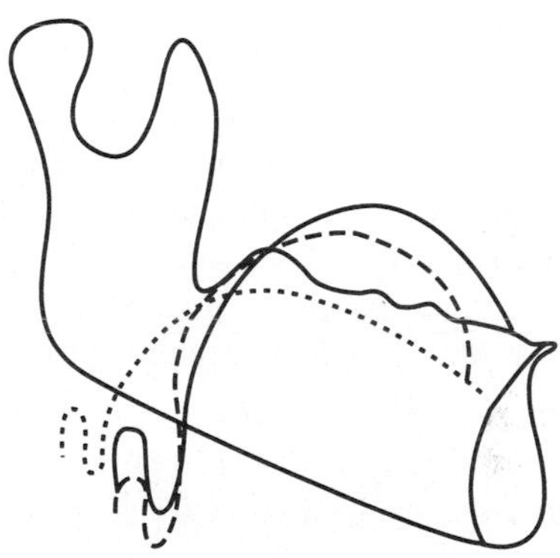

FIGURE 4-27
Three basic tongue shapes for author Kent derived from the shape families illustrated in Figure 4-26.

Lip and Jaw Interaction

The general remarks made about tongue and jaw interaction apply as well to the interaction between lip and jaw. Usually, the position of the jaw during speech is controlled to assist the lips in achieving a desired mouth opening. Hence, when the desired mouth opening is one of narrowing or rounding, the jaw typically is closed or elevated. Conversely, when a wide mouth opening is desired, the jaw usually is open or lowered. However, when the jaw is not free to move, as in the case of a pipe smoker, the lips can function independently to make the appropriate changes in mouth opening. In addition, a given phonetic feature of lip articulation can be accomplished while the jaw satisfies one of two opposing articulatory requirements. Consider, for example, the feature of rounding for the back vowels. Because the rounded back vowels have jaw positions ranging from relatively closed (/u/ in *who*) to relatively open (/ɔ/ in *law*), the feature of rounding must be accomplished whether the jaw is elevated or lowered. The photographs in Figure 4-28 give an example. Note that the lips are rounded for both the vowels /o/ (low) and /ɔ/ (law), although the amount of mouth opening, and hence degree of jaw lowering, is quite different between these two vowel productions.

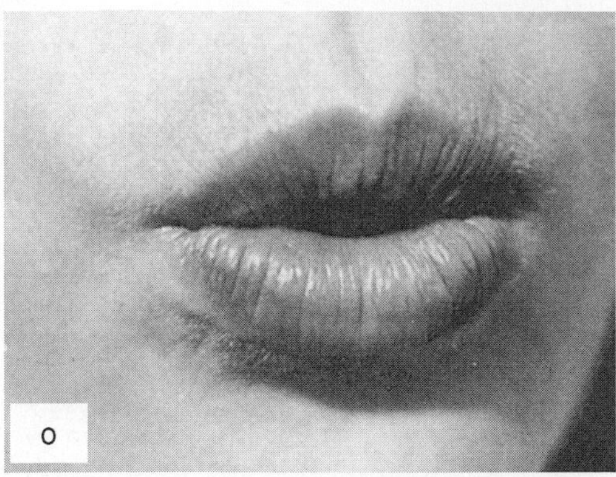

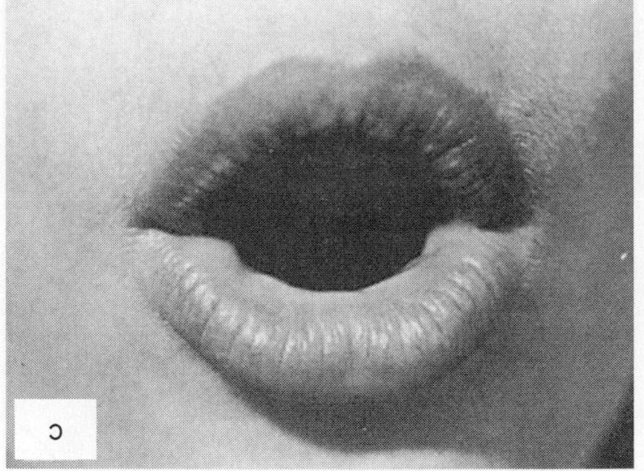

FIGURE 4-28
Photographs of the mouth opening for the vowels /o/ *(low)* and /ɔ/ *(law)*. Notice that the lips can be rounded in association with different degrees of mouth opening (jaw elevation).

SOME COMMON ARTICULATORY MODIFICATIONS OF ENGLISH VOWELS (SEE ALSO CHAPTER 6)

Diphthongization

Diphthongization occurs when a vowel ordinarily produced as a monophthong is articulated with a diphthongal character. For example, speakers of Southern speech sometimes produce *yes* /j ɛ s/ as /j e ə s/ and *cat* /k æ t/ as /k e æ t/. Diphthongization should be noted in a phonetic transcription whenever more than one vowel quality can be heard in a syllable nucleus. This decision is not always easy, especially for vowels like /u/ and /æ/, which often are produced with a slowly changing tongue position by speakers of General American English.

Monophthongization

Monophthongization means that a diphthong is produced as a monophthong, or single-element vowel. For example, a speaker who says /ɑ/ for /ɑ͞ɪ/, as often happens in Southern speech, is monophthongizing diphthong /ɑ͞ɪ/. This modification is transcribed with the symbol of the single vowel element that replaces the diphthong. As noted in the discussion of diphthongs, /e͞ɪ/ and /o͞ʊ/ tend to be produced as the monophthongs /e/ and /o/, respectively, at rapid rates of speech or when they are not strongly stressed. The diphthongs /ɑ͞ɪ/, /ɑ͞ʊ/, and /ɔ͞ɪ/ do not have monophthong allophones in General American English.

Nasalization

Isolated vowels and diphthongs produced by normal speakers of General American English are resonated and radiated orally; that is, sound energy usually passes only through the oral cavity and not through the nasal cavity. This means, in articulatory terms, that the velopharynx is closed as the vowel is produced. But when English vowels and diphthongs are produced in the context of nasal segments, they usually are **nasalized** to some degree. Velopharyngeal opening for a preceding nasal segment is maintained during the vowel or diphthong, and velopharyngeal opening for a following nasal segment is anticipated during the vowel or diphthong. Of course, a vowel or diphthong that is both preceded and followed by nasal segments, like /i/ in *mean*, is influenced from both directions.

Velopharyngeal opening of the anticipatory kind is illustrated for the articulation of diphthong /ɑ͞ɪ/ in Figure 4-29. The black line represents the diphthong onglide and the red line, the diphthong offglide. Because this diphthong was followed by a nasal consonant, the velopharynx begins to open during the diphthongal movement of the tongue. Consequently, the diphthong is nasalized. A conspicuous velopharyngeal opening can be seen for the diphthong offglide. Thus, the velopharynx is already open by the time the oral

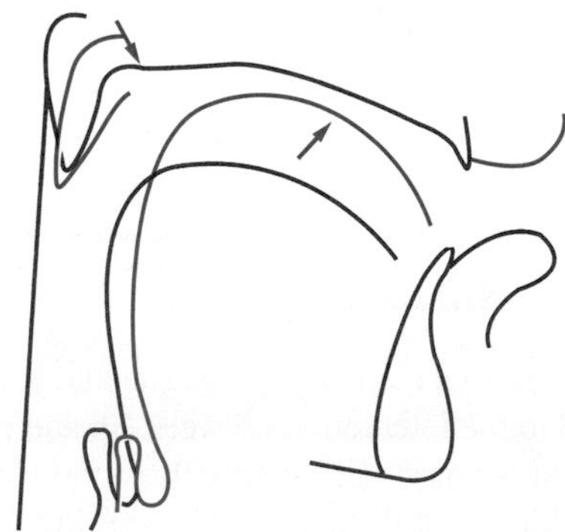

FIGURE 4-29
Velopharyngeal opening during diphthong /ɑ͞ɪ/. Diphthong onglide is shown by black line, and the offglide is shown by red line. Velum begins to open during /ɑ͞ɪ/ in anticipation of a nasal consonant that follows the diphthong; for example, the phrase *I know* /ɑ͞ɪ n o͞ʊ/.

closure is made for the following nasal consonant, in this case /n/. The same pattern can be seen for vowel /ɑ/ in the word *contract* (noun form) in Figure 4-30. The black line in this figure shows the articulatory positions at the instant of release of the consonant /k/, and the red line shows the articulatory positions assumed during the mid-point (in time) of the vowel /ɑ/. Obviously, the vowel will be produced as a nasalized sound because of the velopharyngeal opening during the vowel articulation.

Nasalization of a vowel rarely, if ever, will alter the meaning of an English word. The word *eye* (or *I*), phonetically diphthong /ɑ͡ɪ/, means the same thing to a listener whether the vowel is produced with or without nasal resonance. In other words, vowel nasalization is allophonic in English. Furthermore, the nasalized allophone is in complementary distribution (this term is discussed in Chapter 2) to the oral (nonnasalized) vowel allophone, because the nasal variant normally occurs only in the context of nasal sounds. Because a nasalized vowel is an allophonic member of a family (the vowel phoneme), the feature of nasalization does not change the phoneme symbol. Hence, phoneme /i/ includes both the oral and nasal allophones. The occurrence of nasalization is transcribed by adding a diacritic mark to the phonetic symbol, which is placed within brackets rather than virgules. Diacritic marks are discussed in detail in Chapter 6. For the moment, suffice it to say that the nasal allophone of a vowel phoneme is indicated by the special mark placed over the symbol that identifies the vowel. For example, the nasalized vowel in *mean* is transcribed phonetically as [ĩ].

Reduction

Reduction was discussed in connection with the schwa /ə/, and a general diagram of reduction was shown in Figure 4-14. Reduction occurs as the rate of speaking increases or as the stress on a vowel is decreased. For example, as the stress on the second syllable of the word *educate* is progressively lessened, the vowel tends to change from /u/ to /ʊ/ and from /ʊ/ to /ə/. Reduction can be characterized along the two dimensions of length (duration) and centralization. As a vowel is reduced, its duration decreases, and it is articulated more toward the center of the oral cavity. The schwa vowel /ə/ represents the limit of reduction because it has the shortest duration of all vowels (Klatt [1976] says that unstressed vowels like schwa reach the compression limit of vowel production) and because it is produced with a central tongue position. Generally, centralization can be represented along vectors or lines within the quadrilateral diagram of vowel articulation (Figure 4-14). The vowel changes in the second syllable of *educate* can be represented as articulatory changes along a line that runs from /u/ to /ʊ/ to /ə/. Shortening of vowel duration and centralization of the vowel articulation tend to co-occur because, as the duration of a vowel is decreased, there is less time for the articulators to reach extreme positions (that is, positions near the sides of the quadrilateral diagram). Reduction is a powerful factor in the articulation of vowels in context.

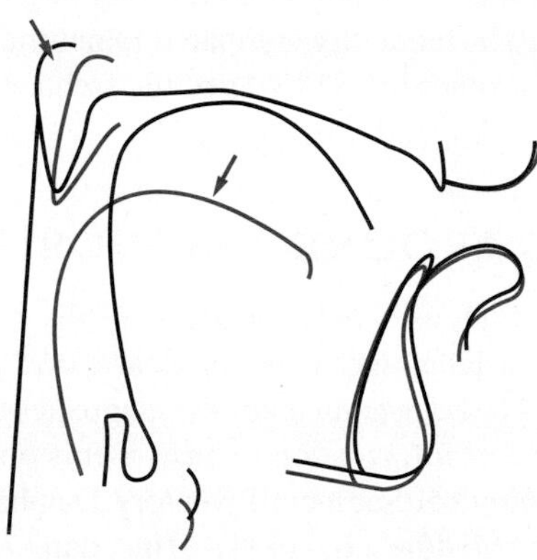

FIGURE 4-30
Velopharyngeal opening in the first syllable of the word *contract* (noun form). The black line represents the articulatory configuration at the beginning of movement from the first consonant (contract) to the following vowel (contract). The red line represents the configuration for vowel /ɑ/, which is nasalized in anticipation of the following nasal consonant (contract).

Rhotacization and Derhotacization

The vowels /ɝ/ and /ɚ/ (f*ur*th*er*) always carry *r* coloring; other vowels can carry *r* coloring when they occur adjacent to /r/. For example, the /ɔ/ in *morning* [m ɔ r n ɪ ŋ] is colored by, or affected by, the following /r/. Following Ladefoged (1975), we refer to this *r* coloring of a vowel as rhotacization (or rhotacism). Thus, a rhotacized vowel is one with *r* coloring, and it occurs in normal speech adjacent to /r/. The term **derhotacization** (or derhotacism) applies to a situation in which a normally *r*-colored vowel loses all or part of the *r* color. See the discussion of /r/ in Chapter 5 for the articulatory correlates of rhotacization.

Other Modifications

A more complete listing of articulatory modifications of vowels is given in Chapter 6, which also defines diacritic marks for transcription.

ALLOGRAPHS OF THE VOWEL PHONEMES OF ENGLISH

In Chapter 2, *allograph* was defined as any one alphabet letter or combination of letters that represents a particular phoneme. Any one phoneme usually can be spelled in a number of ways, and any one alphabet letter often can be used to represent different sounds. Table 4-4 gives the allographs for the vowel phonemes of English. Each allograph is italicized in a sample word. For example, for phoneme /i/, some allographs are the *e* in *be,* the *ee* in *see,* and the *ea* in

TABLE 4-4
Allographs of the Vowel Phonemes of English

Phoneme	Allograph (Italicized in Sample Word)
/i/	b*e*, s*ee*, *ea*t, mar*i*ne, k*ey*, *ei*ther, ch*ie*f, C*ae*sar, p*eo*ple, *ae*on, debr*is*, Ph*oe*nix, qu*ay*
/ɪ/	*i*t, pr*e*tty, h*ea*r, h*y*mn, h*e*re (e-e), sh*ee*r, w*ei*rd, b*ee*n, b*u*sy, s*ie*ve, w*o*men, b*ui*lt, g*i*ve (i-e)
/e/ or /e͡ɪ/	f*a*te, r*ai*n, st*ea*k, r*ei*gn, *eigh*t, pr*ey*, sach*e*t, g*au*ge, s*ay*
/ɛ/	b*e*d, h*ea*d, th*e*re (e-e), c*a*re (a-e), *ai*r, th*ei*r, *ae*rial, *a*ny, s*ay*s, h*ei*fer, l*eo*pard, fr*ie*nd, b*u*ry, *ae*sthetic, gu*e*st
/æ/	h*a*t, pl*ai*d, l*au*gh, h*a*ve (a-e), mer*i*ngue
/ɑ/	t*o*p, w*a*s, p*al*m, h*ea*rt, gu*a*rd, kn*ow*ledge, h*o*nest, baz*aa*r, s*e*rgeant, *ah* (and frequently in words containing *ar,* e.g., b*ar*)
/ɔ/	h*au*nt, y*aw*n, c*augh*t, *ough*t, cl*o*th, *a*ll, G*eo*rge, abr*oa*d (speakers vary in the pronunciation of these words)
/o/ or /o͡ʊ/	b*o*ld, h*o*me (o-e), s*ow*, h*oe*, s*ew*, th*ough*, b*oa*t, br*oo*ch, y*eo*man, b*eau*, ch*au*ffeur, s*ou*l
/ʊ/	b*oo*k, p*u*t, w*ou*ld, b*o*som
/u/	h*oo*t, t*o*, tr*ue*, bl*ew*, sh*oe*, y*ou*, r*u*le (u-e), fr*ui*t, l*o*se (o-e), l*ieu*, Si*oux*, Sa*u*lt, thr*ough*, b*eau*ty (as part of a /ju/ combination), tw*o*, rh*eu*matic, gn*u*, qu*eue*
/ʌ/	c*u*t, d*o*ne (o-e), r*ou*gh, s*o*n, d*oe*s, bl*oo*d
/ə/	Can be spelled by virtually any of the orthographic vowels of English and by many combinations of these orthographic vowels
/ɝ/	h*er*, b*ur*n, b*ir*d, l*ear*n, w*or*m, p*urr*, j*our*ney, M*yr*tle, rest*aur*ant, s*ear*ch, c*ur*d
/ɚ/	fath*er*, lab*or*, tap*ir*, mart*yr*, murm*ur*, acr*e*
/a͡ɪ/	f*i*nd, r*i*de (i-e), b*y*, *ai*sle, *ay*, *eye*, d*ye*, n*igh*t, d*ie*, b*uy*, h*eigh*t, t*y*pe (y-e)
/a͡ʊ/	*ou*t, c*ow*, b*ough*, F*au*st, Macl*eo*d
/ɔ͡ɪ/	*oi*l, t*oy*

eat. In each list of allographs, the most common ones are given first.

FREQUENCY OF OCCURRENCE FOR ENGLISH VOWELS

Data on the frequency of occurrence of English vowels are given in Appendix B, and it is a good idea to spend some time examining the tabled data to learn how unequally different vowels are used in our language. Figure 4-31 summarizes one of the major conclusions. This illustration shows the relative frequency of occurrence of front, central, and back vowels as proportionate areas of a quadrilateral. Note that front vowels are used to a much greater degree than either central or back vowels and that the central vowels occur more frequently than the back vowels. As Figure 4-31 shows, the front vowels make up about 50 percent of the total frequency of occurrence data for English vowels. Because rounded vowels are generally back vowels, it is also implicit from this illustration that lip rounding for vowels is used relatively infrequently compared to neutral or retracted lip shapes. For other breakdowns of the frequency of occurrence data, see Appendix B.

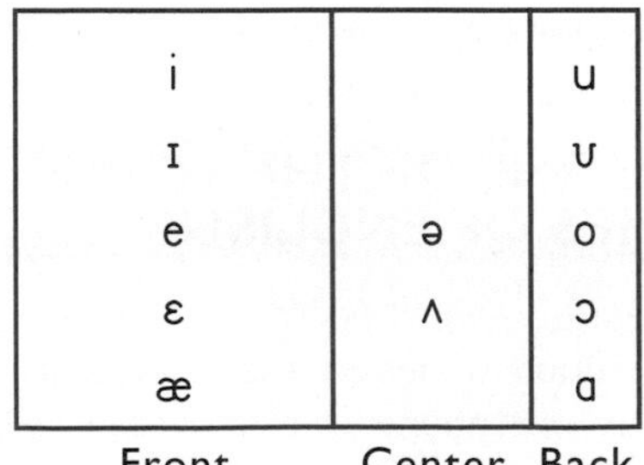

FIGURE 4-31
Relative frequency of occurrence of front, central, and back vowels, shown as proportions of a quadrilateral. Based on the data of Mines, Hanson, and Shoup (1978).

VOWELS AROUND THE WORLD

American English uses only a fraction of the possible vowels in a natural language. It is not clear exactly how many different vowels are used in all of the languages of the world, but one source of information to answer this question is the UCLA Phonological Segment Inventory Database, abbreviated UPSID (Maddieson, 1984). This database provides valuable information on the phonetic inventories of 317 languages. (A more recent version is based on 451 languages; Maddieson and Precoda, 1990.) Schwartz, Boe, Vallee, and Abry (1997) analyzed UPSID to determine the major patterns in the vowel inventories of the represented languages. Figure 4-32 shows the grid for 37 different vowel symbols in UPSID. Although these 37 vowels may not cover all of the possible vowels in the world's languages, they go a long way toward this goal. Schwartz et al. reached several conclusions about vowel inventories, some of which are summarized here:

1. Languages first select vowels from a primary vowel system of three to nine vowels that have a high frequency of occurrence across languages and for which duration (length) is the typical modification. In this primary system, five to seven vowels are particularly favored. Most languages select the three corner vowels /i/, /a/, and /u/. The triangle formed by these vowels is therefore a basic pattern selected by a large number of languages.
2. For languages that have more than about nine vowels, the additional vowels (from one to seven) are selected from a new dimension. Schwartz and colleagues termed these vowels a secondary system. The favored number of vowels in this system is five.
3. The vowels in both the primary and secondary systems are concentrated at the periphery of the vowel grid (i.e., the sides of the vowel quadrilateral), usually with a balance between front and back vowels. American English is a good example of a balanced front–back system. For languages without such a balance, front vowels generally outnumber back vowels.
4. The preferred nonperipheral (i.e., not located on the sides of the quadrilateral) vowel is the schwa. Because the occurrence of schwa apparently does not interact with other vowel selections in a system, it is considered a "parallel" vowel. Selection of schwa may be based on intrinsic principles such as vowel reduction.

The vowel grid in Figure 4-32 is useful for several purposes beyond an inventory of the world's vowels. It can be used to compare different languages and, for example, to understand some of the issues in learning a new language. Consider a child whose first language (L1) is Spanish (a five-vowel system, consisting of the vowels /i e a o u/) but is acquiring American English as a second language (L2). One of the main tasks, then, is to acquire several additional vowels, including some that differ in duration or length from the vowels in the Spanish system. The same general situation would apply to a child whose first language is modern Hebrew or Japanese (both of which are five-vowel systems similar to Spanish). But now consider a child whose L1 is Korean, which has the ten vowels /i ɨ e ɛ ɑ o ø u y ʌ/. In this case, some of the L1 vowels do not carry over to American English as an L2. In particular, the rounded front vowels /ø/ and /y/ do not occur in American English. If we reverse the situation and consider a child whose L1 is American English and who is learning Korean as L2, we see that this child must learn two rounded front vowels.

A general conclusion from studies of L2 vowel acquisition is that the difficulty of learning the new vowels depends on their similarity to vowels in L1. A vowel in L2 is difficult to learn if it is similar, but not identical, to a vowel in L1. Apparently, the similarity creates an interference between the new sound to be learned and a vowel in the original phonetic system. In contrast, a vowel in L2 is relatively easy to learn if it is quite different from any vowel in L1. The new L2 vowel is readily adopted because it does not compete with vowels in L1. The degree of similarity can be expressed in terms of acoustic properties, which are discussed in Chapter 10.

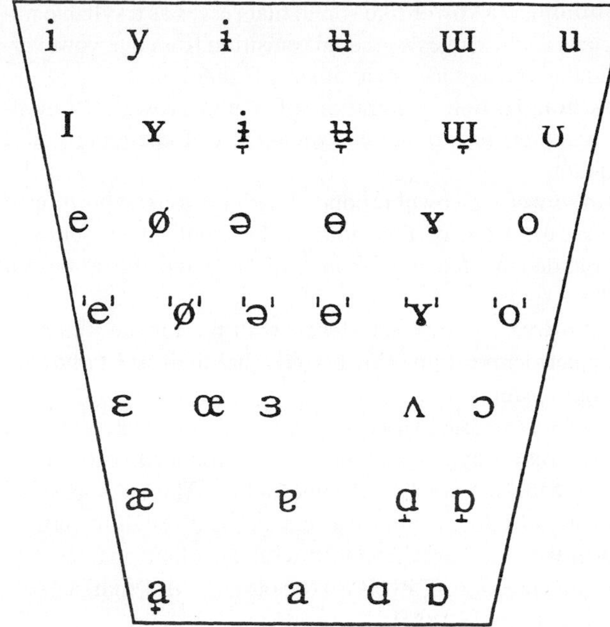

FIGURE 4-32
Grid for representing the 37 vowel symbols in UPSID. Reprinted from J. L. Schwartz, L.-J. Boe, N. Vallee, and C. Abry (1997), "Major trends in vowel system inventories." *Journal of Phonetics,* Volume 25, p. 236. Reprinted with permission of Academic Press. Copyright 1997.

GLOSSARY

Back vowel a vowel produced with the tongue positioned toward the back of the mouth. The back vowel series is bounded by the high-back /u/ (who) and the low-back /ɑ/ (ha).

Central vowel a vowel produced with the tongue positioned in the center of the mouth; for example, the first vowel in *upon.*

Corner vowel (or **point vowel**) a vowel located at any one of the four points of the vowel quadrilateral: high-front /i/ (he), low-front /æ/ (hat), low-back /ɑ/ (ha), or high-back /u/ (who).

Derhotacization partial loss of *r* coloring from a normally rhotacized vowel (/ɝ/ or /ɚ/ in English).

Diphthong a vowel-like sound that serves as a syllable nucleus and involves a gradual transition from one vowel articulation (onglide) to another (offglide).

Diphthongization alteration of a pure vowel (or monophthong) to a dynamic articulation of changing vowel quality.

Front vowel a vowel produced with the tongue positioned near the front of the mouth. The front vowel series is bounded by the high-front /i/ (he) and the low-front /æ/ (hat).

High vowel a vowel produced with the tongue in a high (superior) position. Vowels /i/ (he) and /u/ (who) are high vowels.

Lax vowel (or **short vowel**) a vowel that is relatively short in duration and is assumed to be produced with a relatively relaxed vocal tract musculature. The assumption of laxness (reduced muscular tension) is difficult to verify.

Low vowel a vowel produced with the tongue in a low (inferior) position. Vowels /ɑ/ (hot) and /æ/ (hat) are low vowels.

Monophthong a pure vowel; that is, a vowel of essentially unchanging phonetic quality throughout its duration.

Monophthongization alteration of a diphthong to a pure vowel; that is, loss of the dynamic phonetic quality of a diphthong.

Nasalized vowel a vowel produced with nasal resonances, usually because of an open velopharynx.

Offglide the terminal vowel or vocal tract shape of a diphthong.

Onglide the initial vowel or vocal tract shape of a diphthong.

Point vowel see **corner vowel.**

***r* colored** a sound that carries the phonetic quality of /r/, the rhotic consonant. This quality is best described acoustically, as the articulatory correlate is complex.

Reduction of a vowel generally, a shortening or unstressing of a vowel, which may be accompanied by a change in vowel quality, usually in the direction of centralization.

Retroflex literally "turned back"; this term is used to denote sounds that carry *r* coloring, such as the vowels in the words *bird* and *further*. However, "retroflex" is a misleading and inaccurate articulatory description and is best regarded as an arbitrary label. See **rhotacization.**

Rhotacization a property or process related to *r* coloring. A sound that has *r* coloring, or comes to have it because of contextual influences, is called rhotacized or rhotic. A physiologic definition is complex, so an acoustic definition is preferable.

Rounded vowel a vowel that is produced with rounding or protrusion of the lips; for example, vowels /u/ (who) and /ɝ/ (her). Actually, either protrusion or narrowing of the mouth opening may produce the desired acoustic effects.

Schwa vowel the ultimate reduced vowel /ə/, which is described as unstressed, lax or short, and mid-central. Schwa occupies the center of the vowel quadrilateral and can achieve the minimal duration for a vowel sound.

Tense vowel (or **long vowel**) a vowel that is relatively long in duration and is assumed to be produced with a relatively tense or active musculature of the vocal tract.

Tongue advancement the vowel feature or dimension pertaining to the position of the tongue body along the anterior–posterior aspect. Advancement implies anterior or frontal position.

Tongue height the vowel feature or dimension pertaining to the position of the tongue body along the superior–inferior aspect.

Unrounded vowel a vowel that is produced without rounding or protrusion of the lips; for example, /i/ (he) and /ɑ/ (ha) are unrounded.

Vowel a speech sound that is formed without a significant constriction of the oral and pharyngeal cavities and that serves as a syllable nucleus.

Vowel quadrilateral a four-sided figure having the corner, or point, vowels /i u ɑ æ/ as its vertices. The quadrilateral diagram is useful for describing the tongue position for vowel articulation, as its two basic dimensions are high–low and front–back.

EXERCISES

1. Draw a quadrilateral figure and label on it the articulatory dimensions of front–back and high–low. Then mark on the quadrilateral the locations of the following vowels: /i ɪ e æ u ʊ o ɔ ɑ ʌ ə ɝ/. Practice this exercise until you can easily and quickly construct the vowel quadrilateral.

2. Relying on the General American pronunciation of the following words, classify the vowel in each word with the appropriate articulatory descriptors: high, high-mid, mid, low-mid, low; front, central, back.

   (a) troop ____________
   (b) caught ____________
   (c) beg ____________
   (d) look ____________
   (e) steel ____________
   (f) wand ____________
   (g) shook ____________
   (h) steam ____________
   (i) rib ____________
   (j) track ____________
   (k) cook ____________
   (1) roam ____________
   (m) pearl ____________
   (n) still ____________

3. Each of the following words contains two adjacent vowels. Describe in articulatory terms the movements of the tongue and lips (if any) during the transition from the first vowel to the second. For example, in the word *neon* [n i ɑ n] the tongue moves back and down in going from /i/ to /ɑ/, and the mouth (lip) opening increases.

   (a) piano ______________
   (b) duo ______________
   (c) trio ______________
   (d) rayon ______________
   (e) coerce ______________
   (f) react ______________
   (g) nuance ______________
   (h) noel ______________
   (i) seance ______________
   (j) coeval ______________
   (k) reiterate ______________
   (l) cooperate ______________

4. Each time you read through the following passage, do one or more of the following: (a) underline every letter that represents a front vowel, (b) double-underline every letter that represents a central vowel, (c) draw a vertical line through every letter that represents a back vowel, and (d) overline every letter that represents a diphthong.

   Vowels are early sounds to appear in a child's speech. Front vowels tend to predominate in an infant's early vowel usage. It has been suggested that an infant could produce a set of front vowels by holding the tongue near the front of the mouth and varying the amount of jaw opening. A closed jaw position would yield /i/, and an open jaw position would yield /æ/.

5. Assuming General American dialect, center over each vowel alphabet letter(s) in the following words the phoneme symbol that best fits the vowel pronunciation.

   (a) money
   (b) fencepost
   (c) diplomat
   (d) lamplighter
   (e) suitcase
   (f) library
   (g) overpower
   (h) laundromat
   (i) bookmark
   (j) reinterpret
   (k) knowhow
   (l) mustard
   (m) merciless
   (n) boilerplate
   (o) wanderlust
   (p) rectify
   (q) neologism
   (r) administrate
   (s) luncheonette
   (t) geometry
   (u) utensil
   (v) misunderstood

TRANSCRIPTION TRAINING

Transcription items for vowels are recorded on Tape 1A. A Transcription Sheet and Transcription Key are provided on the following pages. As you listen to each word, write your transcription of the vowel sound in the brackets on the Transcription Sheet. Check your answers on the Transcription Key, which can be masked by a sheet of paper. Notice that the word lists are constructed to train on different groups of vowels as follows:

Transcription List A—corner vowels of vowel quadrilateral /i/, /u/, /æ/, and /ɑ/ (or /ɔ/, which alternates with /ɑ/ in many words, depending on dialect).

Transcription List B—front vowels /i/, /ɪ/, /e/ (or /e͡ɪ/), /ɛ/, and /æ/.

Transcription List C—back vowels /u/, /ʊ/, /o/ (or /o͡ʊ/), /ɔ/, and /ɑ/.

Transcription List D—central vowels /ɝ/, /ʌ/, /ɚ/, and /ə/; diphthongs /ɑ͡ɪ/, /ɔ͡ɪ/, /ɑ͡ʊ/, /e͡ɪ/, and /o͡ʊ/.

PROCEED TO: Clinical Phonetics Tape IA: Transcription Lists A, B, C, D

MODULE TIME	
TOTAL	6:22
ELAPSED	00:00–06:22

Clinical Phonetics Tape IA
Transcription List A

TRANSCRIPTION KEY

1	me	[i]	26	ramp	[æ]
2	on	[ɑ]	27	blue	[u]
3	at	[æ]	28	treat	[i]
4	two	[u]	29	talc	[æ]
5	top	[ɑ]	30	real	[i]
6	keep	[i]	31	ghoul	[u]
7	moon	[u]	32	nude	[u]
8	knee	[i]	33	calm	[ɑ]
9	back	[æ]	34	barn	[ɑ]
10	gap	[æ]	35	rank	[æ]
11	gang	[æ]	36	creed	[i]
12	dot	[ɑ]	37	tool	[u]
13	peaked	[i]	38	bomb	[ɑ]
14	ruined	[u]	39	trapped	[æ]
15	pond	[ɑ]	40	clean	[i]
16	poor	[u]	41	long	[ɔ]
17	boot	[u]	42	rang	[æ]
18	bat	[æ]	43	tank	[æ]
19	drop	[ɑ]	44	group	[u]
20	teamed	[i]	45	keel	[i]
21	league	[i]	46	banged	[æ]
22	loot	[u]	47	lock	[ɑ]
23	wrong	[ɔ]	48	bleed	[i]
24	lagged	[æ]	49	clue	[u]
25	bald	[ɔ]	50	grew	[u]

MODULE TIME	
TOTAL	6:22
ELAPSED	00:00–06:22

Clinical Phonetics Tape IA
Transcription List A

TRANSCRIPTION SHEET

1	me	[ ]	26	ramp	[ ]
2	on	[ ]	27	blue	[ ]
3	at	[ ]	28	treat	[ ]
4	two	[ ]	29	talc	[ ]
5	top	[ ]	30	real	[ ]
6	keep	[ ]	31	ghoul	[ ]
7	moon	[ ]	32	nude	[ ]
8	knee	[ ]	33	calm	[ ]
9	back	[ ]	34	barn	[ ]
10	gap	[ ]	35	rank	[ ]
11	gang	[ ]	36	creed	[ ]
12	dot	[ ]	37	tool	[ ]
13	peaked	[ ]	38	bomb	[ ]
14	ruined	[ ]	39	trapped	[ ]
15	pond	[ ]	40	clean	[ ]
16	poor	[ ]	41	long	[ ]
17	boot	[ ]	42	rang	[ ]
18	bat	[ ]	43	tank	[ ]
19	drop	[ ]	44	group	[ ]
20	teamed	[ ]	45	keel	[ ]
21	league	[ ]	46	banged	[ ]
22	loot	[ ]	47	lock	[ ]
23	wrong	[ ]	48	bleed	[ ]
24	lagged	[ ]	49	clue	[ ]
25	bald	[ ]	50	grew	[ ]

MODULE TIME	
TOTAL	6:03
ELAPSED	06:22–12:25

Clinical Phonetics Tape IA
Transcription List B

TRANSCRIPTION KEY

1	yes	[ɛ]	26	rich	[ɪ]
2	wish	[ɪ]	27	veal	[i]
3	sheep	[i]	28	Yale	[e͡ɪ]
4	faith	[e͡ɪ]	29	jazz	[æ]
5	thanks	[æ]	30	fence	[ɛ]
6	rash	[æ]	31	that	[æ]
7	weaved	[i]	32	whale	[e͡ɪ]
8	this	[ɪ]	33	fish	[ɪ]
9	waste	[e͡ɪ]	34	yeast	[i]
10	when	[ɛ]	35	fizz	[ɪ]
11	fast	[æ]	36	seethe	[i]
12	vest	[ɛ]	37	dwell	[ɛ]
13	wage	[e͡ɪ]	38	vast	[æ]
14	cheese	[i]	39	eighth	[e͡ɪ]
15	thing	[ɪ]	40	hatch	[æ]
16	thief	[i]	41	sting	[ɪ]
17	stretch	[ɛ]	42	hedge	[ɛ]
18	badge	[æ]	43	haze	[e͡ɪ]
19	share	[ɛ]	44	his	[ɪ]
20	they	[e͡ɪ]	45	bear	[ɛ]
21	which	[ɪ]	46	heave	[i]
22	teach	[i]	47	bath	[æ]
23	yams	[æ]	48	freeze	[i]
24	gems	[ɛ]	49	shrill	[ɪ]
25	check	[ɛ]	50	staged	[e͡ɪ]

MODULE TIME	
TOTAL	6:03
ELAPSED	06:22–12:25

Clinical Phonetics Tape IA
Transcription List B

TRANSCRIPTION SHEET

1	yes	[ ]	26	rich	[ ]
2	wish	[ ]	27	veal	[ ]
3	sheep	[ ]	28	Yale	[ ]
4	faith	[ ]	29	jazz	[ ]
5	thanks	[ ]	30	fence	[ ]
6	rash	[ ]	31	that	[ ]
7	weaved	[ ]	32	whale	[ ]
8	this	[ ]	33	fish	[ ]
9	waste	[ ]	34	yeast	[ ]
10	when	[ ]	35	fizz	[ ]
11	fast	[ ]	36	seethe	[ ]
12	vest	[ ]	37	dwell	[ ]
13	wage	[ ]	38	vast	[ ]
14	cheese	[ ]	39	eighth	[ ]
15	thing	[ ]	40	hatch	[ ]
16	thief	[ ]	41	sting	[ ]
17	stretch	[ ]	42	hedge	[ ]
18	badge	[ ]	43	haze	[ ]
19	share	[ ]	44	his	[ ]
20	they	[ ]	45	bear	[ ]
21	which	[ ]	46	heave	[ ]
22	teach	[ ]	47	bath	[ ]
23	yams	[ ]	48	freeze	[ ]
24	gems	[ ]	49	shrill	[ ]
25	check	[ ]	50	staged	[ ]

MODULE TIME	
TOTAL	5:51
ELAPSED	12:25–18:16

Clinical Phonetics Tape IA
Transcription List C

TRANSCRIPTION KEY

1	jaw	[ɔ]	26	shoes	[u]
2	joke	[o͡ʊ]	27	alms	[ɑ]
3	psalm	[ɑ]	28	gold	[o͡ʊ]
4	shoot	[u]	29	crook	[ʊ]
5	should	[ʊ]	30	books	[ʊ]
6	though	[o͡ʊ]	31	cough	[ɔ]
7	could	[ʊ]	32	whole	[o͡ʊ]
8	rouge	[u]	33	thought	[ɔ]
9	shawl	[ɔ]	34	vault	[ɔ]
10	Vaughn	[ɔ]	35	groom	[u]
11	through	[u]	36	looked	[ʊ]
12	wash	[ɔ] or [ɑ]	37	yawn	[ɔ]
13	woods	[ʊ]	38	slew	[u]
14	throw	[o͡ʊ]	39	both	[o͡ʊ]
15	stone	[o͡ʊ]	40	gone	[ɔ]
16	halls	[ɔ]	41	would	[ʊ]
17	strewn	[u]	42	nook	[ʊ]
18	palms	[ɑ]	43	soul	[o͡ʊ]
19	stood	[ʊ]	44	room	[u]
20	salt	[ɔ] or [ɑ]	45	whom	[u]
21	squaw	[ɔ]	46	haunt	[ɔ]
22	flowed	[o͡ʊ]	47	those	[o͡ʊ]
23	shook	[ʊ]	48	swath	[ɑ]
24	food	[u]	49	draw	[ɔ]
25	spot	[ɑ]	50	ought	[ɔ]

MODULE TIME	
TOTAL	5:51
ELAPSED	12:25–18:16

Clinical Phonetics Tape IA
Transcription List C

TRANSCRIPTION SHEET

1	jaw	[ ]	26	shoes	[ ]
2	joke	[ ]	27	alms	[ ]
3	psalm	[ ]	28	gold	[ ]
4	shoot	[ ]	29	crook	[ ]
5	should	[ ]	30	books	[ ]
6	though	[ ]	31	cough	[ ]
7	could	[ ]	32	whole	[ ]
8	rouge	[ ]	33	thought	[ ]
9	shawl	[ ]	34	vault	[ ]
10	Vaughn	[ ]	35	groom	[ ]
11	through	[ ]	36	looked	[ ]
12	wash	[ ]	37	yawn	[ ]
13	woods	[ ]	38	slew	[ ]
14	throw	[ ]	39	both	[ ]
15	stone	[ ]	40	gone	[ ]
16	halls	[ ]	41	would	[ ]
17	strewn	[ ]	42	nook	[ ]
18	palms	[ ]	43	soul	[ ]
19	stood	[ ]	44	room	[ ]
20	salt	[ ]	45	whom	[ ]
21	squaw	[ ]	46	haunt	[ ]
22	flowed	[ ]	47	those	[ ]
23	shook	[ ]	48	swath	[ ]
24	food	[ ]	49	draw	[ ]
25	spot	[ ]	50	ought	[ ]

MODULE TIME	
TOTAL	9:29
ELAPSED	18:16–27:45

Clinical Phonetics Tape IA
Transcription List D

TRANSCRIPTION KEY

1	eyebrow	[a͡ɪ]	[a͡ʊ]	32	ruckus	[ʌ]	[ə]
2	cowboy	[a͡ʊ]	[ɔ͡ɪ]	33	foyer	[ɔ͡ɪ]	[ɚ]
3	rainbow	[e͡ɪ]	[o͡ʊ]	34	murder	[ɝ]	[ɚ]
4	daylight	[e͡ɪ]	[a͡ɪ]	35	hurdle	[ɝ]	
5	highway	[a͡ɪ]	[e͡ɪ]	36	cupboard	[ʌ]	[ɚ]
6	thyroid	[a͡ɪ]	[ɔ͡ɪ]	37	turtle	[ɝ]	
7	lifeboat	[a͡ɪ]	[o͡ʊ]	38	sister	[ɪ]	[ɚ]
8	railroad	[e͡ɪ]	[o͡ʊ]	39	further	[ɝ]	[ɚ]
9	greyhound	[e͡ɪ]	[a͡ʊ]	40	sirloin	[ɝ]	[ɔ͡ɪ]
10	housewife	[a͡ʊ]	[a͡ɪ]	41	surround	[ɝ]	[a͡ʊ]
11	boathouse	[o͡ʊ]	[a͡ʊ]	42	station	[e͡ɪ]	[ə]
12	outside	[a͡ʊ]	[a͡ɪ]	43	acre	[e͡ɪ]	[ɚ]
13	lifeline	[a͡ɪ]	[a͡ɪ]	44	survive	[ɝ]	[a͡ɪ]
14	downspout	[a͡ʊ]	[a͡ʊ]	45	alike	[ə]	[a͡ɪ]
15	hyoid	[a͡ɪ]	[ɔ͡ɪ]	46	buttons	[ʌ]	
16	roadhouse	[o͡ʊ]	[a͡ʊ]	47	rusted	[ʌ] [ə] or [ɪ]	
17	skylight	[a͡ɪ]	[a͡ɪ]	48	annoy	[ə]	[ɔ͡ɪ]
18	daytime	[e͡ɪ]	[a͡ɪ]	49	butter	[ʌ]	[ɚ]
19	townhouse	[a͡ʊ]	[a͡ʊ]	50	certain	[ɝ]	
20	Friday	[a͡ɪ]	[e͡ɪ]	51	cradle	[e͡ɪ]	
21	outline	[a͡ʊ]	[a͡ɪ]	52	surly	[ɝ] [ɪ] or [i]	
22	rowboat	[o͡ʊ]	[o͡ʊ]	53	cousin	[ʌ]	
23	highlight	[a͡ɪ]	[a͡ɪ]	54	lighter	[a͡ɪ]	[ɚ]
24	pie plate	[a͡ɪ]	[e͡ɪ]	55	person	[ɝ] [ə] or [ɪ]	
25	houseboy	[a͡ʊ]	[ɔ͡ɪ]	56	towers	[a͡ʊ]	[ɚ]
26	slurred	[ɝ]		57	subtle	[ʌ]	
27	suburb	[ʌ] [ɝ] or [ɚ]		58	putty	[ʌ]	[ɪ]
28	astound	[ə]	[a͡ʊ]	59	pious	[a͡ɪ] [ə] or [ɪ]	
29	joyous	[ɔ͡ɪ]	[ə]	60	writer	[a͡ɪ]	[ɚ]
30	rubber	[ʌ]	[ɚ]	61	worthy	[ɝ] [ɪ] or [i]	
31	curtain	[ɝ]		62	perturb	[ɝ]	[ɝ]

MODULE TIME	
TOTAL	9:29
ELAPSED	18:16–27:45

Clinical Phonetics Tape IA
Transcription List D

TRANSCRIPTION SHEET

1	eyebrow	[ ]	[ ]	32	ruckus	[ ]	[ ]
2	cowboy	[ ]	[ ]	33	foyer	[ ]	[ ]
3	rainbow	[ ]	[ ]	34	murder	[ ]	[ ]
4	daylight	[ ]	[ ]	35	hurdle	[ ]	
5	highway	[ ]	[ ]	36	cupboard	[ ]	[ ]
6	thyroid	[ ]	[ ]	37	turtle	[ ]	
7	lifeboat	[ ]	[ ]	38	sister	[ ]	[ ]
8	railroad	[ ]	[ ]	39	further	[ ]	[ ]
9	greyhound	[ ]	[ ]	40	sirloin	[ ]	[ ]
10	housewife	[ ]	[ ]	41	surround	[ ]	[ ]
11	boathouse	[ ]	[ ]	42	station	[ ]	[ ]
12	outside	[ ]	[ ]	43	acre	[ ]	[ ]
13	lifeline	[ ]	[ ]	44	survive	[ ]	[ ]
14	downspout	[ ]	[ ]	45	alike	[ ]	[ ]
15	hyoid	[ ]	[ ]	46	buttons	[ ]	
16	roadhouse	[ ]	[ ]	47	rusted	[ ]	[ ]
17	skylight	[ ]	[ ]	48	annoy	[ ]	[ ]
18	daytime	[ ]	[ ]	49	butter	[ ]	[ ]
19	townhouse	[ ]	[ ]	50	certain	[ ]	
20	Friday	[ ]	[ ]	51	cradle	[ ]	
21	outline	[ ]	[ ]	52	surly	[ ]	[ ]
22	rowboat	[ ]	[ ]	53	cousin	[ ]	
23	highlight	[ ]	[ ]	54	lighter	[ ]	[ ]
24	pie plate	[ ]	[ ]	55	person	[ ]	[ ]
25	houseboy	[ ]	[ ]	56	towers	[ ]	[ ]
26	slurred	[ ]		57	subtle	[ ]	
27	suburb	[ ]	[ ]	58	putty	[ ]	[ ]
28	astound	[ ]	[ ]	59	pious	[ ]	[ ]
29	joyous	[ ]	[ ]	60	writer	[ ]	[ ]
30	rubber	[ ]	[ ]	61	worthy	[ ]	[ ]
31	curtain	[ ]		62	perturb	[ ]	[ ]

Clinical Phonetics Tape IA
Transcription List D, Continued

TRANSCRIPTION KEY

63	dirty	[ɝ] [ɪ] or [i]		67	mercy	[ɝ] [ɪ] or [i]	
64	muscle	[ʌ]		68	litter	[ɪ]	[ɚ]
65	sucker	[ʌ]	[ɚ]	69	mutton	[ʌ]	
66	lighter	[a͡ɪ]	[ɚ]	70	tighten	[a͡ɪ]	

Clinical Phonetics Tape IA
Transcription List D, Continued

TRANSCRIPTION SHEET

63	dirty	[ ]	[ ]	67	mercy	[ ]	[ ]
64	muscle	[ ]		68	litter	[ ]	[ ]
65	sucker	[ ]	[ ]	69	mutton	[ ]	
66	lighter	[ ]	[ ]	70	tighten	[ ]	

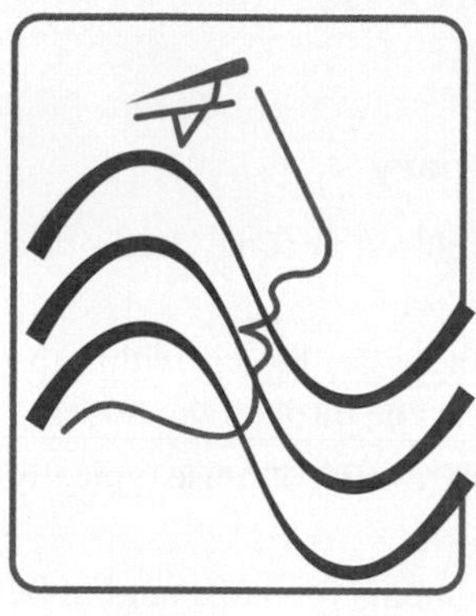

Consonants

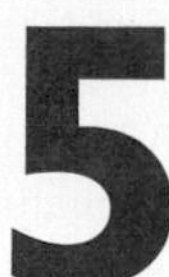

Consonant articulation is described with respect to three basic dimensions: place, manner, and voice. The **place of articulation** tells *where* a sound is formed, the **manner of articulation** tells *how* it is formed, and **voice** tells whether or not the *vocal folds are vibrating* in association with the consonant segment. English consonants can be described by using a modifier or descriptor for each of these three dimensions, as shown in the following list.

Voicing	*Place*	*Manner*
voiced	bilabial	stop
voiceless	labiodental	nasal
	interdental	fricative
	alveolar	affricate
	palatal	liquid
	palatal-velar	(a) lateral
	glottal	(b) rhotic
		glide

Using all these possible combinations of voicing, place, and manner, we would have a total of almost 100 consonants. However, the English language uses only about one-fourth of this number. The number of *possible* consonant sounds is far larger than 100, because other languages have voicing, place, and manner capabilities in addition to those just listed. For example, some languages incorporate whistles, clicks, and sounds formed at other places in the vocal tract. But it also should be noted that not all combinations of the descriptors given above are possible sounds, for some combinations are not pronounceable.

Consonant phonemes in English, then, can be described by specifying the voicing, place, and manner. For instance, the sound *b,* as in *b*ee, a*b*ove, and ru*b*, is described as a voiced, bilabial, stop consonant. This description tells us that the sound is produced with vibrating vocal folds (voiced), with a constriction at the lips (*bi* meaning "two" and *labia* meaning "lips"), and with a complete closure (stopping) at the place of articulation. Given our earlier definition of phonemes with respect to minimal pairs of words, it should be possible to change the voicing, place, or manner features and thereby create other consonants. For example, if we alter only the voicing, changing it to voiceless instead of voiced, we have the sound *p,* as in *p*ea, a*pp*le, and ri*p*. Notice that *b* and *p* are alike in place of articulation (both involving the lips) and manner of articulation (both involving a complete closure or stopping), but that they differ in activity of the vocal folds. Because changes in the voicing, place, and manner may produce different phonemes, they are called the phonemic features of English. That is, these are the modifications of consonant sound production that can be used to create the morphemes of the English language.

A simple model will be used to explain the general properties of consonant production. This model (Figure 5-1) consists of a lung chamber, pharyngeal cavity, oral cavity, and nasal cavity. The lung is separated from the pharyngeal cavity by the vocal folds, and the oral and nasal cavities are separated by the velopharynx. Each open circle in the model represents a valve or opening. The dots represent air pressure contained within a chamber, and the lines ending in the open arrowheads represent airflow.

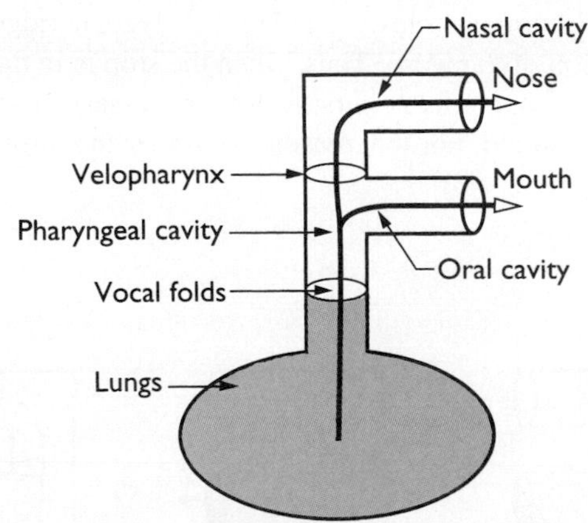

FIGURE 5-1
Simplified model to describe consonant production. Dots represent heightened air pressure, and lines with open arrowheads represent airflow. This drawing illustrates that airflow resulting from an overpressure in the lungs can escape through both the oral and nasal cavities.

MANNER OF ARTICULATION: STOPS

Although there is no one place of articulation at which all manners of articulation are used in English, there is one place at which *almost all* manners apply, and that is the lingua-alveolar articulation. Therefore, we will use this place of articulation to contrast the basic manner types. **Lingua** means tongue, and **alveolar** refers to the prominent ridge just behind the upper central teeth. This place of articulation normally is used for the initial sounds in the words *too, dew, sue, zoo, Lou,* and *new.* Say these words to yourself and note the similarity in place of articulation for the initial consonants. To produce these sounds, a speaker places the tongue tip close to or in contact with the alveolar ridge. The degree of closure depends on the manner of articulation.

Let us concentrate first on the words *too* and *dew.* By saying these words, you should be able to affirm that the tongue tip presses tightly against the alveolar ridge, stopping the egressive airflow momentarily. These two sounds, which are given the phonemic symbols /t/ and /d/, are the lingua-alveolar (or just alveolar) **stop consonants.** *A stop consonant, regardless of where it is made, is formed by a complete closure of the vocal tract, so that airflow ceases temporarily and air pressure builds up behind the point of closure.* This manner of articulation is illustrated in Figure 5-2(*a*). Because air is impounded behind the closure, the cavity becomes a pressure chamber. When the impounded air is released, it produces a short burst of noise, called the **stop burst.** Because the release of the stop is associated with an audible burst, some phoneticians call sounds like /t/ a stop plosive or plosive (*plosive* referring to the small explosion of escaping air). However, the plosive phase does not always occur in the production of sounds like /t/. For example, the word *tot* can be produced with an intelligible final /t/ even if the tongue tip remains closed against the alveolar ridge at the completion of the word. Thus, when the stop is in the word-final position, a release burst is not a necessary characteristic of this sound. For that reason, we prefer the term **stop** to *stop plosive* or *plosive.*

Stops—Articulatory Summary

1. The oral cavity is completely closed at some point for a brief interval.
2. The velopharynx is closed (otherwise, the air within the oral pressure chamber would escape through the nose).
3. Upon release of the stop closure, a burst of noise typically is heard.
4. The closing and opening movements for stops tend to be quite fast, usually the fastest movements in speech.

A frequently occurring allophone (phonetic variant) of the /t/ and /d/ phonemes occurs in words such as *city, ladder, latter, butter, writer, rider, patty,* and *laddy.* Speakers of English usually produce these words with the allophonic lingua-alveolar **flap** /ɾ/ in the intervocalic position. The flap is a modified stop sound, in which a rapid stroking or flapping motion of the tongue tip contacts the alveolar ridge very briefly. The flap also is known by the names **tap** and **one-tap trill.** In a sense, the flap may be regarded as a reduced version of /t/ and /d/, as it can replace both of these phonemes in pairs such as *latter–ladder, writer–rider,* and *knotting–nodding.* Some phoneticians give the flap full phonemic status as a manner of production, but we prefer to view it as a variant or modification of the more general stop category.

The stop phonemes of English are represented by the initial sounds in the words *pill, bill, till, dill, kill, gill.* Say these words to yourself and attempt to verify the similarity in manner, but not place, of production. Note in particular the four features described above: oral closure, velopharyngeal closure, noise burst associated with release, and rapid articulatory movement.

MANNER OF ARTICULATION: FRICATIVES

The initial sounds of *sue* and *zoo* are lingua-alveolar **fricatives.** They are produced by bringing the tongue tip up to the alveolar ridge but not pressing tightly against it. Because the

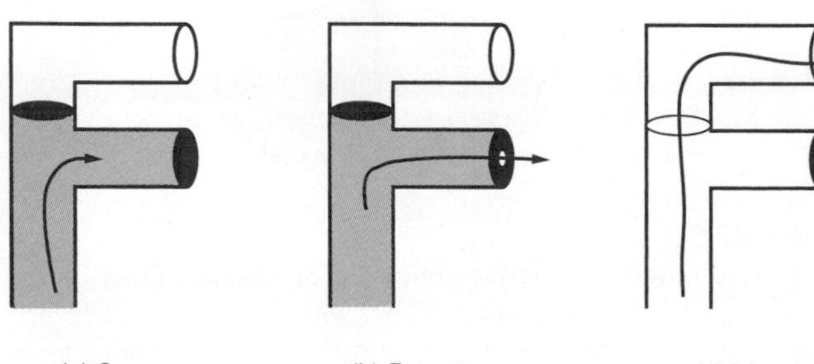

FIGURE 5-2
Simplified model shown in Figure 5-1 adapted for production of (*a*) stops, (*b*) fricatives, and (*c*) nasals. A blackened port indicates closure, and a partially blackened port indicates frication constriction.

closure is incomplete, air escapes with a hissing noise through a narrow central groove in the tongue. All fricatives are made with a continuous noise production (called frication). *Thus, a fricative is defined as a sound that is produced with a narrow constriction through which air escapes with a continuous noise.* The intensity of the noise varies with place of articulation. The lingua-alveolar fricatives are among the most intense. Although both stops (as in *too, due*) and fricatives (as in *sue, zoo*) can have associated noise segments, the noise burst segment for stops (10 to 20 ms) is much briefer than that for fricatives (100 ms or so). The nature of fricative production is illustrated schematically in Figure 5-2*(b)*, which shows the air pressure chamber behind the constriction and the narrow constriction or passageway. Noise energy is generated as air escapes through the passage.

Fricatives—Articulatory Summary

1. The articulators form a narrow constriction through which airflow is channeled. Air pressure increases in the chamber behind the constriction.
2. As the air flows through the narrow opening, a continuous frication noise is generated.
3. Because effective noise production demands that all of the escaping air be directed through the oral constriction, fricatives are produced with a closed velopharynx.

The nine fricatives of English are represented by the final sounds in the words *leaf, leave, teeth, teethe, bus, buzz, rush,* and *rouge* and the initial sound of *he* (this sound does not occur word-finally). Say these sounds and attempt to verify the three articulatory features just listed.

MANNER OF ARTICULATION: NASALS

The first sound in *new* is a lingua-alveolar nasal consonant. For **nasal** consonants, the sound energy created by pulses of air from the vibrating vocal folds must radiate (pass) through the nasal cavities, with the oral tract usually being completely closed. To demonstrate to yourself that this sound involves the nasal tract, try saying the words *new, no, knee,* and *nay* while pinching your nose tightly with your fingers. The resulting sounds will not be acceptable *n* sounds, although they will bear some similarity to them.

By definition, a nasal consonant is produced with a complete oral closure (like a stop), but with an open velopharynx, so that voicing energy travels out through the nose. In most languages, including English, the characteristic of nasal sound transmission also affects vowel sounds adjacent to nasal consonants. In the words *no* and *on,* the vowels following and preceding the *n* sound tend to be nasalized (sound energy passes through both the nose and mouth). Figure 5-2*(c)* illustrates the salient features of nasal consonant production.

Nasals—Articulatory Summary

1. The oral tract is completely closed, as it is for a stop.
2. The velopharyngeal port is open to permit sound energy to radiate outward through the nasal cavities.
3. Even if the oral closure is broken, sound may continue to travel through the nose as long as the velopharynx remains open.

The nasals of English are represented by the final consonants in the words *ram, ran,* and *rang.* Verify the nasal manner by saying each word with your nostrils alternately open and closed.

MANNER OF ARTICULATION: LIQUIDS

There are two types of **liquids: lateral** sounds and **rhotic** sounds. Here we will discuss both only briefly, as a more detailed analysis will be presented later. The lateral sound occurs initially in the words *Lou, Lee, law,* and *low.* The tongue tip makes a midline, or central, closure with the alveolar ridge, but an opening is maintained at the sides of the tongue. Therefore, sound energy generated in the larynx radiates laterally, or around the sides of the tongue. *Hence, a lateral sound has midline closure and lateral opening for sound transmission,* as shown in Figure 5-3.

The rhotic liquid consonant is the *r* consonant, as in *rue, raw,* and *ray.* This is a complex sound, to be considered in depth later in this chapter. *For the present, it is sufficient to note that the common ways of producing the rhotic, or* r, *sound are to (1) hold the tongue tip so it is curled back slightly and not quite touching the alveolar ridge or the adjoining palatal area, and (2) bunch the tongue in the palatal area of the mouth.* (See Figure 5-4.) Sound energy from the vibrating vocal folds then passes through the opening between tongue and palatal vault.

Both the lateral sound, as in *Lou,* and the rhotic sound, as in *rue,* are liquids. *A liquid is a vowel-like consonant in which voicing energy passes through a vocal tract that is constricted only somewhat more than for vowels. The shape and location of the constriction is a critical defining property, being distinctive for a given type of liquid.*

Liquids—Articulatory Summary

1. Sound energy from the vocal folds is directed through a distinctively shaped oral passage, one that can be held indefinitely for sustained production of the sound, if required.
2. The velopharynx is always (or at least almost always) closed.
3. The oral passageway is narrower than that for vowels but wider than that for stops, fricatives, and nasals.

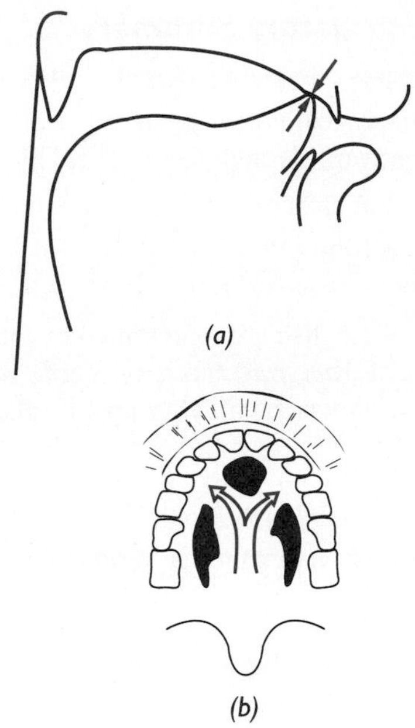

FIGURE 5-3
Articulation of the lateral consonant /l/. A lateral-view articulatory configuration is shown in *(a)*, and an inferior view of the roof of the mouth is shown in *(b)*. Lateral opening around the point of tongue contact shown in *(a)* allows sound energy to pass through the mouth. Regions of tongue contact are shown in *(b)* as dark areas.

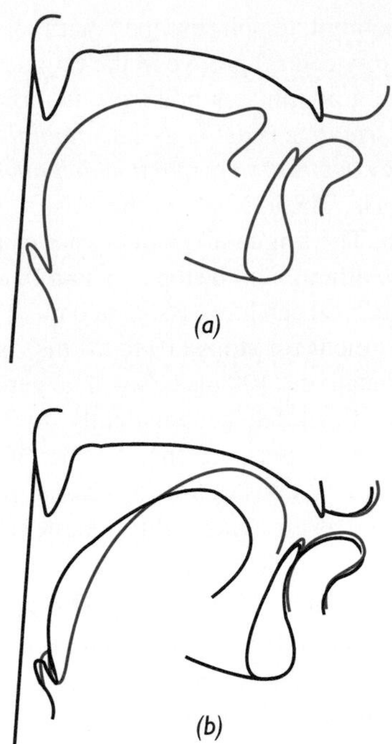

FIGURE 5-4
Articulations of the rhotic /r/. The retroflex articulation is shown in *(a)* and the bunched articulation in *(b)*. The black and red lines in *(b)* represent the bunched /r/ in two different vowel contexts.

The lateral /l/ in *Lou* and the rhotic /r/ in *rue* occur at only one place of articulation in General American English. However, in some dialects and in some speech disorders, lateralized or rhotic modifications occur for other sounds, as discussed in Chapter 6.

MANNER OF ARTICULATION: GLIDES

Glide sounds, also known as **semivowels,** are made at two places in English: lingua-palatal and labio-lingua-velar. The lingua-palatal glide (symbolized phonemically as /j/) occurs in the words *you, yes,* and *yawn.* The voiced labio-lingua-velar /w/ occurs in the words *woo, we,* and *one,* and the voiceless labio-lingua-velar /ʍ/ is used by some speakers in the words *why, which,* and *when. A glide sound has a vocal tract constriction somewhat narrower than that for vowels but less severe than that for stops and fricatives and is characterized by a gliding motion of the articulators from a partly constricted state to a more open state for the following vowel.* (A glide is always followed by a vowel.) The gliding motion from the constricted state to the following vowel is the distinguishing and defining property of glides. These gliding movements are slower than the closing and opening movements for stops. An illustration of glide production is given in Figure 5-5.

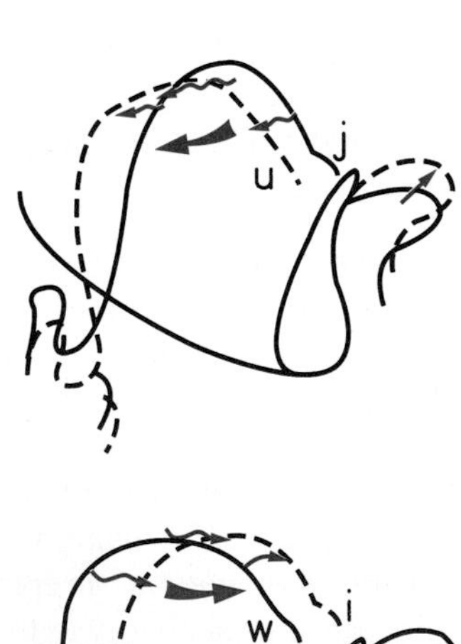

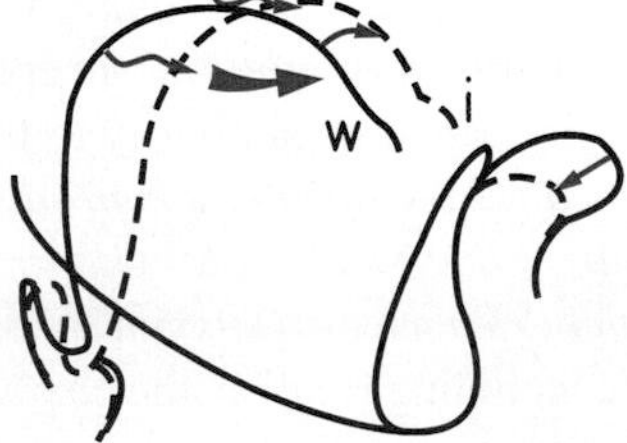

FIGURE 5-5
Articulations for the glide consonants /j/ and /w/ in the words *you* and *we*, respectively. The drawings show lip and tongue movements relative to the jaw. Notice that the glide articulations for *you* are essentially opposite to those for *we.*

Glides—Articulatory Summary

1. The constricted state for the glide is narrower than that for a vowel but wider than that for stops and fricatives.
2. The articulators make a gradual gliding motion from the constricted segment to the more open configuration for the following vowel.
3. The velopharynx is generally, if not always, closed.
4. The sound energy from the vocal folds passes through the mouth, in a fashion similar to that for vowels.

There are only three glides in English, represented by the initial sounds in *you* (/j/), *we* (/w/), and *while* (/ʍ/ in some but not all pronunciations).

MANNER OF ARTICULATION: AFFRICATES

Affricates *are best viewed as combination sounds involving a stop closure followed by a fricative segment.* Air pressure built up during the stop phase is released as a burst of noise, similar in duration to that for fricative sounds. The affricates of English are produced only at the palatal place of production, as in the words *church* and *judge.* In these words, both the initial and final segments are affricates. The basic properties of affricates are illustrated schematically in Figure 5-6.

Affricates—Articulatory Summary

1. Affricates are a combination of a stop closure and a fricative segment, with the frication noise closely following the stop portion.
2. Affricates are made with complete closure of the velopharynx.

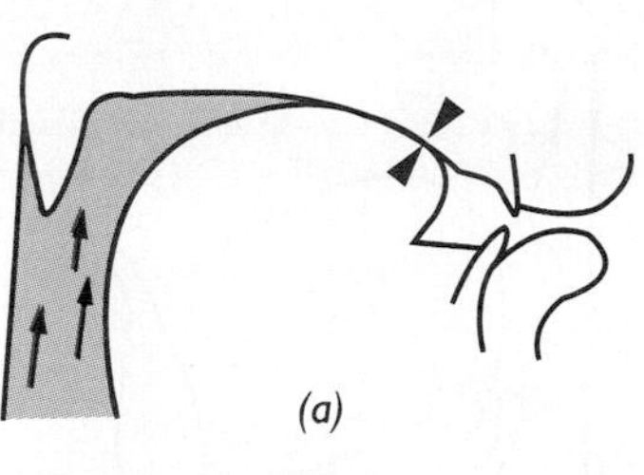

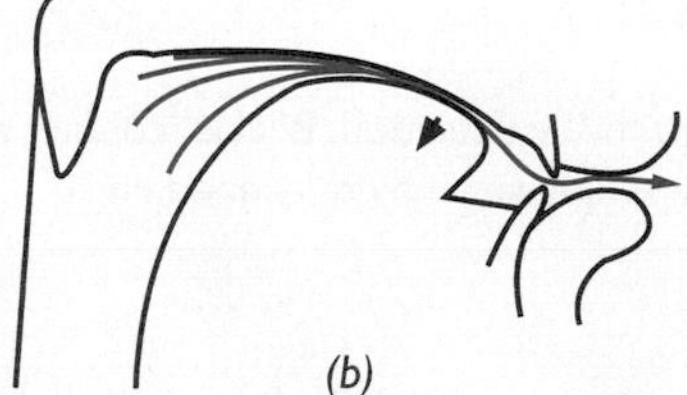

FIGURE 5-6
Schematic illustration of affricate production, showing *(a)* the buildup of air pressure during the stop portion and *(b)* the release of air through a narrow passage during the fricative portion.

PLACE OF ARTICULATION

It should be apparent by now that most consonants are formed by completely or nearly closing the vocal tract at some point. Place of articulation describes where the point of closure or constriction is located. An intuitive impression about place of articulation can be gained by reciting the words listed under each place of articulation in Table 5-1 and noting where the italicized sound is produced. The phonetic symbol for each of these sounds is given after the key word. The words *why* and *way* are placed in parentheses to indicate that, for the sound in question, two articulators are involved. The /w/, as in *way* and *wag,* involves constrictions of both lips and tongue, as does the /ʍ/, the voiceless counterpart to /w/.

PLACE OF ARTICULATION: BILABIALS /b/ /p/ /m/ /w/ /ʍ/

Sounds formed at the **bilabial** place of articulation are the voiced and voiceless stops /b/ and /p/, the nasal /m/, and the voiced and voiceless glides /w/ and /ʍ/. The latter two sounds are described as having two places of articulation because they are produced with rounding of the lips and with the tongue in a high-back (/u/-like) position. The tongue-positioning requirement for /w/ and /ʍ/ should be emphasized, because in our experience students sometimes fail to recognize its significance. Notice that no English fricatives or affricates are made at the bilabial place of production.

Two basic lip articulations are needed to produce the five sounds /p b m w ʍ/. The first articulation, lip closure, is required for the bilabial stops /b/ and /p/ and the bilabial nasal /m/. Usually, this articulation consists of a closing phase, a closed phase, and a releasing or opening phase. Both the closing and releasing phases are accomplished in about 50 to 75 ms. These articulations are among the briefest (fastest) in speech. Bilabial closure for /b/ is illustrated in Figure 5-7. Notice that the tongue can take different positions during the bilabial closure; in this illustration, the tongue takes the position for the vowel that follows the /b/. The articulation for /m/ is similar to that for /b/; thus, some phoneticians regard /m/ as a "nasalized bilabial stop." The voiced and voiceless /b/ and /p/ have basically the same labial articulation, although some authorities describe /p/ as having a forceful articulation involving greater muscular activity. These authorities describe /p/ as tense and /b/ as lax (see, for example, Chomsky and Halle, 1968). The reality of a tense–lax distinction for voiced and voiceless stops is still a matter of some controversy, but physiologic studies should resolve the issue.

TABLE 5-1
Place of Articulation for English Consonants

Place of Articulation						
Bilabial	Labiodental	Interdental	Alveolar	Palatal	Velar	Glottal
Both lips	Lips and teeth	Tongue tip and teeth	Tongue tip and ridge behind teeth	Tongue blade and palate	Tongue dorsum and velum	Vocal folds
*p*ie /p/	*f*ear /f/	*th*aw /θ/	*t*wo /t/	ru*sh* /ʃ/	ra*ck* /k/	*h*igh /h/
*b*ye /b/	*v*eer /v/	*th*e /ð/	*d*ue /d/	rou*ge* /ʒ/	ra*g* /g/	
*m*y /m/			*s*ue /s/	ri*ch* /ʧ/	ra*ng* /ŋ/	
(*w*ay) /w/			*z*oo /z/	ri*dge* /ʤ/	(*w*ay) /w/	
(*wh*y) /ʍ/			*n*ew /n/	*r*aw /r/	(*wh*y) /ʍ/	
			Lou /l/	*y*aw /j/		
			bu*tt*er /ɾ/			

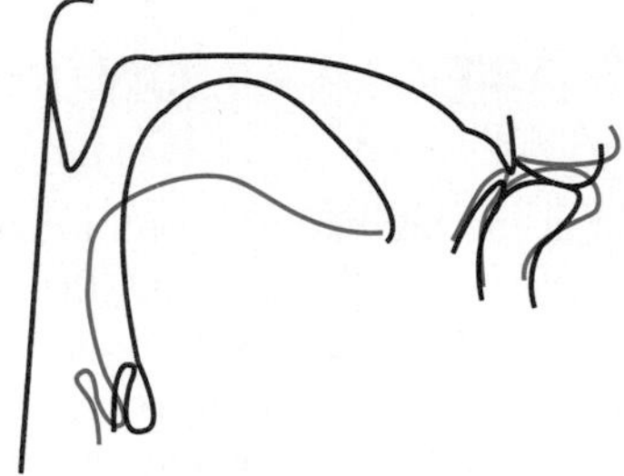

FIGURE 5-7
X-ray tracings of the bilabial closure in /b a/ (black line) and /b u/ (red line). During the bilabial closure for /b/, the tongue assumes the position for the following vowel.

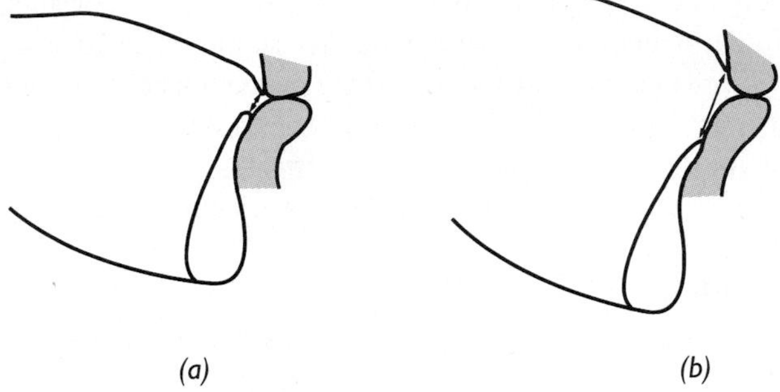

(a) *(b)*

FIGURE 5-8
Bilabial closure for a closed jaw position in *(a)* and an open jaw position in *(b)*.

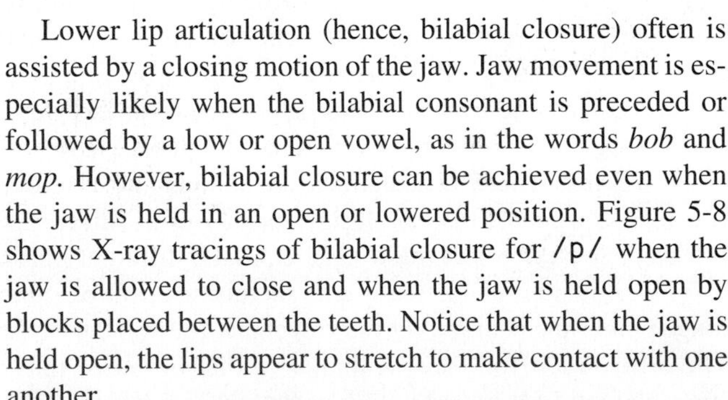

Lower lip articulation (hence, bilabial closure) often is assisted by a closing motion of the jaw. Jaw movement is especially likely when the bilabial consonant is preceded or followed by a low or open vowel, as in the words *bob* and *mop*. However, bilabial closure can be achieved even when the jaw is held in an open or lowered position. Figure 5-8 shows X-ray tracings of bilabial closure for /p/ when the jaw is allowed to close and when the jaw is held open by blocks placed between the teeth. Notice that when the jaw is held open, the lips appear to stretch to make contact with one another.

The stops /b/ and /p/ are oral consonants, produced with velopharyngeal closure to permit the containment of air within the oral cavity. The nasal /m/ is produced with an open velopharynx (Figure 5-9), so that sound energy is radiated through the nasal cavities rather than the oral cavity. Otherwise, the articulatory configuration for /m/ is like that for /b/ and /p/.

The other lip articulation is one variously known as rounding, narrowing, protrusion, or lengthening. Actually, the different names are justified in that different speakers have somewhat different articulations. Whereas some speakers protrude the lips (pushing them forward from the teeth), other speakers have primarily a narrowing movement in which the lips move toward, but do not reach, closure. The gesture of rounding or protrusion is shown in Figure 5-10,

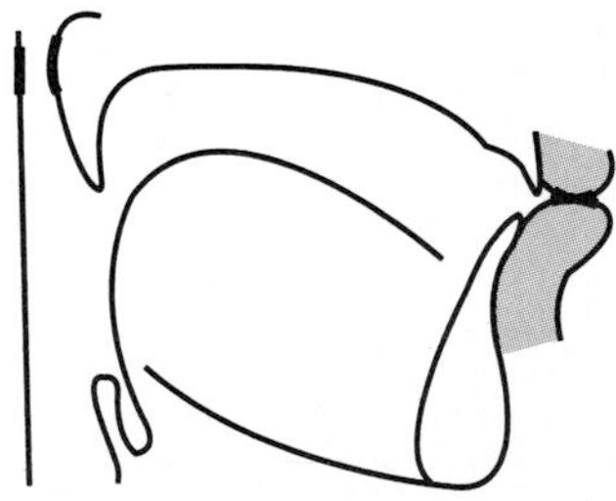

FIGURE 5-9
X-ray tracing of /m/ articulation. Bilabial contact and velopharyngeal opening are emphasized by thickened lines.

which is based on X-ray tracings of the /w/ articulation in the word *we*. Photographs of lip rounding are presented in Figure 4-4. The rounding or protrusion articulation is slower than for bilabial closure and generally takes 75 to 100 ms or more.

PLACE OF ARTICULATION: LABIODENTALS /f/ /v/

Only the fricatives /f/ (voiceless) as in *fat* and /v/ (voiced) as in *vat* are made as **labiodental** sounds. The basic articulation, shown in Figure 5-11, involves a constriction between the lower lip and the upper teeth (incisors). The fricative energy for /f/ and /v/ is weak compared to that for /s/ and /z/. Because the lower lip is attached to the jaw, the constricting movement of lower lip to upper teeth often is assisted by jaw movement. The lower lip movement for the labiodental constriction is somewhat like that for bilabial closure. The velopharynx is closed, as it is for all consonants except the nasals.

PLACE OF ARTICULATION: INTERDENTALS (OR DENTALS) /θ/ /ð/

Only fricatives are formed at the **interdental** (or **dental**) location: the voiceless interdental /θ/ as in *thin* and the voiced interdental /ð/ as in *this*. Figure 5-12 illustrates the articulation, which takes two major forms, interdental and dental. For the interdental, the tongue tip is protruded slightly between the front teeth (incisors), so that a narrow constriction is formed between the tongue and the cutting edge of the teeth. For the dental articulation, the tongue tip contacts the back of the front teeth, so that the constriction is between the tongue and the inside surface of the teeth. The noise energy is weak, comparable to that for /f/ and /v/. In many speakers, the tip of the tongue is visible during /θ ð/ production. Although the jaw often closes somewhat to aid formation of the constriction, it cannot close completely, or there would not be adequate interdental opening for the tongue tip. These sounds tend to be made with a dental, rather than interdental, constriction in rapid speech.

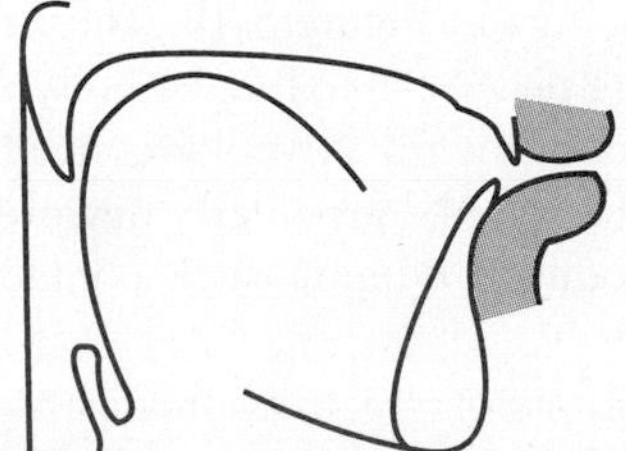

FIGURE 5-10
Lip protrusion, or lip rounding, for the first sound in we. Notice the forward extension of lips and the narrow mouth opening.

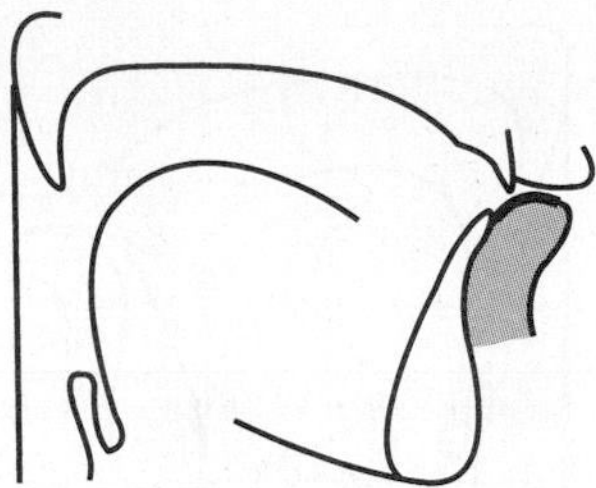

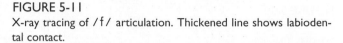

FIGURE 5-11
X-ray tracing of /f/ articulation. Thickened line shows labiodental contact.

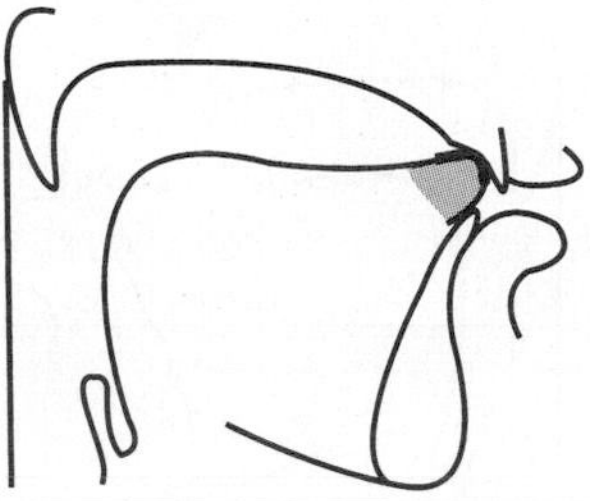

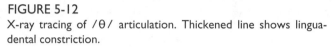

FIGURE 5-12
X-ray tracing of /θ/ articulation. Thickened line shows linguadental constriction.

PLACE OF ARTICULATION: ALVEOLARS /t/ /d/ /s/ /z/ /l/ /n/

Lingua-Alveolar Stops: /t/ and /d/

X-ray tracings of the **lingua-alveolar** consonant closure for /t/ (two) and /d/ (dew) are shown in Figures 5-13 and 5-14. Note the similarity in articulation. Because both of these sounds are stops and require the development of air pressure behind the point of oral closure, the velopharynx is closed. The jaw often closes partially to aid the lingual contact against the alveolar ridge. The site of lingual contact is nearly identical for /d/ and /t/, but /t/ may have a firmer contact and a more rapid release, both of which are related to the fact that /t/ has a greater air pressure than /d/. In addition, /t/ tends to have a longer duration of closure than /d/. These differences are discussed in the section on voicing later in this chapter.

The exact position and shape of the tongue for articulation of /t/ and /d/ varies with phonetic context. One of the most conspicuous contextual effects is that associated with a following dental fricative, as in the words *width* and *eighth*. Because of the influence of the dental fricative, the /d/ and /t/ in these words are made with a dental, rather than alveolar, contact, as illustrated in Figure 5-15. Another fairly frequent modification occurs in the context of palatal sounds, like the /j/ in some pronunciations of *Tuesday* /t j u z d e͡ɪ/. The following palatal causes the /t/ to be

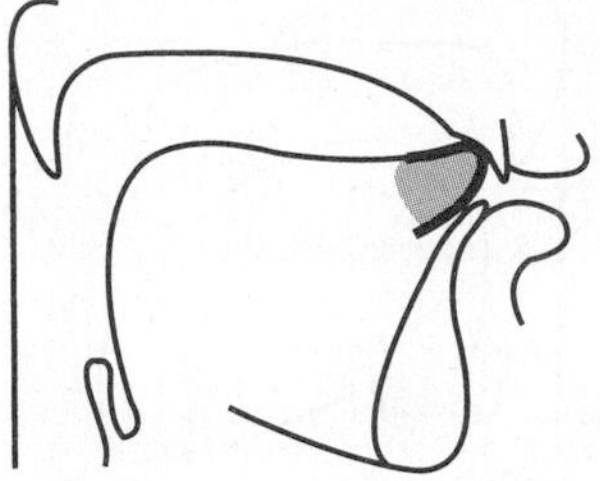

FIGURE 5-13
X-ray tracing of /t/ articulation. Thickened line shows lingua-alveolar contact.

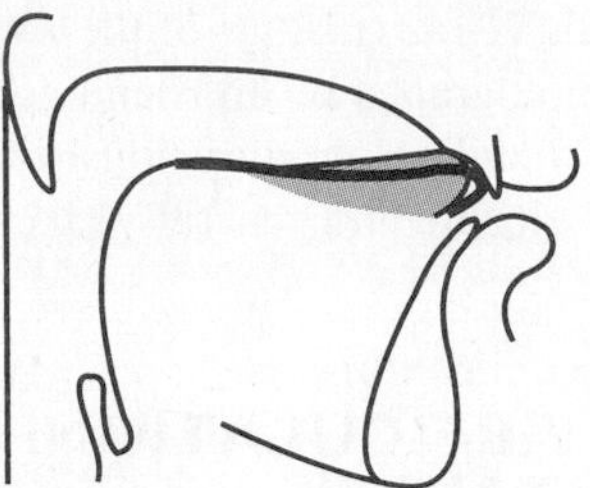

FIGURE 5-15
Alveolar (thin line) and dental (thick line) articulation of /t/.

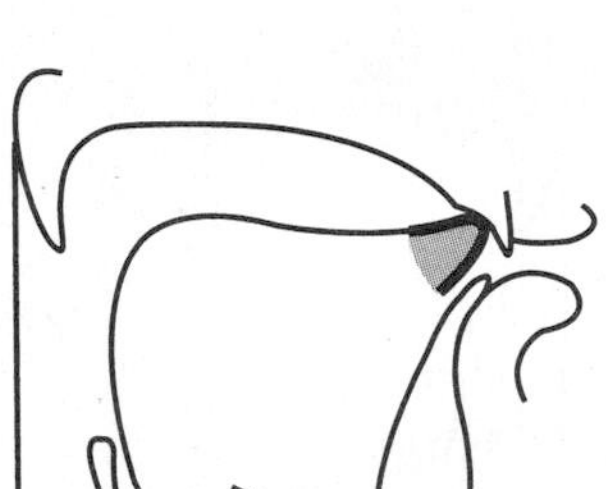

FIGURE 5-14
X-ray tracing of /d/ articulation. Thickened line shows lingua-alveolar contact.

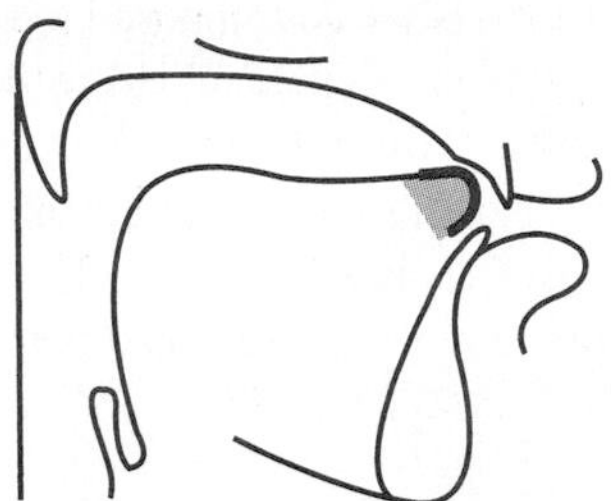

FIGURE 5-16
X-ray tracing of /s/ articulation. Thickened line shows lingua-alveolar constriction.

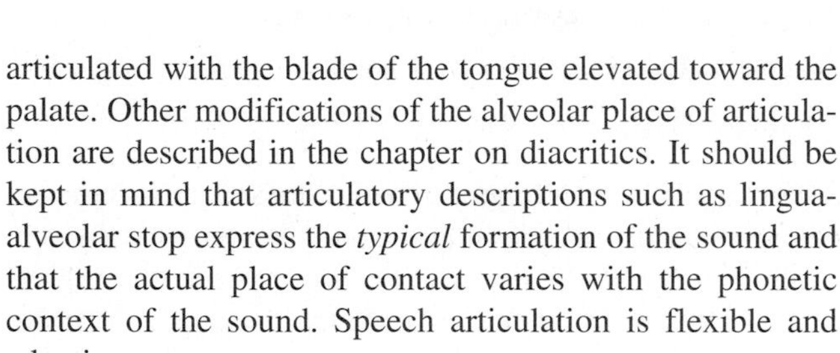

articulated with the blade of the tongue elevated toward the palate. Other modifications of the alveolar place of articulation are described in the chapter on diacritics. It should be kept in mind that articulatory descriptions such as lingua-alveolar stop express the *typical* formation of the sound and that the actual place of contact varies with the phonetic context of the sound. Speech articulation is flexible and adaptive.

Lingua-Alveolar Fricatives: /s/ and /z/

These sounds are depicted by the X-ray tracing in Figure 5-16. Because /s/ (sue) and /z/ (zoo) have the same place and manner of articulation, separate X-ray tracings are not shown. For both /s/ and /z/, the velopharynx is closed to allow air pressure to build up in the mouth. The jaw usually assumes a fairly closed position. The /s/ and /z/ are sometimes called groove fricatives, because a midline groove is formed in the tongue as a narrow passageway for escaping air. Some phoneticians describe /s/ and /z/ as having a blade articulation, because the constriction can be made between the alveolar ridge and the part of the tongue just behind the tip.

The lingual articulation for /s/ and /z/ varies somewhat with phonetic context and with speaker. Some speakers consistently use a **dentalized** constriction, in which the tongue makes a constriction with the area just behind the upper front teeth (incisors). These modifications are discussed in detail later in this book.

Lingua-Alveolar Lateral: /l/

The X-ray tracing in Figure 5-17 illustrates the most common articulation of the /l/ (Lou) in American English. The tongue tip makes contact with the alveolar ridge, and the dorsum of the tongue assumes a position similar to that for vowel /o/ (low). The contact is midline only, so that sound energy radiates through the sides of the mouth, around the midline closure. This sound derives its manner classification from the feature of lateral resonance. The similarity of dorsal tongue position between /l/ and /o/ is shown by the composite X-ray tracings in Figure 5-18. The /l/ might be described as having an /o/-like tongue body and dorsum but a midline contact of the tip. Alveolar contact is not a necessary feature of the sound. Particularly in word-final position, /l/ may be produced without such contact, as shown in Figure 5-19.

Most descriptions of /l/ in phonetics books distinguish between "light *l*" (or "clear *l*") and "dark *l*." However, there is considerable disagreement about the articulatory differences that underlie the distinction of "light" and "dark." The following quotations are illustrative.

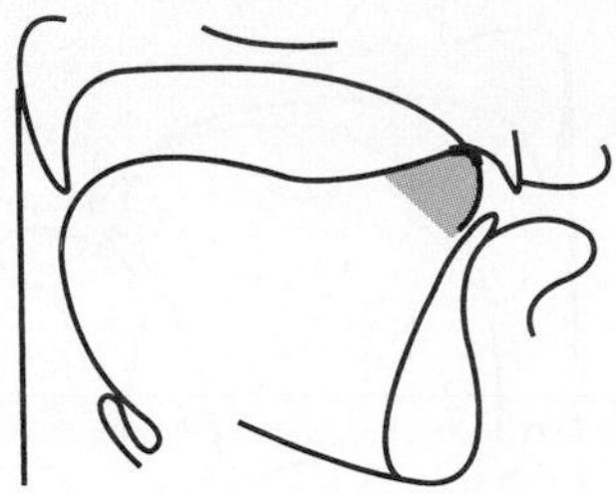

FIGURE 5-17
X-ray tracing of /l/ articulation. Thickened line shows lingua-alveolar contact. (See also Figure 5.3.)

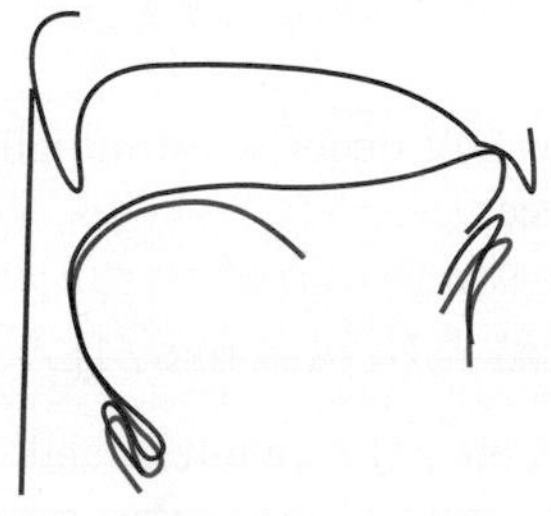

FIGURE 5-18
X-ray tracings of /l/ articulation (black line) and /o/ articulation (red line), showing similarity in root and dorsal positions of the tongue.

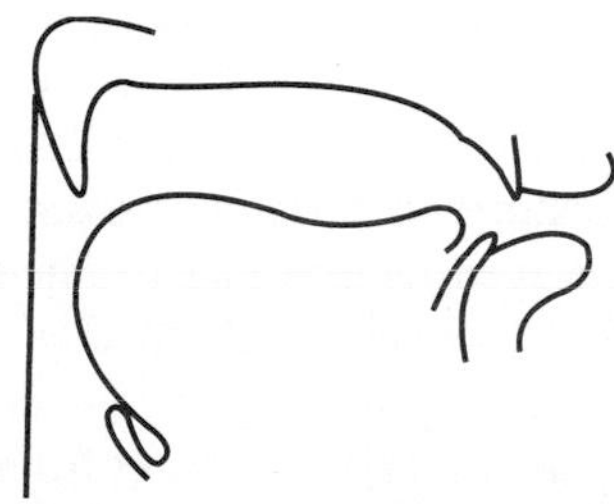

FIGURE 5-19
X-ray tracing of postvocalic /l/ articulated without lingua-alveolar contact.

> *When [l] is made with the tongue against the teeth, it is referred to as dental [l], or, more often, as clear [l]. When it is made alveolarly, it is called "dark l." In Southern, British, and Eastern English, [l] before a front vowel, particularly a high front vowel, is clear. In General American all [l]'s are dark.* (Wise, *Applied Phonetics,* 1957, p. 131)

> *We should point out here that the so-called "lightness" or "clearness" of an* l *is not entirely dependent upon the position of the forepart of the tongue. In other words, the terms "front* l*" and "light* l*" are not exactly synonymous. A little experimentation will demonstrate that it is possible to keep the tip of the tongue on the upper teeth and produce* l*'s of varying degrees of lightness and darkness.* (Kantner and West, 1941, p. 120)

Kantner and West went on to state that two other factors, besides the point of highest elevation of the tongue, determine the degree of lightness or darkness of /l/. First, increased lip spreading was said to result in a lighter /l/. Second, the back of the tongue was said to be flattened and lowered for a very light /l/ but raised for dark /l/.

Giles (1971) studied /l/ articulation by X-ray motion pictures and concluded that the position of the tongue dorsum distinguishes among three general types of /l/: prevocalic, postvocalic, and syllabic. The postvocalic and syllabic /l/ were quite similar except for the timing of movements for /l/ with respect to the preceding vowel. Postvocalic /l/ differed from the prevocalic variety in having a more posterior (farther back) position of the dorsum. Occasionally, contact of the tongue tip was not made for the postvocalic allophones in words like *Paul* (see Figure 5-19). The only other major variation that was observed in Giles's speech sample was dentalization of /l/ when followed by a dental sound, as in *health* /h ɛ l θ/.

The failure of some normal adult speakers to make tongue tip contact for /l/ in word-final or postvocalic position should be remembered when evaluating /l/ production in children. We frequently hear children produce an /o/-like sound for final /l/ in words like *seal.* Apparently, this "substitution" is not necessarily unusual or deviant, and caution should be observed in evaluating the child's proficiency for /l/ articulation. It is prudent to test /l/ production in more than one context or syllabic position before ascribing the /o/-like sound to an articulatory error.

Lingua-Alveolar Nasal: /n/

As the X-ray tracing in Figure 5-20 shows, /n/ (new) is made with a lingua-alveolar contact like that for /t/ and /d/, but with the velopharynx open. Sound energy from the larynx radiates outward through the nasal cavity. Articulatory (allophonic) modifications of the oral closure are similar to those for /t/ and /d/. For example, /n/ is dentalized (made with tongue contact against the upper teeth rather than the alveolar ridge) in words like *ninth,* where it is followed by a dental fricative.

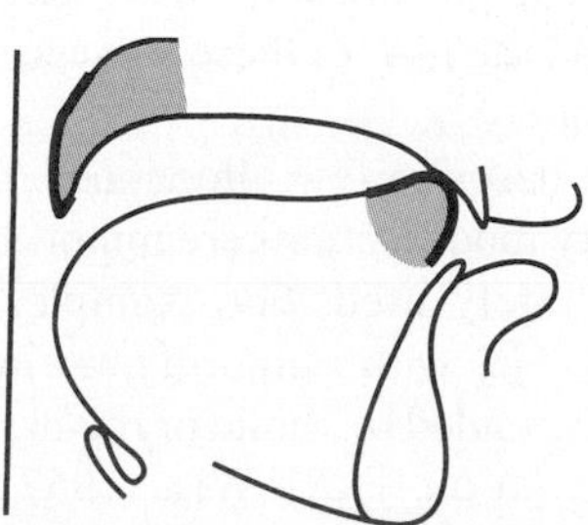

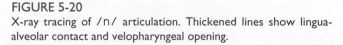

FIGURE 5-20
X-ray tracing of /n/ articulation. Thickened lines show lingua-alveolar contact and velopharyngeal opening.

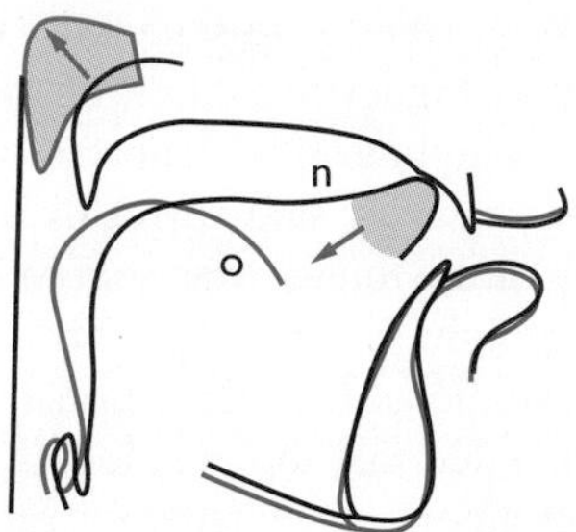

FIGURE 5-21
Articulatory configurations during the word-initial /n/ (black line) and following vowel /o/ in *no one.*

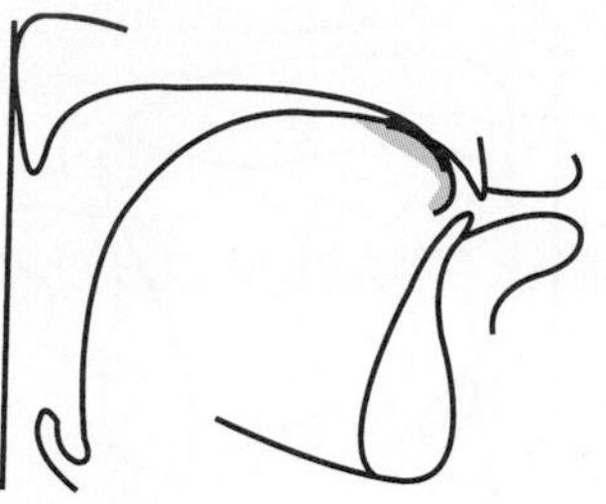

FIGURE 5-22
X-ray tracing of /ʃ/ articulation. Thickened line shows lingua-palatal constriction.

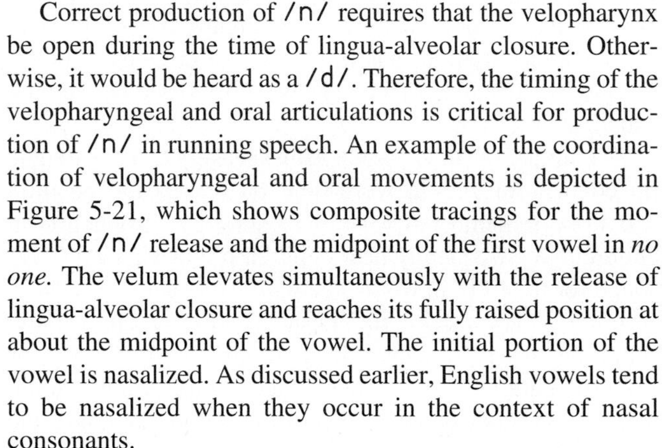

Correct production of /n/ requires that the velopharynx be open during the time of lingua-alveolar closure. Otherwise, it would be heard as a /d/. Therefore, the timing of the velopharyngeal and oral articulations is critical for production of /n/ in running speech. An example of the coordination of velopharyngeal and oral movements is depicted in Figure 5-21, which shows composite tracings for the moment of /n/ release and the midpoint of the first vowel in *no one.* The velum elevates simultaneously with the release of lingua-alveolar closure and reaches its fully raised position at about the midpoint of the vowel. The initial portion of the vowel is nasalized. As discussed earlier, English vowels tend to be nasalized when they occur in the context of nasal consonants.

PLACE OF ARTICULATION: PALATALS /ʃ/ /ʒ/ /tʃ/ /ʤ/ /r/ /j/

Lingua-Palatal Fricatives: /ʃ/ and /ʒ/

As shown by Figure 5-22, /ʃ/ (shoe) and /ʒ/ (rouge) are produced by elevating the tip and blade of the tongue toward the palate, hence, **palatal.** Fricative noise is generated as air passes through the channel between tongue and palate. The noise is quite intense, similar in total energy to that for /s/ and /z/. Thus, the intense fricatives are /s/, /z/, /ʃ/, and /ʒ/, and the weak fricatives are /f/, /v/, /θ/, /ð/, and /h/. Although /ʃ/ and /ʒ/ can be produced with a variety of lip positions, there is a general tendency for speakers to round the lips for these sounds, especially in isolated production.

Phoneticians describe few allophones of /ʃ/ and /ʒ/. Most articulatory modifications are minor. In addition, some allophones are rarely used. For example, the retroflex or rhotacized [ʃ], /ʃ/ with *r* coloring, normally occurs only when /ʃ/ is surrounded by rhotic or rhotacized sounds, as in the word *harsher* [h ɑ r ʃ ɚ]. Wise (1957) notes in *Applied Phonetics* that /ʒ/ is the least frequently used of all English sounds and that it is not originally an English sound but was introduced "partly from adoption from Norman French and partly by assimilation within the older cluster [z j]" (p. 137). /ʒ/ does not occur word-initially in English, except in proper names.

Lingua-Palatal Affricates: /tʃ/ and /ʤ/

The palatal affricates /tʃ/ (church) and /ʤ/ (judge) are produced with an articulation similar to that for the palatal fricatives /ʃ/ and /ʒ/. The major difference is in the manner of production. The affricates are formed by first stopping the flow of air by contacting the tip (and perhaps blade) of the tongue against the palate. Then the stop is released gradually into an immediately following fricative. As explained earlier, it is the two-phase articulation that gives rise to the digraph symbols, /t/ + /ʃ/ = /tʃ/ and /d/ + /ʒ/ = /ʤ/. Chomsky and Halle (1968) distinguished the stops from the affricates by a feature of delayed release. Affricates were said to have a delayed release that resulted in a relatively long noise segment. Stops were said to have an instantaneous release that resulted in a short noise segment. But it should be remembered that /t/ and /d/ differ from /tʃ/ and /ʤ/ in *both* place and manner.

Palatal Rhotic: /r/

Despite years of phonetic research, a careful articulatory description of /r/ (rue) is still wanting. Examples of /r/ articulation are shown in the X-ray tracings of Figure 5-23, but we stress the word *examples.* This sound can be produced with a number of different tongue and lip articulations by the same speaker. Comparisons across a large number of talkers may reveal an even greater articulatory variability.

Generally, the articulation of /r/ falls into two classes, which we term **retroflex** and **bunched.** Retroflex means "turning or turned back" (the morpheme *retro* means "back" and the morpheme *flex* means "turn") and is intended to describe the action of the tip of the tongue, as shown in Figure 5-23*(a).* Although the tongue tip does not really "turn backward," the positioning of the tongue is quite striking in an X-ray film, as no other English sound has this type of articulation. The tongue body assumes a mid-central position, and the lips often (but not necessarily) are rounded.

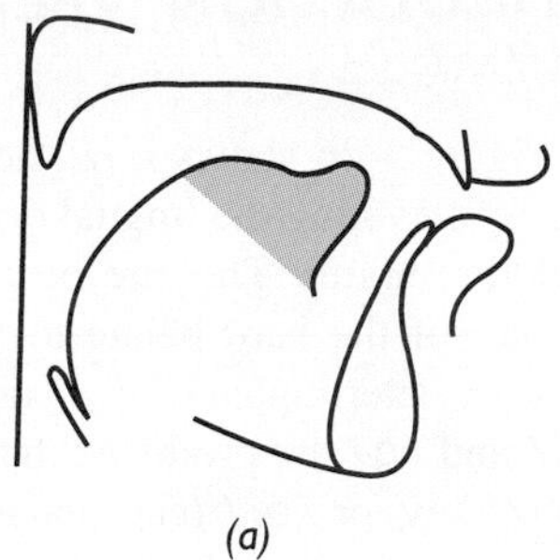
(a)

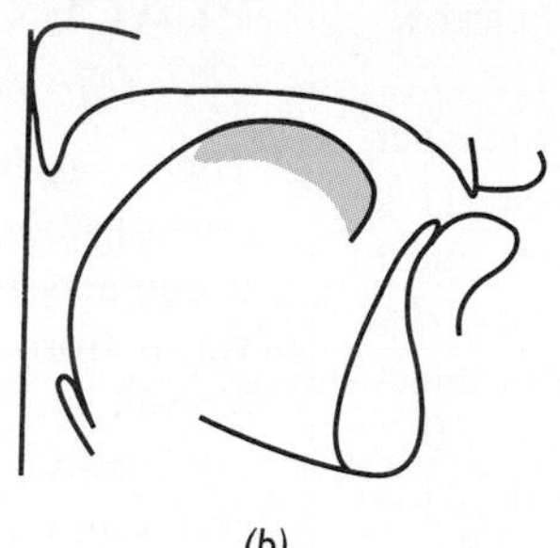
(b)

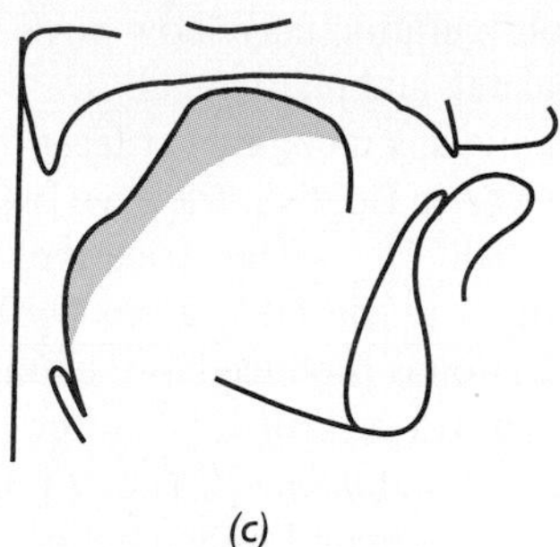
(c)

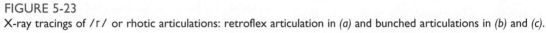

FIGURE 5-23
X-ray tracings of /r/ or rhotic articulations: retroflex articulation in *(a)* and bunched articulations in *(b)* and *(c)*.

The bunched articulation, shown in Figure 5-23*(b)*, is produced with an elevation of the blade toward the palate but with the tip turned down. The position of the tongue body appears to vary with vowel context, and the lips often are rounded. Sometimes the bunched articulation is accompanied with a bulging of the tongue root in the lower pharynx and with a flattening or depression of the dorsum, as in Figure 5-23*(c)*.

It is not clear how these different articulations are associated with phonetic context and syllable position, except that the bunched articulation may be favored postvocalically by some speakers. All the articulations represented in Figure 5-23 are prevocalic. It is clear that /r/ articulation is accommodated to the lingual articulation of the surrounding elements. For example, Figure 5-24 shows how /r/ is produced in the word *true* [t r u]. Upon release of the /t/, the tongue tip is drawn back and downward as the blade is elevated to form a bunched articulation. In the transition from /r/ to /u/, the blade is lowered. The composite drawing illustrates the smooth, flowing motions of the articulators during speech. Because the movements associated with /r/ tend to be slow and glidelike, it can be difficult to determine any one tongue position that represents the /r/. The comments of Kantner and West are instructive:

> r *is a sound that, even more than* t, k, *and* l, *is influenced by neighboring sounds. We will not be far wrong if we think of* r *as being dragged all over the mouth cavity by the various sounds with which it happens to be associated. This means that different sounds that we recognize as* r *are sometimes produced by fundamentally different movements.* (Kantner and West, 1941, pp. 152–153)

In an X-ray study of three speakers, Zawadzki and Kuehn (1980) observed two basic types of /r/: prevocalic /r/ for syllable initiation, and postvocalic /r/ for terminating a syllable or for forming a syllabic nucleus. Compared to the postvocalic /r/, the prevocalic allophone was described as having "a greater lip rounding, a more advanced [fronted] tongue position, and less tongue dorsum grooving" (p. 253). Earlier, Delattre and Freeman (1968) identified six different tongue shapes associated with /r/, but most of these six shapes could be classified as bunched articulations. Zawadzki and Kuehn (1980) commented on an important, and often overlooked, feature of the /r/ articulation in the Delattre and Freeman study: All the /r/ allophones had a narrowing of the vocal tract in the pharyngeal region. Some degree of pharyngeal narrowing is evident for most of the /r/ articulations shown in Figures 5-4 and 5-23. It is difficult to determine if this same feature characterizes the /r/ articulations observed by Zawadzki and Kuehn because their X-ray tracings did not include the lower part of the pharyngeal cavity. But pharyngeal narrowing may not be a *necessary* feature of /r/ production, given that one bunched /r/ in Figure 5-4 has an advanced tongue root. In general, /r/ articulations seem to be associated with a narrowing in both the palatal and pharyngeal regions, and the X-ray tracings in Figure 5-23 are good examples of how these two types of narrowing can be accomplished simultaneously. In addition, many speakers produce /r/ with lip rounding, so that the

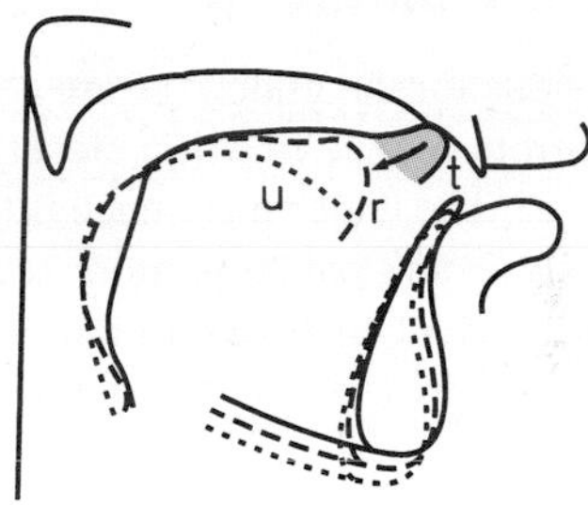

FIGURE 5-24
Composite of articulatory configurations for the three phonetic segments in *true*: /t/—solid lines; /r/—dashed lines; /u/—dotted lines. Because lip positions changed slightly, only one position is shown.

vocal tract configuration may show *three* regions of narrowing: labial, palatal, and pharyngeal.

Most phoneticians recognize at least three major manner allophones of /r/ in English: fricative [ɹ] or [r̝]; trilled [r̆]; and one-tap trill [ɾ]. The fricative [ɹ] occurs most frequently after /t/ or /d/, as in *try* [t ɹ a͡ɪ] and *dry* [d ɹ a͡ɪ]. Frication is produced as the tongue breaks contact with the alveolar ridge. Trilled [r̆] often is heard after /θ/, as in *three* [θ r̆ i] and *throw* [θ ɾ̆ o ʊ]. One-tap trill [ɾ] is not common in American English but occurs in British English intervocalically, as in *very* [v ɛ ɾ ɪ], which sounds like "veddy." Other variants are discussed later in this text. Because a variety of lingual and labial modifications are possible, it is best to represent their occurrence with appropriate diacritic marks introduced in the following chapter.

Lingua-Palatal Glide: /j/

The tongue motions for the glide /j/ are depicted in Figure 5-25. The high-front tongue position closely resembles that for vowel /i/ (he). The major difference is that the constriction between tongue and palate is more severe for /j/, so that it is described as a consonant articulation. Jaw position also is similar for the two sounds, being relatively closed (elevated).

Glide /j/ in English always precedes a vowel. Therefore, its articulation takes the form of a tongue movement from palatal constriction (high-front tongue body) to the tongue position for the following vowel. The articulatory motion is slower than that observed for stops and fricatives. Because of its resemblance to /i/ and its vowel-like properties, /j/ sometimes is called a semivowel. But /j/ differs from the vowels in that it cannot be used as a nucleus of a syllable and can occur only prevocalically.

A tongue motion similar to that for /j/ occurs in words in which another palatal consonant precedes /u/, for example, *shoe, chew, June.* Usually, the /j/ is not used to transcribe these words: /ʃ u/, not /ʃ j u/. Notice how difficult it is to say a word like *shoe* with a clearly audible /j/ between the /ʃ/ and the /u/.

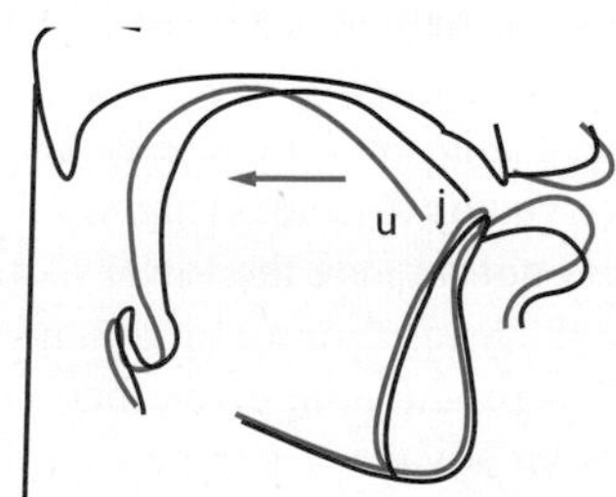

FIGURE 5-25
X-ray tracing of articulation of glide /j/, showing movement from /j/ (black line) to vowel /u/ (red line). Note high-front, or palatal, tongue position for /j/.

PLACE OF ARTICULATION: VELARS /k/ /g/ /ŋ/ /w/ /ʍ/

The X-ray tracing in Figure 5-26 shows how the **velar** (or dorsal) stops are made by elevating the lingual dorsum until it contacts the roof of the mouth. The site of articulation varies from the back part of the hard palate to the velum. Vowel context is the major determinant of the exact place of articulation. When /k/ and /g/ are produced in the context of a front vowel, like /i/ (key) or /æ/ (cat), the articulation is made frontally. But when these sounds are produced in the context of a back vowel, like /u/ (coo) or /ɑ/ (calm), the articulation is made farther back, near the velum. This variation, illustrated in Figure 5-27, is a good example of the articulatory interaction between sounds.

Jaw position for the velars is quite variable, apparently being determined primarily by the vowel context. Jaw motion does not assist the tongue articulation for velars as much as it does the articulations for dental, alveolar, and palatal

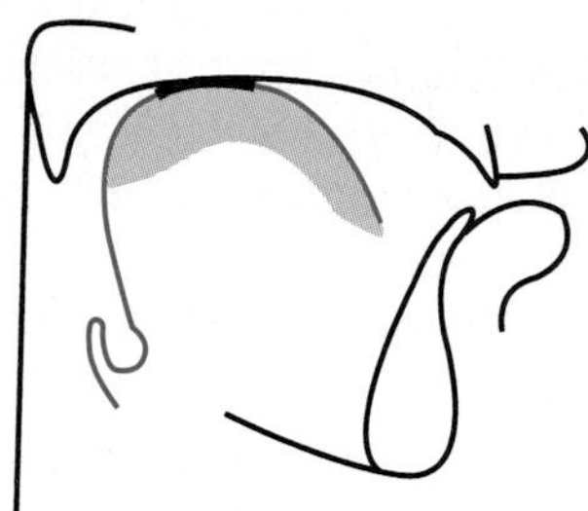

FIGURE 5-26
X-ray tracing of /k/ articulation. Thickened line shows lingua-velar contact.

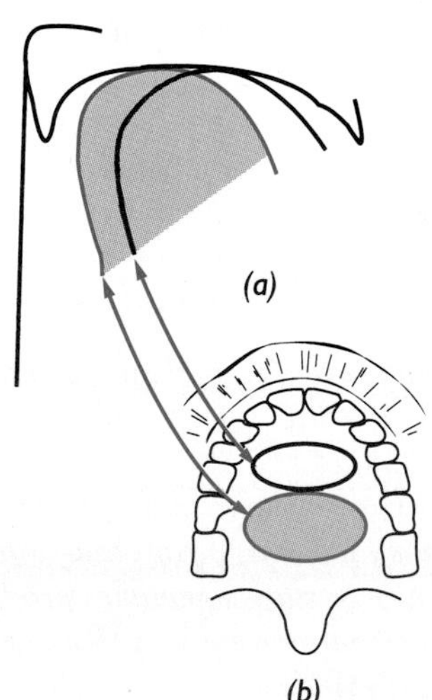

FIGURE 5-27
Variation in place of articulatory contact for the lingua-velar consonants. Contact site varies from front to back over the roof of the mouth. A lateral view is shown in *(a)* and an inferior view of the roof of the mouth is shown in *(b)*.

sounds. Because the hinge of the jaw is located toward the back of the head, the mechanical advantage that jaw movement gives to lingual consonants declines as the point of articulation moves back in the mouth. Therefore, jaw motion is less helpful in making a velar contact than it is for more frontal contacts. Measurement of the degree of jaw closure for lingual consonants in the same vowel context, that is, /ɑ θ ɑ/, /ɑ s ɑ/, /ɑ ʃ ɑ/, and /ɑ k ɑ/, show that the smallest degree of jaw closing occurs for the velar sound (Kent and Moll, 1972).

Although /k/ and /g/ are classified as stops along with /p/, /b/, /t/, and /d/, the velar stops are less stoplike than the bilabial and alveolar stops. /k/ and /g/ frequently are made with a sliding contact of the dorsum against the roof of the mouth. Figure 5-28 illustrates this sliding contact. This figure is based on the movements of small metal markers attached to the surface of the tongue. The movement paths of the markers were observed in an X-ray motion picture. Note that the markers first move upward, then forward during the sliding contact, and finally downward to the positions for the vowel. Because the vowel context was the same on either side of the velar consonant, the beginning and ending points of the movement paths are nearly the same.

Because of the sliding tongue contact and also because the tongue release for /k/ and /g/ is not so abrupt as that for the other stops, the velars tend to generate more noise energy. That is, the noise burst for /k/ and /g/ is longer than that for the other stops. There is little risk that the velar stops will be heard as fricatives because English does not have any velar fricatives.

The velar nasal /ŋ/ (sing) has an articulation like that for /k/ and /g/ except that the velopharynx is open (Figure 5-29). The exact site of contact varies with context, especially the surrounding vowels. The tongue elevation for the velars is somewhat higher than that for vowel /u/, as illustrated in Figure 5-30. The overall similarity between the /ŋ/ and /u/ articulations should be kept in mind when evaluating articulatory distinctions between consonants and vowels.

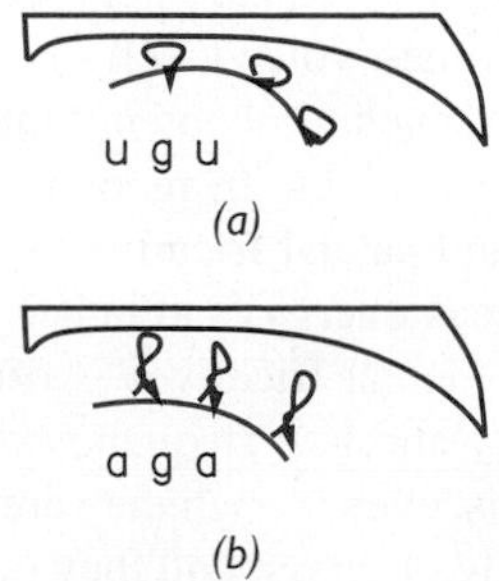

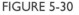

FIGURE 5-28
The lines ending in arrowheads show the motion paths of small pellets attached to the tongue during articulation of /u g u/ in *(a)* and /ɑ g ɑ/ in *(b)*. The motion paths are roughly circular or elliptical because of a sliding motion during articulatory contact for /g/.

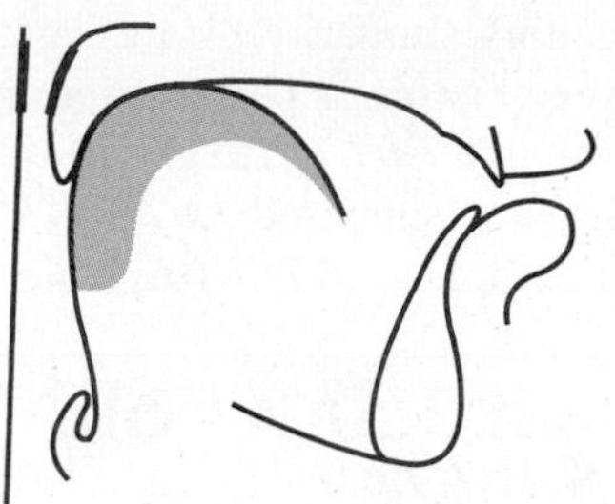

FIGURE 5-29
X-ray tracing of /ŋ/ articulation. Thickened lines show linguavelar contact and velopharyngeal opening.

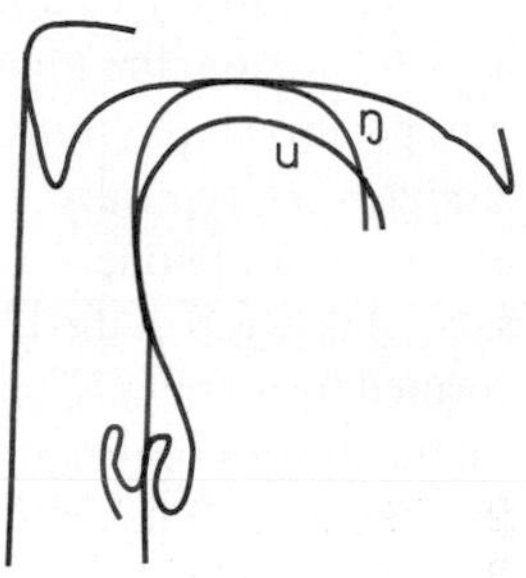

FIGURE 5-30
Composite drawing to show similarity in tongue positions for /ŋ/ (red line) and /u/ (black line). To simplify the drawing, only the closed velopharyngeal port is shown.

Some authors (e.g., Perkell, 1969), state that consonants and vowels use a different musculature, with the larger muscles being used to position the tongue body for vowels. However, it would appear that these larger muscles also could be used for many consonants, including /w/, /j/, /ʃ/, /r/, /k/, /g/, /ŋ/.

The labio-velar glides /w/ and /ʍ/ (also transcribed /hw/) are produced with a rounding of the lips and an arching of the tongue in the area of the velum. In fact, the articulatory configuration for /w/ (Figures 5-5 and 5-10) closely resembles that for the high-back vowel /u/. Many speakers use the voiceless /ʍ/ rarely, if at all. MacKay (1978) commented that /ʍ/ does not appear in most American dialects, and Tiffany and Carrell (1977) observed that the /w/–/ʍ/ contrast may be in the process of disappearing.

One reason we discuss /w/ and /ʍ/ under the velar place of articulation is to emphasize that these sounds are produced with a high-back tongue position, a fact that quite a few of our students have neglected in quizzes of articulatory description. The participation of both lips and tongue in the articulation of /w/ is particularly important clinically because of the frequent occurrence of /w/ for /r/ substitutions noted in clinical reports. It should be clear from comparisons of the labio-velar articulation in Figures 5-5 and 5-10 with the rhotic (especially bunched allophone) articulation in Figures 5-4 and 5-23 that /w/ and /r/ have at least a general articulatory similarity. At the same time, we suggest that not every /r/ error perceived as a /w/ is in fact produced as a genuine /w/ in the client's phonetic system. We believe that many supposed /w/ for /r/ substitutions are examples of derhotacized /r/ (see Chapter 6).

PLACE OF ARTICULATION: GLOTTALS /h/ /ʔ/

The **glottals** are sounds formed at the vocal folds and include the glottal fricative /h/ (who) and the glottal stop /ʔ/. The /h/ is formed as air passes through a slit between the vocal folds and into the upper airway, thus creating turbulence noise. Because /h/ does not require a supralaryngeal constriction for its formation, the tongue, jaw, and lips are free to assume any positions except those that close off the oral cavity. Although /h/ typically is voiceless, some phoneticians hear a voiced allophone in words like *Ohio.* This allophone is transcribed /ɦ/ in the IPA.

The stop /ʔ/ is formed by a brief closure at the folds. Although /ʔ/ is not a phoneme of English, it occurs frequently in the speech of many people and has allophonic and junctural functions. The /ʔ/ can be hard to hear, but a good example of its occurrence is the phrase *Anna Adams,* in which the glottal stop separates the final vowel of *Anna* from the initial vowel in *Adams.* Thus, *Anna Adams* might be transcribed phonetically as [æ n ə ʔ æ d ə m z].

SUMMARY BY MANNER OF ARTICULATION

The purpose of this review section is to give a unified summary of the information on place of articulation. At the same time, summary comments are made concerning manner of articulation, which is used as the basic outline of discussion.

Stop consonants, which involve a complete blockage of the airstream and an abrupt release of the blockage, are produced at four places: bilabial, alveolar, velar, and glottal. These places of articulation are schematically summarized in Figure 5-31. Voiced and voiceless pairs are produced at the bilabial (/b/–/p/), alveolar (/d/–/t/), and velar (/g/–/k/) sites. The glottal stop /ʔ/ is made by a complete closure of the vocal folds. Although some phoneticians regard /ʔ/ as a voiceless sound because the folds are not vibrating during its production, the requirement that the vocal folds be brought together gives it at least one point of similarity to the voiced sounds. Generally, the stop manner implies that the articulator makes a temporary tight contact that can be released to produce a short burst of noise energy. However, the burst is not a necessary feature of the stops. Furthermore, the velar stops frequently are articulated with a sliding motion of the lingual dorsum against the roof of the mouth; and this property, together with the fact that the articulatory release is somewhat more gradual than that for the bilabial and alveolar stops, causes the velars to be more fricative-like. This difference has perceptual consequences, as listeners confuse velar stops with fricative sounds more often than they confuse the bilabial and alveolar stops with fricatives (Klatt, 1968).

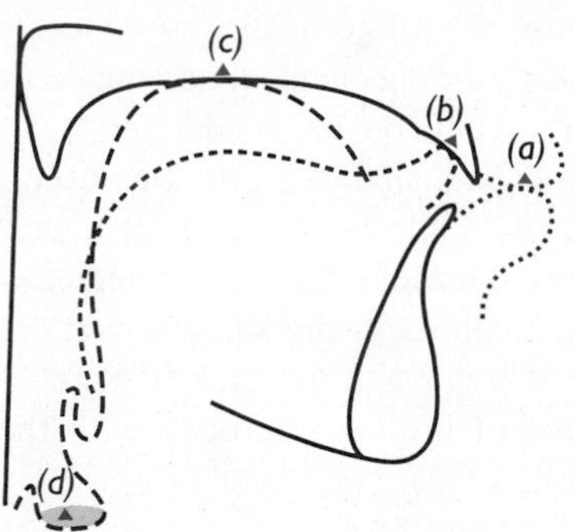

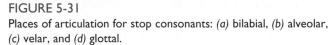

FIGURE 5-31
Places of articulation for stop consonants: *(a)* bilabial, *(b)* alveolar, *(c)* velar, and *(d)* glottal.

Nasal consonants, produced with complete blockage at some point in the oral cavity but with an open velopharynx, are made at the bilabial (/m/), alveolar (/n/), and velar (/ŋ/) sites of contact. The oral articulation is quite similar to that for the homorganic stop; that is, /m/ resembles /b/, /n/ resembles /d/, and /ŋ/ resembles /g/. The places of oral closure are the same as those shown in Figure 5-31 except that the glottal stop usually is not considered as a nasal because the site of articulation is below that of the oral–nasal division, the velopharynx.

Fricative consonants, produced with an airway constriction sufficiently narrow to generate continuous noise (frication or turbulence noise), are made at the labiodental, dental, alveolar, palatal, and glottal sites of articulation. At each site except the glottal, voiced and voiceless cognates are produced: /v/–/f/, /ð/–/θ/, /z/–/s/, /ʒ/–/ʃ/. For that matter, even the glottal place of articulation has an allophonic voice alternation, for the intervocalic /h/ in words like *Ohio* is sometimes voiced (/ɦ/). The alveolar and palatal fricatives are much more intense than the labiodental, dental, and glottal fricatives. In recognition of this difference, the alveolar and palatal fricatives are called **stridents** or **sibilants.** The weak energy, and hence low audibility, of the labiodental and dental fricatives is offset by their relatively high visibility and low frequency of occurrence (see Appendix B). That is, even though they are not always easily heard, they are easily observed and they occur infrequently.

Affricate consonants, characterized by a two-phase articulation of stop (complete closure) followed by frication (noise segment), occur in English only at the palatal site. The two palatal affricates /ʤ/ and /ʧ/ are voiced and voiceless, respectively.

Liquid consonants, vowel-like sounds that have narrower constrictions than true vowels, are made at the alveolar and palatal places of articulation. Following Ladefoged (1993), we use the term *liquid* as a cover term for the lateral /l/ and the rhotic /r/. The lateral is made with a midline alveolar contact but lateral opening. The tongue dorsum usually assumes an /o/-like position, and this feature may be more constant than the alveolar contact, which does not always occur in postvocalic position. Rhotic /r/ has a palatal constriction that results from either a retroflex articulation of the tongue tip (turned up and slightly back) or a bunched articulation of the tongue body with the tip turned down and the blade elevated.

Glide consonants, which have gliding movements originating from articulatory constrictions somewhat narrower than for vowels but not as narrow as for fricatives and stops, are produced as the palatal /j/ and the labio-velars /w/ and /ʍ/. Palatal /j/ closely resembles the high-front vowel /i/ but has a narrower constriction. Labio-dental /w/ closely resembles the high-back vowel /u/ but again has a narrower constriction. Labio-velar /ʍ/ is the voiceless cognate of /w/.

SUMMARY BY PLACE OF ARTICULATION

Obviously, the tongue is used for a number of places of articulation, and these possibilities are shown in Figure 5-32. Part *(a)* of this illustration shows the articulations of the tongue tip: interdental, dental, alveolar, and retroflex. Part *(b)* shows the articulation of blade and palate, and part *(c)* shows the articulation of dorsum and roof of the mouth (velar). Labial articulations are depicted in Figure 5-33, which shows rounding, bilabial closure, and labiodental constriction. Figure 5-34 shows the articulations of the velopharynx, depicted as elevation of the velum for oral consonants and lowering of the velum for nasal consonants. The other structures involved in velopharyngeal closure are not shown, but it should be recalled that the lateral walls of the pharynx can have an important role in velopharyngeal articulation. The larynx serves as an articulator in the production of fricative /h/ and the stop /ʔ/. For the fricative, the folds are separated sufficiently so that frication noise is generated. For the stop, the folds are brought together tightly so that airflow is blocked (and vocal fold vibrations cease) for a period of time. Finally, the jaw is indirectly related to place of articulation in its role as skeletal support for the tongue and lower lip and in its contribution to the movement of these structures.

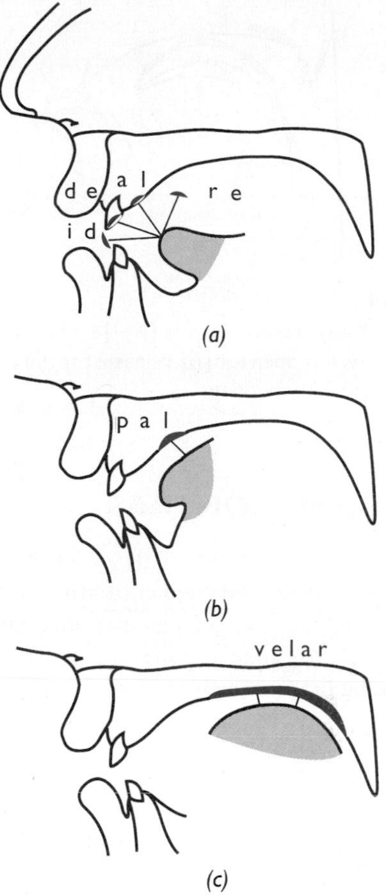

FIGURE 5-32
Places of articulation for lingual consonants: *(a)* interdental (id), dental (de), alveolar (al), and retroflex (re) articulations; *(b)* palatal (pal) articulation; *(c)* major sites (front and back) of velar articulation.

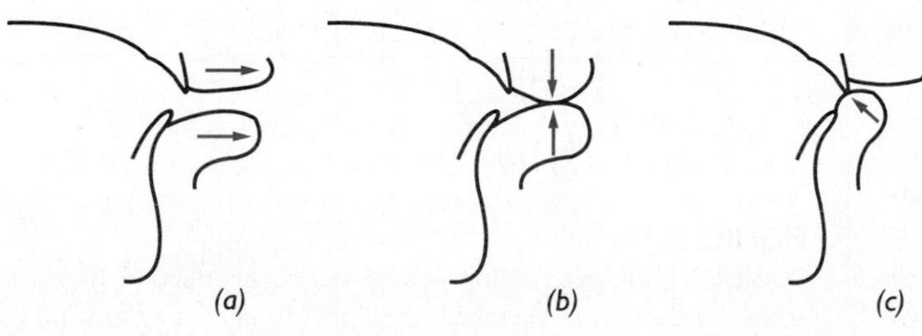

FIGURE 5-33
Lip articulations: *(a)* rounding or protrusion, *(b)* bilabial closure, and *(c)* labiodental constriction.

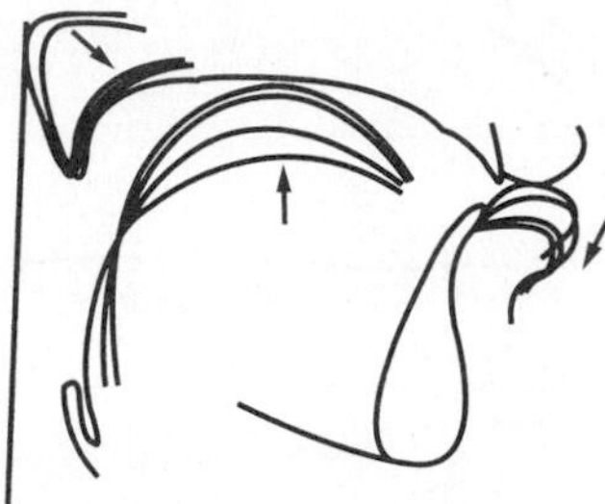

FIGURE 5-34
Composite of X-ray tracings for the [p]–[ɪ]–[ŋ] sequence in the word *camping.* As lips open for [p] release, tongue elevates for [ɪ] and [ŋ], and velopharynx opens.

THE VOICING CONTRAST

The voicing contrast is most easily described for pairs of sounds that share place and manner of articulation but differ in the voicing feature. Such pairs are called **cognates.** The **voiced** and **voiceless** cognate pairs of English are presented in the following list.

	Voiced	*Voiceless*	*Examples*
Bilabial stop	/b/	/p/	bay–pay
Labial-velar glide	/w/	/ʍ/	witch–which
Labiodental fricative	/v/	/f/	vat–fat
Interdental fricative	/ð/	/θ/	thy–thigh
Alveolar stop	/d/	/t/	doe–toe
Alveolar fricative	/z/	/s/	zip–sip
Palatal fricative	/ʒ/	/ʃ/	rouge–rush
Palatal affricate	/ʤ/	/ʧ/	gin–chin
Velar stop	/g/	/k/	gap–cap

The basic distinction between each member of these cognate pairs is that one member is associated with vocal fold vibration and the other is not. Thus, /b/ in *bay* is said to be voiced, but /p/ in *pay* is said to be voiceless. However, the superficial simplicity of the voicing contrast is deceiving. For example, we will discuss in this section the fact that vocal fold vibration actually can *cease* during some *voiced sounds* and the fact that the *voicing distinction* for some word-final consonants is carried perceptually by the *length of the vowel* that precedes the consonants. Thus, it is an oversimplification to say that the vocal folds vibrate during voiced sounds and do not vibrate during voiceless sounds.

First, we consider some of the physiological implications of the voicing contrast. It is important to recognize that special adjustments are required to keep the vocal folds vibrating during a period of vocal tract closure. The need for these adjustments can be appreciated by performing a simple experiment: Close your lips tightly, pinch your nostrils closed with your fingers, and try to make a voiced sound, like a sustained /m/. You will notice that phonation is possible only for a short time, and you might puff out your cheeks in an effort to sustain the phonation. Voicing or phonation is difficult under these circumstances because the vocal folds vibrate only if air passes between them. When the vocal tract is closed, airflow eventually ceases (because the air has nowhere to go), and so does voicing. Puffing the cheeks helps to maintain voicing for a short interval because the puffing expands the oral chamber and allows air to pass from the lungs into the mouth. In short, it is difficult to voice sounds when the vocal tract is closed. Voicing is most easily maintained when the vocal tract is open, as in the case of vowels.

How then can a speaker maintain voicing during a period of closure for the italicized sounds in a*b*out, a*bd*icate, a*g*ain, and O*gd*en? There are two general possibilities: (1) Allow a small leakage of air from the vocal tract (for example, through the velopharyngeal port); or (2) increase the volume of the supralaryngeal cavity. Most speakers seem to use the second alternative. The supralaryngeal cavity can be enlarged in several ways, but the two primary means are shown in Figure 5-35, parts *(b)* and *(c)*.

1. The larynx position drops during the period of vocal tract closure so that the vocal tract is lengthened. As the drawing in Figure 5-35 shows, the hyoid bone and larynx may move downward together. You can test this possibility yourself by placing your finger on the larynx while attempting to phonate with the lips and nostrils tightly closed. Do you feel a depression of the larynx?
2. The pharynx expands through a forward motion of the tongue during the vocal tract closure. Pharyngeal expansion is illustrated in Figures 5-35 and 5-36. Figure 5-36 shows X-ray tracings of stop closure for /k/ and /g/. Notice that the size of the pharynx is greater for the voiced stop than it is for the voiceless stop.

Both of these mechanisms result in an increase in the supralaryngeal volume. The increase in volume is function-

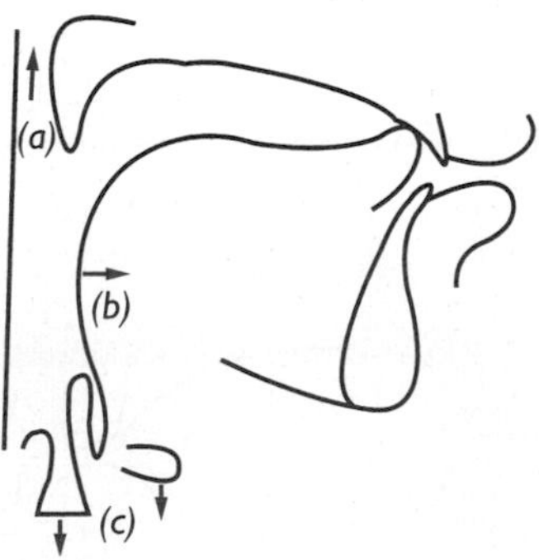

FIGURE 5-35
Possibilities for maintaining voicing during production of voiced stops: *(a)* opening of velopharyngeal port to permit airflow, *(b)* expansion of pharynx, and *(c)* lowering of larynx.

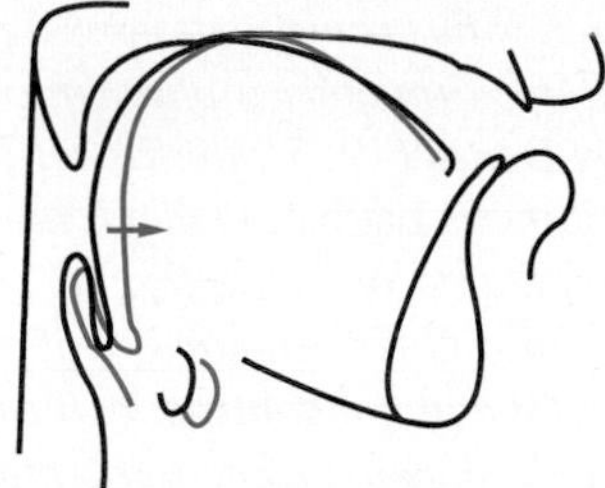

FIGURE 5-36
Composite X-ray tracings for voiced /g/ (black line) and voiceless /k/ (red line). Pharynx width expands for /g/, as shown by arrow.

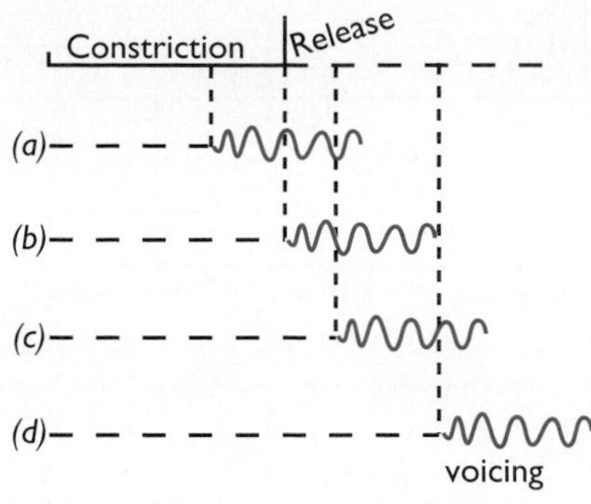

FIGURE 5-37
Timing patterns of supralaryngeal and laryngeal events to explain variations in voice onset time. Onset of voicing (sawtooth line) is described relative to instant of release of consonant articulation.

ally the same as a leak of air from the oral or pharyngeal cavity. Hence, voicing is maintained during vocal tract closure by a small increase in the volume of the vocal tract, allowing air to move from the lungs into the pharynx.

The need for special vocal tract adjustments to sustain voicing during articulatory closure may explain why young children frequently devoice consonants; that is, *dog* is produced with a final consonant that is more like /k/ than /g/. Consonant devoicing, especially in final position, frequently has been noted as characteristic of developing speech (Ingram, 1989).

Another complication in the phonetic study of voicing is that the sound cues by which we make phonetic judgments of voicing vary with word position and consonant type. For a stop consonant in word-initial position, say, *bat* versus *pat,* the effective difference very often is the **voice onset time** (VOT), which is the time difference between the release of the stop closure and the beginning of the vocal fold vibrations. The timing patterns are illustrated schematically in Figure 5-37. If the vocal fold vibrations begin before the stop is released, the stop is said to be **prevoiced** (or, it has a voicing lead), and the VOT in ms has a negative sign. For example, a VOT of –30 ms means that the voicing began 30 milliseconds before the stop release. If the vocal vibrations begin after the stop release, the stop is said to have a voicing lag, and the VOT in ms is a positive value (for example, VOT = 50 ms). If the vocal vibrations begin simultaneously with the stop release, the VOT is zero. Generally, an initial stop in English is perceived as voiced if (1) voicing precedes articulatory release, as in Figure 5-37*(a);* (2) voicing begins simultaneously with articulatory release, as in part *(b);* or (3) voicing begins shortly after, within 25 ms or so, articulatory release, as in part *(c).* An initial stop is perceived as voiceless if voicing begins significantly later (usually more than 50 ms) than articulatory release, as in part *(d).* Hence, whether an initial stop is heard as voiced or voiceless depends upon the *relative timing* of vibration in the larynx and articulatory release of the stop.

A feature that is related to voicing for stops is aspiration. **Aspiration** is a friction noise (like that for /h/) generated as air flows through the vocal folds and into the upper cavities. Stops are said to be aspirated if an interval of aspiration, or frication, precedes voicing. Stops are said to be unaspirated if such an interval does not occur. In English, released voiceless stops are aspirated unless they follow /s/. Only when these stops occur after /s/ in the same syllable are they unaspirated. Voiced stops are unaspirated in English. The occurrence of aspiration is controlled by the glottal opening present when the articulatory closure for the stop is released. If the folds are sufficiently separated, aspiration will occur. If the glottal opening is negligible when the stop is released, aspiration will not occur. The occurrence of unaspirated voiceless stops following /s/ seems to be related to the relative timing of vocal fold movement and the oral articulations. That is, if the folds begin to come together during the stop, the glottal opening may be quite small at the moment of stop release.

In the word-medial or intervocalic position, the voicing contrast is associated with a difference in vocal fold vibration and sometimes with a difference in duration of consonant constriction. For example, in the word pair *ribbing–ripping,* the vocal fold vibrations continue throughout the word *ribbing* (all segments being voiced), but they cease for a short time during the bilabial closure for /p/ in *ripping.* In addition, the duration of bilabial closure often is longer for the voiceless consonant, so that the lips may remain closed longer for /p/ than for /b/. Still another possible cue for the word-medial voicing contrast is that the release burst will be stronger for the voiceless stop than for the voiced stop. Finally, it should be noted that the voiced velar stop /g/ sometimes is momentarily devoiced in medial and intervocalic positions. Figure 5-38 shows the envelope of the voicing signal obtained from a contact microphone strapped to the neck tissue over the larynx. The vertical dimension (y-axis) shows the amplitude of voicing, and the horizontal dimension (x-axis) is time. For /ɑ k ɑ/ in the top trace, vocal fold vibration ceases for a considerable period of time, corresponding roughly to the interval of stop closure. But vocal

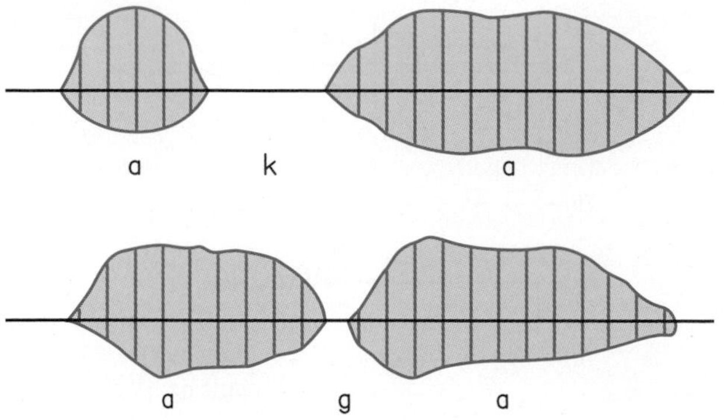

FIGURE 5-38
Envelope of voicing signal recorded by a throat microphone. Voicing signal ceases for a long interval during /k/ (upper trace) and for a brief interval during /g/ (lower trace). Hence, /g/ is not necessarily continuously voiced.

fold vibration also ceases for /ɑ g ɑ/, though for a much shorter time.

Word-finally, the duration of the vowel preceding the consonant is the most important factor in determining whether the consonant will be heard as voiced or voiceless. Vowels preceding voiced consonants are longer than vowels preceding voiceless consonants. For example, it has been shown that the noun and verb forms of the word *use,* /j u s/ and /j u z/, may end in an essentially identical *voiceless* segment. The difference in voicing perceived by a listener depends on the fact that the vowel is longer for the verb form than for the noun form (Denes, 1955).

The tendency for vowels to be longer before voiced than voiceless consonants is common to all languages, but some languages, like English, have capitalized on this difference to make it the voicing contrast for final-position consonants. That is, although all languages have longer vowels before the voiced consonant, English has accentuated this difference in vowel length to make it a reliable cue for voicing of the consonant. Chen (1970) reports the following ratios, calculated as the average length of vowels before voiceless consonants divided by the average length of vowels before voiced consonants (the smaller the ratio, the larger the difference in vowel duration):

English	0.61
French	0.87
Russian	0.82
Korean	0.78
Spanish	0.86
Norwegian	0.82

In view of the peculiarities of the voicing contrast in English, Hyman offers an interesting observation:

> *Since there is a tendency in English to devoice final voiced obstruents (such as in the word* bad*), the vowel-length discrepancy has come to assume a phonological role, and perhaps ultimately a phonemic role. As has been shown by Denes (1955), the vowel-length difference in such pairs as* bat:bad *is much more important perceptually than any voicing difference which may be present in the final C [consonant]. It is also relevant here to note that the initial contrast in the minimal pair* pat:bat *has been shown to be, perceptually, one of aspirated vs. unaspirated, rather than voiceless vs. voiced. It thus appears that English is in the process of losing its voice contrast in consonants (note the loss of the /t/–/d/ contrast in most intervocalic positions): the final voice contrast is being replaced with a length contrast and the initial contrast is being replaced with an aspiration contrast.* (Hyman, 1975, p. 173)

This comment is a good reminder that spoken languages are not dead and fixed. Rather, languages change as they are spoken. A Rip van Winkle who sleeps through a century of change in the language habits of his own country might awake to discover that the people around him speak with a strange dialect.

ALLOGRAPHS OF THE CONSONANT PHONEMES OF ENGLISH

Recall from Chapter 2 that an *allograph* is any one alphabet letter or combination of letters that represents a given phoneme. The allographs of the consonant phonemes of English are presented in Table 5-2. For each phoneme, the allographs are italicized in a sample word. For example, the allographs for the phoneme /b/ are the *b* in *but,* the *bb* in *rabbit,* and the *pb* in *cupboard.*

FREQUENCY OF OCCURRENCE AND PLACE OF ARTICULATION

Appendix B summarizes data on the frequency of occurrence of consonants in American English. Obviously, because consonants do not appear with equal frequency, some places of articulation are much more heavily used than others. The unequal use of different places of articulation is represented graphically in Figure 5-39, which is based on data for the 20 most frequently occurring consonants in the study by Mines, Hanson, and Shoup (1978). The sections in the circle graph are sized in proportion to the frequency of use of each place of articulation. The alveolar place of production is used as frequently as all other places combined.

Recognizing that the front vowels occur more frequently than central or back vowels and that the alveolar place is the most frequently occurring in consonant production, we can represent what should be the most frequently occurring tongue shape and position by a composite of a front vowel (say /ɛ/ for sake of illustration) and an alveolar consonant. This composite is shown in Figure 5-40. Interestingly, the

TABLE 5-2
Allographs of the Consonant Phonemes of English

Phoneme	Allograph (italicized in a sample word)
/b/	*b*ut, ra*bb*it, cu*pb*oard
/p/	*p*ay, su*pp*er, hiccou*gh* (/p/ also may occur as an intrusive in words containing the combinations *mf, mph, mt, mth,* and *ms;* for example, *comfort* may be pronounced [k ʌ m p f ɚ t], and *warmth* may be pronounced [w ɔ r m p θ])
/d/	*d*oll, a*dd,* rais*ed,* cou*ld*
/t/	*t*ail, bu*tt*er, walk*ed,* dou*bt,* recei*pt,* indi*ct,* *Th*omas, *pt*omaine (/t/ also may occur as an intrusive in words containing the combination *nce* or *ns;* for example, *dance* may be pronounced [d æ n t s])
/g/	*g*o, e*gg,* va*gue,* *gu*ess, *gh*ost, e*x*ist (when pronounced with /g z/ rather than /k s/)
/k/	ba*ck,* *c*ut, *ch*emical, o*cc*ur, s*q*uall, bouti*que,* *kh*aki, yo*lk,* fi*x* (as part of a /k s/ cluster), *qu*ay (/k/ also may occur as an intrusive in words containing the combination *ngth;* for example, *length* may be pronounced [l ɛ ŋ k θ])
/v/	*v*ine, sa*vv*y, o*f,* Ste*ph*en (some pronunciations)
/f/	*f*an, o*ff,* *ph*one, enou*gh,* hal*f*
/ð/	*th*is (both /ð/ and /θ/ occur as *th*)
/θ/	*th*in
/z/	*z*oo, bu*zz,* i*s,* sci*ss*ors, di*s*cern, a*s*thma, *x*ylophone, e*x*ist (when pronounced with /g z/ rather than /k s/)
/s/	*s*ay, mi*ss,* *c*ity, *sc*ent, *ps*alm, walt*z,* *sc*hism, li*st*en, bo*x* (as part of a /k s/ cluster)
/ʒ/	plea*s*ure, rou*ge,* bi*j*ou, a*z*ure, apha*s*ia, bra*z*ier
/ʃ/	*sh*e, *s*ugar, ac*t*ion, o*c*ean, *ch*ef, pre*c*ious, pa*ss*ion, *sch*ist, fu*chs*ia, con*sc*ious, nau*se*ous, an*x*ious (as part of a /k ʃ/ cluster)
/h/	*h*appy, *wh*o, Mona*gh*an
/m/	*m*an, su*mm*er, wo*mb,* hy*mn,* psal*m,* diaphra*gm*
/n/	*n*ow, fu*nn*y, *kn*ife, *gn*ome, *pn*eumatic, si*gn,* *mn*emonic
/ŋ/	thi*ng,* thi*n*k, fi*n*ger, si*ng*er, ton*gue,* a*n*xious
/l/	*l*aw, a*ll,* litt*le,* kenn*el,* i*sl*and, ki*ln*
/r/	*r*ed, ca*rr*y, *wr*ong, *rh*yme, co*rps,* mo*r*tgage, cata*rrh*
/ʤ/	*j*am, *g*em, a*dj*acent, bri*dg*e, cor*d*ial, Geor*ge,* gra*d*ual, exa*gg*erate
/tʃ/	*ch*ief, ca*tch,* *c*ello, righ*te*ous, ques*t*ion, na*t*ure, man*si*on
/w/	*w*on, *o*ne, q*u*een, ch*o*ir
/ʍ/	*wh*ich
/j/	*y*es, on*i*on, hallelu*j*ah, *u*se (as part of a /j u/ combination), poi*gn*ant (also occurs in words like *few, fuel, feud* as part of a /j u/ combination)

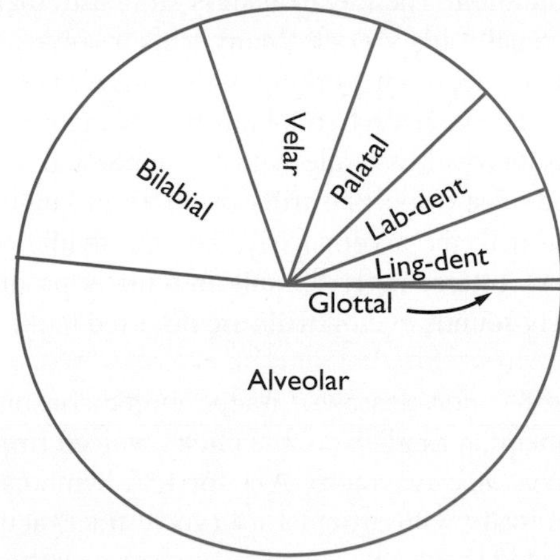

FIGURE 5-39
Circle graph showing relative frequency of occurrence of different places of articulation. Based on data for the 20 most frequently occurring consonants reported by Mines, Hanson, and Shoup (1978).

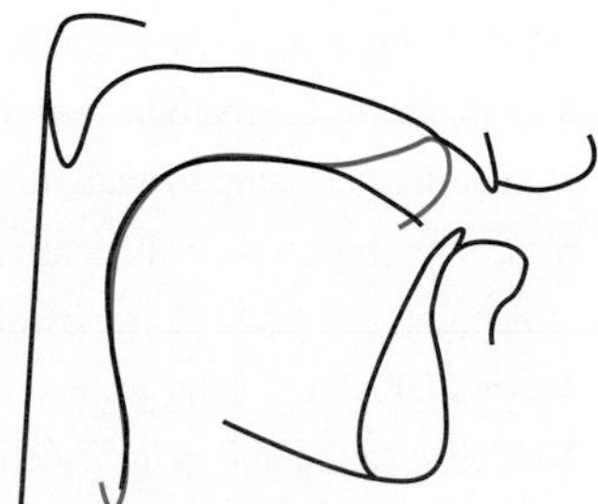

FIGURE 5-40
Composite drawing of articulatory configuration for front vowel /ɛ/ (black line) and alveolar consonant (red line) produced in isolation. Notice overall similarity of tongue shape.

overall shape of the tongue for the front vowel and for the alveolar consonant is highly similar, except of course for the position of the tongue tip. Because alveolar consonants tend to be produced with a fronted tongue body position, the frequently occurring front vowels and the frequently occurring alveolar consonants can be produced with basically the same positioning of the tongue body.

SUMMARY CLASSIFICATION OF CONSONANTS

Table 5-3 summarizes the consonants of American English using the terms introduced in this chapter. Note that each sound is uniquely described by descriptions of voicing, place of articulation, and manner of articulation. When two or more sounds share the same place of articulation, they are called **homorganic.** For example, the initial sounds in the following words are homorganic because they are produced with a common lingua-alveolar articulation: *dip, not, tack.* When two or more sounds share the same manner of articulation, they are called **homotypic.** For example, the initial sounds in the following words are homotypic because they are all fricatives: *four, thick, sour, she.* Sometimes several manners of articulation are grouped into a single category. An **obstruent** is a sound made with a complete or narrow constriction at some point in the vocal tract. The obstruents include the stops, fricatives, and affricates. As mentioned earlier, the class of liquids includes the rhotic and the lateral. Also mentioned earlier, cognates are pairs of sounds that are distinguished by a particular phonetic feature, such as voicing.

TABLE 5-3
Classification of the Consonants of American English

IPA Symbol	Description
[b]	Voiced bilabial stop
[p]	Voiceless bilabial stop
[d]	Voiced lingua-alveolar (apical) stop
[t]	Voiceless lingua-alveolar (apical) stop
[g]	Voiced lingua-velar (dorsal) stop
[k]	Voiceless lingua-velar (dorsal) stop
[m]	Bilabial nasal
[n]	Lingua-alveolar (apical) nasal
[ŋ]	Lingua-velar (dorsal) nasal
[l]	Lingua-alveolar lateral
[ɾ]	Lingua-alveolar flap (one-tap trill)
[r]	Alveolar rhotic or retroflex
[v]	Voiced labiodental fricative
[f]	Voiceless labiodental fricative
[ð]	Voiced lingua-dental fricative
[θ]	Voiceless lingua-dental fricative
[z]	Voiced lingua-alveolar fricative
[s]	Voiceless lingua-alveolar fricative
[ʒ]	Voiced lingua-palatal fricative
[ʃ]	Voiceless lingua-palatal fricative
[j]	Voiced palatal glide (semivowel)
[w]	Voiced labial and velar glide (semivowel)
[hw] or [ʍ]	Voiceless labial and velar fricative/glide
[ʤ]	Voiced palatal affricate; see component sounds
[ʧ]	Voiceless palatal affricate; see component sounds
[ʔ]	Glottal stop
[h]	Voiceless glottal fricative

CONSONANTS AROUND THE WORLD

Compared to other languages, American English is about average in its number of consonants. But as you probably can attest if you have tried to learn other languages, there are many possible consonants that American English does not use.

First, there are manner classes of consonants in other languages that are not used at all in American English. To understand these classes, it is helpful to follow the International Phonetic Association in classifying consonants as pulmonic and nonpulmonic. The pulmonic consonants are produced with a pulmonic (typically egressive) airstream, and the nonpulmonic consonants are not.

The major class of pulmonic consonant not used in American English is the **trill,** defined as a sound made with a supraglottal vibration. The vibration requires a flow of air (hence pulmonic airstream) directed between two articulators that are held together with just enough muscle tension to produce vibration. The mechanism is similar to that used to make the vocal folds vibrate. Many trills involve actions of the lips or tongue, often working with some other part of the vocal tract. The raspberry (bilabial trill), sometimes used to express disapproval, is made with the upper and lower lips. Among the most important trills in different languages are the bilabial trill, the alveolar trill, and the uvular trill (Appendix A-1). Interestingly, infants frequently produce trills in their early sounds even if trills are not used in the ambient language.

The three major classes of nonpulmonic consonants not used in American English are the **clicks, voiced implosives,** and **ejectives** (see Appendix A-1 for IPA symbols). These sounds are made with articulatory (vocal tract) actions that generate sound in the absence of an egressive airstream from the lungs. A click is a stop produced with an ingressive velaric airstream. The back of the tongue closes against the velum simultaneously as another closure is formed at some forward point in the vocal tract. The two closures trap a pocket of air between them. Once this closed space is formed, a downward or backward movement of the tongue enlarges the volume of the space so that a negative air pressure is created. When the articulatory closure is released, air flows to equalize the pressure, and a click is generated.

A voiced implosive (sometimes called ingressive) is a stop made with an ingressive glottalic airstream. To produce this sound, the larynx is pulled rapidly downward while the vocal folds are adducted but not tightly closed. The rapid descent of the larynx causes air to flow ingressively through the glottis, resulting in vocal fold vibration.

An ejective is a stop made with a glottalic egressive airstream. The articulation is a rapid upward movement of the larynx while the vocal folds are closed tightly. In effect, the larynx acts like a piston to produce a positive pressure change in the vocal tract. Ejectives are also known as glottalized or checked, recursives, or abruptives. The IPA diacritic [ʼ] is used to mark an ejective.

American English also does not use all possible places of articulation for the manner categories of stop, nasal, flap, fricative, affricate, and glide. For example, American English does not use: retroflex, palatal, or uvular stops; labiodental, retroflex, palatal, or uvular nasals; retroflex, velar, uvular, or pharyngeal fricates; labiodental or velar glides; or retroflex, palatal, or velar laterals. Some of these place variations do occur clinically, especially for individuals who have anatomic abnormalities. Some people with cleft palate may use pharyngeal stops to substitute for the velar stops /k g/ and palatal stops to substitute for the alveolar stops /t d/ and the velar stops /k g/ (Trost, 1981).

GLOSSARY

Affricate a manner of articulation; an affricate is a consonant sound formed by a stop + fricative sequence. The only English affricates are /ʤ/ (judge) and /ʧ/ (church).

Alveolar a place of articulation pertaining to the alveolar ridge, or alveolus; alveolar consonants are formed by articulation of the tongue against the alveolar ridge.

Aspiration a fricative noise generated as air escapes through partly adducted vocal folds and into the upper cavities.

Bilabial a place of articulation pertaining to the two lips; bilabial consonants are produced by articulations of the lips.

Bunched /r/ an allophone of the consonant /r/ for which the tongue assumes a bunched or humped shape close to the palatal region.

Click a stop produced with an ingressive velaric airstream.

Cognate a member of a pair of sounds that are opposed or distinguished by a particular phonetic feature. For example, /d/ (do) and /t/ (to) are voiced and voiceless cognates.

Dental place of articulation pertaining to the teeth; dental consonants are formed by articulations of the lips or tongue with the upper teeth.

Dentalized articulated with the teeth; a dentalized consonant has a modified articulation that involves dental contact or constriction.

Ejective a stop made with an egressive glottalic airstream.

Flap a manner of articulation in which a sound is formed by a quick tapping movement of an articulator against a surface. In English, flaps are allophones of stops.

Fricative a manner of articulation in which a continuous noise is generated as air is channeled through a narrow articulatory constriction.

Glide a manner of articulation that involves a gliding movement from a partly constricted vocal tract to a more open vocal tract shape. Glides resemble diphthongs in their dynamics but cannot serve as syllable nuclei.

Glottal place of articulation pertaining to the glottis or the vocal folds; a glottal consonant is one formed by glottal (vocal fold) articulation.

Homorganic having the same place of articulation (*homo* = "same" and *organic* = "relating to an organ or structure"). For example, /m/ and /b/ are homorganic because they share a bilabial articulation.

Homotypic having the same manner of articulation (*homo* = "same" and *typic* = "relating to type or manner"). For example, /m/ and /n/ are homotypic because they share the nasal manner.

Interdental a place of articulation involving insertion of the tongue tip into the space between the upper and lower incisors (the interdental space).

Labiodental a place of articulation involving the lower lip and upper teeth.

Lateral a manner of articulation in which sound escapes around the sides of the tongue.

Lingua pertaining to the tongue.

Lingua-alveolar a place of articulation in which the tongue completely or nearly closes against the alveolar ridge.

Liquid a cover term (manner of articulation) for the rhotic /r/ and lateral /l/, both of which have a vocal tract that is constricted only somewhat more than that for vowels. Unlike glides, which are similar, liquids do not require a movement for their auditory identification.

Manner of articulation an aspect of articulatory phonetics pertaining to how a sound is formed, that is, the *means* of sound generation. Whereas place of articulation describes *where* in the vocal tract a sound is formed, manner of articulation describes how the sound is made.

Nasal a manner of articulation in which sound energy radiates into the nasal cavity; nasal sounds are associated with an open velopharynx.

Obstruent a sound formed with a complete or narrow constriction of the vocal tract; a stop, fricative, or affricate.

One-tap trill another name for **flap.**

Palatal a place of articulation pertaining to the palatal area, which lies behind the alveolar ridge. Palatal sounds are made with articulations of the tongue against the palate.

Place of articulation an aspect of articulatory phonetics pertaining to where in the vocal tract a sound is formed. Ordinarily, place of articulation is described by reference to the articulators and associated vocal tract surfaces; for example, lingua-alveolar, labiodental.

Prevoiced a condition of voicing, usually applied to obstruents, in which voicing or vocal fold vibration begins sometime before an articulatory event, such as release of a constriction or onset of frication noise.

Retroflex /r/ an allophone of the consonant /r/ for which the tongue tip is turned up to point toward the palate. Although *retroflex* literally means "turned back," the tongue tip rarely can be said to assume such a shape.

Rhotic a manner of articulation pertaining to *r* coloring; the rhotic consonant /r/ has several allophones and a complex and variable articulation. The two major allophones, bunched and retroflex, involve vocal tract constrictions in two or three places: labial, palatal, and pharyngeal.

Semivowel see **glide.**

Sibilant a speech sound characterized by an intense, high-pitched noise; for example, the fricatives /s/ (see) and /ʃ/ (she).

Stop a manner of articulation in which the vocal tract is completely closed for some interval, so that airflow ceases.

Stop burst a brief explosion of air that occurs when a stop closure is released and the impounded air escapes. Stop bursts usually are about 5 to 20 milliseconds in duration.

Stop consonant a consonant that is made with complete closure at some point in the vocal tract, so that airflow is temporarily interrupted and air pressure builds up behind the point of closure.

Strident a speech sound characterized by an intense frication noise, such as that heard for /s/ (see) and /ʃ/ (she). Sibilants and stridents are similar except that some phoneticians classify the nonsibilants /f/ (five) and /v/ (vine) as stridents.

Tap another name for **flap.**

Trill a pulmonic consonant made with a supraglottal vibration.

Velar a place of articulation pertaining to the undersurface of the hard and soft palate. Velar consonants are made with articulations of the dorsum of the tongue against the velar surface. Velars are also known as dorsal sounds.

Voice the sound produced by vocal fold vibration.

Voice onset time (VOT) the interval between an oral articulatory event (often the release of a stop) and the onset of voicing. If onset of voicing precedes the articulatory event, the sound is said to be prevoiced or to have a voicing lead (negative value of VOT), and if onset voicing follows the articulatory event, the sound is said to have a voicing lag.

Voiced associated with vocal fold vibration. A sound is said to be voiced if the vocal folds vibrate during its production.

Voiced implosive also called voiced ingressive; a stop made with an ingressive glottalic airstream.

Voiceless not associated with vocal fold vibration. A sound is said to be voiceless if the vocal folds do not vibrate during its production.

EXERCISES

1. Shown in Figure 5-41 are drawings of a side view of the vocal tract and the roof of the mouth. The ellipses (flattened circles) represent points of articulation. For both parts, identify by proper term the place of articulation represented by each ellipse.

2. For each consonant in the following word list, circle each letter for a consonant made with the tongue and underline each letter for a consonant made with the lips. Remember that two alphabet characters sometimes represent a single consonant phoneme, in which case you should circle or underline both letters.

(a) c o u g h	(i) p h o n e m e
(b) s c i s s o r s	(j) f i f t e e n
(c) p u f f	(k) b o o k m a r k
(d) m a n n i n g	(l) b a s e b a l l
(e) r a b b i t	(m) s h u f f l e
(f) v a l e n t i n e	(n) f e r v o r
(g) t h i c k e s t	(o) s n o w m a n
(h) w r i t h i n g	(p) o c e a n

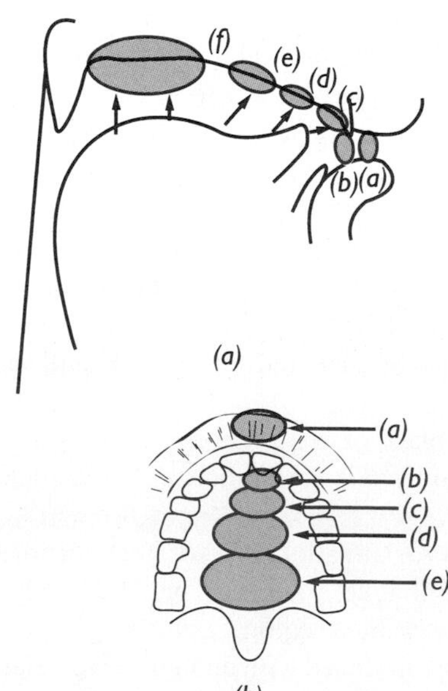

FIGURE 5-41
Ellipses showing places of consonant articulation: *(a)* lateral view of vocal tract; *(b)* view from below roof of mouth.

3. Verify the phonetic transcriptions provided for the standard pronunciation of the following words. Some of the transcriptions are in error because of incorrect consonant symbols. Circle each incorrect consonant and write the correct symbol above it.

Word	*Transcription*
(a) finger	[f ɪ n g ɚ]
(b) toothpaste	[t u ð p e͡ɪ s t]
(c) hammer	[h æ m ɚ]
(d) wristwatch	[r ɪ s t w ɔ ʃ]
(e) curtains	[c ɝ t n s]
(f) gasoline	[g æ s ə l i n]
(g) teenager	[t i n e͡ɪ ʤ ɚ]
(h) telephone	[t ɛ l ə p h o n]
(i) bookshelf	[b ʊ k ʃ ɛ l f]
(j) thanksgiving	[ð æ ŋ k s g ɪ v ɪ n g]

4. Classify and group each of the following words according to the manner of articulation of the *first* consonant. List the words in six columns having the headings Stop, Nasal, Fricative, Affricate, Liquid, and Glide.

can	this	red	job	nose	pot	wine
keep	saw	choose	man	wail	show	lamb
wheel	name	bed	ring	phone	thigh	yes
gin	chorus	zipper	happy	knew	fate	

5. Write next to each word the phonetic symbol or symbols corresponding to the italicized letter(s). *Example:* tha*nks* [ŋ k s]

(a) fi*fths* [ ]
(b) mea*s*ure [ ]
(c) wi*nd*ow [ ]
(d) la*mpsh*ade [ ]
(e) tra*ct*or [ ]
(f) *squ*eal [ ]
(g) be*nch* [ ]
(h) nu*dged* [ ]
(i) swi*ms*uit [ ]
(j) *th*us [ ]
(k) boo*ked* [ ]
(l) fini*sh* [ ]
(m) thi*stle* [ ]
(n) *sw*eet [ ]
(o) cru*nched* [ ]
(p) we*st* [ ]
(q) *c*ute [ ]
(r) *str*eak [ ]
(s) wi*thdr*aw [ ]
(t) wai*stl*ine [ ]

6. Write a phonetic transcription for each of the following words and then review the number of morphemes in the word.

Word	*Transcription*	*Morphemes*	*Comment*
(a) girl	[ ]	1	
(b) mission	[ ]	1	2 syllables but only one morpheme
(c) boys	[ ]	2	boys + s (plural)
(d) women's	[ ]	3	woman + (plural) + (possessive)
(e) svelte	[ ]	1	note violation of a phonetic sequencing constraint: English does not permit [sv] as a word-initial cluster except in borrowed words
(f) conceive	[ ]	2	note that second morpheme does not stand alone as a word
(g) reptilian	[ ]	2	reptile + ian
(h) demoted	[ ]	3	de + mote + (past tense)
(i) encryption	[ ]	3	en + crypt + ion
(j) transmission	[ ]	3	trans + mit + ion

TRANSCRIPTION TRAINING

The items for transcription training are recorded on audiocassette tape 1A. They are the same lists that were used previously for vowel transcription. Transcribe the entire word and check your transcription against the key. Notice that each word list gives practice with a different group of consonants as follows:

TRANSCRIPTION LIST A—stops /b d g p t k/
nasals /m n ŋ/
liquids /r l/

(Most of these phonetic symbols use the alphabet letter ordinarily associated with the sound; only /ŋ/ does not have a corresponding alphabet character.)

TRANSCRIPTION LIST B—fricatives
/v f ð θ z s ʒ ʃ h/
affricates /ʤ ʧ/
glides /w ʍ j/

TRANSCRIPTION LIST C—all consonants introduced in lists A and B

TRANSCRIPTION LIST D—consonant review and introduction of syllabic consonants (see Chapter 6) and the alveolar flap

PROCEED TO: Clinical Phonetics Tape 1A:
Transcription Lists A, B, C, D

MODULE TIME	
TOTAL	6:22
ELAPSED	00:00–06:22

Clinical Phonetics Tape 1A
Transcription List A

TRANSCRIPTION KEY

1	me	[m i]	26	ramp	[r æ m p]
2	on	[ɑ n]	27	blue	[b l u]
3	at	[æ t]	28	treat	[t r i t]
4	two	[t u]	29	talc	[t æ l k]
5	top	[t ɑ p]	30	real	[r i l]
6	keep	[k i p]	31	ghoul	[g u l] or [g u ə l]
7	moon	[m u n]	32	nude	[n u d]
8	knee	[n i]	33	calm	[k ɑ m]
9	back	[b æ k]	34	barn	[b ɑ r n]
10	gap	[g æ p]	35	rank	[r æ ŋ k]
11	gang	[g æ ŋ]	36	creed	[k r i d]
12	dot	[d ɑ t]	37	tool	[t u l] or [t u ə l]
13	peaked	[p i k t]	38	bomb	[b ɑ m]
14	ruined	[r u n d]	39	trapped	[t r æ p t]
15	pond	[p ɑ n d]	40	clean	[k l i n]
16	poor	[p u r]	41	long	[l ɔ ŋ]
17	boot	[b u t]	42	rang	[r æ ŋ]
18	bat	[b æ t]	43	tank	[t æ ŋ k]
19	drop	[d r ɑ p]	44	group	[g r u p]
20	teamed	[t i m d]	45	keel	[k i l] or [k i ə l]
21	league	[l i g]	46	banged	[b æ ŋ d]
22	loot	[l u t]	47	lock	[l ɑ k]
23	wrong	[r ɔ ŋ]	48	bleed	[b l i d]
24	lagged	[l æ g d]	49	clue	[k l u]
25	bald	[b ɔ l d]	50	grew	[g r u]

MODULE TIME	
TOTAL	6:22
ELAPSED	00:00–06:22

Clinical Phonetics Tape 1A
Transcription List A

TRANSCRIPTION SHEET

1	me	[ ]	26	ramp	[ ]
2	on	[ ]	27	blue	[ ]
3	at	[ ]	28	treat	[ ]
4	two	[ ]	29	talc	[ ]
5	top	[ ]	30	real	[ ]
6	keep	[ ]	31	ghoul	[ ]
7	moon	[ ]	32	nude	[ ]
8	knee	[ ]	33	calm	[ ]
9	back	[ ]	34	barn	[ ]
10	gap	[ ]	35	rank	[ ]
11	gang	[ ]	36	creed	[ ]
12	dot	[ ]	37	tool	[ ]
13	peaked	[ ]	38	bomb	[ ]
14	ruined	[ ]	39	trapped	[ ]
15	pond	[ ]	40	clean	[ ]
16	poor	[ ]	41	long	[ ]
17	boot	[ ]	42	rang	[ ]
18	bat	[ ]	43	tank	[ ]
19	drop	[ ]	44	group	[ ]
20	teamed	[ ]	45	keel	[ ]
21	league	[ ]	46	banged	[ ]
22	loot	[ ]	47	lock	[ ]
23	wrong	[ ]	48	bleed	[ ]
24	lagged	[ ]	49	clue	[ ]
25	bald	[ ]	50	grew	[ ]

MODULE TIME	
TOTAL	6:03
ELAPSED	06:22–12:25

Clinical Phonetics Tape 1A
Transcription List B

TRANSCRIPTION KEY

1	yes	[j ɛ s]	26	rich	[r ɪ tʃ]
2	wish	[w ɪ ʃ]	27	veal	[v i l] or [v i ə l]
3	sheep	[ʃ i p]	28	Yale	[j e͡ɪ l]
4	faith	[f e͡ɪ θ]	29	jazz	[ʤ æ z]
5	thanks	[θ æ ŋ k s]	30	fence	[f e n s] or [f ɛ n t s]
6	rash	[r æ ʃ]	31	that	[ð æ t]
7	weaved	[w i v d]	32	whale	[w e͡ɪ l]
8	this	[ð ɪ s]	33	fish	[f ɪ ʃ]
9	waste	[w e͡ɪ s t]	34	yeast	[j i s t]
10	when	[ʍ ɛ n]	35	fizz	[f ɪ z]
11	fast	[f æ s t]	36	seethe	[s i ð]
12	vest	[v ɛ s t]	37	dwell	[d w ɛ l]
13	wage	[w e͡ɪ ʤ]	38	vast	[v æ s t]
14	cheese	[tʃ i z]	39	eighth	[e͡ɪ t θ]
15	thing	[θ ɪ ŋ]	40	hatch	[h æ tʃ]
16	thief	[θ i f]	41	sting	[s t ɪ ŋ]
17	stretch	[s t r ɛ tʃ]	42	hedge	[h ɛ ʤ]
18	badge	[b æ ʤ]	43	haze	[h e͡ɪ z]
19	share	[ʃ ɛ r]	44	his	[h ɪ z]
20	they	[ð e͡ɪ]	45	bear	[b ɛ r]
21	which	[ʍ ɪ tʃ]	46	heave	[h i v]
22	teach	[t i tʃ]	47	bath	[b æ θ]
23	yams	[j æ m z]	48	freeze	[f r i z]
24	gems	[ʤ ɛ m z]	49	shrill	[ʃ r ɪ l]
25	check	[tʃ ɛ k]	50	staged	[s t e͡ɪ ʤ d]

MODULE TIME	
TOTAL	6:03
ELAPSED	06:22–12:25

Clinical Phonetics Tape 1A
Transcription List B

TRANSCRIPTION SHEET

1	yes	[ ]	26	rich	[ ]
2	wish	[ ]	27	veal	[ ]
3	sheep	[ ]	28	Yale	[ ]
4	faith	[ ]	29	jazz	[ ]
5	thanks	[ ]	30	fence	[ ]
6	rash	[ ]	31	that	[ ]
7	weaved	[ ]	32	whale	[ ]
8	this	[ ]	33	fish	[ ]
9	waste	[ ]	34	yeast	[ ]
10	when	[ ]	35	fizz	[ ]
11	fast	[ ]	36	seethe	[ ]
12	vest	[ ]	37	dwell	[ ]
13	wage	[ ]	38	vast	[ ]
14	cheese	[ ]	39	eighth	[ ]
15	thing	[ ]	40	hatch	[ ]
16	thief	[ ]	41	sting	[ ]
17	stretch	[ ]	42	hedge	[ ]
18	badge	[ ]	43	haze	[ ]
19	share	[ ]	44	his	[ ]
20	they	[ ]	45	bear	[ ]
21	which	[ ]	46	heave	[ ]
22	teach	[ ]	47	bath	[ ]
23	yams	[ ]	48	freeze	[ ]
24	gems	[ ]	49	shrill	[ ]
25	check	[ ]	50	staged	[ ]

MODULE TIME	
TOTAL	5:51
ELAPSED	12:25–18:16

Clinical Phonetics Tape 1A
Transcription List C

TRANSCRIPTION KEY

1	jaw	[ʤ ɔ]	26	shoes	[ʃ u z]
2	joke	[ʤ o͡ʊ k]	27	alms	[ɑ m z]
3	psalm	[s ɑ m]	28	gold	[g o͡ʊ l d]
4	shoot	[ʃ u t]	29	crook	[k r ʊ k]
5	should	[ʃ ʊ d]	30	books	[b ʊ k s]
6	though	[ð o͡ʊ]	31	cough	[k ɔ f]
7	could	[k ʊ d]	32	whole	[h o͡ʊ l]
8	rouge	[r u ʒ]	33	thought	[θ ɔ t]
9	shawl	[ʃ ɔ l]	34	vault	[v ɔ l t]
10	Vaughn	[v ɔ n]	35	groom	[g r u m]
11	through	[θ r u]	36	looked	[l ʊ k t]
12	wash	[w ɔ ʃ] or [w ɑ ʃ]	37	yawn	[j ɔ n]
13	woods	[w ʊ d z]	38	slew	[s l u]
14	throw	[θ r o͡ʊ]	39	both	[b o͡ʊ θ]
15	stone	[s t o͡ʊ n]	40	gone	[g ɔ n]
16	halls	[h ɔ l z]	41	would	[w ʊ d]
17	strewn	[s t r u n]	42	nook	[n ʊ k]
18	palms	[p ɑ m z]	43	soul	[s o͡ʊ l]
19	stood	[s t ʊ d]	44	room	[r u m]
20	salt	[s ɔ l t]	45	whom	[h u m]
21	squaw	[s k w ɔ]	46	haunt	[h ɔ n t]
22	flowed	[f l o͡ʊ d]	47	those	[ð o͡ʊ z]
23	shook	[ʃ ʊ k]	48	swath	[s w ɑ θ]
24	food	[f u d]	49	draw	[d r ɔ]
25	spot	[s p ɑ t]	50	ought	[ɔ t]

MODULE TIME	
TOTAL	5:51
ELAPSED	12:25–18:16

Clinical Phonetics Tape 1A
Transcription List C

TRANSCRIPTION SHEET

1	jaw	[ ]	26	shoes	[ ]
2	joke	[ ]	27	alms	[ ]
3	psalm	[ ]	28	gold	[ ]
4	shoot	[ ]	29	crook	[ ]
5	should	[ ]	30	books	[ ]
6	though	[ ]	31	cough	[ ]
7	could	[ ]	32	whole	[ ]
8	rouge	[ ]	33	thought	[ ]
9	shawl	[ ]	34	vault	[ ]
10	Vaughn	[ ]	35	groom	[ ]
11	through	[ ]	36	looked	[ ]
12	wash	[ ]	37	yawn	[ ]
13	woods	[ ]	38	slew	[ ]
14	throw	[ ]	39	both	[ ]
15	stone	[ ]	40	gone	[ ]
16	halls	[ ]	41	would	[ ]
17	strewn	[ ]	42	nook	[ ]
18	palms	[ ]	43	soul	[ ]
19	stood	[ ]	44	room	[ ]
20	salt	[ ]	45	whom	[ ]
21	squaw	[ ]	46	haunt	[ ]
22	flowed	[ ]	47	those	[ ]
23	shook	[ ]	48	swath	[ ]
24	food	[ ]	49	draw	[ ]
25	spot	[ ]	50	ought	[ ]

MODULE TIME	
TOTAL	9:29
ELAPSED	18:16–27:45

Clinical Phonetics Tape 1A
Transcription List D

TRANSCRIPTION KEY

1	eyebrow	[a͡ɪ b r a͡ʊ]	32	ruckus	[r ʌ k ə s]
2	cowboy	[k a͡ʊ b ɔ͡ɪ]	33	foyer	[f ɔ͡ɪ ɚ]
3	rainbow	[r e͡ɪ n b o͡ʊ]	34	murder	[m ɝ d ɚ]
4	daylight	[d e͡ɪ l a͡ɪ t]	35	hurdle	[h ɝ d l̩][a]
5	highway	[h a͡ɪ w e͡ɪ]	36	cupboard	[k ʌ b ɚ d]
6	thyroid	[θ a͡ɪ r ɔ͡ɪ d]	37	turtle	[t ɝ t l̩][a]
7	lifeboat	[l a͡ɪ f b o͡ʊ t]	38	sister	[s ɪ s t ɚ]
8	railroad	[r e͡ɪ l r o͡ʊ d]	39	further	[f ɝ ð ɚ]
9	greyhound	[g r e͡ɪ h a͡ʊ n d]	40	sirloin	[s ɝ l ɔ͡ɪ n]
10	housewife	[h a͡ʊ s w a͡ɪ f]	41	surround	[s ɝ a͡ʊ n d]
11	boathouse	[b o͡ʊ t h a͡ʊ s]	42	station	[s t e͡ɪ ʃ ə n]
12	outside	[a͡ʊ t s a͡ɪ d]	43	acre	[e͡ɪ k ɚ]
13	lifeline	[l a͡ɪ f l a͡ɪ n]	44	survive	[s ɚ v a͡ɪ v]
14	downspout	[d a͡ʊ n s p a͡ʊ t]	45	alike	[ə l a͡ɪ k]
15	hyoid	[h a͡ɪ ɔ͡ɪ d]	46	buttons	[b ʌ t n̩ z][a]
16	roadhouse	[r o͡ʊ d h a͡ʊ s]	47	rusted	[r ʌ s t ɪ d]
17	skylight	[s k a͡ɪ l a͡ɪ t]	48	annoy	[ə n ɔ͡ɪ]
18	daytime	[d e͡ɪ t a͡ɪ m]	49	butter	[b ʌ ɾ ɚ]
19	townhouse	[t a͡ʊ n h a͡ʊ s]	50	certain	[s ɝ t n̩][a]
20	Friday	[f r a͡ɪ d e͡ɪ]	51	cradle	[k r e͡ɪ d l̩][a]
21	outline	[a͡ʊ t l a͡ɪ n]	52	surly	[s ɝ l ɪ]
22	rowboat	[r o͡ʊ b o͡ʊ t]	53	cousin	[k ʌ z n̩][a]
23	highlight	[h a͡ɪ l a͡ɪ t]	54	lighter	[l a͡ɪ t ɚ]
24	pie plate	[p a͡ɪ p l e͡ɪ t]	55	person	[p ɝ s ə n]
25	houseboy	[h a͡ʊ s b ɔ͡ɪ]	56	towers	[t a͡ʊ ɚ z]
26	slurred	[s l ɝ d]	57	subtle	[s ʌ t l̩][a]
27	suburb	[s ʌ b ɚ b]	58	putty	[p ʌ ɾ ɪ]
28	astound	[ə s t a͡ʊ n d]	59	pious	[p a͡ɪ ə s]
29	joyous	[ʤ ɔ͡ɪ ə s]	60	writer	[r a͡ɪ t ɚ]
30	rubber	[r ʌ b ɚ]	61	worthy	[w ɝ ð ɪ]
31	curtain	[k ɝ t n̩][a]	62	perturb	[p ɝ t ɝ b]

MODULE TIME	
TOTAL	9:29
ELAPSED	18:16–27:45

Clinical Phonetics Tape 1A
Transcription List D

TRANSCRIPTION SHEET

1	eyebrow	[ ]	32	ruckus	[ ]
2	cowboy	[ ]	33	foyer	[ ]
3	rainbow	[ ]	34	murder	[ ]
4	daylight	[ ]	35	hurdle	[ ]
5	highway	[ ]	36	cupboard	[ ]
6	thyroid	[ ]	37	turtle	[ ]
7	lifeboat	[ ]	38	sister	[ ]
8	railroad	[ ]	39	further	[ ]
9	greyhound	[ ]	40	sirloin	[ ]
10	housewife	[ ]	41	surround	[ ]
11	boathouse	[ ]	42	station	[ ]
12	outside	[ ]	43	acre	[ ]
13	lifeline	[ ]	44	survive	[ ]
14	downspout	[ ]	45	alike	[ ]
15	hyoid	[ ]	46	buttons	[ ]
16	roadhouse	[ ]	47	rusted	[ ]
17	skylight	[ ]	48	annoy	[ ]
18	daytime	[ ]	49	butter	[ ]
19	townhouse	[ ]	50	certain	[ ]
20	Friday	[ ]	51	cradle	[ ]
21	outline	[ ]	52	surly	[ ]
22	rowboat	[ ]	53	cousin	[ ]
23	highlight	[ ]	54	lighter	[ ]
24	pie plate	[ ]	55	person	[ ]
25	houseboy	[ ]	56	towers	[ ]
26	slurred	[ ]	57	subtle	[ ]
27	suburb	[ ]	58	putty	[ ]
28	astound	[ ]	59	pious	[ ]
29	joyous	[ ]	60	writer	[ ]
30	rubber	[ ]	61	worthy	[ ]
31	curtain	[ ]	62	perturb	[ ]

MODULE TIME	
TOTAL	9:29
ELAPSED	18:16–27:45

Clinical Phonetics Tape 1A
Transcription List D, Continued

TRANSCRIPTION KEY

63	dirty	[d ɝ ɾ ɪ]	67	mercy	[m ɝ s ɪ]
64	muscle	[m ʌ s l̩][a]	68	litter	[l ɪ t ɚ]
65	sucker	[s ʌ k ɚ]	69	mutton	[m ʌ t n̩][a]
66	lighter	[l a͡ɪ t ɚ]	70	tighten	[t a͡ɪ t n̩][a]

[a]Syllabic sounds [n̩] and [l̩] will be discussed in Chapter 6.

MODULE TIME	
TOTAL	9:29
ELAPSED	18:16–27:45

Clinical Phonetics Tape 1A
Transcription List D, Continued

TRANSCRIPTION SHEET

63	dirty	[ ]	67	mercy	[ ]
64	muscle	[ ]	68	litter	[ ]
65	sucker	[ ]	69	mutton	[ ]
66	lighter	[ ]	70	tighten	[ ]

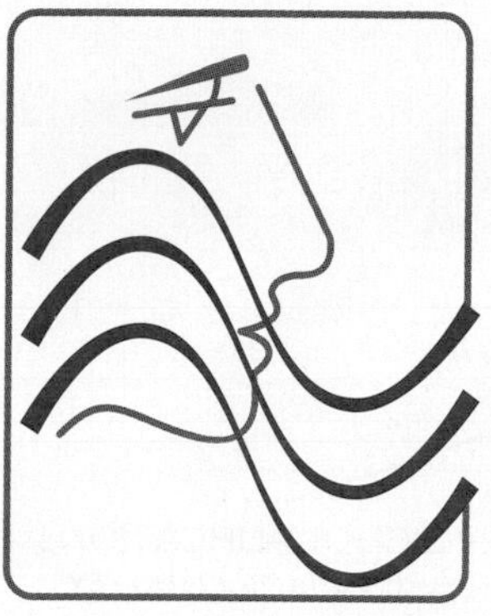

Diacritics and Sounds in Context

6

SUPRASEGMENTALS: PROSODY AND PARALINGUISTICS

Segmental transcription is essential to identify the phonemic or allophonic content of a speaker's message, but this information does not stand alone. Rather, it is accompanied by prosodic and paralinguistic information. The term **prosody** is defined in a number of different ways in the phonetics literature, but most writers agree that it pertains to some of the so-called suprasegmental aspects of speech. Included in this category are intonation, stress pattern, loudness variations, pausing, and rhythm. **Paralinguistics** includes aspects such as voice quality, vocal adjustments, and emotion. Phonetic transcription as considered so far in this book identifies the basic segments, or phonetic units, of an utterance. But each utterance is produced with a number of characteristics that go beyond the identification of a series of phonetic segments. These characteristics are often called **suprasegmental** because they bridge across phonetic segments. In a sense, these suprasegmental characteristics are superimposed on the segmental properties of an utterance, and they may have boundaries defined by syllables, words, phrases, sentences, and even discourses.

Try reading aloud the following transcription:

[a͡ɪ wud la͡ɪk tu tak wɪθ ju]

Most people would read it with a declarative intonation, that is, as a statement of fact and in a neutral emotional tone. But it could also be read as one of the following:

- A slow, measured reading of barely contained anger.
- A joyous, expectant expression with large shifts of vocal pitch.
- A hesitant, quiet voice (as though you were not at all comfortable in approaching the person to whom you need to talk).
- A fairly loud voice with emphasis on the word *talk* (as though the listener didn't understand you the first time).
- A rushed statement with the final word drawn out (as if seeking a response from the other person).
- An ironic sentiment (as though the last thing you really would like is to talk with the person in question).

These variants encompass different prosodic and paralinguistic aspects of speech. They are obviously important in understanding a speaker's true intention, and they are essential to the accurate transcription of speech for some purposes.

Unfortunately, there is much disagreement about how these characteristics should be identified and classified. The account in this book is a very general one that is compatible with some published clinical materials on prosody (Hargrove and McGarr, 1993). Writing about suprasegmentals is also complicated because of major changes sweeping through the study of phonology; for example, the theories of autosegmental and metrical phonology (Goldsmith, 1990). It is outside the scope of this chapter to consider phonological theory, but the concepts developed here should provide the phonetic tools needed for various phonological applications.

Figure 6-1 gives an overview of suprasegmentals. The suprasegmentals are subdivided into the two major components of prosody and paralinguistics. Prosody consists of the various elements listed in Figure 6-1, which will be discussed individually in this chapter. The figure also shows the elements grouped under paralinguistics.

Prosody

A speaker conveys prosodic information by controlling three general aspects of the acoustic signal of speech. These are: vocal fundamental frequency (perceived primarily as vocal **pitch**), vocal intensity (perceived primarily as loudness), and duration (perceived primarily as length). Chapter 10 discusses these acoustic concepts in more detail, but for present purposes it is enough to know that pitch, loudness, and length are the basic dimensions by which prosody is expressed. Some writers use the term *prosody* interchangeably with **intonation.** But we will follow Johns-Lewis (1986) in defining intonation as a part of prosody that pertains to the patterns of pitch rises and falls and to the patterns of stress in a given language. Prosody includes these intonational effects as well as tone, tempo (pause, lengthening, and speaking rate), and loudness. Prosody gives shape to speech on several different levels of linguistic or communicative structure. We will now examine some prosodic effects across several levels of organization, including discourse, sentences, phrases

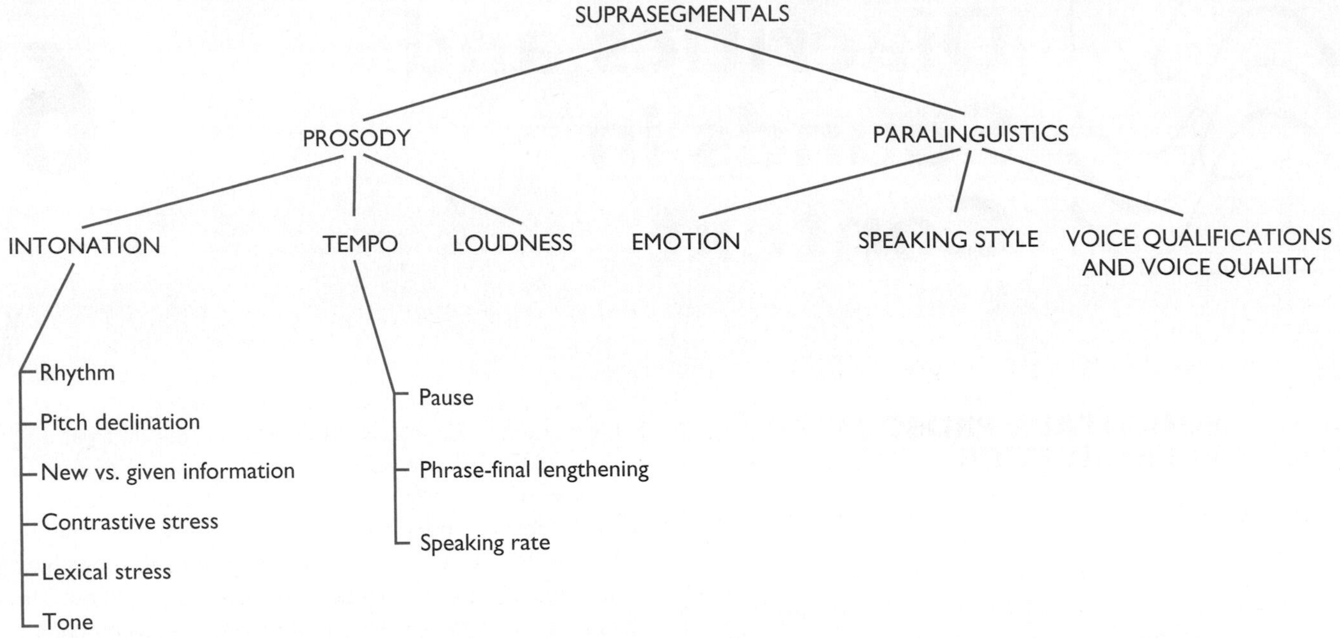

FIGURE 6-1
Tree diagram showing the various suprasegmental components of speech. The two primary subdivisions are prosody and paralinguistics, each of which is further subdivided.

within sentences, and individual words of the speaker's lexicon. The discussion will follow the hierarchical organization in Figure 6-1, beginning with intonation.

Intonation. Intonation embraces a number of phenomena that determine the patterns of pitch rises and falls as well as the stress patterns of a language. The discussion begins with a look at rhythm.

Rhythm. It is a common belief that spoken language has a rhythm or melody. The rhythm may not be as pronounced as in the recitation of poetic verse, but some kind of rhythm seems to be present. **Rhythm** is the distribution of various levels of stress across a syllable chain. **Stress** is the degree of prominence associated with a particular syllable. Languages differ in their rhythmic characteristics and are sometimes classified as stress-timed, syllable-timed, or mora-timed. English is considered to be stress-timed, meaning that it is temporally structured in relation to the stressed syllables of an utterance. In fact, English rhythm has been characterized as an alternating pattern of strong-weak syllables (SWSWSW. . . , where S = strong and W = weak). This should be understood as a general pattern or tendency, not as an absolute. Spanish is said to be a syllable-timed language. In such a language, the temporal pattern is based on successive syllables and their inherent temporal properties. The rhythm of Japanese is based on the mora. The mora is a timing unit which has a beginning that is not necessarily coincident with the beginning of a syllable. A word in Japanese can have two syllables and two mora, or two syllables and three mora. These differences in rhythm across languages are reflected in the temporal adjustments of speech (Hoequist, 1983), and they may even be evident in infant vocalizations during the babbling period (De Boysson-Bardies, Sagart, and Durand, 1984). They are one reason why some languages often seem to have different melodies.

Rhythm is important in the understanding of speech, in part because it enables the listener to predict upcoming elements in the speech stream. Prediction of upcoming information makes for an efficient perceptual processing (Martin, 1972). If the rhythmic pattern of speech is largely predictable, then the listener in a sense knows "when" to listen for essential acoustic information.

Pitch Declination. How does a listener identify major linguistic units such as clauses and sentences? One major cue is **pitch declination.** *Declination* means "fall." Vocal pitch (or its physical correlate, the fundamental frequency contour) typically declines across clauses or sentences. That is, the pitch or fundamental frequency begins at a relatively high value on the first word or syllable of the sentence and then gradually falls to lower values across the remaining words. However, there are disputes in the literature on how this overall tilt is regulated (Cohen, Collier, and t'Hart, 1982). Two influential interpretations have been advanced. One view, which we will call the linear declination theory, is that fundamental frequency falls gradually and linearly throughout a sentence (Maeda, 1976; Sorensen and Cooper, 1980; Thorsen, 1985). This may even be a universal property of spoken language, insofar as all languages tend to have sentences with pitch declination. Lieberman (1967) proposed another view, called the breath-group theory. According to this theory, a declarative sentence can be divided into nonterminal and terminal parts, and variation in fundamental frequency is permitted only in the nonterminal part of the fundamental frequency contour. The nonterminal part can assume different patterns of fundamental frequency change, but the terminal part usually has a rapid fall in fundamental frequency. Some studies have shown that an important acoustic cue for syntactic structure is the fall in fundamental frequency and intensity at the end of the breath group (Landahl, 1980; Lieberman and Tseng, 1981; Lieberman, Katz, Jongman, Zimmerman, and Miller, 1985).

Theoretical disagreements aside, the important point is that a falling pitch within the clause or sentence is a major perceptual cue that helps the listener to recognize major syntactic groupings of words. If the declination extends to the entire clause or sentence, then it would give a basic form to the prosody of a multisyllable utterance. Pitch is not necessarily the only kind of declination that occurs in speech. It is possible that declination effects can also occur for overall amplitude and for the range of articulatory movements in speech. In a sense, utterances tend to start "big" (high fundamental frequency, high amplitude, and large range of tongue or jaw movement) and then get smaller.

New Versus Given Information. Speakers also use prosody to highlight words that present new information in a message. When radio or television announcers introduce a new topic, they usually cue the listener to the key word or words. This is known as the distinction between new and given information (Figure 6-1). An example comes from a study by Behne (1989), who described prosodic effects in a mini-discourse such as the following:

1. "Someone painted the fence."
2. "Who painted the fence?"
3. "PETE painted the fence."

In this exchange, the new information in sentence 3 is "Pete," who is identified as the individual who painted the fence. Try rehearsing this little exchange, and try to identify how you might say "Pete" in sentence 3. Did you say it relatively longer and with a higher vocal pitch? That is what the subjects in Behne's study did. New information is often spoken with a lengthening of the critical word and with a higher fundamental frequency. Behne also showed that the same cues are used in French, but they are deployed somewhat differently. Languages differ in their use of prosodic characteristics, much as they differ in their segmental characteristics.

Contrastive Stress. Stress can be used for a variety of purposes in speaking. To illustrate contrastive stress, suppose that two persons are driving to a house in an unfamiliar part of a city, relying on instructions they received from a friend. The problem is that they remember the instructions differently. The exchange might go like this:

Pat: "Now we turn left at the drive-in bank."

Terry: "I know for certain that he said to turn *right* at the drive-in bank."

Pat: "No, we're supposed to turn right at the *laundromat.*"

Terry: "It was *right* at the *bank.*"

This kind of conversation typically uses contrastive stress to mark a word, phrase, or clause that contradicts or contrasts with one that was previously stated or implied in the discourse. In this conversational sample, the words printed in italics represent the use of contrastive stress. Acoustically, the element receiving contrastive stress may have a longer duration, a higher fundamental frequency, and a greater intensity. If Pat and Terry continue this discussion, both may add to their voices still another modification—impatience or anger. But that is another story to be taken up later in the discussion of paralinguistics.

Lexical Stress. Prosody can distinguish words in the lexicon. Particularly good examples are English words that form noun/verb pairs: *IMport* versus *imPORT, PROtest* versus *proTEST,* and *INsert* versus *inSERT.* In each pair, stress pattern is the major spoken contrast, and the stressed syllable is printed in uppercase letters. Notice that a segmental transcription would not distinguish these words. Another example of word-level prosody is the stress pattern on compounds versus phrases. Say the following to yourself and try to describe the difference in their production:

Compound Noun	*Noun Phrase*
blackboard	black board
blackbird	black bird

Stress pattern contrasts the compound noun (e.g., *BLACKboard*) with the noun phrase (e.g., *black BOARD*).

These examples illustrate that prosodic effects are woven into several levels of spoken English. Furthermore, these effects may interact. One word in an utterance may receive more than one type of prosodic influence. Consider this example: "I didn't say *IMpact,* I said *COMpact.*" In this sentence, the italicized words have a specified lexical stress, are given contrastive stress, and fit into the overall intonational pattern of the sentence (including declination).

Tone. Most of the world's languages are tone languages. In these languages, tone is part of the phonemic structure used to distinguish words. Tone denotes the regulation of fundamental frequency to produce contrasts, such as level (no change in vocal pitch), falling (falling pitch), rising (rising pitch), or rising-falling (a rising segment followed by a falling segment). Depending on which tonal pattern is used, a different word is specified. A good example comes from the Mandarin dialect of Chinese. In this dialect, the phonetic sequence [m ɑ] can mean at least four different words, depending on the tone that is used by the speaker. A level tone is used for the word *mother,* a rising tone for *hemp,* a falling-rising tone for *horse,* and a falling tone for *to scold.* English is not a tone language and, therefore, little will be said about tone in this book. However, clinicians need to be aware that speakers with a language background other than English may use tonal contrasts. See Appendix F for further discussion of foreign dialects.

Tempo.

Tempo includes pause, lengthening, and speaking rate. These aspects have in common a primary effect on the temporal pattern of speech. The rhythm of a language, discussed earlier under the heading of intonation, also affects its tempo. The description of English as a stress-timed language carries implications for the temporal pattern of its syllable durations.

Pause (Juncture). It may seem strange that silence carries communicative value, but pauses are part of the informational structure of speech, and it is sometimes important that an accurate phonetic transcription notes the occurrence and relative duration of pauses. Pauses serve several functions, including (1) marking boundaries between units such as phrases or clauses, (2) indicating hesitations while a speaker retrieves words or plans utterances, and (3) increasing the sense of anticipation as a listener waits for information to follow (Green and Ravizza, 1995; Mukherjee, 2000). Internal open juncture, discussed later in this chapter, refers to pauses and related phenomena that help to mark the location of major syntactic boundaries. But speech patterns often involve pauses that go beyond the marking of internal open juncture. Therefore, it is helpful to have a way of indicating pauses that are considered to be an important aspect of a speech pattern.

Consider the sentence *I saw her at the airport and I could hardly believe what she was wearing.* To illustrate some of the functions of pausing, let us examine this sentence with pauses identified for the three purposes just described: *I saw her at the airport* [pause to delimit the first clause of the sentence] *and* [hesitation while speaker finds the words to complete the sentence] *I could hardly believe what she was* [pause for stylistic effect—to enhance the listener's anticipation of the concluding words] *wearing.* The symbol of one or more periods within parentheses is recommended as a convenient way of indicating pause phenomena in speech. Depending on the purposes of transcription, this symbol may be used for all notable pauses, or only for those considered to reflect hesitations or deliberate exaggerations of normal pausing. Pauses can be especially notable in the speech of young children and individuals with communicative disorders. These pauses often seem to occur as the speaker tries to retrieve a particular word or to formulate a linguistic structure.

The word *pause* generally refers to silences of at least 200 ms duration. Shorter intervals of silence occur frequently in speech, and many of these are related to individual phones, such as stops and affricates. Usually, the duration of silence for a stop or affricate gap is no longer than 50 to 100 ms. These short intervals of silence carry informational value, because they are part of the essential nature of stops and affricates.

Pause duration also is affected by a host of cognitive, affective-state, and social interaction variables, to be discussed in a later section on paralinguistics.

Phrase-Final Lengthening. At the level of sentence structure, juncture and pause phenomena are used to mark multiword units. An important example in English is known as **phrase-final** (or **prepausal**) **lengthening.** This refers to a lengthening of the last stressable syllable in a major syntactic phrase or clause. For example, contrast your productions of these two sentences:

1. Red, green, and blue were the decorator's colors.
2. Blue, green, and red were the decorator's colors.

Do you hear a difference in your productions? Most speakers produce the word *blue* in sentence 1 longer than the same word in sentence 2. Similarly, they produce the word *red* in sentence 2 longer than the same word in sentence 1. The word preceding the noun clause boundary is lengthened. The following analysis identifies the key features, where the bar (———) represents lengthening of the word it follows, and the slash (/) indicates a phrase boundary:

Red, green, and blue———/ were the decorator's colors.

Blue, green, and red———/ were the decorator's colors.

This kind of prosodic information helps listeners to recognize the structure of spoken sentences. This process is called **parsing** and consists essentially of the assignment of meaning to words as they are heard. Phrase-final lengthening and pitch declination are two major cues that enable listeners to identify syntactic groupings in spoken language.

Read and Schreiber (1982) believed that children rely on this prosodic cue to a greater degree than adults do. They also noted that prosody supplies the young language learner with an accessible starting point for interpreting the complex syntactic structures of language. Moreover, a similar phenomenon may characterize the utterances of infants in the babbling stage of speech development. The phenomenon, called **final syllable lengthening,** is defined as a lengthening of the final syllable in a syllable group or phrase. For example, when an infant babbles [d ɑ d ɑ d ɑ d ɑ], the fourth syllable may be lengthened relative to its predecessors in the babbling string. Oller and Smith (1977) did not find significant evidence of final syllable lengthening in the multisyllable productions of 8- to 12-month-old infants, but Zlatin-Laufer (1980) and Mitchell (1988) both reported that this effect occurred in the vocalizations of infants in the second half of the first year of life. It appears that final syllable lengthening is more likely to occur in disyllables (e.g., [da da]) than in long strings of multisyllabic babbling. A similar pattern holds for adult speech, in which phrase-final lengthening is less apparent in longer utterances or connected discourse (Klatt, 1976).

Speaking Rate. Looking again at Figure 6-1, we now turn to the prosodic variable of speaking rate. As speaking rate increases, the durations of the components of speech necessarily get smaller. The speaker has to produce more segments, syllables, or words per unit of time. Inversely, as speaking rate decreases, the durations of the components of speech necessarily get longer. What is not entirely clear is how the changes in temporal pattern are distributed across the components. Studies have shown that the reduction for increased rate or the lengthening for decreased rate is not constant or linear across all segments. Generally, in fast speech, pauses and steady-state segments for vowels and consonants tend to be sacrificed more than transitional or dynamic aspects of the speech signal. Stressed vowels tend to be preserved better than unstressed vowels. At very fast speaking rates, segments and unstressed syllables may be deleted. Rapid rates also tend to be accompanied by **undershoot,** which is a reduction in the articulatory movements for a particular sound. Vowels especially can be produced at rapid speaking rates in a manner that deviates from the production for an isolated production of the sound. Some examples of changes in fast speech follow.

Deletions in Fast Speech (Dalby, 1984):

camera: [k æ m ə r ə] → [k æ m r ə]
definite: [d ɛ f ɪ n ɪ t] → [d ɛ f n ɪ t]
support: [s ə p o r t] → [s p o r t]
surprise: [s ɚ p r a͡ɪ z] → [s p r a͡ɪ z]

Phonetic Change:

going to → gonna
want to → wanna

Articulatory change (Adams, Weismer, and Kent, 1993) involves articulatory adjustments that are different for opening and closing movements and for movements of the lower lip and tongue. That is, the adjustments are not made in a simple, invariant manner across different sounds.

Apparently, speakers and listeners know "fast rate" rules that permit understanding of sentences even when entire syllables are dropped at rapid speaking rates. Attempts to use acoustic measures to study the effect of speaking rate obviously must be used with recognition of changes in the phonetic structure of the speech signal. Interestingly, some speech synthesizers (machines that produce speech artificially) accomplish changes in speaking rate simply by making proportionate reductions in all phonetic segments. Although this pattern is unlike that used by human speakers, the synthesized speech maintains good intelligibility even at fast rates (Gunderson, 1992). Listeners seem to be quite flexible in their adjustments for speaking rate.

Loudness. Loudness is the perceived magnitude or strength of a sound. It varies along a perceptual dimension of weak to strong, or soft to loud. In general, the loudness of a sound varies with the amplitude of the acoustic signal, as discussed in Chapter 10. There is no generally accepted transcriptional device for loudness, although some symbols for discourse transcription will be mentioned later in this chapter. See Chapter 10 for a discussion of a related attribute, vocal effort.

The Bases of Prosody

Speech Production Correlates. The lay listener, when asked to describe what stressed units in speech "sound like," usually says that a stressed syllable or word is "louder." Given that loudness is most directly related to sound intensity, we might expect that sound intensity is the physical correlate of our perception of stress. However, experimental studies show that stress perception is related to three acoustic parameters—duration, intensity, and fundamental frequency. It is questionable which of these is the most important, and it is possible that different speakers weight the acoustic cues differently. Generally, increased stress is associated with longer syllable durations, greater intensity of sound, and an elevation of the fundamental frequency. There are also acoustic changes in individual sound segments; for example, stressed vowels may assume a more distinctive acoustic structure. The literature on the acoustic correlates of prosody is too vast to be considered here, but it should be noted that the correlates are not simply specified and may vary across speakers and types of utterances. For further discussion, see the works of Fry (1955, 1958) and De Jong (1991).

It is important for clinical purposes that stress can alter vowel and consonantal articulation (Kent and Netsell, 1971; De Jong, 1991). When a syllable is stressed, its articulatory movements tend to become larger, so that the movements in stressed syllables are more contrastive. Both vowels and consonants are produced with more extreme articulatory positions. For instance, a strongly stressed production of the high-front vowel /i/ can be more fronted than a weakly stressed version of this vowel. The stressed production also has a longer duration. These are important considerations in speech training programs, many of which recommend the use of stressed forms for early training of a speech sound.

As noted earlier, tempo or speaking rate also affects articulation. As tempo increases, movements tend to be smaller in magnitude, and, in some speakers, the velocity of individual movements may increase.

Developmental Perspective. Many writers have concluded that infants and young children use prosodic characteristics of a language before they master the segmental aspects. It is possible that prosodic structure is particularly important to young language learners because it provides a structure for the phonetic interpretation of adult utterances. This may be why caregivers tend to use an exaggerated intonational pattern ("motherese") when talking to their young children (Fernald and Mazzie, 1991).

Baltaxe, Simmons, and Zee (1984) summarized several interesting roles of prosody in speech and language development:

1. In the early stages of language development, prosody often is more advanced than phonological, syntactic, or semantic development.
2. Early prosodic units may play a facilitating role for both the perceptual and productive aspects of language. In particular, they may function as "frames" for other units of language.
3. These early prosodic "frames" seem to be more stable than the segmental characteristics that may accompany them.
4. The maturation of the control of speech may proceed in the developmental order of fundamental frequency first, then timing, and lastly segmental contrasts.
5. The developing prosodic system interacts with the other aspects of language and appears to reach adult characteristics only at puberty.

These observations suggest that a "prosody calendar" may be a useful way to view the general process of speech development.

Stress patterns in a language could also provide important organizational clues to the infant. One of the things an infant must learn to do is to recognize words in the flow of speech. How do infants recognize words in the fast flow of adult speech? Could prosody help? It may. If English does in fact have a basic alternation of strong and weak syllables as its underlying rhythm, then the infant can use this expectation to process the temporal pattern of speech. With this temporal background, a simple strategy to recognize words could follow a basic principle: Segment speech at the onsets of strong syllables as a first step in recognizing words. In English, content words tend to be either monosyllabic or polysyllabic with stress on the first syllable (Cutler, 1992). Adults also are highly sensitive to stress patterns in English. For example, they can use this information even when segmental information is eliminated by auditory masking (Smith, Cutler, Butterfield, and Nimmo-Smith, 1989).

Syllables and Prosody. The syllable plays a major role in most discussions of prosody. In fact, it is difficult to discuss prosody without referring to syllables. Edwards and Beckman (1988) concluded that the syllable is a necessary unit to describe stress patterns and the phonetic characteristics of larger units, such as phrases or clauses. The syllable would then appear to be central to the description of prosodic phenomena. But what is the syllable? Chapter 2 discussed the difficulties of defining it but left the real chore to this chapter. Most people have an intuitive sense of what a syllable is. Most of us can agree on the number of syllables contained in words like *bookshelf* (2), *territory* (4), and *computer* (3). Unhappily, intuition is not matched by an ease of formal definition. The syllable is not easy to define, and lengthy treatises have been written on this troublesome subject (Fudge, 1969; Hooper, 1972; Venneman, 1972; Kahn, 1980; Goldsmith, 1990). The following discussion is a selective review of a complicated literature.

Two general approaches have been taken to define the syllable. First, the syllable is recognized by many writers as a phonological constituent that is made up of phonetic segments. In other words, the syllable has an internal structure. Goldsmith (1990) condensed the outcome of traditional work on the syllable's internal structure as follows: "The syllable is a phonological constituent composed of zero or more consonants, followed by a vowel, and ending with a shorter string of zero or more consonants" (p. 108). This rather abstract statement describes how phonetic segments are combined to make syllables. But it is not fail-safe. One shortcoming is that it excludes syllabic consonants, such as the nasal /n/ used by many speakers to form the second syllable of the word *button.* To take account of these sounds, we might revise Goldsmith's statement as follows: "The syllable is a phonological constituent composed of (a) zero or more consonants, followed by a vowel, and ending with a shorter string of zero or more consonants, or (b) a sonorant consonant serving as a syllabic nucleus." This definition, however, would not win a prize in lexicography. Can we do better?

In the second general approach, the syllable has been described in relation to the overall sound pattern of the speech stream in which it occurs. Bloomfield ([1933] 1984) wrote of syllabicity in terms of the "force" that sounds have upon the ear. He used the term **sonority** in reference to this auditory force: "Evidently some of the phonemes are more sonorous than the phonemes (or the silence) which immediately precede or follow. . . ." (p. 120). Phonemes having a crest of sonority were said to be syllabic; other phonemes were considered nonsyllabic. Sonority is not without problems of its own. This concept has been criticized because of the difficulty of providing a suitable definition. The suggested correlates of sonority include: degree of perceptual prominence, total acoustic energy, vocal tract openness, or the physiological effort given by the speaker to sound production. Highly sonorant sounds tend to be prominent perceptually, are associated with strong acoustic energy, have an open vocal tract, and involve a certain combination of respiratory and phonatory activity. These are relative terms, so that determination of degree of sonority depends on a sound's phonetic environment. For additional discussion, see the works of Christman (1992), Clements (1990), Keating (1983), Ladefoged (1993), and Price (1980).

If these two general approaches are combined, we could conclude that the syllable has a loosely specified internal structure and an auditory impact in the flow of speech. Any definition of the syllable must reconcile these internal and external criteria. The following comments work toward this goal.

As a further step toward a definition, Figure 6-2 shows the internal structure of the syllable commonly recognized in modern phonological theory. Hierarchically beneath the syllable are the components of **onset** and **rhyme.** The onset is either null (zero) or is realized as one or more consonants. The rhyme has two components, the **nucleus** (vowel element) and an optional **coda** (consonant or consonant cluster). This diagram roughly accords with the definition given earlier of a syllable's internal structure. But it goes further by proposing not only that the syllable is composed of phonetic segments, but that the syllable has the subdivisions of onset and rhyme, with the rhyme being composed of a nucleus and coda. This syllable structure helps to account for a variety of phonological and psychological phenomena, ranging from syllabic influences on phonological patterns to slips of the tongue in everyday speech.

Understanding the internal structure of syllables is important because syllables are linked to their constituent segments through language-specific rules. Within a particular language, phonetic segments are regulated by principles that are based on syllable type and position of the segment within the syllable. A speaker of American English knows that *gvise* and *tleen* are not likely to be English words, because the initial consonant clusters violate the phoneme sequencing constraints of the language. Many important phonological principles are based on how segments relate to their parent syllables.

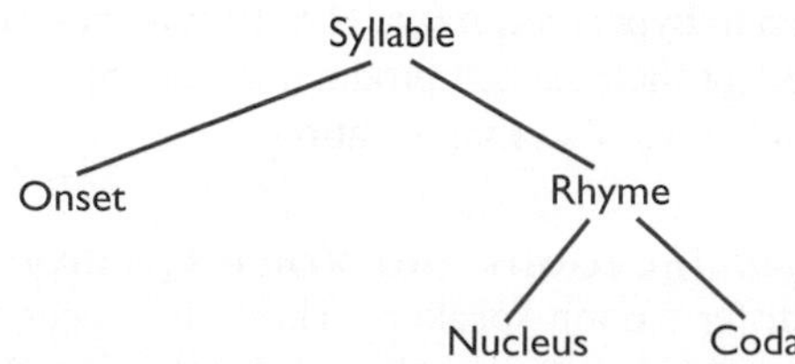

FIGURE 6-2
Basic structure of the syllable, as recognized by many linguists.

Now for the second part of the definition. Recall that syllables are identified within the prosodic flow of an utterance. Many linguists categorize syllables as heavy or light, depending on their prominence in this flow. A popular way of scaling this prominence is in terms of sonority. As Bloomfield ([1933] 1984) observed, some sounds are associated with a crest of sonority; these are syllabic sounds. This formulation suggests that there are two classes of sounds: sonorants and nonsonorants. However, sonority is perhaps better regarded as a scalar rather than a binary feature, meaning that sounds are not simply sonorant or nonsonorant, but that they have **degrees** of sonority. Sounds can be scaled according to the degree of sonority they typically have, as shown in Table 6-1.

Sonority values are important not only for understanding the relative prominence of a sound in the flow of speech but also for understanding the way in which phonetic constituents are arranged within the syllable. According to a principle called the Sonority Principle, consonant clusters are usually formed so that different manners of articulation are sequenced to allow one sonority peak for each syllable. For example, if the sounds [i], [t], [r], and [z] are to be arranged within a syllable, then [t r i z] is a good arrangement, providing for a sequence of sonority that builds up from [t] to [r] to [i] and then declines again to [z]. Think of the ideal pattern of speech as a series of triangular peaks. Each peak is a sonorant crest and, thus, the nucleus of a syllable. Vowels are usually the sonorant crests because they are the most sonorant of all sounds. But sonorant consonants can also occur as crests. In a word such as *button,* the nasal /n/ can be a sonorant crest following the sonorant dip for [t]. There are certainly exceptions to the Sonority Principle in syllable structure; for example, words like *axe* and *lapse* do not conform to this principle. But it has general application to the syllables of English and most languages.

TABLE 6-1
Sonority Values Assigned to Selected Phonemes

Phoneme(s)	Value
/ɑ/	10
/e/, /o/	9
/i/, /u/	8
/r/, /w/	7
/l/	6
/m/, /n/	5
/s/	4
/v/, /z/, /ð/	3
/f/, /θ/	2
/b/, /d/, /g/	1
/p/, /t/	0.5

As noted in Chapter 2, the concept of sonority as the basis of syllabification encounters difficulties with some phonetic sequences. Consider vowel + vowel sequences in words like *trio, piano,* and *chaos.* The abutting vowels are not necessarily associated with two distinct crests of sonority but instead may be produced as one prolonged interval of sonority. The solution may take two different forms. One is to acknowledge that the prolonged sonority interval is related to two distinct sound patterns. That is, the interval contains two segments of high sonority that can potentially be separated by a short pause or a glottal stop without destroying the form of the word. The other solution is to allow segments of high sonority to occur in a single syllable only if they form a diphthong.

We take sonority as the *sine qua non* of syllabicity. Syllabic phonemes are relatively sonorous in the flow of speech, and segments within syllables are generally arranged to form a single sonorant peak within the syllable. The concept of sonority helps to explain the two major facets of a syllable, its internal organization and its identification in the flow of speech. Therefore, a syllable is a sonorant crest in the auditory pattern of speech. There are several advantages to this definition, but one in particular is that it affords a way to match up prosodic and segmental features of speech. Silverman and Pierrehumbert (1990) observe that associating prosodic specifications with sonority peaks is an effective way of coordinating prosodic and segmental features. Prosodic structure may be important to infants in their early learning about speech. Prosody, and its rhythmic base, is a possible foundation on which the infant can learn about the phonetic structure of a language (Kent, Mitchell, and Sancier, 1991).

Paralinguistic Aspects

Emotional State. A speaker's affect (attitude, commitment, mood, emotion) can interact with prosodic characteristics. One example is the occurrence of rising intonation on what is intended as a declarative utterance—a pattern that may suggest a lack of certainty, a desire to elicit a response from the listener, or even a lower social status than one's listener. Various emotional states can be signaled in a speaker's voice, and the acoustic cues for these states are combined with the various cues that signal prosodic distinctions and voice quality. According to Hollien (1980), acoustic changes associated with different emotional states are as follows:

1. Anger—increase in vocal fundamental frequency, increase in vocal intensity, and moderate increase in tempo.
2. Fear—moderate increases in vocal fundamental frequency, vocal intensity, and tempo.
3. Grief, sorrow, or depression—moderate decreases in vocal fundamental frequency, vocal intensity, and tempo.

Paralinguistic factors also can affect the tempo of speech. The following general patterns are drawn from a review by Rochester (1972) on pause durations in speech:

1. Pause duration increases with the complexity of a communicative task. For example, pauses tend to be longer in explanations than in descriptions. This result holds for both silent and filled (voiced) pauses.
2. Highly variable results have been reported on the effects of affective states, although a few studies indicate that pause durations consistently increase under anxiety.
3. Social interaction variables that have been reported to affect pauses are the presence versus the absence of an audience as well as audience sensitivity.

Speaking Style. There are many variations in style of speaking. Individuals often adjust their style to communicative setting. For instance, a formal style is typically used while giving a lecture, but a casual style is adopted while talking privately with a close friend. One particular style variation is important in clinical phonetics. It concerns the distinction between ordinary conversational speech and **clear speech.** Clear speech refers to the kind of speech that is used in a deliberate attempt to increase intelligibility or understanding. Clear speech might be used over a poor telephone connection or in speaking to a very young child or to an individual with a severe hearing impairment who appears to have difficulty in understanding speech. Compared to conversational speech, clear speech is (1) slower (longer pauses between words and lengthening of some speech sounds), (2) more likely to avoid modified or reduced forms of consonant and vowel segments, and (3) characterized by a greater intensity of obstruent sounds, particularly stop consonants (Picheny, Durlach, and Braida, 1986). All in all, these modifications make the speech slower and more acoustically contrastive. Vowels in ordinary conversational speech frequently are modified or reduced, which causes them to lose some of their acoustic distinctiveness. Likewise, stops occurring in word-final position in conversation often are not released, so that the burst cue is not available to listeners. But in clear speech, vowels are not likely to be modified or reduced, and stop consonants (and consonants in general) tend to be released. More detailed articulatory differences between casual and clear speech are described by Adams (1990) in a study using an X-ray microbeam.

Lindblom (1990) proposed a theory that accounts for some of the variations that speakers introduce according to communicative settings and needs. The theory contends that speakers vary their speech output along a continuum from hypospeech to hyperspeech (the H & H hypothesis). That is, speakers adapt their speech production patterns to the various circumstances of communication.

Voice Qualifications and Voice Quality. Voice qualities differ among speakers. These differences are one reason we can identify people just by the sound of their voices. Individuals also can have different voice qualities, either by intentional modification or because of a physical condition, such as a cold. This book cannot cover voice quality in any depth, but it is important to recognize that the quality of voice is relevant to phonetic transcription. An extremely hoarse or breathy voice may affect the speaker's ability to make voicing adjustments in speech. Young children may use a variety of voice qualities, some of which can make transcription difficult. Children with developmental disabilities, such as Down syndrome or cerebral palsy, frequently have voice qualities that hinder phonetic distinctions. Therefore, it can be important to note a persistent voice quality as part of a phonetic transcription.

Several different rating systems have been developed for voice qualifications and voice quality. These systems are concerned with identifying and rating the severity of phonatory features, such as roughness, hoarseness, strain, tremor, loudness or pitch instability, and pitch or loudness level. It is beyond the scope of this book to discuss the various possibilities. The reader is referred especially to Laver (1980), who describes a detailed system for the phonetic classification of voice. His system was adopted by the Working Party for Pathological Speech and Voice, established at the 1989 meeting of the International Phonetics Association Congress in Kiel (Duckworth, Allen, Hardcastle, and Ball, 1990). Simpler systems, however, may suffice for certain applications, such as indicating the presence of hoarseness. One such system is included in the following section.

Clinical Assessment of Suprasegmentals

This section mentions briefly some approaches for the clinical assessment of suprasegmental features. In the main, assessment of prosody traditionally has been accomplished within the general framework of assessment for specific disorders, such as aphasia, deafness, autism, and second language learning. Few general-purpose methods of prosodic assessment have been introduced.

Crystal's *Prosody Profile (PROP)*. One of the few general-purpose assessments of prosody is Crystal's (1982) *Prosody Profile (PROP)*, which was specifically designed to profile prosodic disability. Crystal's system is compatible with the view that prosodic disability is basically a phonological deficit in which the speaker makes inappropriate or inaccurate use of prosodic features. PROP is a single-page chart that summarizes linguistic uses of pitch, loudness, speaking rate, pause, and rhythm. Prosodic analysis reflects three primary ways in which pitch patterns are used in a language: (1) **Tone units** describe the organization of connected speech into structures such as clauses, phrases, and words. A tone unit is defined as a "finite set of pitch movements, grouped into a distinctive contour and uttered with a distinctive rhythm" (Crystal, 1982, p. 114). (2) **Tones** are the elemental components from which tone units are constructed. Every syllable in a given tone unit has a tone. (3) **Tonicity** is tonic placement, or the selection of one syllable to stand out from all the others in a tone unit. This syllable is called the tonic syllable, and it is said to carry the nuclear tone. Nuclear tones are of three major types: simple (unidirectional pitch movements of falling, rising, and level), complex (change in direction of pitch movement within the syllable), and compound (combinations of tones acting as a single tone). For a related discussion, see Brewster (1989).

Shriberg, Kwiatkowski, and Rasmussen's *Prosody-Voice Screening Profile (PVSP)*. Approaches to *describe* deviations in prosody, such as the PROP procedure and the systems presented in the following two sections, can be contrasted with approaches used to *quantify* deviant prosody and voice. Figures 6-3 and 6-4 illustrate the basic elements of one quantified approach, titled *Prosody-Voice Screening Profile (PVSP)* (Shriberg, Kwiatkowski, and Rasmussen, 1990). The following brief description of the PVSP illustrates how this approach is used in communicative disorders.

PVSP data are based on a sample of natural conversational speech between an examiner and a speaker. In practice, one audiorecorded speech sample can be used to assess language production, speech production (e.g., phonetic transcription), and prosody-voice. A set of exclusion codes (Figure 6-4) is first applied to identify those utterances that cannot be coded for prosody or voice. The relative occurrence of each of these codes provides useful information on paralinguistic and nonlinguistic aspects of a person's communication. For example, speech samples from adults with cognitive disabilities have been shown to include a high frequency of certain behaviors (e.g., lip smacks) that are seldom present in samples from other speakers (Shriberg and Widder, 1990).

The examiner proceeds to code each utterance in the sample as *appropriate* or *inappropriate* on each of the 31 prosody-voice variables shown in Figure 6-4. Standards for these judgments are provided by audio training exemplars, much like the tutorial materials in this text are used to teach phonetic transcription. Prosody includes codes for utterances that meet criteria for inappropriate phrasing, rate, or stress. Voice includes codes for utterances that meet criteria for inappropriate loudness, pitch, or laryngeal or resonance quality. Note how these categories extend the prosodic variables discussed earlier in this chapter.

Figure 6-5 illustrates one clinical research use of the PVSP measure (Shriberg, 1993). The graphs shown in Figure 6-5 were produced by a computer program that compares prosody-voice "profiles" of different speakers. In this example, the filled circles indicate the averaged performance of a group of children with developmental speech delay of unknown origin. The open triangles are the averaged performance of a group of children whose speech delays were suspected to involve deficits in linguistic-motor processing. As shown in the top left panel, the children with the

Prosody-Voice Screening Profile (PVSP) Scoring Form

Identification

Name_______	Tape Label_______	☐ Telegraphic Speech ☐ Respiratory Involvement		
Age_______ M___ F___	_______	**Screening Outcome**		
Sample Date_______	Side A_____ B_____		**Pass**	**Fail**
Sample Type_______	**Counter Number**	Phrasing	____	____
		Rate	____	____
Examiner_______	Beginning of Sample ____	Stress	____	____
Scoring Date_______	First Coded Utterance ____	Loudness	____	____
		Pitch	____	____
Scorer_______	Last Coded Utterance ____	Quality	____	____

Profile

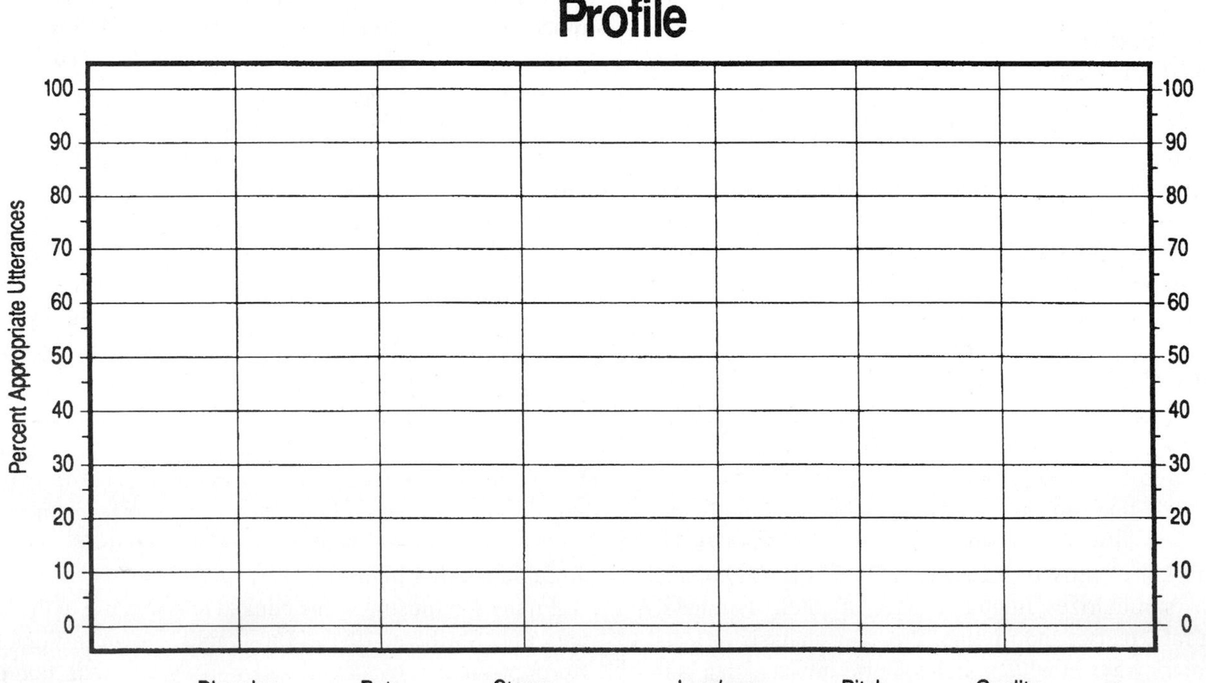

FIGURE 6-3
Cover page from *Prosody-Voice Screening Profile (PVSP)*. Shriberg, Kwiatkowski, and Rasmussen (1990). Tucson, AZ: Communication Skill Builders Inc. Reproduced with permission of the publisher.

Exclusion Codes

Content/Context	Environment	Register	States
C1 Automatic Sequential ___	E1 Interfering Noise ___	R1 Character Register ___	S1 Belch ___
C2 Back Channel/Aside ___	E2 Recorder Wow/ Flutter ___	R2 Narrative Register ___	S2 Cough/Throat Clear ___
C3 I Don't Know ___	E3 Too Close to Microphone ___	R3 Negative Register ___	S3 Food in Mouth ___
C4 Imitation ___	E4 Too Far from Microphone ___	R4 Sound Effects ___	S4 Hiccup ___
C5 Interruption/ Overtalk ___		R5 Whisper ___	S5 Laugh ___
C6 Not 4 (+) Words ___			S6 Lip Smack ___
C7 Only One Word ___			S7 Body Movement ___
C8 Only Person's Name ___			S8 Sneeze ___
C9 Reading ___			S9 Telegraphic ___
C10 Singing ___			S10 Yawn ___
C11 Second Repetition ___			
C12 Too Many Unintelligibles ___			

Prosody-Voice Codes

Prosody

Phrasing	Rate	Stress
1 Appropriate ___	1 Appropriate ___	1 Appropriate ___
2 Sound/Syllable Repetition ___	9 Slow Articulation/Pause Time ___	13 Multisyllabic Word Stress ___
3 Word Repetition ___	10 Slow/Pause Time ___	14 Reduced/Equal Stress ___
4 Sound/Syllable and Word Repetition ___	11 Fast ___	15 Excessive/Equal/ Misplaced Stress ___
5 More than One Word Repetition ___	12 Fast/Acceleration ___	16 Multiple Stress Features ___
6 One Word Revision ___		
7 More than One Word Revision ___		
8 Repetition and Revision ___		

Voice

Loudness	Pitch	Quality: Laryngeal Features	Quality: Resonance Features
1 Appropriate ___	1 Appropriate ___	1 Appropriate ___	1 Appropriate ___
17 Soft ___	19 Low Pitch/Glottal Fry ___	23 Breathy ___	30 Nasal ___
18 Loud ___	20 Low Pitch ___	24 Rough ___	31 Denasal ___
	21 High Pitch/Falsetto ___	25 Strained ___	32 Nasopharyngeal ___
	22 High Pitch ___	26 Break/Shift/ Tremulous ___	
		27 Register Break ___	
		28 Diplophonia ___	
		29 Multiple Laryngeal Features ___	

FIGURE 6-4
Exclusion codes and prosody-voice codes from *Prosody-Voice Screening Profile (PVSP)*. Shriberg, Kwiatkowski, and Rasmussen (1990). Tucson, AZ: Communication Skill Builders Inc. Reproduced with permission of the publisher.

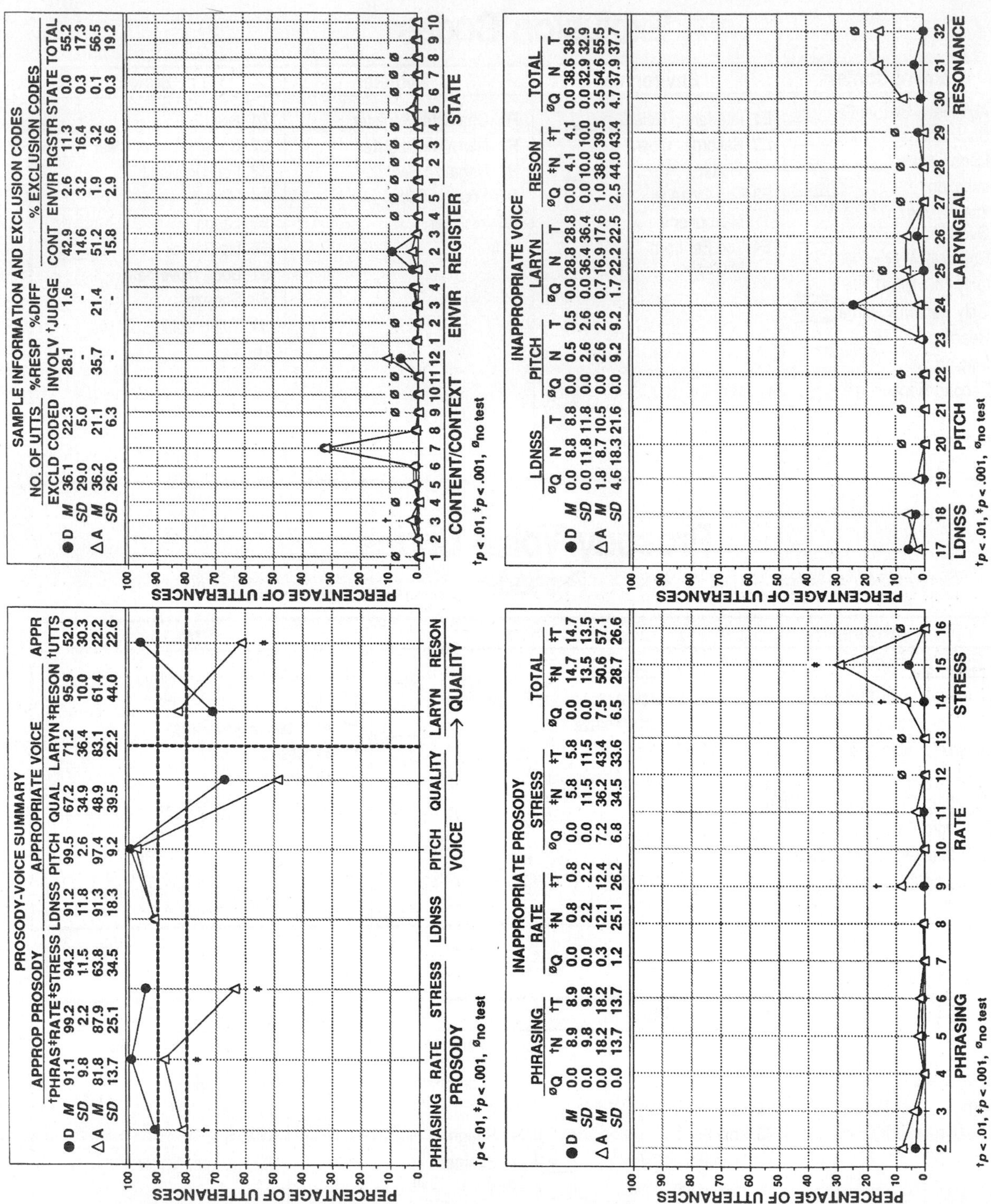

FIGURE 6-5
Illustration of clinical research use of *Prosody-Voice Screening Profile (PVSP)*. See Figure 6-4 for the key to each of the 31 exclusion codes and 31 prosody-voice codes. Shriberg (1993). Reproduced with permission of the publisher.

suspected linguistic-motor deficits had significantly lower scores on each of the three prosody variables and on vocal resonance. The two lower panels provide comparative information for each of the individual prosody and voice codes listed in Figure 6-4. Just as articulation tests are used to quantify and profile segmental aspects of speech (see Chapter 9), prosody-voice data are used to quantify and profile a speaker's suprasegmental status (cf. McSweeny and Shriberg, 2001).

Selected Extensions to the International Phonetic Alphabet. As noted earlier, a special working party established by the International Phonetics Association adopted Laver's system for the transcription of voice quality. Laver's system affords a detailed description but requires some effort to learn and apply. Some of the IPA extensions for atypical speech (Duckworth et al., 1990) may suffice for some transcription purposes. Some examples of the extensions follow. In each example, the symbol **x** represents a phonetic symbol in a transcription.

Pausing is indicated by periods placed within parentheses, with the number of periods indicating the relative length of a pause:

[**x**(.)**x**]—short pause

[**x**(..)**x**]—medium-length pause

[**x**(...)**x**]—long pause

Loudness is indicated with the symbols **f** *(forte)* and **p** *(piano)* placed as subscripts around the affected portion of the transcription (bold letters are used in the examples here):

[xxx{$_{\mathbf{f}}$xxx$_{\mathbf{f}}$}xxx]—loud speech

[xxx{$_{\mathbf{ff}}$xxx$_{\mathbf{ff}}$}xxx]—louder speech

[xxx{$_{\mathbf{p}}$xxx$_{\mathbf{p}}$}xxx]—soft speech

Rate of speech is shown by use of the terms *allegro* and *lento:*

[xxx{$_{\mathbf{allegro}}$xxx$_{\mathbf{allegro}}$}xxx]—fast speech

[xxx{$_{\mathbf{lento}}$xxx$_{\mathbf{lento}}$}xxx]—slow speech

Voice quality is noted similarly with labeled braces. For example, use of falsetto voice is represented by the symbol **F:**

[xxx{$_{\mathbf{F}}$xxx$_{\mathbf{F}}$}xxx]

Symbols for Conversational Analysis. Transcription of conversational samples may require the use of symbols for situations that do not arise, or do not arise frequently, in other kinds of speech samples. Some conventions for conversational analysis are described as follows (drawn from French and Local, 1986):

=	Shows that one utterance follows immediately (no delay) from another.
(.)	marks a pause of less than a tenth of a second, which is a rather short pause in speech. Longer pauses can be noted quantitatively by entering the estimated duration of the pause within parentheses; e.g., (2.5) indicates a pause of 2.5 seconds.
:	indicates lengthening of the sound it follows.
.h (or h.)	represents outbreath. The symbol can be repeated to indicate longer outbreaths.
[	shows the point at which overlapping talking begins. A slash (/) is used to indicate where the overlapping talking ends.
<f>	is placed below an interval of talk to show that it is produced more loudly *(forte)* than is normal for the speaker.
<p>	is placed below an interval of talk to show that it is produced more quietly *(piano)* than is normal for the speaker.
<cr>	is placed below an interval of talk to show that it is produced with increasing loudness *(crescendo).*
<l>	is placed below an interval of talk to show that it is produced more slowly *(lento)* than is normal for the speaker.
...	marks an omission of a stretch of talk.
***	indicates an obscure or unintelligible utterance. Each asterisk represents one syllable.

Referring to these symbols, interpret the following conversational sample:

Well **<1.0>** I think that the problem is clear **h.h.h.**

|———————— f ————————|

They didn't read the directions = They just went on with it. **h.**

|———————— f ————————|

|———————— cr ————————|

No: wonder:, then, that it didn't work as expected. **h.**

This is the last time I will let them be unsupervised. **h.**

|———————— p ————————|

COARTICULATION

Consider the sentence, "Could you keep her stew steaming hot?" As produced by a speaker of General American English, this sentence would have a phonetic transcription like the following:

[kud ju kip hɚ stu stimɪŋ hɔt]

If we studied this utterance in detail with acoustic analysis (discussed in Chapter 10) or with an X-ray motion picture, we would discover these facts:

1. The [k] in *could* is produced with a back tongue articulation, but the [k] in *keep* is articulated with a relatively front tongue position.
2. The [h] in *her* is produced with an [ɝ]-like vocal tract configuration, but the [h] in *hot* has an [ɔ]-like vocal tract configuration.
3. The [s] in *stew* is produced with lip rounding, but the [s] in *steaming* is not.
4. The vowels in *steaming* are nasalized, but the vowel in *stew* is not.

These observations indicate that what we consider to be the same phonetic segment is not necessarily produced in the same way in different utterances. Actually, speech is replete with these modifications. Sounds are adapted to their phonetic contexts to make speech easier and faster. Many of these modifications are grouped together under the term **coarticulation,** which means that the production of a sound is influenced by other sounds around it, that is, by its phonetic context.

What are the contextual factors that cause coarticulation in items 1–4 of the list just identified?

In item 1, the [k] in *keep* is followed by the front vowel [i], whereas the [k] in *could* is followed by the back vowel [ʊ]. The exact place of articulation for the stop [k] is accommodated to the following vowel. If the vowel is front, then the [k] is made near the front of the oral cavity. But if the vowel is back, then the [k] also is made more as a back sound.

In item 2, the vocal tract configuration during the production of [h] anticipates the configuration of the following vowel. This is possible because the [h] sound does not have a highly specified position for the tongue, jaw, or lips. Therefore, the [h] in *her* can be produced with lip rounding and rhotic articulation suitable for vowel [ɝ]. Similarly, the [h] in *hot* can be produced with an open jaw and a low-back tongue position suitable for vowel [ɔ]. We can say that the [h] is *coproduced* with the following vowel.

In item 3, the [s] in *stew* is produced with lip rounding because this labial articulation is needed for the following vowel and does not interfere with production of the [s]. Lip rounding is not observed for the [s] in *steaming* because the following vowel [i] is not a rounded vowel. The fricative [s] can be rounded or not, depending on the following vowel.

In item 4, the vowels [i] and [ɪ] in *steaming* are both nasalized because they either precede a nasal consonant (in the case of [i]) or occur between two nasals (in the case of [ɪ]). Vowels can assume the nasalization of a neighboring consonant.

In each instance, the articulatory modification of a sound can be explained by a consideration of the phonetic context. These modifications give speech articulation a complex, highly overlapping character. The segments of speech interact, so that some of their features or properties are coarticulated (articulated together). Coarticulation refers to the various events in speech in which the vocal tract has simultaneous adjustments that are appropriate for two or more sounds. The direction of a coarticulatory effect can be described as forward (anticipatory) or backward (retentive). In forward coarticulation, an articulatory feature for a phonetic segment is evident in the production of an earlier segment. Nearly all the examples discussed above are forward coarticulation.

Backward coarticulation is illustrated with the utterance, "Please give me a cup of tea." An X-ray motion picture of most speakers would reveal that the velopharynx is open during the [i] of *me* but not during the [i] of *tea.* How do we explain this difference? Notice that the coarticulated property of velopharyngeal opening (nasalization) is attributable to the [m] that precedes the [i] in *me.* In this case, the direction of the coarticulatory effect is backward in the speech stream—hence, backward coarticulation.

Coarticulation usually is explained in terms of the concepts of spreading, shingling, or blending of articulatory properties across neighboring speech sounds. Although these three terms have a general similarity in their meaning, they are not identical in their implications for understanding the mechanisms of coarticulation.

Spreading (also called feature spreading) denotes an expansion or stretching of an articulatory feature. This concept seems especially appropriate if we think of features as being extendable to reach from one segment to another. This idea was often implemented as a spreading of binary feature values (e.g., spreading of nasalization as a [+nasal] and spreading of lip rounding as a [+round]) (Moll and Daniloff, 1971; Benguerel and Cowan, 1974). As applied to item 3 discussed earlier, the lip rounding feature for the vowel [u] would be spread or stretched to the preceding consonants [s] and [t]. As Boyce and Espy-Wilson (1997) explain, this account implies that "the underlying articulatory plan (including trajectory of movement, placement of movement in the vocal tract, etc.) for producing the target segment has been altered from the form it would take if it were bordered by different neighboring segments; in other words, *articulatory plan varies by segmental context"* (p. 3742; emphasis added). Shingling is a similar idea but denotes an overlapping such that a feature from one sound overlies an adjacent sound segment, rather like one roof tile covering another. Shingling allows a sound segment to be penetrated by a particular feature from another segment. For example, some accounts of nasalization propose that a nasality feature is shingled from a nasal phone to its preceding or succeeding phone.

Blending (also called coproduction) does not alter the segmental articulatory plan but rather supposes that coarticulation results from the overlap and blending of unaltered articulatory plans for adjacent segments. That is, the articulation is reshaped to accommodate the segment's phonetic neighbors, but the segment itself is not altered. The result is an articulation that takes into account the overall nature of one segment vis-à-vis the nature of the segments that surround it. Therefore, a modified movement is produced that can be intermediate to the movements for the two sounds in question.

These different accounts of coarticulation hold implications for the development of speech in children. The spreading and shingling accounts suggest that children must construct different articulatory plans for different segmental contexts. Blending, however, implies that children can rely on stable articulatory plans for individual segments but learn to overlap and blend these unchanged plans for adjacent segments. It is relevant to note that coarticulation may differ across individual speakers (Van den Heuvel, Cranen, and Rietveld, 1996), which may also favor the blending account, on the assumption that individual speakers develop unique strategies for blending segments. Coarticulation is one consideration in explaining why children may produce a given sound correctly in one phonetic context but not in another. By drawing on principles of coarticulation, it is possible to design contexts that facilitate correct sound production (Kent, 1982).

Coarticulation is limited primarily by the compatibility of two sounds. A common way of determining compatibility is to compare the phonetic features of the two sounds in question. Consider a consonant sound C and a vowel sound V that form a syllable CV. First, let us assume that C is the bilabial consonant /b/ and V is any vowel. Because the bilabial consonant can be produced with virtually any tongue position (so long as the vocal tract is not obstructed by the lingual articulation), the tongue is free to anticipate the lingual articulation for the vowel. Therefore, [b] in the word *bee* will be produced with an [i]-like tongue position, and the [b] in the word *boo* will be produced with an [u]-like tongue position. That is, /b/ offers very little coarticulation resistance to the vowel's lingual articulation. Both the bilabial stops and the labiodental fricatives have minimal coarticulation resistance (Recasens, 1985; Fowler and Brancazio, 2000). Coarticulation resistance depends especially on articulatory constraints that limit the physiological adjustments for a particular phone (Recasens, Pallares, and Fontdevila, 1997; Tabain, 2001). But now consider that consonant C is the lingua-palatal consonant /ʃ/. Because this consonant has a highly specified tongue position, it is not free to accommodate the lingual articulation of the following vowel. In other words, it has a high coarticulation resistance.

Keating (1990) proposed a window model of coarticulation that defines a permissible variation for an individual articulator, depending on the phonetic context. The "window" is the range of values that can be assumed by a particular articulatory dimension for a given feature. The window defines the allowable contextual variability for a phonetic feature; it specifies a range of possible positions. For example, the jaw has a certain range of positions that can be assumed for a given feature such as closed or open. Similarly, the velum has a certain range of positions that it can take for a feature such as closed (nonnasal). For some segments, the window is narrow, so that little contextual variation can occur. For other segments, the window is wide, so that contextual variation is considerable. According to this model, a speaker discovers the allowable tolerance for an articulatory dimension that is associated with a particular feature.

DIACRITIC MARKS: AN [æ̃] IS NOT AN [æ̤] IS NOT AN [æː]

To this point in the book, we have been concerned with **broad transcription,** which makes use of phonemic symbols only. But when we transcribe the diverse allophonic variations (and misarticulations) that occur in speech, we have to use a finer, more detailed system than the set of phonemic symbols. For this kind of transcription, **narrow transcription,** it is necessary to use special modifiers called **diacritic marks.**

As a simple example, consider the speaker who tends to nasalize his speech. This speaker may produce the word *bad* with a nasalized vowel /æ̃/. This nasalization does not alter the selection of a phoneme symbol for the vowel, because in the English language, a nasalized /æ̃/ is still recognized as an [æ]. To indicate in the phonetic transcription that such a change in production has occurred, the diacritic mark [˜] is placed directly over the /æ/ symbol: [b æ̃ d]. Suppose that another speaker tends to produce vowels with a breathy voice, so that her production of the word *bad* has a conspicuous breathy quality. We can indicate this aspect of production by using the diacritic mark [̤], which is placed directly under the vowel symbol: [b æ̤ d].

The conventions for diacritic marks used in this book are not exactly the same as those of the International Phonetic Alphabet (IPA). We have departed slightly from the IPA system in favor of a system that we believe to be easier to learn and easier to use, especially as applied to communicative disorders. For the most part, our departures from the IPA system do not change the marks themselves but rather have to do with where the marks are placed. In the system used here, we have tried to be uniform by putting all the marks of a given category in a given position. For example, all the diacritic marks that refer to tongue position are placed directly under the phonemic symbol being modified, and all the diacritic marks that refer to lip position are placed directly over the phonemic symbol being modified.

The entire set of diacritic marks, or diacritics, is presented in Figure 6-6. Note that most of the diacritics are marked in one of six positions, represented by the numbers in Figure 6-6. A few miscellaneous marks are noted at the bottom right corner of the figure. Each numbered position is specified relative to the main symbol (IPA phonemic or phonetic symbol that is modified by the diacritic). The diacritic positions are as follows:

1. Onglide symbols, placed to the *upper left* of the main symbol.

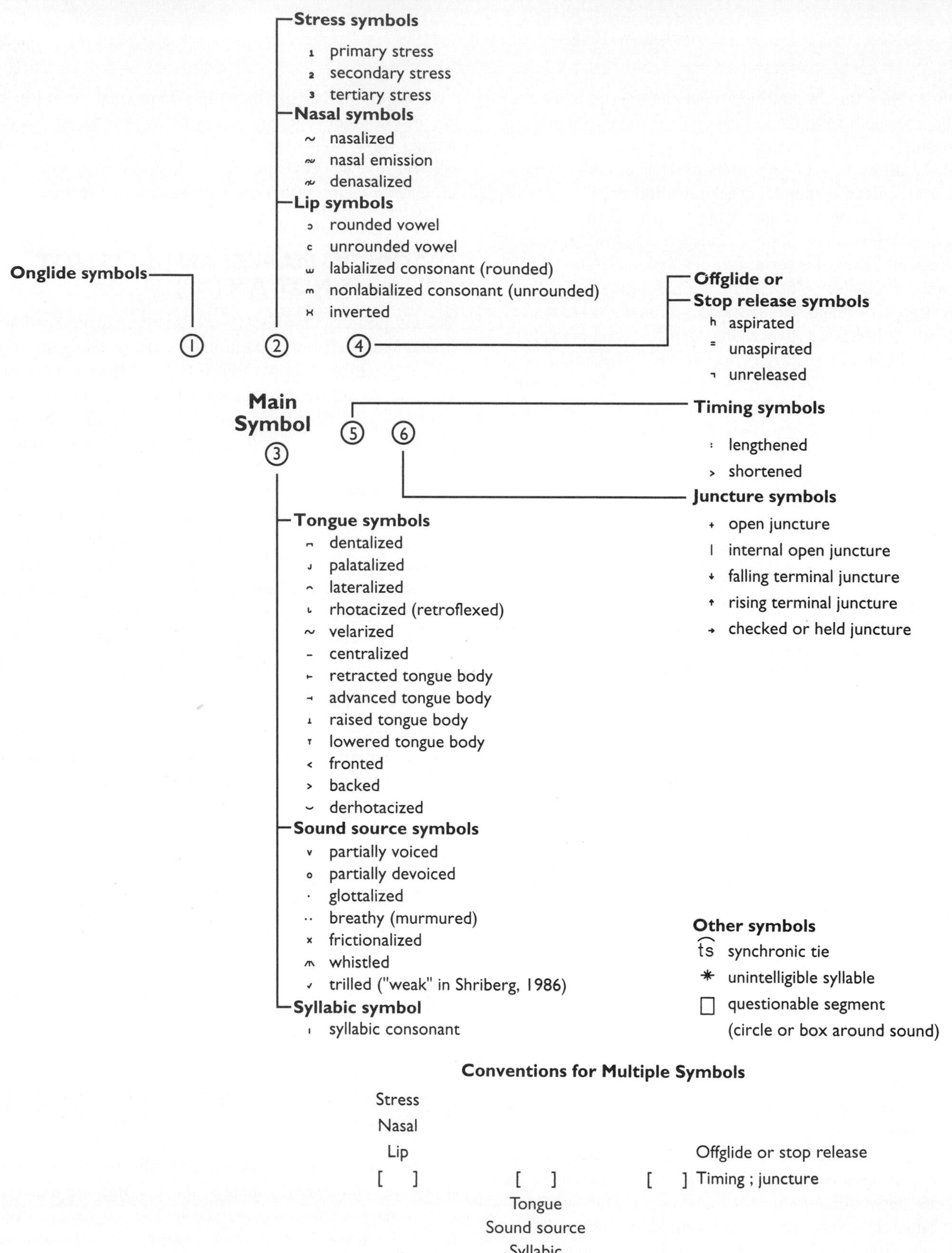

FIGURE 6-6

Diacritic marks for phonetic transcription. The numerals 1–6 show the placement of marks within a given category. For example, marks having to do with tongue position or adjustment are located under the phonemic symbol to be modified. When multiple diacritics are used, follow the conventions shown at the bottom of the figure (the brackets represent the main symbol). For example, when diacritics are to be used for both tongue and sound source, the tongue diacritic is written above that for sound source. Thus, a partially voiced, dentalized /s/ would be transcribed [s̪̬]. When diacritics from the same category are used together, they are written side by side; for example, a partially devoiced, trilled /r/ is transcribed [ɾ̥̌].

2. Stress symbols, placed *over* the main symbol.
2. Nasal symbols, placed *over* the main symbol (and directly under the stress symbol if both are used).
2. Lip symbols, placed *over* the main symbol (and directly under any stress or nasal symbols).
3. Tongue symbols, placed *under* the main symbol.
3. Sound source or larynx symbols, placed *under* the main symbol (and directly under any tongue symbols that are used).
3. Syllabic symbol, placed *under* the main symbol (and directly under any tongue or source symbols).
4. Offglide symbols, placed to the *upper right* of the main symbol.
4. Stop release symbols, placed to the *upper right* of the main symbol.
5. Timing symbols, placed directly *to the right* of the main symbol.
6. Juncture symbols, placed directly *to the right* of the main symbol (and following any timing symbols).

The diacritic marks, together with the definitions of their associated terms, are discussed within each major category as follows. Later, we will suggest that you return to these descriptions as you listen to examples on the audio sample.

ONGLIDE SYMBOLS

Onglide symbols represent a brief or fragmentary sound that precedes the main symbol in a transcription. For example, if a very brief [ə] is heard at the onset of a fricative [s], then the transcription would be [ᵊ s].

STRESS SYMBOLS

Stress marking is discussed in some detail elsewhere in this chapter. For the present, note that three degrees of stress are marked with the numerals 1, 2, or 3 placed above the main symbol, which must be a vowel. When stress is marked with this number system, the top line of the transcription is reserved for stress marks.

Primary Stress [t u b ə] (numeral 1 over u)

The numeral 1 is placed over a vowel that is judged to carry **primary,** or first-level, **stress.** This is the highest degree of stress in an utterance, although it is possible for more than one syllable in an utterance to carry primary stress.

Secondary Stress [ɛ m b ɑ r k] (numeral 2 over ɛ)

The numeral 2 is placed over a vowel that is judged to carry **secondary,** or second-level, **stress.** It is possible for a multi-syllable utterance to have two or more syllables with secondary stress.

Tertiary Stress [ə b a͡ʊ t] (numeral 3 over ə)

The numeral 3 is placed over a vowel that is judged to carry **tertiary,** or third-level, **stress.** This is the lowest degree of stress in an utterance, but it is possible for more than one syllable in an utterance to carry tertiary stress.

NASAL SYMBOLS

The nasal symbols describe aspects of velopharyngeal function, that is, the valving between the oral cavity and the nasal cavity.

Nasalized [m æ̃ n]

A **nasalized** sound is produced with nasal resonance, which is created by an open velopharyngeal port allowing voicing energy to radiate through the nasal cavity. Velopharyngeal opening is illustrated for a vowel in Figure 4-30. In English, we normally nasalize vowels produced before or after nasal consonants. Compare the [æ] sounds in *man* and *bad,* the former of which is nasalized and the latter of which is not. Nasalization is essentially "talking through the nose."

Nasal Emission [s m a͞ɪ l] (nasal emission mark over s)

The sound of **nasal emission** is characterized by the release of noise energy through the nose. Nasal emission does not commonly occur in normal speech but is frequently noted in the speech of people with a cleft palate or other velopharyngeal incompetence. These speakers, who cannot close the velopharyngeal port tightly, may allow the noise energy of a fricative like /s/ to escape through the nose.

Denasalized [r æ n] (denasalization mark over æ)

A **denasalized** segment is produced without nasalization or without an appropriate degree of nasalization. In normal English speech, this symbol rarely would be used, but it might be used for a speaker who failed to open the velopharyngeal port when it normally would open. If, for example, a child with cerebral palsy did not open the velopharynx for a vowel that is normally nasalized in English, one could mark the vowel as denasalized. In this case, the diacritic mark would indicate a deviation from the normal speech pattern of nasalization. A denasalized quality also may be heard for speakers with nasal congestion, as from a cold.

LIP SYMBOLS

Rounded (or Protruded) Vowel [sw i t] (rounding mark over i)

A **rounded** vowel is produced with a rounding, or protrusion, of the lips. In English, many of the back vowels are normally rounded, as in the case of /u/ and /o/. If you produce an /i/ while keeping the lips in a rounded state like that used for /u/, you should hear a marked difference in vowel quality. If a person uttered the word *sweet* but held the lip rounding needed for the /w/ throughout the word, then the vowel /i/ would be produced as a rounded vowel. The diacritic symbol for rounding may be easier to remember if you recall that ɔ is the symbol for a rounded vowel, phoneme /ɔ/.

Unrounded (or Unprotruded) Vowel [h u͗]

An unrounded vowel is produced without a rounding of the lips. Thus, if a speaker fails to round his or her lips for a vowel that is normally rounded, like /u/, this symbol would describe this deviation from the expected articulation.

Labialized Consonant [k̫ w i n]

A **labialized** consonant is produced with a constriction, or narrowing, of the lips (very much like rounding in the case of a vowel). In English, we tend to labialize many consonants when they are followed by a rounded vowel or by the /w/ sound. Thus, in the word *queen,* it is natural for a speaker to say a labialized /k/ in anticipation of the lip narrowing and protrusion for the /w/. This symbol is easy to remember if you recall that the /w/ is labialized and the diacritic mark is like a small *w* placed over the phonemic segment. Many English consonants tolerate labialization. For example, in the word *stew* /s t u/, lip rounding needed for the /u/ usually begins during the preceding /s/, so that both /s/ and /t/ are produced with lip rounding. Figure 6-7 illustrates the difference in lip configuration for a labialized and nonlabialized /s/.

Nonlabialized Consonant [w͆ i d]

The consonant is not articulated with a constriction, or narrowing, of the lips. If a speaker failed to narrow and protrude the lips for the /w/ in *weed,* the nonlabialization symbol would be appropriate. Try to say *weed* without labialization.

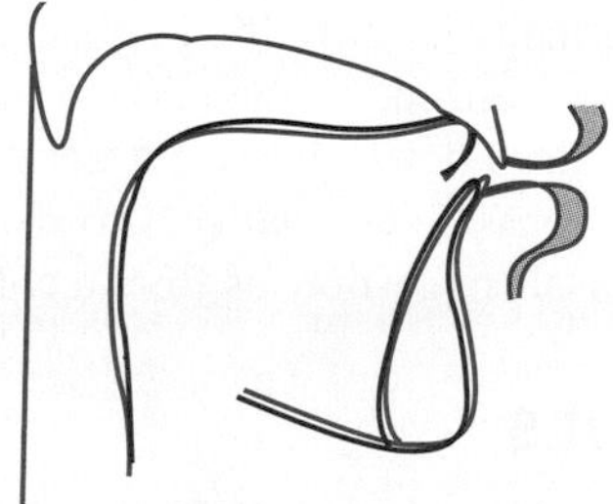

FIGURE 6-7
Articulatory configurations for a labialized (black line) and nonlabialized (red line) /s/. The shaded region shows the difference in lip position. For the labialized production, the vocal tract is lengthened in the forward direction.

Inverted Lip [b̆ i n]

Inversion, as illustrated in Figure 6-8, involves a curling back of the lip. In extreme inversion, the lip may be pulled back over the teeth. Inversion is not a common articulatory modification and is observed more often in neurologically or structurally impaired speakers than in normal speakers. Figure 6-8 is derived from an X-ray film of a child with cerebral palsy.

TONGUE SYMBOLS

The tongue symbols describe modifications of lingual articulation. Most of these symbols describe a modification in the place of articulation, but a few of them describe modifications in the manner of articulation.

Dentalized [w ɪ d̪ θ]

A **dentalized** consonant is articulated with the tip of the tongue against the back of the upper teeth (more precisely, the upper central incisors). Dentalization is illustrated in Figure 6-9. We normally dentalize the stop /d/ in words like *width,* where a dental fricative follows the stop. You should be able to feel a difference in the position of your tongue for

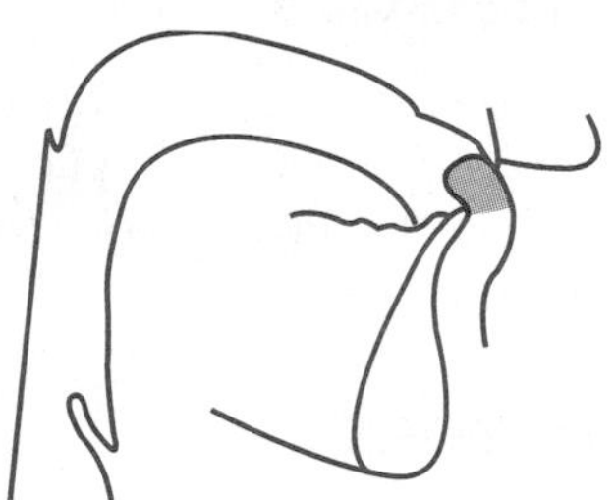

FIGURE 6-8
X-ray tracing of a child with cerebral palsy showing inversion of lower lip. Note that the lower lip is curled back behind the incisors.

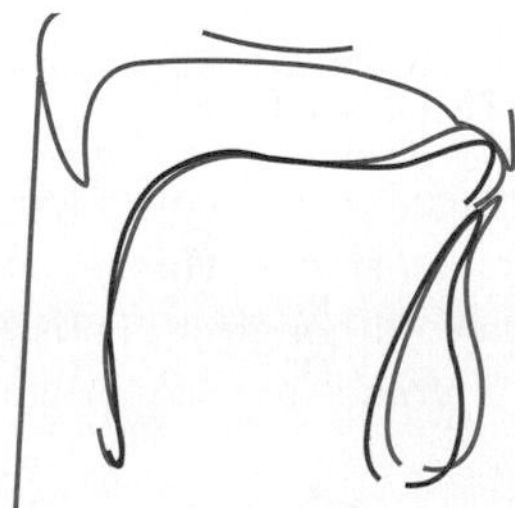

FIGURE 6-9
Articulatory configurations of an alveolar (black line) and dentalized (red line) consonant made with tongue tip contact. In the dentalized production, the tongue tip is farther forward, making contact with the area behind the upper frontal incisors.

the /d/ in *width* and the /d/ in *lid.* Of course, normally the /d/ is articulated as a lingua-alveolar stop. The dental allophone [d̪] is in complementary distribution with the more usual alveolar [d]. Some children dentalize many or all of the sounds that are alveolar in adult speech. Note that dentalization of a normally alveolar sound is an example of fronting, or forward movement of place of articulation.

Palatalized [s̡ i l]

In **palatalized** consonant articulation, the blade, or front part of the tongue minus the tip, is close to the palatal area just behind the alveolar ridge. Perhaps the simplest way of viewing this modification is in its similarity to the normal articulation for the palatal fricative /ʃ/. A sketch of a palatalized and a normal (nonpalatalized) /s/ articulation is given in Figure 6-10. In Russian, which has both palatalized and nonpalatalized consonants, the former are called *soft* and the latter *hard* consonants, to signify the difference in auditory quality.

Lateralized [s̭ l i p]

The distinguishing property of a **lateralized** sound is the release of air through the sides (or at least one side) of the mouth. Thus, a lateralized /s/ is characterized by emission of the fricative air around the sides of the tongue, rather than through a narrow groove or slit in the midline of the articulator. One way of simulating lateral [s] is to place your tongue in position for an [l] and try to produce an [s]. You have succeeded if you produce a sound best described as "slurpy" or "lisping."

Rhotacized (or Retroflexed) [h ɑ r ʃ˞ ɚ]

As mentioned earlier, *r* coloring is a complicated articulation that takes at least two forms. One form is literally **retroflexion,** that is, involving a backward (*retro-*) turning (*flexion*) of the tongue tip. The other form takes the appearance of a bunching of the tongue in the front of the mouth, essentially in the palatal area. Ladefoged (1993) uses the term **rhotacized** to describe *r* coloring, whichever articulation may be involved, and we think this term is a good one because it does not have the inflexible and sometimes misleading articulatory interpretation of a word like retroflexion. At this point, it is sufficient to say that a sound with a retroflex modification has an *r* coloring or *r* similarity. This modification normally occurs in the word *harsher,* for which the /ʃ/ is rhotacized owing to the influence of the preceding and following *r* sounds. Although the difference is subtle to untrained ears, you might be able to perceive the effect of rhotacization by comparing the /ʃ/ sounds in the words *harsher* and *wishy.* It may help to prolong the fricative portions in the two words as you say them.

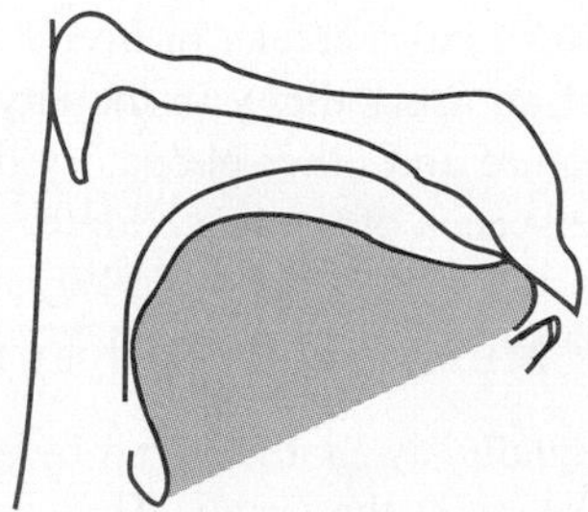

FIGURE 6-10
Articulatory configurations of a normal alveolar /s/ (black line) and a palatalized allophone (red line). In the palatalized production, the blade of the tongue is raised toward the palatal area.

Velarized [f i l̰]

Velarization is a constriction of the vocal tract between the dorsum of the tongue and the posterior palate, or velum. Most speakers of English use a velarized [l̰], the so-called dark *l,* whenever /l/ is in postvocalic position at the end of a word. This /l/ usually is made with an elevated and back tongue body position and frequently without an anterior contact by the tongue tip. See the discussion of /l/ in Chapter 5 and note the drawings of /l/ articulation in that chapter.

Centralized [w ɪ n d o̱]

When a vowel is **centralized,** the tongue body is displaced toward the central region of the oral cavity. In its extreme form, centralization leads to a substitution of the schwa [ə] for the target sound. For example, with progressive centralization of the final vowel in *window,* the word would change from [w ɪ n d o] to [w ɪ n d o̱] to [w ɪ n d ə]. Notice that the particular direction of tongue displacement during centralization depends upon the articulation of the target sound. (See the diagram in Figure 4-14.) A centralized /i/ would move backward and downward (toward the center of the mouth), whereas a centralized /ɑ/ would involve a forward and upward movement. To some degree, centralization is a natural consequence of increased speaking rate or reduced stress. As a shorter period of time is allowed for a vowel articulation, the tongue undershoots, or falls short of its target position for the vowel, and thus exhibits a centralized articulation. Say the word *amputate* first very slowly and deliberately and then gradually faster and faster. You should be able to hear a change from [æm p j u t e͡ɪ t] to [æm p j ʊ t e͡ɪ t] to [æm p j ə t e͡ɪ t].

Retracted [b æ̠ t]

A **retracted** tongue position is one in which the tongue body is drawn back from the vowel target position. For example, a retracted /æ/ has a tongue position drawn back *toward* that for /ɑ/, without of course actually moving as far back as /ɑ/. The sound [æ̠] is intermediate in tongue position between a normal [æ] and a normal [ɑ]. The diacritic mark is easily remembered if you think of it as an arrow pointing toward the back (or right, by convention in this book, meaning back of the mouth).

Advanced [p ɑ̟ t]

An **advanced** tongue body position is forward, or anterior, to the target position. Thus, advanced /ɑ/ is more forward than a normal [ɑ] but not as far forward as a normal [æ]. Notice that the diacritic for advancement is an arrow pointing to the front of the mouth (left means front by the convention adopted in this book).

Raised [b ɛ̝ d]

A **raised** tongue body position is elevated above the usual, or target, position. A raised [ɛ̝] is higher than the usual [ɛ] but not so high as to sound like [ɪ].

Lowered [h ɛ̞ d]

A **lowered** tongue body position is lower than the usual, or target, position for a sound. Lowered [ɛ̞] is lower than the usual [ɛ] but not so low as to sound like [æ].

Fronted [s̟ n o͡ʊ]

A **fronted** consonant is one in which the place of articulation is unusually forward, but the exact modification is difficult to determine. Fronting applies to place of *consonant* articulation, whereas advancement refers to general tongue body position (usually for vowels but also for some consonants, like /k g/, involving the tongue body). In the example [s̟ n o͡ʊ], the transcriber might have been certain that the articulation was more anterior than it should have been but was uncertain as to exactly where the constriction was made. Whenever possible, the most explicit description should be given in the transcription, but a more general description like fronting is preferable to a highly questionable place specification.

Backed [z̠ u]

A **backed** consonant is one in which the place of articulation is unusually back, or posterior, but the exact modification is difficult to determine. See the comments immediately preceding for fronting. A back sound has a constriction that is in some sense farther back than the expected constriction for the phoneme symbol that is being modified.

Derhotacized [r̮ ɛ d]

A **derhotacized** sound is an /r/ consonant or an *r*-colored vowel that is significantly lacking in *r*-ness (rhotic or retroflex quality) but does not fall into another phonemic category of English. For example, a child who misarticulates /r/ may produce a sound that seems to be somewhere in between /r/ and /w/. Rather than assign this error production to the /w/ category, it is better to show by the transcription that the error sound is not a genuine substitution of /w/ for /r/. Hence, a derhotacized sound is one that lacks the expected /r/ quality that is accomplished by bunching or retroflexion of the tongue but is not so far removed from the target sound that a judgment of phonemic substitution is warranted.

SOUND SOURCE SYMBOLS

The symbols in this category pertain to alterations of the source of sound energy; for example, sound generation at the larynx or noise generation at a site of fricative constriction.

Partially Voiced [æ b s̬ ə n t]

This diacritic is most frequently used to mark an unusual degree of voicing for a sound that is normally voiceless. It is not necessary that the segment be totally voiced; indeed, it often is of interest to describe partial voicing. Many normal speakers will voice the [s] in a word like *absurd* or *absent,* owing to the influence of the surrounding voiced sounds.

Partially Devoiced [d ɔ g̊]

In devoicing, a normally or typically voiced segment is partially or totally devoiced. In the example [d ɔ g̊], the [g] symbol might be retained in preference to the voiceless cognate [k] if some degree of voicing is maintained. Children have a tendency to devoice final obstruents; for example, [ʃ u z̥] for *shoes,* [d ɔ g̊] for *dog,* and [k ɑ r d̥] for *card.* Liquids and glides tend to be devoiced in normal adult speech when they follow voiceless sounds; for example, [p l̥ e͡ɪ] for *play,* [t r̥ i] for *tree,* and [t w̥ ɑ͡ɪ s] for *twice.*

Glottalized (or Creaky Voice) [b ɑ̣ k s]

A **glottalized** sound has a creaky or irregular voice quality, often because of an aperiodicity in the laryngeal vibratory pattern. This feature and other phonatory deviations occur frequently in the speech of young children.

Breathy (or Murmured) [p l e͡ɪ ɪ̤ ŋ]

Breathy voice quality is characterized by air wastage, and therefore often noise, at the larynx. The vocal folds vibrate but do not close adequately during the vibratory cycle to prevent a continuous loss of air. The escape of air through the vocal folds causes an [h]-like noise to be combined with the voicing signal.

Frictionalized (or Spirantized) [s t̽ ɑ p]

A **frictionalized** or spirantized stop has noise energy caused by fricative-like airflow through a narrow oral constriction. This feature occurs through a failure of stop formation. In normal speech, the dorsovelars /k g/ often are frictionalized because the tongue makes a sliding contact with the roof of the mouth and does not release the constriction as rapidly as the lips and tongue tip do for /p b/ and /t d/.

Whistled (or Hissed) [s͎ i]

Whistling, almost entirely restricted to fricatives, involves a sharply tuned noise source like that of normal whistling with the lips. This feature is most commonly heard with /s/and /ʃ/.

Trilled [t r̬ ɑɪ]

A **trilled** sound is made with rapid, repetitive movements of alternating opening and closing, essentially vibratory in nature. Although trilled sounds do not commonly occur in English, they may be heard in other languages, such as German.

SYLLABIC SYMBOL

A small number of consonants can serve a syllabic function, meaning that they can serve as the nucleus of a syllable. The consonants most likely to do so are the nasals [m], [n], and [ŋ], the lateral [l], and the rhotic [r]. A syllabic consonant is indicated with a small vertical tic placed under the main symbol. For example, if the second syllable of the word *button* is produced with a syllabic nasal, the word would be transcribed as [b ʌ t n̩].

OFFGLIDE SYMBOLS

An offglide symbol is used to indicate the presence of a brief or fragmentary sound that immediately follows a more dominant, fully articulated sound. For example, if the word *her* is produced with a brief schwa vowel immediately following the vowel [ɝ], then the word would be transcribed as [h ɝ ᵊ].

STOP RELEASE SYMBOLS

These symbols denote laryngeal and supralaryngeal characteristics associated with stop articulation, having to do primarily with (1) the relative timing of articulatory release and laryngeal valving, and (2) whether or not the stop closure is released with an audible burst.

Aspirated [tʰ ɑ p]

An **aspirated** stop has two intervals of noise, both of which typically are audible. The first noise segment is the release burst, the brief (5 to 20 ms) noise produced as the impounded air escapes in a plosive burst. This segment is followed by a generally longer interval of noise generated as air passes through the gradually closing vocal folds and the upper airway (an /h/-like sound). For voiceless stops in English, the vocal folds initially are open during the stop closure, so that the air pressure in the lungs can be fully transmitted to the oral cavity. The vocal folds then must close to allow voicing for a following voiced sound. But as the folds come together, the air passing between them generates a flat noise of rather weak intensity. Table 6-2 helps explain this sequence of events. During phase 1 of the stop articulation, the folds are open so that air from the lungs fills the closed oral cavity. Upon phase 2, the impounded air escapes with an audible explosion or burst. During phase 3, the folds are being brought together while the oral airway is open, so that air escapes through the mouth. This escaping air causes frication, or the aspiration noise. Finally, with phase 4, the folds are approximated so that voicing occurs, and the aspiration noise normally comes to an end.

Unaspirated [s t⁼ɑ p]

An unaspirated stop may have an audible release burst, but it does not have an aspiration interval. In English, unaspirated stops occur normally only when stops immediately follow fricatives, usually the /s/. Other released stops are aspirated. One possible explanation for the occurrence of unaspirated stops following fricatives is that the vocal folds begin their closing movement early during the consonant cluster, so that the folds are nearly approximated shortly after the stop is released. Interestingly, some children with /s/ omission produce the allophonically appropriate unaspirated stop even when the /s/ is judged to be omitted. That is, the child will say [t⁼ɑ p] for the word *stop.*

Unreleased [l æ p˺]

An unreleased stop is one in which the articulatory closure is not broken with an audible burst of air (stop burst). For

TABLE 6-2 Vocal Fold Movements in the Production of Aspirated Stops

Phase 1	Phase 2	Phase 3	Phase 4
Folds are open.	Folds are open.	Folds begin to close.	Folds are brought together for voicing.
Stop closure is made.	Stop closure is released.	Oral airway is open.	Oral airway is open.

example, the final [p] in the word *lap* is not necessarily released. In fact, the lips can remain closed for a considerable period of time, virtually indefinitely, because the release burst is not a critical perceptual cue for the perception of an utterance-final stop. This fact can be demonstrated easily by saying the following words as you prolong the articulatory closure for the final stop: *rob, stop, road, seat, dog, trick.*

TIMING AND JUNCTURE SYMBOLS

These symbols are used to note variations in temporal pattern and intonation. For example, they may indicate that a sound is lengthened or prolonged, a pause occurs during an utterance, or a response is spoken as a question. Timing is concerned with durations, that is, whether sounds are long or short in their articulation. Juncture might be called "oral punctuation." Speech is produced with a number of cues that function somewhat like the commas, periods, and other punctuation marks used in writing. Juncture marks are used to indicate separation, pausing, and termination within speech. For example, a speaker can say *yes* in several ways: with finality, indicating an end to a conversation; with thoughtful prolongation and pause, as though he or she is still thinking about something; or with an interrogative intonation (questioning), to ask for repetition or clarification. The entertainer Victor Borge had a popular comical sketch in which he introduced special punctuation sounds (pops, splurts, raspberries, and the like) in conversational speech. For example, he used a special sound to show where an exclamation point might appear in a written transcript. Actually, a speaker normally uses a variety of sound pattern modifications to convey "punctuation" as well as attitudes, feelings, and other paralinguistic properties of speech.

Lengthened [s iː]

Lengthening means that a sound is prolonged; the duration of its articulation is conspicuously great or at least greater than what might ordinarily be expected. The transcription example indicates that vowel [i] is lengthened, that is, that the speaker held or maintained the vowel sound. In Southern speech, words like *lark* [l ɑ r k] may be produced without *r*-coloring but with a lengthened vowel so that the speaker still makes a phonetic distinction between *lock* [l ɑ k] and *lark* [l ɑː k]. Lengthening also occurs for some productions of geminate (double) consonants; for example, *that time* [ð æ tː a͡ɪ m], *sad day* [s æ dː e͡ɪ], *some more* [s ʌ mː ɔ r]. Some phoneticians distinguish a single point [ˑ] from a double point [ː]. The single point is used to indicate a smaller degree of lengthening. However, we have found that such a distinction is difficult to teach and to use reliably; therefore, we recommend that the double-point symbol be used for most purposes. However, if you hear an extremely lengthened sound, such as a prolongation in stuttered speech, you can represent it with iterated double-point symbols; for example [sːːː iːː], for prolonged /s/ and prolonged /i/.

Shortened [w e ˃]

Shortening is indicated whenever a sound is conspicuously brief in duration. In the transcription example, the vowel [e] is marked as shortened. Shortening is appropriately marked for sounds that are abbreviated, truncated, or rushed in some respect. As another example, we sometimes hear children produce [s] segments that are almost so short as to sound like exploded [t]. But because the segment is perceptually identifiable as [s], the shortening mark is used rather than to transcribe the modification as a substitution of [t] for [s]: [s ˃].

Close Juncture [a͡ɪ d ɪ d ɪ t] (I Did It)

Close juncture is not marked in a phonetic transcription because it implies that no special time separation occurs between elements; the transition between phones is made in a way that is physiologically convenient and should not interfere with the communication of meaning. Hence, close juncture is a kind of default juncture and occurs when no other junctural conditions apply. It does not alter a phonetic transcription.

Open Juncture [ə n a͡ɪ s + mæn] Versus [ə n + a͡ɪ s mæn]

Open juncture is a short pause or gap that separates phone boundaries of syllables in ambiguous or confusable utterances. For example, the transcription examples distinguish *a nice man* from *an ice man.* Note that the segmental or phonemic content of these two phrases is identical but that they differ in timing or phrasing. Open juncture, which is represented phonetically by + or by a graphic space, is used in these transcriptions to show where a pause occurs. Open juncture also distinguishes confusable pairs like *nitrate* and *night rate. Nitrate* [n a͡ɪ + t r e͡ɪ t] differs from *night rate* [n a͡ɪ t + r e͡ɪ t] in pause or gap location.

Internal Open Juncture [l ɛ t s h ɛ l p | ʤ e͡ɪ n]

Internal open juncture generally is used to represent phrasing and is similar to commas, semicolons, and interjections in writing. The pause or gap indicated by internal open juncture usually is longer than that for the syllabic open junctures just discussed. In the transcription example of *Let's help, Jane,* the pause associated with the comma is represented in the phonetic transcription by the vertical line symbolic of internal open juncture. Notice that this juncture distinguishes the helper from the helpee.

Falling Terminal Juncture [t ʊ d e͡ɪ ↓]

Terminal juncture marks the end of an utterance (sentence, sentence fragment, or single-word response). Falling terminal juncture is associated with declarative statements in general and is conveyed acoustically by a falling fundamental frequency (voice pitch) on the last syllable. For example, the transcription example of *today* might be a reply to the question "When are you leaving for vacation?" The vertical arrow points downward to signify the falling fundamental frequency.

Rising Terminal Juncture [t ʊ d e͡ɪ ↑]

Rising terminal juncture generally represents interrogatives or questions. Questions are often signaled acoustically by a rise of fundamental frequency (voice pitch) on the final syllable. Thus, the transcription example of *today* indicates a question, "(Are you leaving) today?" The direction of the arrow indicates the rising fundamental frequency.

Checked or Held Juncture [t ʊ d e͡ɪ →]

Checked or held juncture may indicate either a speaker's intention to continue talking after a pause or an expression of continued interest in another speaker's utterance. For example, if a speaker is describing a list of activities for a week of vacation, *today* might be uttered with checked juncture to introduce the activities for the first day of the week. This type of juncture is frequently used by teachers when calling upon students to answer a question; [ʤ ɑ n →] (John . . .) identifies the student by name, and the checked juncture indicates that the teacher is waiting for the student's response. Checked juncture is expressed acoustically by a relatively flat or fixed fundamental frequency on the final syllable, often in association with a lengthening of that syllable.

OTHER SYMBOLS

Synchronic Tie [d͡z u]

A synchronic tie is used when two distinct articulations are linked or tied together in one segment. For example, the transcription [d͡z u] indicates that the [d] and [z] are produced synchronically, like an affricate. The tie symbol is used to represent this quality of linking or combination. The word *synchronic* literally means "together in time" or "at the same time" and is used here to denote that two sounds appear to occur together as one segment.

Unintelligible Syllable [*]

Clinical transcription often presents situations in which a person's speech is not intelligible. For example, a child with a speech disorder might say a word or several words that the clinician fails to understand. An asterisk [*] is used to represent each syllable in such words, for example, [* *** **]

Questionable Segment ⓐ or ⓘ?

A circle is used around each segment in a transcription about which the transcriber is unsure. Either the questionable sound or sounds are circled (for example, (k) ɑ t, (k ɑ) t, (k ɑ t)) or a question mark representing questionable segments is circled (for example, k (?) t, (? ?) t, (? ? ?)). In computer fonts, circles are replaced by rectangles.

STRESS AND OTHER SUPRASEGMENTAL FEATURES

Stress Marking in the IPA

The importance of stress can be shown by asking someone who can read phonetic transcription to say aloud the following utterances:

[ɛ s k ɔ r t] [p r o t ɛ s t] [ɪ n k l a͡ɪ n]

Note that each of these words can be either a noun (having a greater level of stress on the first syllable) or a verb (having a greater level of stress on the second syllable). However, the segmental transcription alone does not indicate which form, noun or verb, is to be used. To make this distinction, some kind of stress marking is needed. The IPA convention is to mark the primary (highest level) stress with a small vertical mark above the line and before the affected syllable. Secondary (the next highest level) stress is marked with a similar vertical mark located below the line and before the affected syllable. The noun and verb forms of the words *escort, protest,* and *incline* are stress-marked as follows in the IPA:

Nouns	*Verbs*
[ˈɛsˌkɔrt]	[ˌɛsˈkɔrt]
[ˈproˌtɛst]	[ˌproˈtɛst]
[ˈɪnˌkla͡ɪn]	[ˌɪnˈkla͡ɪn]

A third (tertiary) level of stress is indicated in the IPA by the absence of a stress mark. For example, the weak second syllable of the words *father, city,* and *sofa* carries no special mark in the transcriptions [ˈf ɑ ð ɚ], [ˈs ɪ ɾ ɪ], and [ˈs o͡ʊ f ə]. The three levels of stress (primary, secondary, and tertiary) are represented in the words *ratify* [ˈr æ ɾ ɪ ˌf a͡ɪ] and *allophone* [ˈæ l ə ˌf o͡ʊ n].

One disadvantage of the IPA stress marks is that they often are difficult to distinguish from the various diacritic marks used in a narrow transcription. Another disadvantage is that the marks are supposed to precede the affected syllable, which means that the transcriber must make decisions about syllabification (where one syllable ends and another begins). Syllabification decisions are not always obvious, so the requirement of syllable segregation for stress marking can stand in the way of transcription.

Stress Marking by Number

Because of these disadvantages in the IPA system of stress marking, we favor the method described previously in which stress level is represented simply as a number above the nucleus of the syllable (the nucleus being the vowel, diphthong, or syllabic consonant core of the syllable). Thus, the noun and verb forms of the word *incline* are represented as [$\overset{1}{\text{ɪ}}$ n k l $\overset{2}{\text{aɪ}}$ n] and [$\overset{2}{\text{ɪ}}$ n k l $\overset{1}{\text{aɪ}}$ n], respectively. The numerals for stress marking are placed above any diacritics used in narrow transcription, such placement reflecting the suprasegmental nature of stress. The words *ratify* and *allophone* are stress marked as follows: [r $\overset{1}{\text{æ}}$ ɾ $\overset{3}{\text{ɪ}}$ f $\overset{2}{\text{aɪ}}$] and [$\overset{1}{\text{æ}}$ l $\overset{3}{\text{ə}}$ f $\overset{2}{\text{oʊ}}$ n].

The determination of stress level sometimes is a difficult judgment, as it requires that each syllable in an utterance be compared against others. Hence, stress is a relational feature, involving comparisons across syllables. We recommend that the beginning student first identify the syllable with primary stress and then make decisions about secondary and tertiary levels. Say each of the following words and place a "1" over the orthographic spelling of the syllable with primary stress. The correct answer is shown at the right.

telephone	tel
ocean	o
building	build
Wisconsin	con
Nebraska	bras
salad	sal
again	gain
window	win
dinosaur	di
Wyoming	o
greyhound	both syllables have primary stress

Usually, only one syllable in a word has primary stress, but some words, like *greyhound,* typically have primary stress on both syllables. Two-syllable words having equal (primary) stress on both syllables are called **spondees;** other examples are the words *hothouse, horseshoe,* and *pathway.*

Polysyllabic words or phrases may contain more than one syllable of secondary or tertiary stress. For example, the word *relativity* has primary stress on the third syllable, secondary stress on the first syllable, and tertiary stress on the second, fourth, and fifth syllables.

[r $\overset{2}{\text{ɛ}}$ l $\overset{3}{\text{ə}}$ t $\overset{1}{\text{ɪ}}$ v $\overset{3}{\text{ɪ}}$ ɾ $\overset{3}{\text{ɪ}}$]

Syllabification [b ʌ t n̩] [b æ t l̩] [r ʌ b m̩]

A special kind of reduced syllable is produced when the nucleic function ordinarily served by a vowel or diphthong is accomplished by a consonant, usually /m/, /n/, or /l/, but infrequently /r/. These consonants can, under certain conditions, become syllabic, meaning that they constitute in themselves a syllable. The syllabic function is indicated by a short vertical line directly under the consonant symbol. In the transcription examples, /n/, /l/, and /m/ are syllabic in *button, battle,* and *rub (the)m* ("rub'm"), respectively. **Syllabification** does not necessarily or always occur in these utterances, as they could be produced with the schwa vowel in the reduced syllable: [b ʌ t ə n], [b æ t ə l], and [r ʌ b ə m]. Syllabic consonants are most likely to occur when the consonant is homorganic (similar in place of articulation) with the boundary consonant in the preceding syllable. In the examples here, the homorganic pairings are /tn/, /tl/, and /bm/. When the homorganic condition is not satisfied, as in *tackle, trouble, siphon,* and *knock (the)m* ("knock'm"), a schwa vowel is more likely to be heard because the point of articulation necessarily changes between the consonants. In homorganic pairings, the articulatory contact can be maintained across the two sounds, and thus an open vocal tract (that is, a potential vowel) does not intervene. Some phoneticians use a syllable /r/ in words like *taper, tighter,* and *roller,* but we prefer the schwar /ɚ/ in these sequences.

ABBREVIATORY DEVICES IN PHONETIC DESCRIPTION

On occasion, the clinician may not want to take the time to record a detailed phonetic description of a client's speech. For example, it may be sufficient simply to listen to the client's conversational speech or a sample of reading and to record some general impressions about the phonetic behavior. For such an application, the clinician may proceed as follows.

First, to obtain phonetic information on at least broad categories of speech behavior, the clinician might consider the phonetic classes of stop, fricative, nasal, glide, liquid, and vowel-diphthongs, abbreviated S, F, N, G, L, and V, respectively. Then, upon hearing sounds in each category, the clinician notes errors, especially frequent or pervasive errors, for the major diacritic categories presented in this chapter, namely, lip articulation features, nasalization, tongue articulation features, source features, stop release features, and prosodic features. Because each of these categories of diacritics has a specified location in the diacritic marking system, a tally of errors can be kept by the diacritic location of the errors detected. Examples of an abbreviated phonetic description follow.

S̥ F̥	Devoicing of stops and fricatives.
Ṽ G̃	Nasalization of vowels and glides.
S͔ F͔	Fronting of stops and fricatives.
V̥ V̤ Ṿ	Abnormal phonation of vowels: devoicing, breathiness, glottalization.

$\underset{\times}{S}$ Spirantization of stops.

$\underset{\lrcorner}{S}$ $\underset{\lrcorner}{F}$ Palatalization of stops and fricatives.

$\underset{\sqcap}{S}$ $\underset{\sqcap}{F}$ Dentalization of stops and fricatives.

$\underset{\vdash}{V}$ Retraction of tongue body for vowels.

Consider the following abbreviated phonetic description of a child's speech:

$$\underset{\circ}{\underset{<}{S}}\ \underset{\circ}{\underset{<}{F}}\ \underset{..}{\underset{\vdash}{V}}$$

This description indicates that the child makes errors of tongue placement (fronting) for stops and fricatives, and errors of tongue body position (retraction) for vowels. In addition, the child frequently devoices segments and tends to use a breathy voice quality.

One reason for the modified system of diacritics in this book is that the system simplifies the tally of phonetic errors and allows a fairly easy and quick interpretation of the results with respect to major categories of error. In contrast, the diacritics used in the IPA to denote modifications of tongue articulation are variously placed with respect to phoneme symbols, so it is rather difficult to keep a record of these errors separate from errors of lip articulation, phonation, or nasalization. With the modified system used in this book, all errors of tongue articulation are marked in the same place, directly under the phoneme symbol. Therefore, a large number of errors affecting tongue position would be signified by the frequent appearance of diacritics in the slot directly under the phoneme symbol; for example, $\underset{\sqcap<\sqcap\lrcorner<}{S}$ $\underset{<<\sqcap\sqcap\lrcorner<<}{F}$ would indicate multiple errors of fronting, dentalization, and palatalization detected in a speech sample.

A system of abbreviation (we might call it phonetic shorthand) is especially important when the clinician is listening to conversational speech or reading. Phonetic decisions have to be made quickly, and there may not be time to write descriptive remarks such as "dentalized stops and fricatives." To use the shorthand system, the clinician might bear in mind the following configuration for diacritic marking. The blackened space is the position for a phonetic element or class symbol (such as V, S, F), and the bracketed words indicate positions for diacritics:

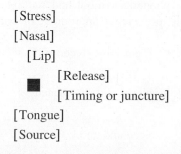

[Stress]
[Nasal]
[Lip]
■ [Release]
[Timing or juncture]
[Tongue]
[Source]

Whether a phonemic element or a class abbreviation is used in the black space depends on the degree of abstraction or generalization required. For example, if a phonetic modification applies to a class of sounds, like stops, then the abbreviation S (for stop) should be used. On the other hand, if the modification applies only to one stop, like [t], then the phonemic symbol [t] should be used.

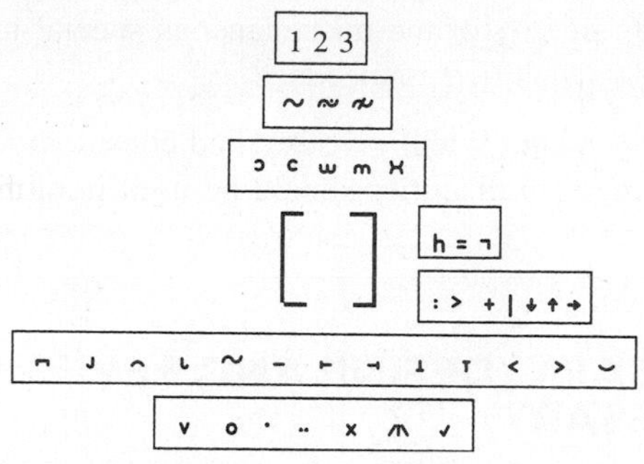

FIGURE 6-11
Complete set of diacritic marks arranged by placement relative to phonemic symbol (brackets). This composite diagram might be useful in early transcription practice using the diacritic system.

In using the diacritic system for the first time, it may be helpful to circle the suitable diacritics from a list such as that shown in Figure 6-11. In this configuration, all diacritics of a particular kind (for example, tongue modifications) are bracketed and placed in the appropriate location with respect to the symbol (phonetic element or class abbreviation) being modified. After some practice with the listed diacritic configuration, the clinician should acquire sufficient familiarity to rely on memory for the diacritics.

SOME GUIDELINES FOR USING DIACRITIC MARKS

The following questions might be useful to ask when using diacritic marks.

1. Which phonetic symbol best represents the sound in question? (Write the symbol in brackets: [æ], [s], [t].)
2. Is the sound produced with any modification of source? If so, write the appropriate diacritic *under* the phonetic symbol: [æ̤], [$\underset{\wedge}{s}$], [$\underset{\times}{t}$].
3. Is the sound a stop consonant? If so, is it unreleased [t˺]? If it is released, is it aspirated [tʰ] or unaspirated [t⁼]?
4. Is the sound produced with any modification of place of articulation? That is, is there any modification of lingual or labial articulation? If so, place the lingual [$\underset{\frown}{z}$] or labial [$\overset{w}{j}$] diacritic in the appropriate place.
5. Is there any modification of velopharyngeal function, such as nasalization, nasal emission, or denasalization? If so, mark accordingly.
6. Is there any aspect of juncture or duration that should be indicated? Is there a pause or inflection (both are manifestations of juncture)? Is the sound abruptly terminated or prolonged? If so, mark appropriately.

7. Finally, are any of the miscellaneous special marks for stress of syllabification needed?

Chapters 7, 8, and 9 will give detailed consideration to the question of *when* diacritics should be used in clinical phonetics.

GLOSSARY (DEFINE AND REVIEW IF NECESSARY)

Because the format of this chapter is basically a series of definitions, we simply list these terms as a study guide rather than repeat the definitions given systematically in the chapter.

advanced
aspirated
backed
breathy
broad transcription
centralized
checked or held juncture
clear speech
close juncture
coarticulation
coda
denasalized
dentalized
derhotacized
diacritic marks
final syllable lengthening
frictionalized
fronted
glottalized
internal open juncture
intonation
inversion of the lip
labialized
lateralized
lengthening
lowered
narrow transcription
nasal emission
nasalized
nucleus
onset
open juncture
palatalized
paralinguistics
phrase-final lengthening
pitch
pitch declination
prepausal lengthening
primary stress
prosody
raised
retracted
retroflexion
rhotacized
rhyme
rhythm
rounded
secondary stress
shortening
sonority
spondee
stress
suprasegmental
syllabification
terminal juncture (falling and rising)
tertiary stress
tone units
tones
tonicity
trilled
undershoot
velarization
whistling

EXERCISES

1. Describe where diacritic marks are placed for the following speech sound characteristics:

 (a) Modifications of tongue movement or position

 ____

 (b) Velopharyngeal function

 ____

 (c) Modifications of sound at the larynx

 ____

 (d) Features of stop release

 ____

 (e) Juncture

 ____

 (f) Lip configuration

 ____

2. For each phonetic description, provide the phonetic symbol and appropriate diacritic mark. *Example:* Voiceless lingua-alveolar fricative with nasal emission—[s͌]

 (a) Nasalized high-front, tense vowel [ ]
 (b) Unaspirated voiceless bilabial stop [ ]
 (c) Labialized voiced lingua-dental fricative [ ]
 (d) Lengthened low-back, tense vowel [ ]
 (e) Lowered mid-front, lax vowel [ ]
 (f) Glottalized high-mid-back, lax vowel [ ]
 (g) Trilled voiceless lingua-alveolar stop [ ]
 (h) Devoiced bilabial nasal [ ]
 (i) Retroflex voiceless palatal fricative [ ]
 (j) Dentalized voiced lingua-alveolar fricative [ ]

3. For each phonetic symbol and multiple modifications given here, provide the appropriate diacritic marks.

 Example: [k̬ʷ], partially voiced and labialized

 (a) [æ], nasalized and lengthened

 (b) [d], devoiced and unreleased

 (c) [s], dentalized and lengthened

(d) [ɪ], breathy and raised

(e) [u], unrounded and nasalized

(f) [l], velarized and devoiced

(g) [t ʃ], retroflexed and partially voiced

(h) [t], aspirated and frictionalized

4. Using the number system for stress marking, transcribe the following words (General American pronunciation) and indicate the stress pattern.
   (a) transcribe ____________
   (b) satisfy ____________
   (c) legislature ____________
   (d) furniture ____________
   (e) Arizona ____________
   (f) Chicago ____________
   (g) overload ____________
   (h) skyscraper ____________
   (i) typewriter ____________
   (j) Lithuania ____________
   (k) masterpiece ____________
   (l) Mississippi ____________

5. Briefly describe the meaning of each diacritic in the following transcription.
   (a) [j e ᵊ→] ____________
   (b) [w a͡ɪ̃ ↑] ____________
   (c) [h ɛ̤ l õ] ____________
   (d) [p l̥ iː z →] ____________
   (e) [k $\overset{2}{\text{ʌ}}$ p $\overset{3}{\text{ə}}$ k $\overset{1}{\text{ɔ}}$ f $\overset{3}{\text{ɪ}}$] ____________
   (f) [g ʊ̞ d m ɔ̃ r n ɪ̃ ŋ] ____________
   (g) [a͡ɪ d ɪ ʔ n o͡ʊː ð æᶦ t̚] ____________

6. The following is an exercise in reading transcription—a linguistic potpourri. Try reading each transcription, referring to the International Phonetic Alphabet chart (inside cover) to guide your pronunciation of unfamiliar symbols. Stress is marked using the IPA system.

Spanish

jota	['x o t a]
pegar	[p e 'ɣ a r]
la boca	[l ɑ 'β o k a]

French

peu	[p ø]
faim	[f ɛ̃]
Chopin	[ʃ ɔ ' p ɛ̃]
monsieur	[m ə ' s j ø]

German

Tag	[t ɑ ː x]
Zug	[t s uː x]
spielen	[' ʃ p iː l ə n]

Italian

Signori	[s i ' ɲ ɔ r ɪ]
grazie	[' g r ɑ t s j e]

Russian

(trick)	[' ʃ t u k ə]
(good welfare)	[' b l a ɣ ə]

Norwegian

dryppe	[' d r y pː ə]
dod	[d oː]

Finnish

kiitos	[' k i t o s]
yksi	['y k s i]

TRANSCRIPTION TRAINING

Transcription List E

Tape 1B, List E, provides practice in marking stress. Use the stress marking by number system above the phonetic transcription.

PROCEED TO: Clinical Phonetics Tape 1B: Transcription List E

MODULE TIME	
TOTAL	5:00
ELAPSED	00:00–05:00

Clinical Phonetics Tape 1B
Transcription List E

TRANSCRIPTION KEY

1	gasoline	[gæsəlin]	21	ratify	[ræɾɪfaɪ]
2	stationary	[steɪʃənɛrɪ]	22	tobacco	[tʊbæko]
3	bookshelf	[bʊkʃɛlf]	23	typewriter	[taɪpraɪɾɚ]
4	Arizona	[ɛrɪzoʊnə]	24	community	[kəmjunɪɾɪ]
5	vacation	[vekeɪʃən]	25	quarterback	[kwɔrtɚbæk]
6	sanctuary	[sæŋktʃuɛrɪ]	26	thesaurus	[θisɔrəs]
7	adjustment	[ədʒʌstmənt]	27	united	[junaɪɾəd]
8	Ohio	[ohaɪo]	28	dedication	[dɛdɪkeɪʃən]
9	Miami	[maɪæmɪ]	29	California	[kælɪfɔrnjə]
10	edition	[ɛdɪʃən]	30	atmosphere	[ætməsfɪr]
11	relinquish	[rɪlɪŋkwɪʃ]	31	substance	[sʌbstəns]
12	Chicago	[ʃɪkɑgo]	32	geography	[dʒiɑgrəfɪ]
13	university	[junɪvɝsɪɾɪ]	33	Wyoming	[waɪomɪŋ]
14	boisterous	[bɔɪstrəs]	34	dictionary	[dɪkʃənɛrɪ]
15	redeemer	[ridimɚ]	35	reduction	[rɪdʌkʃən]
16	rotation	[roteɪʃən]	36	multiply	[mʌltɪplaɪ]
17	decision	[disɪʒən]	37	television	[tɛləvɪʒən]
18	Seattle	[siætl̩]	38	Argentina	[ɑrdʒəntinə]
19	irritation	[ɪrɪteɪʃən]	39	profession	[profɛʃən]
20	Wisconsin	[wɪskɑnsɪn]	40	religion	[rɪlɪdʒɪn]

MODULE TIME	
TOTAL	5:00
ELAPSED	00:00–05:00

Clinical Phonetics Tape 1B
Transcription List E

TRANSCRIPTION SHEET

1	gasoline	[ ]	21	ratify	[ ]
2	stationary	[ ]	22	tobacco	[ ]
3	bookshelf	[ ]	23	typewriter	[ ]
4	Arizona	[ ]	24	community	[ ]
5	vacation	[ ]	25	quarterback	[ ]
6	sanctuary	[ ]	26	thesaurus	[ ]
7	adjustment	[ ]	27	united	[ ]
8	Ohio	[ ]	28	dedication	[ ]
9	Miami	[ ]	29	California	[ ]
10	edition	[ ]	30	atmosphere	[ ]
11	relinquish	[ ]	31	substance	[ ]
12	Chicago	[ ]	32	geography	[ ]
13	university	[ ]	33	Wyoming	[ ]
14	boisterous	[ ]	34	dictionary	[ ]
15	redeemer	[ ]	35	reduction	[ ]
16	rotation	[ ]	36	multiply	[ ]
17	decision	[ ]	37	television	[ ]
18	Seattle	[ ]	38	Argentina	[ ]
19	irritation	[ ]	39	profession	[ ]
20	Wisconsin	[ ]	40	religion	[ ]

Transcription List F

Audio sample 1B provides practice in transcribing casual speech, including terminal juncture symbols.

PROCEED TO: Clinical Phonetics Tape 1B: Transcription List F

MODULE TIME	
TOTAL	2:34
ELAPSED	05:00–07:34

Clinical Phonetics Tape 1B
Transcription List F

TRANSCRIPTION KEY

(Note: These samples represent casual, slurred speech.)

1	Where did you go?	[wɛrdʒəgo͡ʊ↑]
2	He isn't here.	[hiɪznhɪr↓]
3	I don't know.	[a͡ɪɾono͡ʊ↓]
4	What are you going to do?	[wʌtʃəgɔnədu↑]
5	It's something new.	[ɪtsʌmʔm̩nu↓]
6	She's around the corner.	[ʃizəra͡ʊnəkɔrnɚ↓]
7	What's the time?	[wʌtsəta͡ɪm↑]
8	How do you spell it?	[ha͡ʊjəspɛlɪt→]
9	It's in the red car.	[ɪtsɪnərɛkɑr↓]
10	Didn't you know that?	[dɪntʃəno͡ʊæt↑]
11	I'm going now.	[a͡ɪgoɪnːa͡ʊ↓]
12	Want to stay here?	[wɑnəste͡ɪhɪr↑]
13	Up and away.	[ʌpm̩əwe͡ɪ↓]
14	I've got to write it.	[a͡ɪgɑɾəra͡ɪɾɪt↓]
15	Did you finish?	[dɪdʒufɪnɪʃ↑]

MODULE TIME	
TOTAL	2:34
ELAPSED	05:00–07:34

Clinical Phonetics Tape 1B
Transcription List F

TRANSCRIPTION SHEET

(Note: These samples represent casual, slurred speech.)

1	Where did you go?	[ ]
2	He isn't here.	[ ]
3	I don't know.	[ ]
4	What are you going to do?	[ ]
5	It's something new.	[ ]
6	She's around the corner.	[ ]
7	What's the time?	[ ]
8	How do you spell it?	[ ]
9	It's in the red car.	[ ]
10	Didn't you know that?	[ ]
11	I'm going now.	[ ]
12	Want to stay here?	[ ]
13	Up and away.	[ ]
14	I've got to write it.	[ ]
15	Did you finish?	[ ]

Vowels and Diphthongs Quiz

The next two audio sample training modules test phonetic transcription skills with children's speech. Each word was said by a child with normally developing speech. For this first quiz, transcribe only the vowels and diphthongs. Although you may hear some sound modifications that could be transcribed with diacritics, enter only the phoneme symbols in the brackets provided.

PROCEED TO: Clinical Phonetics Tape 1B: Vowels and Diphthongs Quiz

MODULE TIME	
TOTAL	5:53
ELAPSED	07:34–13:27

Clinical Phonetics Tape 1B
Vowels and Diphthongs Quiz

TRANSCRIPTION KEY

1	grass	[æ]	16	toes	[o͡ʊ]
2	house	[a͡ʊ]	17	twins	[ɪ]
3	man	[æ]	18	bird	[ɝ]
4	bed	[ɛ]	19	teeth	[i]
5	witch	[ɪ]	20	brush	[ʌ]
6	egg	[ɛ]	21	third	[ɝ]
7	book	[ʊ]	22	knife	[a͡ɪ]
8	five	[a͡ɪ]	23	saw	[ɔ] or [ɒ]
9	can	[æ]	24	play	[e͡ɪ]
10	keys	[i]	25	stove	[o͡ʊ]
11	flower	[a͡ʊ]	26	first	[ɝ]
12	box	[ɑ]	27	clown	[a͡ʊ]
13	cup	[ʌ]	28	boy	[ɔ͡ɪ]
14	hat	[æ]	29	fish	[ɪ]
15	tail	[e͡ɪ]	30	smoke	[o͡ʊ]

MODULE TIME	
TOTAL	5:53
ELAPSED	07:34–13:27

Clinical Phonetics Tape 1B
Vowels and Diphthongs Quiz

TRANSCRIPTION SHEET

1	grass	[ ]	16	toes	[ ]
2	house	[ ]	17	twins	[ ]
3	man	[ ]	18	bird	[ ]
4	bed	[ ]	19	teeth	[ ]
5	witch	[ ]	20	brush	[ ]
6	egg	[ ]	21	third	[ ]
7	book	[ ]	22	knife	[ ]
8	five	[ ]	23	saw	[ ]
9	can	[ ]	24	play	[ ]
10	keys	[ ]	25	stove	[ ]
11	flower	[ ]	26	first	[ ]
12	box	[ ]	27	clown	[ ]
13	cup	[ ]	28	boy	[ ]
14	hat	[ ]	29	fish	[ ]
15	tail	[ ]	30	smoke	[ ]

Transcription Quiz

For this second introduction to children's speech, transcribe the entire word. Again, for clarity, possible diacritic modifications are not included in the key.

PROCEED TO: Clinical Phonetics Tape 1B: Transcription Quiz

MODULE TIME	
TOTAL	7:28
ELAPSED	13:27–20:55

Clinical Phonetics Tape 1B Transcription Quiz

TRANSCRIPTION KEY

1	rabbit	[ræbɪt]	21	monkey	[mʌŋkɪ]
2	glasses	[glæsɪz]	22	boat	[bo͡ʊt]
3	chair	[tʃe͡ɪr] or [tʃɛr]	23	wagon	[wegɪn] or [we͡ɪgɪn]
4	teeth	[tiθ]	24	smooth	[smuð]
5	shoe	[ʃu]	25	fish	[fɪʃ]
6	this	[ðɪs]	26	measuring cup	[mɛʒɚɪŋkʌp]
7	ladder	[lædɚ]	27	jumping	[ʤʌmpɪŋ]
8	station	[ste͡ɪʃɪn]	28	husky	[hʌskɪ]
9	seal	[sil]	29	matches	[mætʃəz]
10	pages	[pe͡ɪʤɪz]	30	hat	[hæt]
11	hanger	[he͡ɪŋɚ]	31	toast	[to͡ʊst]
12	beige	[be͡ɪʒ] or [pe͡ɪʒ]	32	cage	[ke͡ɪʤ]
13	toes	[to͡ʊz]	33	thumb	[θʌm]
14	garage	[gərɑʤ]	34	household	[ha͡ʊsho͡ʊld]
15	valentine	[vælɛnta͡ɪn]	35	carrots	[kɛrɪts]
16	baby	[be͡ɪbɪ]	36	pages	[pe͡ɪʤɪz]
17	feather	[fɛðɚ]	37	boat	[bo͡ʊt]
18	car	[kɑr]	38	bus	[bʌs]
19	toothache	[tuθe͡ɪk]	39	pipe	[pa͡ɪp]
20	dishes	[dɪʃɪz]	40	toothache	[tuθe͡ɪk]

MODULE TIME	
TOTAL	7:28
ELAPSED	13:27–20:55

Clinical Phonetics Tape 1B Transcription Quiz

TRANSCRIPTION SHEET

1	rabbit	[ ]	21	monkey	[ ]
2	glasses	[ ]	22	boat	[ ]
3	chair	[ ]	23	wagon	[ ]
4	teeth	[ ]	24	smooth	[ ]
5	shoe	[ ]	25	fish	[ ]
6	this	[ ]	26	measuring cup	[ ]
7	ladder	[ ]	27	jumping	[ ]
8	station	[ ]	28	husky	[ ]
9	seal	[ ]	29	matches	[ ]
10	pages	[ ]	30	hat	[ ]
11	hanger	[ ]	31	toast	[ ]
12	beige	[ ]	32	cage	[ ]
13	toes	[ ]	33	thumb	[ ]
14	garage	[ ]	34	household	[ ]
15	valentine	[ ]	35	carrots	[ ]
16	baby	[ ]	36	pages	[ ]
17	feather	[ ]	37	boat	[ ]
18	car	[ ]	38	bus	[ ]
19	toothache	[ ]	39	pipe	[ ]
20	dishes	[ ]	40	toothache	[ ]

Diacritics Examples

The last training module on audio sample tape 1B provides examples of sound modifications marked by diacritics. The following table provides a list of the 24 diacritic modifications, which are simulated here by two adult speakers. For each example, a speaker will say two sounds or words twice. Each sound or word will be said first with normal articulation, then with a sound modification. For example, the first set, which demonstrates nasalized vowels, is:

Normal	Nasalized
[æ]	[æ̃]
[i]	[ĩ]

As you listen to each example, follow the text descriptions beginning on page 115. These simulations also generally follow the ordering of symbols in Figure 6-6. Beginning in Chapter 8, you will have the opportunity to transcribe children's sound modifications as they occur in a clinical environment.

PROCEED TO: Clinical Phonetics Tape 1B: Diacritics Examples

MODULE TIME	
TOTAL	7:05
ELAPSED	20:55–28:00

Clinical Phonetics Tape 1B
Diacritics Examples

TRANSCRIPTION KEY

	NORMAL SOUND	MODIFIED SOUND	DISTORTION	COMMENTS[1]
1	[æ]	[æ̃]	Nasalized vowel	
	[i]	[ĩ]		
2	[s]	[s͌]	Fricative with nasal emission	
	[ʃ]	[ʃ͌]		This distortion is typically difficult to perceive.
3	ran [ræn]	ran [ræ͊n]	Denasalized vowel	The nasal consonant is also denasalized.
	mean [min]	mean [mi͊n]		The nasal consonants are also denasalized.
4	[eɪ]	[e͗ɪ]	Rounded vowel	(Diphthong)
	[i]	[i͗]		
5	[u]	[u͑]	Unrounded vowel	
	[oʊ]	[o͑ʊ]		(Diphthong)
6	[s]	[sᷱ]	Labialized fricative	Somewhat whistled [͎] as well
	she [ʃi]	shoe [ʃᷱu]		
7	we [wi]	we [wͫi]	Nonlabialized consonant	
	way [weɪ]	way [wͫeɪ]		
8	see [si]	see [s̪i]	Dentalized /s/	
	ice [aɪs]	ice [aɪs̪]		
9	see [si]	see [s̡i]	Palatalized /s/	
	ice [aɪs]	ice [aɪs̡]		
10	see [si]	see [s̭i]	Lateralized /s/	
	ice [aɪs]	ice [aɪs̭]		
11	see [si]	see [s̢i]	Retroflexed /s/	
	ice [aɪs]	ice [aɪs̭]		Hear the whistle [͎].
12	law [lɔ]	law [l̰ɔ]	Velarized /l/	
	all [ɔl]	all [ɔl̰]		
13	[eɪ]	[e̠ɪ]	Centralized vowel	(Diphthong)
	sit [sɪt]	sit [sɪ̠t]		

[1]Some of these exemplars sound "unnatural" or forced, relative to the way they sound in the examples from speakers with disorders to follow. You may want to write in your own comments and questions at this point, in preparation for the training modules in Chapters 8 and 9.

MODULE TIME	
TOTAL	7:05
ELAPSED	20:55–28:00

Clinical Phonetics Tape 1B
Diacritics Examples, Continued

TRANSCRIPTION KEY

14	[æ]	[æ̠]	Retracted vowel	
	her [hɚ]	her [hɚ̠]		
15	[o͡ʊ]	[o͡ʊ̟]	Advanced vowel	(Diphthong)
	paw [pɔ]	paw [pɔ̟]		
16	[æ]	[æ̝]	Raised vowel	
	men [mɛn]	men [mɛ̝n]		
17	[e͡ɪ]	[e̞͡ɪ]	Lowered vowel	(Diphthong)
	hid [hɪd]	hid [hɪ̞d]		
18	see [si]	see [s̬i]	Partially voiced consonant	
	ice [ɑ͡ɪs]	ice [ɑ͡ɪs̬]		
19	zoo [zu]	zoo [z̥u]	Partially devoiced consonant	
	is [ɪz]	is [ɪz̥]		
20	[ɑ]	[ɑ̣]	Glottalized vowel	
	man [mæn]	man [mæ̣n]		
21	[ɑ]	[ɑ̤]	Breathy vowel	
	[i]	[i̤]		
22	key [ki]	key [k͓i]	Frictionalized stop	
	stay [ste͡ɪ]	stay [st͓e͡ɪ]		
23	[pɑ]	[p⁼ɑ]	Unaspirated stop	
	too [tu]	too [t⁼u]		
24	up [ʌp]	up [ʌp̚]	Unreleased stop	
	sat [sæt]	sat [sæt̚]		

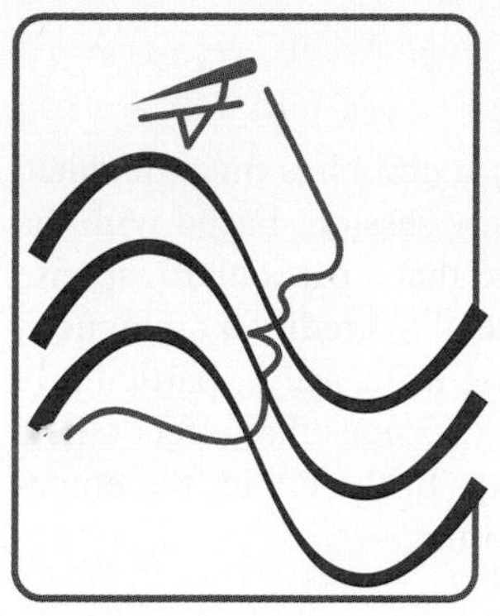

Clinical Scoring and Transcription 7

We are nearing the clinical training sections of this book. But some concepts and procedural issues require discussion before you tackle the text and audio materials in the next chapter. This chapter and associated appendixes should serve as a source for answers to questions that undoubtedly will arise as you attempt clinical phonetics.

Figure 7-1 illustrates the sequence of activities associated with scoring or phonetic transcription. These activities may be divided into three phases: (1) sampling and recording a child's speech, (2) playback and scoring or transcription, and (3) phonological analyses. This chapter is concerned primarily with events in the second phase, although we will discuss briefly issues in obtaining speech samples. Detailed procedures for audio recording and speech sampling are provided in Appendix E.

Let us look first at some factors that influence scoring and transcription.

FACTORS THAT INFLUENCE SCORING AND TRANSCRIPTION

Client Factors

Do characteristics of the person whose speech is being sampled affect the ease and accuracy of scoring and transcription? Unquestionably, they do. Some of the major individual differences are the person's age, dialect, and physical and personality characteristics.

Age. Children present many problems in transcription. For one thing, younger children have trouble understanding directions. The younger the child, the more difficult it is to have the child respond to formal testing. As an examiner, you need to devise effective and efficient ways to obtain speech samples for particular purposes. Procedures and findings for five types of speech samples—ranging from "nondirected" to "directed"—are described in Shriberg and Kwiatkowski (1985).

Children also behave in ways that interfere with transcription. For example, they frequently vary such voice characteristics as loudness and pitch, and they often fail to keep a fixed distance from the microphone of the recorder. They relish kicking tables and playing with microphone cords—all of which create noise on a recording. Occasionally, audio samples in this program will contain such child-generated noises.

The major reason that even the most well-mannered youngster is hard to score or transcribe is, of course, incomplete speech development. In fact, during the speech development period, children often produce sounds that are perceptually ambiguous. For example, Costely and Broen (1976) present acoustic data for a child whose voicing of alveolar stops /t/ and /d/ was indeterminate. Transcribers were baffled as to which stop consonant symbol was appropriate to use. Many studies since this one have shown that children produce sounds that do not clearly fall into adult categories. In the training tapes to follow, we will be concerned with just these sorts of problems.

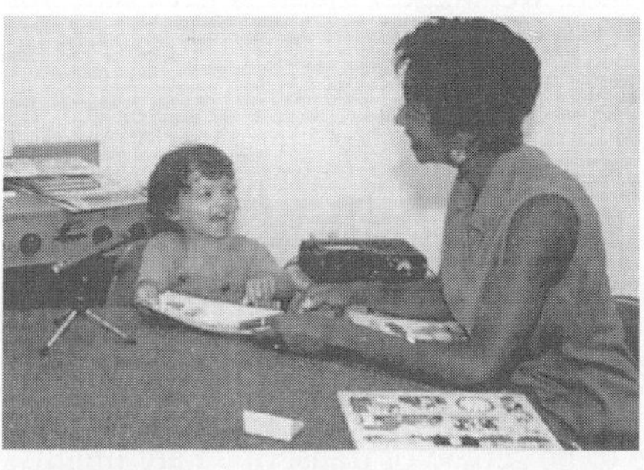
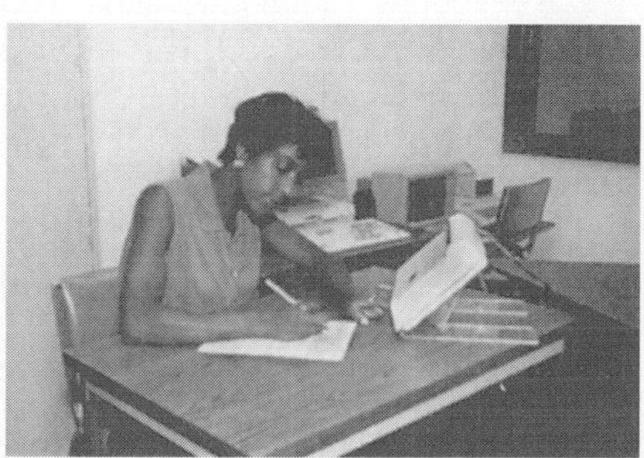
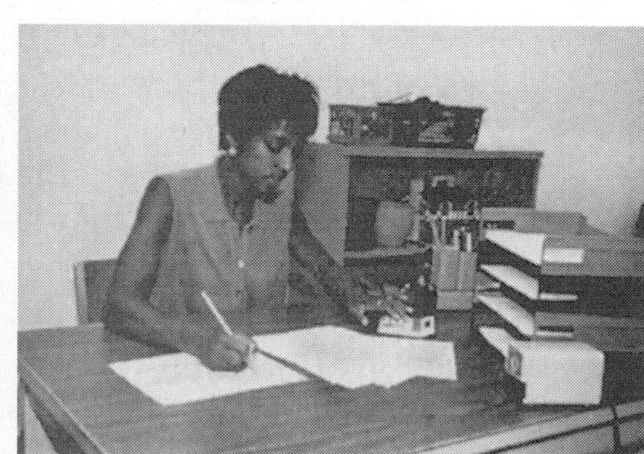

FIGURE 7-1
Obtaining, transcribing, and analyzing a speech sample.

Dialect. Another speech characteristic to consider is the client's dialect. In this text, as in most other American phonetics texts, General American speech is used as the reference dialect. Throughout the United States there are many regional dialects, as well as varieties of English spoken by those for whom English is a second language. For clinical work in communicative disorders, clinicians must learn to transcribe appropriately the dialect of the person with whom they will be working. Clinicians must learn both the phonological rules of the dialect and the boundaries for acceptable production of each allophone. The point to underscore is that dialect differences between speaker and transcriber must be placed in proper perspective. Appendix F is a detailed consideration of dialectal issues as they impact phonetic transcription in the clinical environment.

Physical and Personality Characteristics. Included in this last category of individual differences among speakers are the many physical and personal factors that make one person's speech easier to score or transcribe than another's. A person who uses larger lip movements, for example, may be easier to transcribe than one who speaks with tight lips or clenched teeth. The term "easier" includes concepts of reliability and efficiency. It may be much more tedious and time-consuming to transcribe the speech of certain talkers, even though it is accomplished successfully in the end. Rate of speech is another critical variable. Some talkers speak or read so fast that transcription is extremely difficult, if not impossible.

Transcription may also be biased by more subtle speaker characteristics. For example, Stephens and Daniloff (1974) reported that one of their speakers who had normal *articulation* was perceived by a transcriber working from audiotape as making some /s/ distortions. Stephens and Daniloff suggested that perhaps this subject's atypical *voice quality* had influenced articulation judgments. One of our student clinicians noted a similar problem when transcribing tapes of some children. This student commented: "Sometimes it was hard to separate [the client's] articulation from laryngeal or resonant voice quality. This was especially true [on tapes] where there was a hypernasal resonant quality overriding the articulation." Such observations suggest that a person's voice quality can influence transcription of articulation. Studies suggest that 25 to 50 percent of children with developmental speech disorders—the clinical group used for most of the samples in this text—have notable differences in voice quality (Shriberg and Kwiatkowski, 1994). Therefore, in the training samples to follow, you will hear many examples of children with deviant voice quality.

The interpersonal relationship between client and clinician is yet another source of bias that may affect transcription data. Diedrich and Bangert (1981) found that when the examiner is also the child's clinician, the child will often be judged as more competent. Experienced clinicians will readily acknowledge this tendency to give their client "the benefit of the doubt," especially after a child has misarticulated several items in a row in a therapy session. Faced with the task of continuing to tell the child that a particular response was "wrong," the clinician will tend to credit an ambiguous response as "right." Interpersonal influence is particularly hard to guard against; perceptual decisions that affect others directly are hard to make reliably. In the clinic, the empathetic clinician must remain impartial.

Summary. Clients who are hard to test, who have many speech errors, or whose speech differs from the transcriber's are generally more difficult to score or transcribe reliably. The clinician must be aware of possible speaker characteristics, as well as interpersonal factors, that can bias perception and transcription reliability.

Task Factors

In addition to the client factors just reviewed, several characteristics of the speech task itself should be considered for possible influence on scoring or transcription.

Intelligibility. One important speech task factor is intelligibility. Do we transcribe differently when meaning can be ascribed to the string of sounds in an utterance, as opposed to when the sounds are "uninterpretable"? Oller and Eilers (1975), in a study of this question, found that knowledge of the intended lexical content of an utterance did alter transcription. Such findings, which have been replicated in several studies (see Appendix D), present a disconcerting problem for clinical transcription. If the expectation of hearing a particular word yields a different transcription from that obtained when there is no such expectation, which transcription is more valid?

A phonetics "purist" might argue that the transcriber who is unaware of the intended sounds is more likely to produce valid transcription. In principle, it is hard to disagree with this view. In practice, however, such a view causes problems. Anyone who has had clinical experience with unintelligible children knows that transcription of speech, even when meaning is *known,* is difficult. When intended targets are unknown, transcription is almost impossible. As described in detail elsewhere (Shriberg, 1986, 1993; Shriberg and Kwiatkowski, 1980), we suggest that it is necessary for clinicians to gloss the child's intended targets (words) while obtaining conversational speech utterances from children with speech delays. Clinicians must attempt to determine, word-for-word, what the child intended to say at the time the sample is obtained. In the following practice transcriptions, a gloss of the child's speech is always provided in the text.

Linguistic Context and Response Requirements. Two other important variables associated with the difficulty of the speech sample to be scored or transcribed are linguistic context and response complexity. These characteristics were introduced briefly in Chapter 1.

Linguistic context refers to the number and type of linguistic units (phonemes, syllables, words, and so forth) in which the target linguistic unit(s) is (are) embedded. Because of certain masking phenomena and memory constraints, it is easier to score or transcribe a sound when it occurs in a relatively simple context. For example, it is generally easier to transcribe a phoneme when it occurs in the context of a syllable, rather than a complete sentence. In the training program that follows, we begin with speech samples of relatively simple linguistic complexity.

Response complexity refers to the number of transcription responses per linguistic unit required of the clinician. Generally, it is easier to transcribe one target sound (or cluster) per unit (word, phrase, sentence, and so forth) than to transcribe two or more targets per unit. A case in point: Some clinical situations require that articulation errors for /r/ sounds only be transcribed; other situations require the clinician to keep track of both the /ɝ/ sounds and the /r/ phonemes. Experience in teaching transcription confirms that response requirements must be approached in steps—gradually increasing the number of responses the transcriber must make per linguistic unit.

These generalizations about hierarchies of linguistic context and response complexity can be overridden. For example, a child with a subtle /s/ distortion may be difficult to transcribe reliably when /s/ sounds are sampled in isolation. In contrast, it may be easy to transcribe reliably *both* /r/ and /s/ sounds in a continuous speech sample, provided the child has obvious substitutions for these sounds and speaks reasonably slowly. This is a case where client factors, as discussed earlier, affect the transcription task. The type of error a client makes may be more crucial than the linguistic context and response requirements of the task. Or, further, given two persons with comparable error types, each person's rate of speech or other speech/voice characteristics may substantially affect overall task difficulty.

Successive Judgments. In addition to intelligibility, linguistic context, and response requirements, a fourth speech task factor concerns the problem of maintaining independent judgment in a succession of perceptual decisions. If a sample contains ten successive target /s/ words and the first nine words are judged correct, the tenth word may have to be markedly "wrong" to be perceived as such. This situation is extremely common in clinical situations that emphasize high rates of target responses from clients. The clinician must make a series of rapid judgments. At some point in the series of judgments, the perceptual standard may become biased. Clinicians and speech aides who work daily with many children in such training programs should monitor their reliability. Routine intrajudge reliability checks as defined and described in Appendix D will provide the needed data.

Summary. We have described four factors that influence task variables in transcription: (1) the need for transcribers to be aware of the intended target behaviors—that is, to have an accurate gloss of the child's utterance; the effects of (2) linguistic context and (3) response complexity on the ease and accuracy of transcription; and (4) the difficulty in keeping rapid successive judgments in a sample independent of one another. To determine if these factors are biasing scoring or transcription, clinicians should routinely obtain an estimate of their reliability, intrajudge and interjudge, as described in Appendix D. Considering the central role of scoring or transcription in both assessment and management, periodic calibration of one's perceptual skills is necessary for "sound" clinical practice (pun intended).

Speech Sampling and Audio-Video Recording

In most clinical settings, a portable recorder is the constant companion of the speech-language clinician. Advancements in technology have made excellent recording equipment available and affordable. Portable videotape recorders are available to clinicians as well, but audio recorders are by far more prevalent.

In view of the widespread use of audio recorders, it is surprising that so few applied studies of recording variables have been undertaken. Two questions in the minds of many clinicians are: Is transcription from a recorded source as valid and reliable as transcription of live speech? And, is transcription from an audio source as valid and reliable as transcription from a video recording? Appendix D pursues the first question, including information from several studies and a comprehensive bibliography. Let us address the second question here. Video recording systems have two major advantages.

First, if certain basic prerequisites are met (adequate lighting, sharp focus, good close-ups) video recording allows us to preserve certain gestures associated with speech production. The necessity for observing such behavior, however, and the status of articulatory gestures for phonological analyses are perennial issues in the literature and depend on the purpose for scoring or transcription. Video recording allows you to see more articulatory behavior, but not all articulatory behavior is linguistically significant. A general argument can be made that phonetic transcription should be based on what you *hear,* not on what you *see.* Later we will offer specific suggestions for how to best use visual information obtained live or from a video recording for certain transcription needs.

A second advantage to video recording is the visibility of the context in which the utterances occur. Utterances that otherwise might not be intelligible on audio media may become so when accompanied by information on eye gaze, gestures, or manipulation of objects. For certain research purposes, such information is vital. As discussed previously, however, we feel that interpretations should be validated immediately following each client utterance and recorded as the gloss spoken by the clinician. Accomplished in this way, audio recordings can be equally valid and certainly more efficient sources for clinical scoring or transcription than video, for certain research needs. Of course, for other clinical research purposes, video recordings may be the method of choice.

To summarize our observations on recording factors, advances in electronics have brought us from the era of disc recorders to wire recorders to the present-day technology of analog and digital recorders, CD-ROMs, and other media. The small amount of data on the accuracy of transcribing live versus from audio or video sources has been equivocal. In the absence of data on audio–video recording effects on the validity of transcription, we can only point out some advantages and disadvantages of each type of recording system. In the following section, we suggest procedures that can minimize the main sources of unreliability introduced by the use of audio recordings. A good recorder is a clinician's trusted companion. Speech-language pathologists are well advised to become completely familiar with procedures that will yield high-quality recordings of the speech of their clients. Appendix E provides technical information and specific procedural guidelines.

PREPARATION FOR CLINICAL TRANSCRIPTION

We have just discussed factors that influence the scoring and transcription process. In this section, the step-by-step preparation for scoring or transcription will be inspected in detail. Preparation involves attention to five needs: (1) selecting a system, (2) selecting a set of symbols, (3) selecting a recording form, (4) determining response definitions, and (5) determining conventions (procedural rules).

Selecting a System

As described in Chapter 1, contemporary speech-language pathologists use three systems of clinical phonetics. We have labeled these systems *two-way scoring, five-way scoring,* and *phonetic transcription* (see Chapter 1, Figure 1-1). Two-way scoring organizes perceptual input into just two output categories—"right" and "wrong." Five-way scoring provides four categories of "wrong," including *deletion* (or *omission*), *distortion* (or *approximation*), *substitution,* and *addition* of another sound. Finally, phonetic transcription uses a large set of symbols to describe both normal and disordered speech.

Unfortunately, there have not been any published studies comparing the three systems of clinical phonetics. It would be interesting to know whether a decision is affected by the procedural system used to make it. For example, are listeners more likely to score a target sound as "wrong" when using a two-way system than when using a five-way system? Our experience in teaching the three systems has given us some insight into this question. A brief historical digression is needed to explain.

When we first attempted to program the learning of clinical phonetics (Shriberg and Swisher, 1972), we assumed that two-way scoring was the easiest of the three systems to learn. Thus, two-way scoring became the first step in our early teaching programs, using common error sounds in increasingly complex linguistic contexts, from sounds in isolation to sounds in words, phrases, and so forth. The results were less than successful. Frankly, our students complained a lot. They told us they liked the idea of programmed teaching, but they disagreed with many of the "right–wrong" decisions on the answer keys. Importantly, they also found it hard to tell us *why* they disagreed with an item. As we began to determine which items in the key the disagreements occurred on, we found ourselves using terms and concepts from phonetic transcription, such as allophone, diacritic marking, and so forth. It finally dawned on us that perhaps we should teach phonetic transcription *first.* Although phonetic transcription of speech errors was more difficult to learn, it provided a firm basis for the other two scoring systems. Using this arrangement in subsequent revisions of our program produced improved results. Although mutterings about the validity of our answer keys will never be entirely extinguished, at least disagreements can now be discussed in a more focused and productive manner.

In the training samples to follow, therefore, you will be taught phonetic transcription of children's speech errors from the start. This will seem difficult to begin with, particularly because we begin with vowels. Ultimately, however, it will prove efficient for the reasons just mentioned. Once you are able to identify feature errors such as lateralization, velarization, and so forth, you easily can sort these perceptions into two-way and five-way scoring decisions, which are used later in the program.

In summary, working clinicians should always be able to *choose* among systems to meet their clinical needs. Unfortunately, clinicians who do not use skills learned early in their training will not have this choice. We hope the audio samples and textual materials in this series will provide clinicians with some alternatives. Retrieving one's clinical skills in phonetic transcription may not be as easy as pedaling away on a bicycle after a long absence from biking. But we have seen many experienced clinicians "reacquire" transcription competence with a little effort. In the 20 years since the first edition of this text, narrow transcription skills have become a requirement for the contemporary clinician working with a variety of child and adult speech disorders.

Selecting a Set of Symbols

Once a system has been selected, the next order of business is to select a set of symbols to be used within that system. Table 7-1 is a list of the types of symbols that have been used in two-way and five-way scoring. Symbols for phonetic transcription were presented earlier in this text. Symbols for use of phonetic transcription are fixed; the symbols should be written exactly in the form presented by the International Phonetic Association and in diacritic systems such as the one used in this book. For two-way or five-way scoring, however, the clinician must select a set of symbols and use them consistently. Choosing a set of symbols should involve considerations of clarity, speed, and visibility to the client.

Clarity. Clarity refers to the amount of degradation a symbol can undergo and still retain its identity. For example, use of "+" for correct and "×" for incorrect could be troublesome for clinicians whose penmanship is not always clear, particularly under the press of rapid scoring. The two symbols might easily be confused later. A better decision would be to use "+" versus "0," or any two symbols sufficiently distinct to withstand a certain amount of degradation in the clinical setting.

Speed. Speed is another major consideration, one which requires the use of a symbol drawn with a brief, continuous stroke. For example, "c" is faster than writing out "correct" or "cor." or "OK" and so forth. People who habitually print find certain symbols easier to make than others. You should experiment with making 20 small "x's" rapidly versus 20 of some other symbol for "wrong." Which symbol permits the fastest scoring? You may wish to use the same symbol in all your work, provided it meets other criteria discussed in this section.

Visibility to Client. Visibility to the client refers to the ease with which a client can discern the symbols used for "correct" and "incorrect" responses. Children and motivated adults (who often view therapy as "back to school") will learn to watch the clinician's pencil to monitor the judgments being made about their responses. Such feedback during a therapy session can be counterproductive and, in a test situation, can invalidate test results. Therefore, the test administrator should avoid letting the client make inferences about the "correctness" of his or her responses by using a set of symbols involving similar hand movements, such as check (✔) and check-tail (✔~) Here, the short tail added to the check to make the "incorrect" symbol is visually less obvious than the difference between a "+" and a "0," for example. If it is important to conceal your scoring of responses from the client, be sure to choose symbols that are made with ambiguous movements. Sometimes, however, the choice of symbols is dictated by the type of recording form used, which is discussed next.

Selecting a Recording Form

The purpose for which a sample is being transcribed will often suggest the type of recording form required. Published forms for scoring formal articulation tests are familiar to practicing clinicians. Figures 7-2, 7-3, and 7-4 are response forms from several published articulation tests. Some of the test manuals for these and other articulation tests suggest how to use scoring symbols. Articulation test forms warrant two comments.

First, the space allotted to record a response is quite small on some forms, such as on the form for the McDonald Screening Deep Test of Articulation (Figure 7-4). When one is forced to write rapidly in such a small space, it is particularly important to use an easily distinguishable symbol system and to write legibly.

A second observation about articulation test forms is that they generally require particular care in five-way scoring of clusters. If the transcriber writes "D" or "distortion" in the box provided for a target cluster, the reader cannot discern which consonants in the cluster were distorted. The distortion could have occurred on one or more members of the cluster. A better practice is to transcribe the entire cluster, using "D" for any distorted segments within the cluster; for example [Dpl], [Dtr], [ntD], and so forth. This may look confusing but it actually gives the reader a clearer picture of what was spoken—whether one or more segments in the cluster were distorted and which ones were distorted.

TABLE 7-1
Some Symbols Commonly Used in Two-Way and Five-Way Scoring of Speech Sound Changes

Correct	Incorrect	Substitution	Deletion	Distortion	Addition
Cor.	Incor.	Subst.	Del.	Dist.	Add.
C	I	X/Y[a]	Om. (omission)	D	$^{x}Y^{a}$
✔	✔~	X/	—	Lat. (lateralization)	Y^{x}
+	X		Ø	Dent. (dentalization)	
OK	—			Etc.	
G (good)	NG (not good)				
R (right)	W (wrong)				
A (acceptable)	NA (not acceptable)				

[a]These letters represent the target sound (Y) and the replacement or new sound (X).

9–62392

THE FISHER-LOGEMANN TEST OF ARTICULATION COMPETENCE

Screening ☐ Complete ☐

Record Form for the Picture Test

Name__________ Date__________ Examiner__________

Age__________ Grade (or Occupation)__________ School (or Employer)__________

Birthdate__________ Home Address__________

Native Dialect__________ Foreign Language in home__________

CONSONANT PHONEMES

Place of Articulation

Card #	IPA Phoneme	Common Spelling	Dev. Age	Place of Articulation	Voicing	Stop			Fricative			Affricate			Glide			Lateral			Nasal		
						Pre.	Inter.	Post.	Pre.	Inter.	Post.	Pre.	Inter.	Post.	Pre.	Inter.	Post.	Pre.	Inter.	Post.	Pre.	Inter.	Post.
1 2 3 4 5	p b ʍ w m	p b wh w m	3 5 3 3	Bilabial	V̶	/p	/p	/p	/ʍ[1]														
					V	/b	/b	/b							/w	/w					/m	/m	/m
6 7	f v	f v	4 7	Labio-dental	V̶				/f	/f	/f												
					V				/v	/v	/v												
8 9	θ ð	th th	7 8	Tip-dental	V̶				/θ	/θ	/θ												
					V				/ð	/ð	/ð												
10 11 12 13	t d l n	t d l n	6 5 6 3	Tip-alveolar	V̶	/t	/t[2]	/t															
					V	/d	/d	/d										/l	/l	/l	/n	/n	/n
14 15	s z	s z	7 7	Blade-alveolar	V̶				/s	/s	/s												
					V				/z	/z	/z												
16 17 18 19	ʃ ʒ tʃ dʒ	sh zh ch j	6 7 6 7	Blade-prepalatal	V̶				/ʃ	/ʃ	/ʃ	/tʃ	/tʃ	/tʃ									
					V					/ʒ	/ʒ[3]	/dʒ	/dʒ	/dʒ									
20	j	y	5	Front-palatal	V̶																		
					V										/j	/j							
21	r	r	6	Central-palatal	V̶																		
					V										/r	/r	/r[4]						
22 23 24	k g ŋ	k g ng	4 4 5	Back-velar	V̶	/k	/k	/k															
					V	/g	/g	/g														/ŋ	/ŋ
25	h	h	3	Glottal	V̶				/h	/h													

SUMMARY OF MISARTICULATION PATTERNS:

MANNER OF FORMATION ERRORS:

PLACE OF ARTICULATION ERRORS:

VOICING ERRORS:

Notes: (These and additional notes are discussed in the Manual under "Dialectal Variations")
1. Either /ʍ/ or /w/
2. Either /t/ or /d/
3. Either /ʒ/ or /dʒ/.
4. Either /r/ or /ə/ or lengthening of the preceding vowel.

FIGURE 7-2
The Fisher-Logemann Test of Articulation Competence: Record Form for the Picture Test. (H. Fisher and J. Logemann, The Fisher-Logemann Test of Articulation Competence. Record Form. Iowa City, IA: The Riverside Publishing Company, 1971. Reproduced with permission of The Riverside Publishing Company.)

CONSONANT BLENDS

CARD & ITEM #	/s/ + CONSONANT	CARD & ITEM #	CONSONANT + /r/	CARD & ITEM #	CONSONANT + /l/
26–1	______/s spoon	28–1	______/r present	30–1	______/l sled
26–2	______/s star	28–2	______/r bread	30–2	______/l blue
26–3	______/s slide	28–3	______/r fruit	30–3	______/l plane
		28–4	______/r frying pan		
26–4	______/s snake	28–5	______/r three	30–4	______/l flag
27–1	______/s skate	29–1	______/r tree	31–1	______/l clown
27–2	______/s swing	29–2	______/r dress	31–2	______/l glass.
27–3	______/s smoke	29–3	______/r cry	31–3	______/l bottle
		29–4	______/r green		
Best Context: ______		Best Context: ______		Best Context: ______	
Worst Context: ______		Worst Context: ______		Worst Context: ______	

VOWEL PHONEMES

	FRONT	CENTRAL	BACK
HIGH	32–1. ______/i key 32–2. ______/ɪ mitten		34–4. ______/u two 34–3. ______/ʊ foot
MID	32–3. ______/e table 32–4. ______/ɛ bell	33–4. ______/ɝ shirt 33–3. ______/ə cup	34–2. ______/o phone
LOW	33–1. ______/æ hat		34–1. ______/ɔ ball 33–2. ______/ɑ sock

PHONEMIC DIPHTHONGS: 35–1. ______/aɪ eye 35–3. ______/ɔɪ boy

35–2. ______/aʊ house 35–4. ______/ju U

ANALYSIS OF VOWEL MISARTICULATIONS:

FIGURE 7-2
(continued)

PAT RECORDING SHEET

		Year	Month	Day
Name______________________	Date	____	____	____
School______________________	Birth	____	____	____
Grade__________	Age	____	____	____

Key: Omission (–); substitution (write phonetic symbol of sound substituted); severity of distortion (D1), (D2), (D3); ability to imitate (circle symbol or error).

Sound	Photograph	1	2	3	Vowels, Diph.		Comments
	I				III		
s	saw, pencil, house				aʊ house		
s bl	spoon, skates, stars						
z	zipper, scissors, keys						
ʃ	shoe, station, fish				u shoe		
tʃ	chair, matches, sandwich						
dʒ	jars, angels, orange						
t	table, potatoes, hat				æ hat		
d	dog, ladder, bed				ɔ dog		
n	nails, bananas, can				ə bananas		
l	lamp, balloons, bell				ɛ bell		
l bl	blocks, clock, flag				ɑ blocks		
θ	thumb, toothbrush, teeth				i teeth		
r	radio, carrots, car						
r bl	brush, crayons, train				e train		
k	cat, crackers, cake				ɚ-ə crackers		
g	gun, wagon, egg				ʌ gun		
	II						
f	fork, elephant, knife						
v	vacuum, TV, stove				ju vacuum		
p	pipe, apples, cup				aɪ pipe		
b	book, baby, bathtub				ʊ book		
m	monkey, hammer, comb				o comb		**SCORE**
w-hw	witch, flowers, whistle				ɪ witch		*Sounds*
	I						I Tongue________
ð	this, that, feathers, bathe						II Lip ________
h-ŋ	hanger, hanger, swing						III Vowels________
j	yes, thank you						Total ________
ʒ	measure, beige				ɔɪ boy		
	(story)				ɜ-ɜ bird		

FIGURE 7-3
PAT (Photo Articulation Test) Recording Sheet. (Kathleen Pendergast et al., Photo Articulation Test. PAT Recording Sheet. Danville, IL: The Interstate Printers & Publishers, Inc., 1969. Reproduced with permission of the publisher.)

CONNECTED SPEECH AND LANGUAGE

(Elicit story and conversation by using items 70 through 72. Note language, intelligibility, voice, fluency.)

ADDITIONAL DIAGNOSTIC INFORMATION

(Hearing loss, motor coordination, perceptual deficiencies, emotional factors, attitude toward disorder and treatment.)

THERAPY GOALS AND PROGRESS

Additional copies of this sheet available in pads of 96 each from
The Interstate Printers & Publishers, Inc., Danville, Illinois 61832
Reorder No. 1065

FIGURE 7-3
(continued)

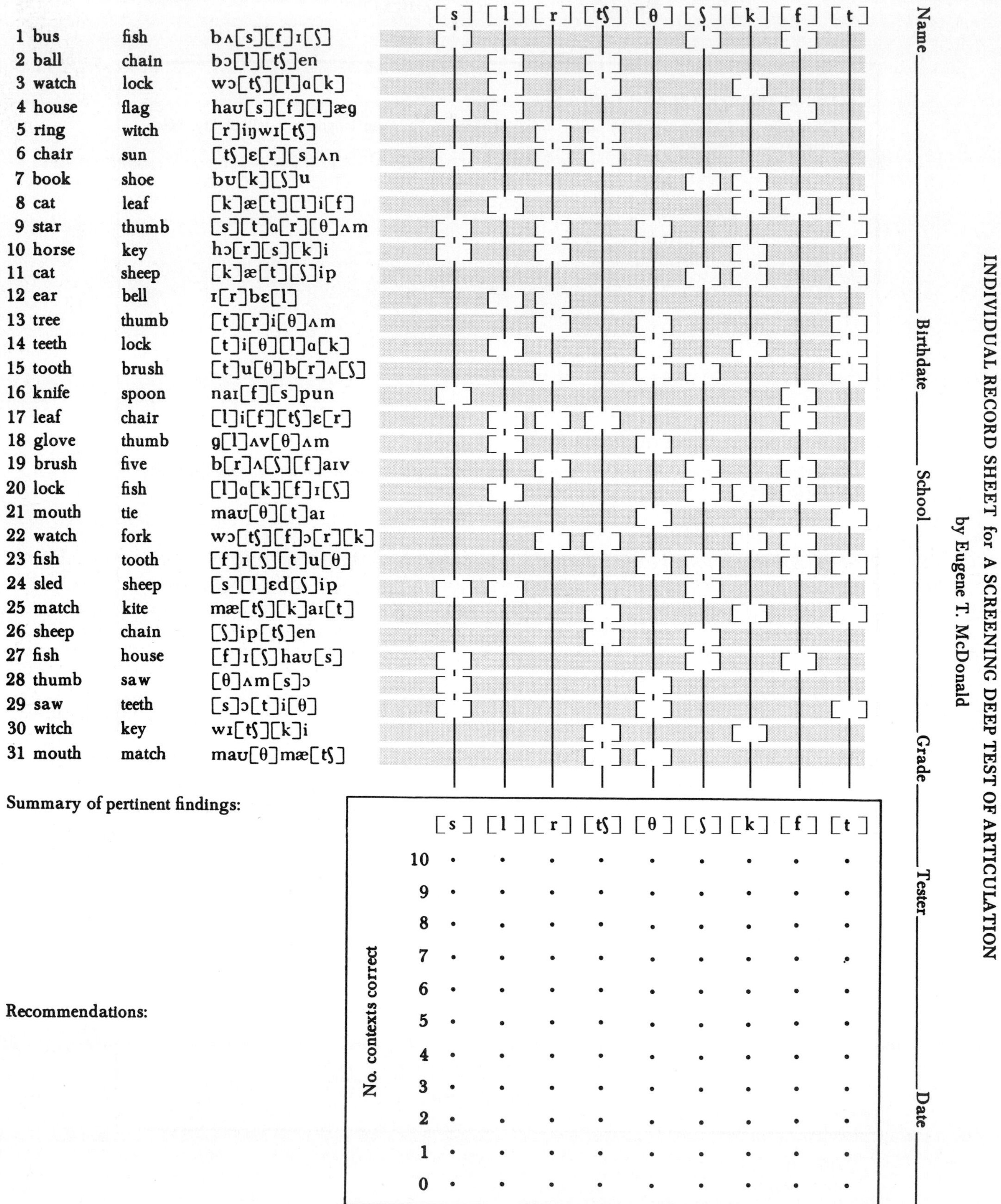

INDIVIDUAL RECORD SHEET for A SCREENING DEEP TEST OF ARTICULATION
by Eugene T. McDonald

Name________ Birthdate________ School________ Grade________ Tester________ Date________

1	bus	fish	bʌ[s][f]ɪ[ʃ]
2	ball	chain	bɔ[l][tʃ]en
3	watch	lock	wɔ[tʃ][l]ɑ[k]
4	house	flag	haʊ[s][f][l]æg
5	ring	witch	[r]iŋwɪ[tʃ]
6	chair	sun	[tʃ]ɛ[r][s]ʌn
7	book	shoe	bʊ[k][ʃ]u
8	cat	leaf	[k]æ[t][l]i[f]
9	star	thumb	[s][t]ɑ[r][θ]ʌm
10	horse	key	hɔ[r][s][k]i
11	cat	sheep	[k]æ[t][ʃ]ip
12	ear	bell	ɪ[r]bɛ[l]
13	tree	thumb	[t][r]i[θ]ʌm
14	teeth	lock	[t]i[θ][l]ɑ[k]
15	tooth	brush	[t]u[θ]b[r]ʌ[ʃ]
16	knife	spoon	naɪ[f][s]pun
17	leaf	chair	[l]i[f][tʃ]ɛ[r]
18	glove	thumb	g[l]ʌv[θ]ʌm
19	brush	five	b[r]ʌ[ʃ][f]aɪv
20	lock	fish	[l]ɑ[k][f]ɪ[ʃ]
21	mouth	tie	maʊ[θ][t]aɪ
22	watch	fork	wɔ[tʃ][f]ɔ[r][k]
23	fish	tooth	[f]ɪ[ʃ][t]u[θ]
24	sled	sheep	[s][l]ɛd[ʃ]ip
25	match	kite	mæ[tʃ][k]aɪ[t]
26	sheep	chain	[ʃ]ip[tʃ]en
27	fish	house	[f]ɪ[ʃ]haʊ[s]
28	thumb	saw	[θ]ʌm[s]ɔ
29	saw	teeth	[s]ɔ[t]i[θ]
30	witch	key	wɪ[tʃ][k]i
31	mouth	match	maʊ[θ]mæ[tʃ]

Summary of pertinent findings:

Recommendations:

No. contexts correct	[s]	[l]	[r]	[tʃ]	[θ]	[ʃ]	[k]	[f]	[t]
10	•	•	•	•	•	•	•	•	•
9	•	•	•	•	•	•	•	•	•
8	•	•	•	•	•	•	•	•	•
7	•	•	•	•	•	•	•	•	•
6	•	•	•	•	•	•	•	•	•
5	•	•	•	•	•	•	•	•	•
4	•	•	•	•	•	•	•	•	•
3	•	•	•	•	•	•	•	•	•
2	•	•	•	•	•	•	•	•	•
1	•	•	•	•	•	•	•	•	•
0	•	•	•	•	•	•	•	•	•

PHONETIC PROFILE

FIGURE 7-4
Individual Record Sheet for A Screening Deep Test of Articulation. (Eugene McDonald, A Screening Deep Test of Articulation. Individual Record Sheet. Pittsburgh, PA: Stanwix House, Inc., 1968. Reproduced with permission of the publisher.)

In addition to forms for commercially available articulation tests, a variety of forms can be helpful for particular scoring or transcription needs. Figure 7-5, for example, is a simple form we have used for two-way scoring of a target sound in continuous speech. Figure 7-6 is a form we use for phonetic transcription of continuous speech. This information is subsequently entered into a computer program for phonetic and phonological analysis (Shriberg, 1986; Shriberg, Allen, McSweeny, and Wilson, 2001). The selection of the proper recording form, as with other decisions that the clinician must make, is an important determinant of the efficiency and effectiveness of any clinical phonetics task.

Determining Response Definitions

Explicit response definitions are needed when using two-way or five-way scoring systems. A good response definition describes the attributes of each response in relation to the target behavior that make it correct, a distortion, a socially acceptable /s/, and so forth. The response definition should allow a clinician to make judgments rapidly and reliably. Good response definitions orient the listener to the crucial aspects of the stimuli requiring attention. Here are some actual response definitions taken from two-way scoring in the clinical literature; note the variety of approaches:

To be scored correct the test phoneme had to look and sound correct. (Paynter, Ermey, Green, and Draper, 1978)

A correct response was defined as a sound production that conformed to Standard General American Speech. (DuBois and Bernthal, 1978)

Subjects were reinforced with tokens when responses were considered 'socially' acceptable (that is, neither drawing attention to the speaker nor interfering with communication). (Irwin, Weston, Griffith, and Rocconi, 1976)

The teeth must be closed. You must not be concerned with the sound of [s] at this point, just the visual features of the mouth, teeth, and tongue. (Mowrer, Baker, and Schutz, 1970)

In these response definitions, listeners are told to attend to visual, acoustic, or articulatory behaviors or combinations of these. By using a common response definition, listeners should be processing the stimuli in similar ways. Also, each will judge the stimuli in the same way on two separate occasions. The choice of response definitions, as seen in these examples, is arbitrary. Variations in response definitions arise from differences in theoretical positions, differences in goals, differences in the stage of clinical management, and so forth.

One component that is missing in the response definitions just listed is a decision logic for dealing with questionable responses, that is, for responses that fall "between the cracks." A good response definition provides a rule for categorizing such behaviors. For some purposes, we might decide to generate a rule that discards questionable stimuli. Alternatively, a rule could assign questionable responses to one or another of the available categories. For example, in a two-way scoring task, the following three response definitions are possible (Figure 7-7):

1. Solution *(a)* is the conservative approach. Responses that seem to be in the "gray area" (shown here in red) are simply discarded from subsequent analyses. Such a response definition could be used to purify data—only unambiguously judged responses will be preserved for some analysis procedure.
2. Solution *(b)* says to score responses correct unless they are heard as incorrect, just as one is "innocent until proven guilty" in jurisprudence. This criterion assumes that the population sampled has a higher probability of being innocent ("correct") *and* that *negative* judgments should not be made unless one is fairly certain of the data on which they are based. When screening a group of college students for errors in speech, for example, we might assign all questionable /s/ responses to "correct" because this is a normally speaking sample.
3. Solution *(c)* assumes the opposite position. Such a response definition might be used for the ultimate benefit of those already enrolled in a speech management program. Here, the approach is to assume that if a person's actual probability of correct responses is lower than 50 percent, questionable responses should be assigned to "incorrect." This criterion, "guilty until proven innocent," might be used constructively in a final phase of management or maintenance when a client benefits from feedback about marginally acceptable production while trying to maintain top performance.

The clinician must clearly formulate response definitions; in turn, response definitions will help the clinician accomplish the job. They should be explicit. They should tell the clinician precisely how to go about making judgments, including a decision rule for handling difficult judgments.

Determining Transcription Conventions

The final need in preparation for clinical transcription—after having selected a system, a set of symbols, a recording form, and response definitions—is to determine some conventions for transcription. Conventions are procedures that participants agree to abide by. Several types of conventions or "rules" are important to establish at the outset of any transcription endeavor.

Which Phonetic Behaviors Are to Be Transcribed and Which Can Be Ignored? A basic decision that will require a convention is whether the clinician must attend

NAME: ______________________ DATE: ______________________

SCHOOL/GRADE: ______________________ TARGET SOUND: ______________________

______________________ EXAMINER/CLINICIAN: ______________________

DESCRIPTION OF SAMPLE: ______________________

____

____

	1	2	3	4	5	6	7	8	9	10	11	12	13	14	15	16	17	18	19	20
Correct																				
Incorrect																				
	21	22	23	24	25	26	27	28	29	30	31	32	33	34	35	36	37	38	39	40
Correct																				
Incorrect																				
	41	42	43	44	45	46	47	48	49	50	51	52	53	54	55	56	57	58	59	60
Correct																				
Incorrect																				
	61	62	63	64	65	66	67	68	69	70	71	72	73	74	75	76	77	78	79	80
Correct																				
Incorrect																				
	81	82	83	84	85	86	87	88	89	90	91	92	93	94	95	96	97	98	99	100
Correct																				
Incorrect																				

No. Correct ______________________

No. Incorrect ______________________

Percentage Correct ______________________

FIGURE 7-5
A simple form for two-way scoring of a target sound in continuous speech.

PEPFORM: Cover Page	Study ______ Peplog No. ______ Page ______

Pepfile Name ______ Sampling Dates ______

Subject ______ Sampling Examiner ______

Age ______ Transcription Date ______

D.O.B. ______ Transcriber ______

Notes ______

Utterance No.	Counter No.	Line	Transcription and Comments
		X	
		Y	
		Z	
		X	
		Y	
		Z	
		X	
		Y	
		Z	
		X	
		Y	
		Z	
		X	
		Y	
		Z	
		X	
		Y	
		Z	

FIGURE 7-6
PEPPER (Programs to Examine Phonetic and Phonological Evaluation Records) Transcription Form—a form for phonetic transcription of continuous conversational speech. The orthographic form of a speaker's intended utterance is entered in the X line, the corresponding intended phonetic forms are entered in the Y line, and the realized phonetic forms are entered in the Z line. (Shriberg et al., 2001.)

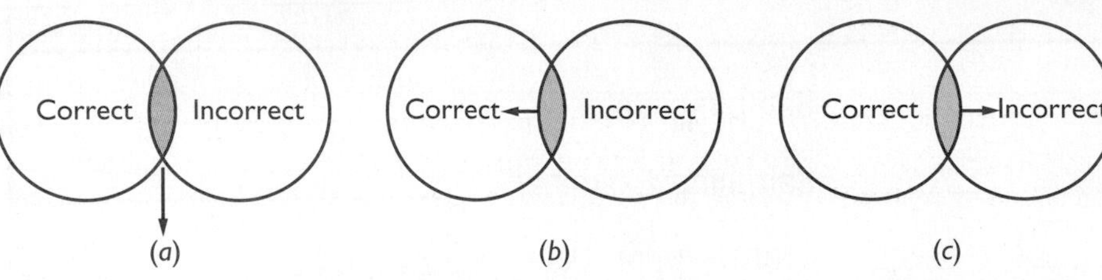

FIGURE 7-7
Three response definitions in a two-way scoring task.

to every bit of the speaker's phonetic behavior. Should every normally occurring allophone, such as the aspiration of initial voiceless stops or assimilative nasality on vowels, be transcribed? Do we want to take the time to transcribe behaviors that are predictable in normal speech? The answer to this question hinges on the purposes of transcription. For the linguist, whose task might be to determine the sound system of an unknown language, it may be necessary to capture such detail. For a particular clinical task, however, such detail may not be of interest. The point is that whether a particular phonetic behavior is to be transcribed or ignored is an arbitrary or situationally determined matter. Confusion will result unless a convention for such decisions is explicit and made available to all parties involved. For example, here is a partial list of the conventions used with clinicians who transcribed continuous speech samples for one clinical research project:

1. Transcribe aspiration/nonaspiration only when it differs from the anticipated allophone.
2. Transcribe hypernasality only when it differs from the anticipated allophone.
3. Transcribe vowel duration only when it differs from the anticipated allophone.
4. Be most precise in your transcription for words that have primary stress; words having secondary stress or that are unstressed will be treated separately in the phonological analysis.
5. If you are undecided between two or more transcriptions of a consonant or consonant cluster, write your best estimate on the line and the alternative(s) above.

How Much of the Data Is to Be Transcribed Live Versus Transcribed Later from Audio or Video Recordings? It is very important to establish a convention for what will be scored or transcribed live as opposed to later from a recording. Stephens and Daniloff's (1974) position on this issue is that scoring of /s/ errors should be made live. As noted earlier in this chapter, these researchers found that live scoring of sibilants compared to audiotape scoring yielded different scores. Shriberg (1972) found that two-way judgments of /s/ errors were only 65 percent reliable from audiotape. Do these unhappy data on audio judgments indicate that we should throw away our recorders? Obviously not. The subject still requires a considerable amount of study. To date, the data are much too limited in scope and methodology to conclude that we should abandon use of the recorder. Furthermore, comparative linguistics has produced much valuable work based on recordings of languages made in the field. A more useful response is to ask what sorts of information are better to transcribe live when it is possible to do so.

One type of information the transcriber should attend to during the live recording session is the visual components of speech. Specifically, the transcriber should pay attention to *lip postures* and *lip closures.* Consider the word *cup* on an audio recording. If the final /p/ of *cup* is unreleased, there will not be an audible burst. If the examiner is audio recording, attention could be paid to transcribing lip closure live, which will resolve later questions about whether or not the child actually produced a final consonant /p/. Similarly, if /r/ is accompanied by lip rounding, such gestures are easier to observe live than to infer from listening to an audio recording.

If video recordings are made, live transcription might focus more on the acoustic characteristics of fricatives and affricates. The assumption is that the video signal will provide a faithful copy of visual information, while the audio signal on a videotape (but not on video disk) is less faithful in reproducing fricative sounds than the audio signal from a good audio recorder.

Summary

Much of the mystique about clinical phonetics is related simply to a lack of understanding about its basic clerical nature. We should not assume that every clinician recalls the symbols learned in the obligatory phonetics course taken in undergraduate programs. Clinicians may be baffled by reports from colleagues simply because they have forgotten how to interpret phonetic symbols rather than due to any other factor. Attention to each of the five preparation tasks described here—selecting a system, a set of symbols, and a response form and determining response definitions and transcription conventions—will provide the necessary base for the efficient use of clinical phonetics.

THE PROCESS OF SCORING OR TRANSCRIPTION

If you have "done your homework"—attended to all the preparatory needs just discussed—the process of scoring or transcription should go smoothly. It is the process itself that we now finally consider.

What takes place in the clinician's mind while doing clinical phonetics? It is tempting to try to model the process of scoring or transcription. Research in speech discrimination, decision theory, information processing, and related areas would provide relevant paradigms. As attractive as such model building would be, we will limit ourselves to a sketch of processes we have observed or readily can infer. Much of what we have learned about transcription comes from simply asking students what went on as they attempted to transcribe and from diaries students have kept while doing transcription tasks.

For ease of communication, we now slip into a "how to" manual style of discourse. Suggestions are made to you, the reader, now as a transcriber. We will assume that scoring or transcription is being accomplished from an audio recording except where otherwise indicated. Moreover, when this edition went to press we did not yet have findings from a study of progress comparing transcription from audiotapes to transcription using CDs. Therefore, all our guidelines to follow (and elsewhere in this text) assume that you are transcribing from portable audiocassette recorders. You may experience some important validity, reliability, and/or efficiency differences transcribing CDs from your computer or portable device, compared to transcription from audiotape devices.

Setting Up

Get Comfortable. Try to find an accommodating place for transcription. The lighting should be good, and the amount of distracting noise and potential visual distractions should be minimized. Be sure that you are comfortable and well oriented toward the playback device. Remote stop-start attachments are especially convenient, but most audiotape recorders require a mechanical, push-button arrangement on the machine itself. Unfortunately, when a recorder is lying flat on a table, you will be poorly oriented toward the loudspeaker. Try to set the recorder on an angle that allows you to manipulate the stop–rewind–start buttons while placing you squarely in front of the speaker. Surprisingly, it is little things like the angle of your wrist and fingers to the equipment that, over the course of a transcription session, begin to take their toll on the efficiency and general satisfaction with clinical transcription. Again, these same guidelines are relevant for playback functions using computer software, a keyboard, and a mouse.

Should I Use Headphones? The choice between using a set of headphones or listening to a recorder or speakers free-field involves several issues. Students we know who have used both generally prefer free-field listening to the use of headphones—especially if a lengthy session of listening is expected. For limited periods of scoring or transcription, headphones do have several advantages. A high-quality set of headphones will deliver excellent sound. By their very feel, headphones create a listening "set" for the student. Moreover, headphones block out competing noise. Especially when your listening place is shared with other students, roommates, and so forth, the headphones have the psychological effect of acting as a barrier to small talk and interruptions. On the negative side, however, headphone use becomes tedious after a certain amount of time, which varies from person to person. If you do use headphones, be sure that they are placed on your head comfortably and that they are in good repair. You will need to take more frequent breaks, but you may find that headphones enhance your overall efficiency.

Previewing the Recording

Undoubtedly, there are some situations where your very first impression of behavior is the most valid. Usually, however, preliminary play of the recording to be transcribed is desirable. Here are some comments from two student clinicians who transcribed speech samples from their clients:

> *It helped to listen to the whole tape once to get set.*
>
> *My approach was to listen to most of the tape without writing to get an idea of what to listen to.*

Note that these students' comments reflect some of the preparation tasks considered earlier. The preplay allows the transcriber to determine some conventions to be followed for the transcription, that is, what types of behaviors are to be transcribed and in what way. A preplay of the recording accomplishes other things: (1) It allows you to set the most appropriate playback level on the audio control and to desensitize yourself to sudden, unexpected intensity changes that invariably occur on speech samples from young children; (2) it allows you to adjust the audio for background noise, such as hiss, to avoid confusing noise with fricative distortions; (3) it allows you to desensitize yourself to any biasing variables, such as voice characteristics of the client; (4) it allows you to adjust to the speech tempo of the client, to determine how much behavior you will be able to score or transcribe at a stretch.

There is one situation in which a preview is absolutely necessary. For unintelligible children or adults, it may be necessary to gloss the sample before a transcription can be made. As described earlier, a gloss is a word-by-word transcription of each word intended by the speaker, including fast speech forms and ungrammatical words. As you may imagine, glossing takes a good deal of time, and clinicians take such trouble only when a phonological analysis of continuous speech is required.

In summary, a preview lets you prepare for the task at hand—to determine what sorts of symbols will be needed and to predict how frequently certain types of behaviors will be occurring on the tape. Too often, if you begin "cold"—without a preview—some or all of the transcription will have to be redone. Guidelines for transcribing persons with dialects (Appendix F) provide especially relevant rationale for previewing the sample.

A preplay may take away some of the drama of simply turning on the playback device and beginning transcription; but, in the long run, the extra time spent in previewing a sample will pay off.

First Presentation of the Target Behavior

After making all the preliminary arrangements covered to this point, you now are ready to score or transcribe. As we have reconstructed it, after you hear the first stimulus to be scored or transcribed, one of two things can happen: Either you score or transcribe it, or you will need to replay it. Let us look at each of these possibilities.

Immediate Recognition. The first possibility is that you may hear the target stimulus, for example, a w/r, an aspirated /k/, a correct /s/, and you instantly "compute." That is, you recognize immediately the scoring or transcription category that you should use to capture this response. Though you may have to pause to be sure you are using the right symbolization, you have made up your mind: it *is* a w/r, it *is* an aspirated /k/, it *is* a correct /s/. No mediation is necessary—at least you are not aware of any mediating processes. With practice, it is this type of instant processing that you will do more and more as you develop competence and confidence in discriminating the types of behaviors trained in this series. It is very similar to sight-reading music. Such symbolic conversions become so rapid that at some point you are not aware of any conscious effort to discriminate the correct symbols. It has become automatic.

Incomplete Recognition. A second possibility is that you will only partially discriminate a response category. Was the behavior a phonemic substitution, or was it a distortion of some sort? The information that we have put together indicates that, invariably, the strategy at this point is to *attempt a simulation of the behavior.* Producing the sound yourself, if you can articulate silently or even out loud a sound that matches the one heard, seems to aid in scoring or transcribing the target sound. The importance to clinical phonetics of being able to imitate deviant speech cannot be overstated. Here are some comments from student diaries:

> *I don't hear symbols. It's still a struggle for me to match my perceptual impressions against graphic representation, especially when I can't imitate it.*
>
> *The stimulus seemed so fleeting that I could not seem to get an accurate auditory image of it. If I was able to produce the child's production myself (what I thought was an accurate production) I was much more able to transcribe it.*
>
> *The better I could imitate, the easier it was to discriminate.*

These comments, particularly the first one, are telling. Clinicians need to learn to make the different types of speech sound errors made by their clients. Distortion-type errors, of course, are the most difficult. This strategy is not foolproof. But as long as a memory for the recorded sound (or live sound) lasts, you should attempt to match your production to that memory. The ability to imitate a child's speech error precisely is also an important skill in management programs when the clinician needs to demonstrate to the child exactly what the child is producing in place of the correct sound.

Second and Subsequent Presentations (Replays)

Replays may be necessary either to confirm the judgment made on the first trial or because a decision was not made as just described. Listeners seem compelled to use replays more often in phonetic transcription than when scoring by two-way or five-way systems. There seems to be an interaction between the level of intelligibility of the speaker, the complexity of the system, and the consequences of making hasty decisions. Ideally, of course, a listener should be equally careful about the discrimination task in all clinical phonetics situations.

One thing we have learned is that the tendency to call for a replay has to be guarded against. One student put it succinctly: "I allowed myself up to *10* repetitions for certain words—this was frustrating!!!" Our experience suggests that the following strategy for replays is best:

1. Play the word or larger sample two or three times without scoring or transcribing.
2. Score or transcribe.
3. Replay only if necessary.

What we are suggesting is that the target response may have to be repeated once or twice to encode it solidly in memory. However, unless it is lengthy, it should be repeated *only* once or twice.

We also suggest that a limitation be placed on the latency of your response, that is, the amount of time between listening and scoring or transcription. If a scoring or transcription response is not made within a given number of seconds, replay the item. If the target behaviors are such that auditory memory does decay with some regularity, such as in a 20-word listening task for /s/, setting an outside limit is useful. It is useful to say, for example, that you will allow no longer than three seconds for a decision or else replay the item. As one student wrote: "After two or three seconds, I just couldn't remember what I had heard."

Strategies for Difficult Words

Another thing that we have observed is that clinicians devise interesting strategies when faced with behavior that is difficult to transcribe. Our diary studies indicate that students approach the transcription of difficult words in one of four ways:

1. Transcribe all the vowels first, then the singleton consonants, then the consonant clusters.
2. Transcribe syllable-by-syllable.
3. Transcribe all phoneme segments first, then add diacritics.
4. Transcribe the easiest behavior first, then go back as often as necessary to transcribe harder sounds.

The first two strategies have the value of forcing the transcriber to look at the syllable peaks, that is, the canonical structures of words (CV, CVC, CVCC, and so forth). The third strategy does most to capture the whole form of the word. Although we have tried all four methods to see which might force more rigor in transcription, the fourth strategy is easily the most used in our poll of students. From one of our student's diaries: "The first time I transcribed what was 'easiest'—what I was sure I heard. Next time, I transcribed what was next easiest. I used the same process until done with the utterance. The longer the utterance was, the more replays." And from another student: "I got the most 'remarkable' features written first."

Overall, then, there are many ways to deal with words that are not immediately transcribed. Try to observe the process you go through as you deal with difficult words. You may find that one or another of these four strategies works best for you.

Four Parameters of Phonetic Transcription

Appendix D provides a review of research findings in phonetic transcription that your instructor may elect to pursue in class. As we conclude this chapter, it is useful to include findings from just one study that will be of interest in the present context.

The information in Table 7-2 was taken from the logbooks of a team of examiners who tested a series of job applicants for positions as research transcriptionists (Shriberg, Hinke, and Trost-Steffen, 1987). The application process used a job sample technique in which applicants were taught some skills in phonetic transcription, followed by criterion testing on those skills. The goal was to select from among all applicants the two persons who could best be trained to work closely with each other as a consensus transcription team for a research project in developmental phonological disorders.

The statements in Table 7-2 are observations about each of the applicants as they proceeded through the training tasks. The observations noted applicants' strengths and weaknesses in four parameters: *perceptual ability, efficiency and productivity, problem-solving ability,* and *interpersonal attitude.* The observations in Table 7-2 vividly convey the perceptual, cognitive, affective, and interpersonal processes that underlie phonetic transcription. Especially when you near the end of your coursework in phonetics, you may find it useful to compare some of your experiences and attitudes about transcription with these observations. Bottom line—would *you* get the job?!

Some Final Suggestions

Here is a roundup of some "do's and don'ts" that may make scoring or transcription successful and satisfying rather than frustrating.

1. Always use a pencil for transcription. Find the lead number that you like best. If you use a hard lead, be sure that it will photocopy (photocopying of clinical materials occurs regularly). Have several pencils available and a good eraser. If ever erasers were needed in adult writing, clinical phonetics is the place.
2. If you are transcribing in a group setting, develop a feeling of self-confidence. Try not to be unduly influenced by others, no matter what your stage of transcription skill (see entries in Table 7-2).
3. Try to keep successive items in a transcription task independent from one another. As discussed earlier, it is difficult to score or transcribe 50 items in a row without being influenced by a cumulative effect of your judgments or transcriptions. It may help to keep in mind that the original purpose for obtaining a series of such length must have included the belief that there would be some variability or inconsistency in production of target responses. Be alert for those new behaviors that may occur within a speech sample.
4. Students tell us that one hour is about as long as they can attend to scoring or transcription. Fatigue undoubtedly sets in even earlier in difficult tasks. The physical activity of stopping and starting a recording alone can be fatiguing. Therefore, breaks should be taken frequently. Learn to recognize your own personal signs of fatigue, be they physical signs or signs in your scoring or transcription that indicate increasingly less precise discriminations.
5. If you are transcribing from an audio recording only, do not become frustrated by the lack of visual information. Being able to watch a person as he or she is talking does help for certain transcription needs; but, for the reasons discussed earlier, the bulk of scoring or transcription across phonetic classes can be accomplished without visual cues. Of course, certain decisions will be just too difficult from an audio recording—particularly if it was not of good quality, if the speaker was not well oriented to the microphone, and so forth. In clinical practice, you will have to decide whether to try to score or transcribe the sample or whether to declare it invalid for such purposes.
6. Do not be worried if you miss some behaviors in a speech sample. Unless you have to account for every bit of speech, it usually is better to leave out questionable scor-

TABLE 7-2
Sample of Examiners' Comments about the Strengths and Weaknesses of Eight Job Applicants for a Consensus Transcription Team[a]

Type	Perceptual Ability	Efficiency and Productivity	Problem-Solving Ability	Interpersonal Attitude
Strengths:	• Seemed to have perceptual skills above what we have seen in other applicants. • Was able to make many of the error sounds, a strategy she used often. • Seemed able to concentrate on hearing what we described. • Seemed able to cross-check her perceptions. • Perception of small differences very good. • Seemed to form perceptual sets very well.	• Very much on task. • Asked questions to clarify what percept we heard. • No doubt she would be a hard worker and stay on task, deal with pertinent issues, etc. • Alert and conscientious. • Well-paced progress throughout the tasks. • Worked diligently to complete the individual sections. • Made lots of good comments focusing on the issues. • Concentrated on segments and seemed "hungry" to keep going. • Comments were consistently focused on primary issues. • Attitude reflected "get down to business" approach. • Comments reflected the pairing of prior learning with new information.	• Strong conceptual framework. • Used strategies to refresh memory and separate out how we were using diacritics. • Conceptually she seemed right on. • Even when her transcription was different from ours, it was very reasonable. • The way she described the process of coming to a decision was very logical.	• Seemed to care very much about the results. • Did not seem bothered by transcription that differed from hers. • Enthusiasm in the consensus process as well as in the transcription task. • She is the type of person it would be great to work with. • She said she loved transcription. • Although she could not hear differences, she said she felt very good about the session as a learning experience. • Eager to learn. • Felt that she would stick with her percept but was not defensive about someone else doing the same. • Enthusiastic and good dynamics in conversation. • Nice give-and-take in the consensus process. • Evidenced a flexible attitude about disagreements. • Took seriously all the components of the session. • Showed confidence but reasonable discussion when her percept didn't match the key.
Weaknesses:	• May experience fatigue more quickly. • Never seemed to use the training information to establish perceptual sets. • Never produced sounds herself for comparison. • Did not seem to be able to cross-check her perceptions. • Did not seem to be able to maintain a perceptual set for later use. • Did not seem to be able to tune in to small perceptual differences. • Changed percepts radically. • Weakness in ability to concentrate. • Evidence of not working at listening. • Could hear some differences but did not seem to work hard at hearing the difficult sounds.	• Her comments were not exactly tangential, but they did not reflect a lot of depth. • Did not ask questions that would probe our rationale for decisions. • Wasn't off task, but she didn't seem as though she would be productive at this type of task.	• Often remarked that she could not come up with any way to describe what she was hearing. • Used no apparent strategies to solve novel problems. • Seemed as if she was guessing instead of drawing logical conclusions. • When her transcriptions differed from ours, it did not always have a "reasonableness" to it. • The fricative distortions that she used did not follow any logical pattern. • It seemed that conceptually it was difficult for her to pull things together as we gave feedback. • Conceptual framework was there, but I'm not sure how often she used it. • Verbalizing strategies were there, but she didn't seem to have strategies to help in difficult situations.	• Give-and-take during consensus practice was skimpy. • Commented that the "test" was "no big deal." • In general, did not seem to exhibit much enthusiasm for the process. • Did not seem to be interested in why there were disagreements. • Perceived some defensiveness in some of her responses. • Didn't seem motivated or interested.

[a]The comments are lightly edited for clarity. (Shriberg, Hinke, and Trost-Steffen, 1987. Reproduced with permission of the publisher.)

ing or transcription decisions—at least to set them aside by circling them or using some other convention. Certain analysis procedures may be confounded because of some puzzling data that are unsupported anywhere else in the corpus. The advice is—try not to be "compulsive" about every bit of speech behavior. Avoid lingering on task decisions. Do what you can, then move on.

7. Finally, to score or transcribe efficiently, you must have absorbed the information discussed in this chapter and in the preceding chapters. To the extent that you do not really know the symbols or have not really established response definitions for yourself, scoring or phonetic transcription will be frustrating. If you cannot readily recreate in your mind where each vowel is made or where to place diacritic symbols, you will have persistent problems in clinical phonetics. Such deficits will increase your latency of transcription, and, in the extra time needed to recall a particular symbol, your memory of the stimulus itself will decay. For a period of time, you may need to work with a sheet listing all of the symbols needed for a particular task directly in front of you. Eventually, however, you must memorize all the symbols and their placements. Such preparation will pay off as you begin the discrimination training in the next chapter.

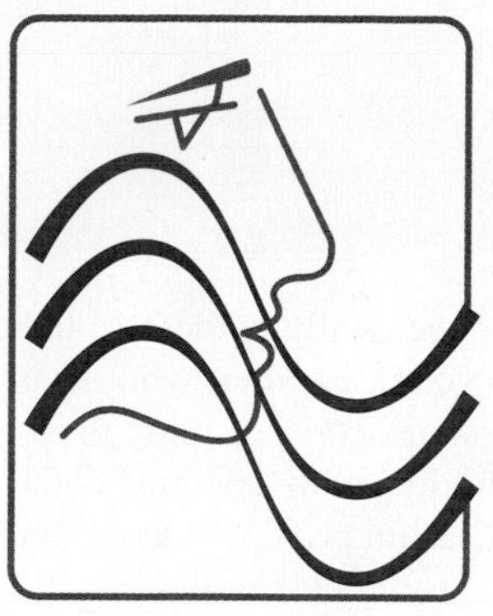

Transcription Training 8

What follows is the first of five parts that provide training in discriminating speech sound changes. The parts are: (a) vowels/diphthongs, (b) stops, (c) fricatives/affricatives, (d) liquids/glides, and (e) nasals. Each part is divided into two sections. A background information section provides some relevant facts and observations about the sound class. A training modules section teaches the transcription skills for the sounds in the class that are most frequently needed in clinical practice. Training modules practice requires access to Clinical Phonetics Tapes #2, #3, and #4. Transcription keys, which include comments for each training module, are provided within the text on the left-hand page. You should cover this page while writing answers in the spaces provided on the right-hand page transcription sheet. Discrimination skills may be practiced in many ways by creative use of these tapes and keys. You should experiment with various possibilities as you proceed through the tapes, adjusting your practice to the inherent difficulty of each module.[1]

PART A: TRANSCRIPTION OF VOWEL AND DIPHTHONG SOUND CHANGES

BACKGROUND INFORMATION

As described in detail in Chapter 4, vowels (and diphthongs) are distinguished from one another by (1) position of tongue body within the oral cavity, (2) tenseness of tongue musculature or vowel duration, and (3) lip posture. Ready knowledge of how vowels and diphthongs differ on each of these features, as described in Chapter 4, is basic to transcription competence. One particular feature, lip rounding, warrants attention before proceeding to some distributional and frequency of occurrence facts.

[1]Appendix D is a discussion of reliability, including procedures to assess your agreement with the answer keys. Before proceeding through the training modules, you should read this section thoroughly. If these materials are used in connection with class assignments, you will need to check with your instructor to see how agreement will be assessed.

The Problem of Transcribing Lip Rounding–Unrounding

Of the 13 vowels in English, only 7 are normally rounded. Only vowels that have a relatively elevated jaw and mid or back tongue body are rounded. Such facts reflect universals of speech production as well as historical facts about the English vowel system. Certain clinical situations require accurate phonetic description of lip postures. For example, a young child who deletes final consonants may, by his or her lip postures on the preceding vowel, reveal his or her developing acquisition of the final consonant. This is discussed in more detail later. Lip posture information may also be useful when working with individuals who have neuromotor problems, for example, to describe the lip inversions seen in some types of cerebral palsy. Also, information on lip postures during vowels by children with severe hearing impairment may be useful in determining progress in speech development. For needs like these, symbols in addition to the five introduced in the diacritics chapter ([ᵓ], [ᶜ], [ᵚ], [ᵐ], [ˣ]) may be required.

A problem with transcribing lip postures, as discussed in Chapter 7, is the availability of visual information, either live or from video sample. In our studies, diacritics indicating lip position on vowels and consonants were not transcribed reliably from audio samples alone. Therefore, the transcription of lip rounding has not been selected for training in this text. You may "hear" lip rounding or unrounding on the audio samples, and you will see lip posture symbols used here and there in the transcription keys. But we do not believe that transcription skills in lip posture diacritics can be learned solely from audio samples. Try to observe lip rounding–unrounding during live transcription sessions or transcription from video sample. When working with clients whose lip postures require modification, the clinician may need to adapt a system of lip gesture symbols that can be discriminated reliably by both the clinician and the client. A clinical example of the use of special lip diacritics is described in Woodard (1991); see Appendix A for annotated references.

Distribution and Frequency of Occurrence Data for Vowels and Diphthongs: Implications for Clinical Transcription

Tables B-1 to B-15 in Appendix B contain many interesting facts about English vowels and diphthongs. For example:

1. Tense vowels occur in stressed syllables and in open syllables (syllables that are not closed by a consonant or a consonant cluster); lax vowels (excepting [ʌ, ə]) do not. Our language has words like *me* [mi] but not *mi* [mɪ], *two* [tu] but not *tuh* [tʊ]. Also, vowels occur in medial word position more frequently than initial or final word position (Table B-6).
2. Children use different vowels in the same proportion as adults do (Tables B-4, B-5). Schwa /ə/ is the most frequent of vowel sounds, about three times as frequent as the next most frequent vowel sound, /ɪ/. The vowel /ɪ/ is also used much more often than other vowels (Table B-8).

How are such data important for clinical transcription? For one thing, it is practical to become competent in transcribing sounds that occur frequently in English. According to these data in Table B-8, we should expect to hear a lot of front vowels, schwas, and centralized sounds. Therefore, the transcription training that follows will use these vowels more than the less frequently occurring vowels.

Another aspect of the statistics in Appendix B is their implications for management. Interestingly, vowels and diphthongs have received little attention by clinical speech-language pathologists. In the past, children who turned up in the clinics seldom had vowel or diphthong errors. As younger children are being served in public schools, however, statistical facts about vowels and diphthongs are becoming increasingly more useful (Pollock and Keiser, 1990; Stoel-Gammon and Harrington, 1990; Pollock, 1991; Otomo and Stoel-Gammon, 1992). To increase a child's intelligibility, it is prudent to select for management sounds that are distributed widely and occur frequently.

In sum, facts about vowels and diphthongs deserve close study, as is the case with all the data available in the tables in Appendix B. These tables contain the technical information needed for a variety of clinic decisions and for construction of management tasks. As introduced in Chapter 1, a primary goal of this book is to impress on student-clinicians the importance of such knowledge for the day-to-day practice of clinical speech-language pathology.

TRAINING MODULES

Overview

Transcription training is directed specifically to those sound changes that occur frequently in young children who have delayed speech. Importantly, this series concerns only those changes ("errors") that occur in children with developmental phonological delays. The series does not provide training on errors made by individuals with neuromotor, hearing, or orofacial involvement, although passing reference is made to sound changes that are relevant to involvements in these areas.

Before beginning practice on the audio samples, you should have immediate recall of each of the vowel and diphthong symbols introduced in the earlier chapters, as well as firm knowledge of the location and perceptual correlates of the following diacritics: [̞], [̝], [̠], [̟], [̄], [ː], and [̃]. Each diacritic describes a change in place or manner. As described in Chapter 6, each diacritic is always positioned above, below, or after the symbol it modifies. You should know these symbols and their conventional position well enough that you do not have to take time to look them up while you are working on the discrimination modules.

Training on the audio samples is divided into six vowel/diphthong sound changes: (1) substitutions, (2) modifications, (3) central vowels, (4) multiple element changes, (5) lengthening, and (6) nasalization. A total of eight transcription training modules, six covering the different changes plus two summary modules, are provided for you to learn to transcribe vowel and diphthong sound changes in children's speech. Here is how to proceed for each training module:

1. Read the text and be sure you understand what to listen for.
2. Proceed to the appropriate portion of the audio sample and transcribe items using the space provided on the transcription sheet (right-hand page). Be sure to write an alternative choice whenever you are undecided. Space is also provided for writing notes to yourself for later reference. The left-hand page, the transcription key, should be masked from view, using a sheet of paper or some other device.
3. When you have finished a training module, check your answers with those given in the transcription key. Note the "Alternatives," "Comments," and "Notes" sections provided in each module.
4. What you choose to do after the first time through each module is entirely up to you. Using transcription key materials, you may wish to repeat the module with or without the transcription key in front of you, discuss your

answers with a friend or the instructor, or complete remaining modules and return to particular modules later. These matters may be decided in conjunction with your instructor. Or, if you are proceeding through this series on your own, you may want to experiment until you find what works best for you.

Vowel and Diphthongs Module #1: Vowel and Diphthong Substitutions

Children's substitutions of one vowel for another usually follow closely the vowel quadrilateral (inside front cover). Substitutions generally involve a sound near the target sound, that is, in an adjacent cell (front, back, high, low, mid, etc.) on the quadrilateral. For example, [o] (mid-back) is a likely substitute for [ʊ] (mid-high-back).

PROCEED TO: Clinical Phonetics Tape 2A: Vowels and Diphthongs Module #1: Vowel and Diphthong Substitutions

MODULE TIME	
TOTAL	3:14
ELAPSED	00:00–03:14

Clinical Phonetics Tape 2A
Vowels and Diphthongs Module #1: Vowel and Diphthong Substitutions

TRANSCRIPTION KEY

	STIMULUS WORD	INTENDED	CONSENSUS	ALTERNATIVES	COMMENTS
1	sheep	[i]	[ɪ]		Make no mistake about the [p]!
2	penny	[ɛ]	[ʌ]		
3	bib	[ɪ]	[ʌ]	[æ], [æ̞], [æᵊ]	
4	wagon	[æ]	[æ]	[æ̞], [ɛᴵ]	
5	book	[ʊ]	[ʌ]		
6	light	[ɑ͡ɪ]	[ɑ͡ɪ]		
7	house	[ɑ͡ʊ]	[ɔ]		
8	feather	[ɛ]	[ɑ]		
9	fish	[ɪ]	[ʌ]	[ɛ]	
10	rabbit	[æ]	[ʌ]	[a], [ɔ]	
11	toothache	[u]	[u]		
12	behind	[ə] or [ɪ]	[i]		Normally unstressed . . . as a preposition!
13	potatoes	[e͡ɪ]	[ɑ͡ɪ]	[e͡ɪ]	
14	chair	[e]	[ɛ]	[e̝], [ɛ̞]	
15	baby	[e͡ɪ]	[i]	[i̝]	
16	crackers	[æ]	[ɑ]		

Notes: Students typically do well on this first module. If you did not, you may want to review the vowel and diphthong symbols. You will have difficulty with the vowel and diphthong modules that follow if you are not yet comfortable with all vowel and diphthong symbols. Try to arrange for a practice session with someone else to be sure you are symbolizing all the vowels and diphthongs correctly. Differences in dialectal background may be a factor. Before proceeding to the remaining modules, be sure you can discriminate and symbolize each of the vowels and diphthongs.

MODULE TIME	
TOTAL	3:14
ELAPSED	00:00–03:14

Clinical Phonetics Tape 2A Vowels and Diphthongs Module #1: Vowel and Diphthong Substitutions

TRANSCRIPTION SHEET

	STIMULUS WORD	INTENDED	PERCEIVED	ALTERNATIVES	COMMENTS
1	sheep	[i]	[ ]		
2	penny	[ɛ]	[ ]		
3	bib	[ɪ]	[ ]		
4	wagon	[æ]	[ ]		
5	book	[ʊ]	[ ]		
6	light	[a͡ɪ]	[ ]		
7	house	[a͡ʊ]	[ ]		
8	feather	[ɛ]	[ ]		
9	fish	[ɪ]	[ ]		
10	rabbit	[æ]	[ ]		
11	toothache	[u]	[ ]		
12	behind	[ə] or [ɪ]	[ ]		
13	potatoes	[e͡ɪ]	[ ]		
14	chair	[e]	[ ]		
15	baby	[e͡ɪ]	[ ]		
16	crackers	[æ]	[ ]		

Vowels and Diphthongs Module #2: Vowel and Diphthong Modifications

Clinicians typically are more concerned with the consonant systems of children with delayed speech than with children's articulation of vowels. For certain clinical applications, however, close transcription of vowels and diphthongs may be required: for example, for analysis of phonological development, for an analysis of essentially "vowel speech," or for intelligibility programming for individuals with severe structural or functional deficits.

For example, clinicians may want to transcribe whether a child's /i/ is articulated appropriately as a high, tense sound [i] or as a somewhat lowered sound [i̞]. The diacritic symbols [̝], [̞], [̘], [̙], and [̠] are used to locate sounds relative to their customary positions within the vowel quadrilateral. Tongue raised [̝] and tongue lowered [̞] symbols may be used more often than tongue fronted [̘], tongue backed [̙], or tongue centralized [̠]. One reason for this difference is that changes in the front–back direction often are toward the *center* of the mouth, where the central vowels /ʌ/ and /ə/ are available to describe such perceptions.

One point of information before you begin this module—the task is going to be difficult! Transcribing vowel modifications is one of the most trying, least reliable tasks in all of phonetic transcription. Do the best you can. As you will see in the transcription key, even the "experts" have great difficulty agreeing on one best transcription for vowel modifications.

PROCEED TO: Clinical Phonetics Tape 2A: Vowels and Diphthongs Module #2: Vowel and Diphthong Modifications

Clinical Phonetics Tape 2A
Vowels and Diphthongs Module #2: Vowel and Diphthong Modifications

TRANSCRIPTION KEY

MODULE TIME	
TOTAL	5:07
ELAPSED	03:14–08:21

EXAMPLES

NORMAL	[æ] [hɝ]	RETRACTED	[æ̘] [hɝ̘]
NORMAL	[o] [pɑ]	ADVANCED	[o̙] [pɑ̙]
NORMAL	[æ] [mɛn]	RAISED	[æ̝] [mɛ̝n]
NORMAL	[e] [hɪd]	LOWERED	[e̞] [hɪ̞d]
NORMAL	[e] [sɪt]	CENTRALIZED	[e̠] [sɪ̠t]

	STIMULUS WORD	INTENDED	CONSENSUS	ALTERNATIVES	COMMENTS
1	pages	[e͡ɪ]	[e͡ɪ]	[i̞]	
2	bed	[ɛ]	[ɛ̞]	[æ̝], [æ]	
3	matches	[æ]	[æ̘]	[a]	
4	hat	[æ]	[æ̘]	[ʌ]	
5	home	[o͡ʊ]	[o͡ʊ]		
6	car	[ɑ]	[ɑ]	[ɑ̙]	
7	hammer	[æ]	[æ̝]	[e͡ɪ̞]	
8	dog	[ɔ]	[ɔː]		Lengthened (see Module #6)
9	witch	[ɪ]	[ɪ]	[ɪ̞], [ɛ̝]	Centralized: [̠]
10	fork	[ɔ]	[ʊ]	[ʊ̝], [o]	
11	cat	[æ]	[ɑ]	[ɑ̙], [ɔ̙], [a]	
12	can	[æ]	[æ̘]	[ɑ], [ɑ̙]	Slightly lengthened; breathy
13	top	[ɔ]	[ɔ]	[ɑ]	Dialectal variants [ɔ] versus [ɑ]
14	watch	[ɔ]	[ʌ]	[ʌ̘], [ɔ̙]	Notable
15	nails	[e͡ɪ]	[e͡ɪ]	[æ], [ɑ͡ɪ°]	Lower and retracted
16	pencil	[ɛ]	[ɪ̞]	[ɛ̝]	
17	baby	[e͡ɪ]	[e͡ɪ]		Almost [ɪ]
18	bed	[ɛ]	[æ̝]	[ɛ̞]	
19	blocks	[ɑ]	[ɑ]	[ɑ̙]	Normal for this dialect
20	lamp	[æ]	[æ̝]		

Notes: As you can see, agreement among transcribers for vowel–diphthong modification is seldom very high. A good way to review these materials is to replay the tape, repeating out loud after each item what you transcribed and the consensus judgment. Another helpful procedure is to say the target vowel and the vowel closest to the modification—then try to make the consensus intermediate vowel. Be sure to assess your agreement by a "liberal" criterion, using the concept of *functional equivalence* described in Appendix D.

Clinical Phonetics Tape 2A
Vowels and Diphthongs Module #2: Vowel and Diphthong Modifications

TRANSCRIPTION SHEET

MODULE TIME	
TOTAL	5:07
ELAPSED	03:14–08:21

EXAMPLES

NORMAL	[æ] [hɝ]	RETRACTED	[æ̠] [hɝ̠]
NORMAL	[o] [pɑ]	ADVANCED	[o̟] [pɑ̟]
NORMAL	[æ] [mɛn]	RAISED	[æ̝] [mɛ̝n]
NORMAL	[e] [hɪd]	LOWERED	[e̞] [hɪ̞d]
NORMAL	[e] [sɪt]	CENTRALIZED	[ë] [sɪ̈t]

	STIMULUS WORD	INTENDED	PERCEIVED	ALTERNATIVES	COMMENTS
1	pages	[e͡ɪ]	[ ]		
2	bed	[ɛ]	[ ]		
3	matches	[æ]	[ ]		
4	hat	[æ]	[ ]		
5	home	[o͡ʊ]	[ ]		
6	car	[ɑ]	[ ]		
7	hammer	[æ]	[ ]		
8	dog	[ɔ]	[ ]		
9	witch	[ɪ]	[ ]		
10	fork	[ɔ]	[ ]		
11	cat	[æ]	[ ]		
12	can	[æ]	[ ]		
13	top	[ɔ]	[ ]		
14	watch	[ɔ]	[ ]		
15	nails	[e͡ɪ]	[ ]		
16	pencil	[ɛ]	[ ]		
17	baby	[e͡ɪ]	[ ]		
18	bed	[ɛ]	[ ]		
19	blocks	[ɑ]	[ ]		
20	lamp	[æ]	[ ]		

Vowels and Diphthongs Module #3: Central Vowels

As developed in Chapter 4, unstressed vowels in English are symbolized with /ə/, termed **schwa**. The schwa symbol occurs often in transcription to describe the unstressed vowels of polysyllabic words and of words in unstressed positions of phrases, sentences, and so forth. Only in very precise or unnaturally stressed speech are *all* vowels given full articulation. For example, the underlined vowels in the sentence "Alw<u>a</u>ys <u>e</u>nunciate pr<u>e</u>cisely" would be given full value ([e͡ɪ], [i], [i]) only in overarticulated, careful speech. In normal speech they often are centralized to schwas.

Individuals with speech disorders may use /ə/ as a centralized vowel even more often than normal speakers. In listening to adults with motor speech disorders or children with delayed speech, for example, the effect of frequent /ə/ substitution is, in a cumulative way, quite pronounced. If vowels are centralized extensively, as they might be if we talked with teeth clenched, speech will lose much of its clarity. Ogilvie and Rees (1969) describe the nature of schwa: "neutral, indeterminate, unstressed, *indefinite, weak*" (emphasis added). Many speakers we transcribe do, indeed, produce "indefinite" central vowels rather than the appropriate high-low-front-back vowels.

Transcription of /ə/ generally is not difficult; one problem does exist, however, which forms the basis of this module. It often is difficult to discriminate /ə/ and /ɪ/. Consider the word *mystic*. Do you hear a /ə/ or an /ɪ/ in the second syllable? The sound is very brief and indeterminate, and it could be transcribed either way. Most phoneticians prefer /ɪ/ in this position because the tongue is high and front as it travels between /t/ and /k/. Therefore the higher /ɪ/ is more likely to be produced in this context than the low /ə/.[2]

When you are unsure of which unstressed vowel you hear, /ə/ versus /ɪ/, two guidelines may be followed:

1. /ɪ/ is somewhat more likely to occur when the original vowel is /i/; for example, "*be*fore" [b ɪ f ɔ r], "*be*cause" [b ɪ k ɔ z], "*re*hearse" [r ɪ h ɝ s], "beaut*i*ful" [b j u t ɪ f ə l], "Bill*y*" [b ɪ l ɪ].
2. Use /ɪ/ as the unstressed vowel before velars; for example, "majest*ic*" [m ʌ ʤ ɛ s t ɪ k], "cosm*ic*" [k ɔ z m ɪ k], "*be*gin" [b ɪ g ɪ n].

If neither of these contexts applies, and you are still unsure of which symbol to use, use /ə/.

[2]The symbol [ɨ] is used by some phoneticians for a centralized /ɪ/. In this text, it is transcribed [ɪ̠].

PROCEED TO: Clinical Phonetics Tape 2A: Vowels and Diphthongs Module #3: Central Vowels

MODULE TIME	
TOTAL	1:46
ELAPSED	08:21–10:07

Clinical Phonetics Tape 2A
Vowels and Diphthongs Module #3:
Central Vowels

TRANSCRIPTION KEY

	STIMULUS WORD	INTENDED	CONSENSUS	ALTERNATIVES	COMMENTS
1	lion	[ə] or [ɪ]	[ɪ]		[l ɑ ɪ n]
2	scissors	[ɚ]	[ɪ]	[ɪ̞], [ɪ̠], [ɛ̠]	
3	flower	[ɚ]	[ʌ]	[ɑ̙]	Note final stress.
4	behind	[ə] or [ɪ]	[ɪ]	[ɪ̝], [ɪ̞]	
5	garage	[ə]	[ə]		
6	glasses	[ə] or [ɪ]	[ə]	[ɪ̠]	
7	carrots	[ə]	[ɪ]	[ɛ̠]	
8	dishes	[ə] or [ɪ]	[ə]		

Notes: As discussed in the text, discrimination of vowels in unstressed syllables is difficult. However, these discriminations do become of interest diagnostically in the case of people who have difficulty acquiring the stress patterns of English. Suggestions for "hearing" these modifications are the same as those for the preceding module.

MODULE TIME	
TOTAL	1:46
ELAPSED	08:21–10:07

Clinical Phonetics Tape 2A Vowels and Diphthongs Module #3: Central Vowels

TRANSCRIPTION SHEET

	STIMULUS WORD	INTENDED	PERCEIVED	ALTERNATIVES	COMMENTS
1	lion	[ə] or [ɪ]	[ ]		
2	scissors	[ɚ]	[ ]		
3	flower	[ɚ]	[ ]		
4	behind	[ə] or [ɪ]	[ ]		
5	garage	[ə]	[ ]		
6	glasses	[ə] or [ɪ]	[ ]		
7	carrots	[ə]	[ ]		
8	dishes	[ə] or [ɪ]	[ ]		

Vowels and Diphthongs Module #4: Vowel–Diphthong Substitutions, Modifications, and Central Vowels

To this point, you have practiced three types of speech sound changes individually—substitutions, modifications, and central vowels. This module provides an opportunity to discriminate among these three changes in children's intended vowels and diphthongs. Before trying this module, be sure that you understand the bases for the transcription choices in each of the three previous keys.

PROCEED TO: Clinical Phonetics Tape 2A: Vowels and Diphthongs Module #4: Vowel–Diphthong Substitutions, Modifications, and Central Vowels

MODULE TIME	
TOTAL	3:44
ELAPSED	10:07–13:51

Clinical Phonetics Tape 2A
Vowels and Diphthongs Module #4: Vowel–Diphthong Substitutions, Modifications, and Central Vowels

TRANSCRIPTION KEY

	STIMULUS WORD	INTENDED	CONSENSUS	ALTERNATIVES	COMMENTS
1	cake	[e͡ɪ]	[e͡ɪ]		
2	bed	[ɛ]	[ʌ]		
3	table	[e͡ɪ]	[a͡ɪ]	[ɛᶦ]	
4	blocks	[ɑ]	[ʌ]		
5	light	[a͡ɪ]	[a͡ɪ]		
6	book	[ʊ]	[ʌ]		
7	dishes	[ɪ], [ə]	[ɪ], [ɪ]	[ɛ], [ɪ̞]	Said with equal stress
8	gun	[ʌ]	[ʌ]		
9	angels	[e͡ɪ]	[e͡ɪ]		[ẽ͡ɪndʒo͡ʊz̥]
10	ladder	[æ]	[ɑ]	[æ̙]	
11	hat	[æ]	[a]	[ʌ̘], [æ̙]	For discussion, see page 33.
12	apple	[æ]	[ɑ]	[ɑ̘], [æ̙]	
13	bunny likes carrots	[ɛ], [ə]	[ɛ], [ʌ]		[bʌnɪ lak kɛwʌ]
14	elephant	[ɛ], [ə]	[ɛ̞], [ɛ]	[ɛ]	[ɛ̞l̰fɛnt]
15	scissors	[ɪ], [ɚ]	[ɪ], [ə]		
16	plane	[e͡ɪ]	[a͡ɪ]	[e̞͡ɪ], [ɑ̝]	
17	baby	[e͡ɪ], [ɪ]	[e͡ɪ], [ɪ]	[e̝͡ɪ]	
18	ring	[ɪ]	[ɪ̠]	[ɛ]	[rʷɪ̠̃ŋ]

Notes: Here's a good place to calculate your agreement with the transcription key. Appendix D presents the procedures. Try calculating your exact agreement with either the "consensus" entry or any of the alternative entries. How are you doing? Look at those items in which you *disagree.* Can you determine any pattern to your differences with the key? Which types of sound changes will require more practice?

MODULE TIME	
TOTAL	3:44
ELAPSED	10:07–13:51

Clinical Phonetics Tape 2A
Vowels and Diphthongs Module #4: Vowel–Diphthong Substitutions, Modifications, and Central Vowels

TRANSCRIPTION SHEET

	STIMULUS WORD	INTENDED	PERCEIVED	ALTERNATIVES	COMMENTS
1	cake	[e͡ɪ]	[ ]		
2	bed	[ɛ]	[ ]		
3	table	[e͡ɪ]	[ ]		
4	blocks	[ɑ]	[ ]		
5	light	[ɑ͡ɪ]	[ ]		
6	book	[ʊ]	[ ]		
7	dishes	[ɪ], [ə]	[ ], [ ]		
8	gun	[ʌ]	[ ]		
9	angels	[e͡ɪ]	[ ]		
10	ladder	[æ]	[ ]		
11	hat	[æ]	[ ]		
12	apple	[æ]	[ ]		
13	bunny likes carrots	[ɛ], [ə]	[ ], [ ]		
14	elephant	[ɛ], [ə]	[ ], [ ]		
15	scissors	[ɪ], [ɚ]	[ ], [ ]		
16	plane	[e͡ɪ]	[ ]		
17	baby	[e͡ɪ], [ɪ]	[ ], [ ]		
18	ring	[ɪ]	[ ]		

Vowels and Diphthongs Module #5: Multiple Element Changes

Multiple element changes are changes of vowels and diphthongs that involve the *addition* of a sound element to the main vowel or diphthong. Such changes are of two types: on- or offglides, and diphthongization.

Onglides and **offglides,** as described in Chapters 4 and 6, are intrusive sounds. A superscript notation is used to indicate that they sound like "intruders" on the primary pattern of the speech sounds, such as [ᵊ ɑ], [ɛ ᶦ]. Onglides and offglides are not fully realized, in terms of duration or loudness. Rather, they are short, transitional sounds that occur as the tongue travels to or from the target sound. As described in Module #3, the schwa [ə] is the most common realization of such indeterminate sounds. Listen to yourself produce the word *seal,* for example. You should hear a slight onglide just before the /l̄/, [s i ᵊ l], yet Kenyon and Knott (1953), in their pronouncing dictionary of English, list the standard production of *seal* as [s i l] because the /ᵊ/ before the /l/ is predictable in this context. As the tongue travels from [i] to [l], [ᵊ] predictably occurs.

Diphthongization differs from on-/offglides only in degree. The difference between what could be described as an on- or offglide and what could be described as a diphthongized vowel is, in fact, quite slight. If the intrusive sound seems only transitional rather than intentional—if it is brief and unstressed—write it as a superscript as described above for on-/offglides. However, if the additional sound is longer in duration or more stressed, place the symbol on the line to indicate diphthongization. In this text, the class of multiple element sound changes includes both types of sound changes.

Before proceeding to training in discrimination of multiple element vowel/diphthong changes, practice in producing such sound changes should be helpful (recall a discussion of just this learning tactic in Chapter 7). Consider five possible *changes* of the vowel /i/ that have been introduced to this point; here is how each might be transcribed:

1. Vowel substitution /i/ → [ɪ], [ɛ], etc.
2. Vowel modification /i/ → [i̞], [i̠], etc.
3. Vowel centralization /i/ → [ə], [ʌ], etc.
4. Vowel onglide /i/ → [ᵊi]
   Vowel offglide /i/ → [iᵊ]
5. Vowel diphthongization /i/ → [i ɑ], [i ɛ], etc.

Now try to say each of the key words exactly as indicated in the phonetic transcription shown in Table 8-1.

Practice the words in Table 8-1 with a friend or audio record them and play them back to yourself. Can you make these sound changes easily? Rapidly? As discussed earlier, phonetic transcription is more reliable if the transcriber is able to articulate faithfully each of the sound changes to be discriminated. Recall too that in the context of clinical management with a child who makes modification errors, the ability to demonstrate errors to the child is part of a clinician's clinical competence. Practice in making vowel modifications (and later in this series, fricative and liquid modifications) is especially beneficial.

TABLE 8-1

Key Word	Substituted Vowel	Modified Vowel	Centralized Vowel	Onglide to Vowel	Offglide from Vowel	Vowel Diphthongization
help	[h ɪ l p]	[h ɛ̝ l p]	[h ʌ l p]	[h ᶦ ɛ l p]	[h ɛ ᶦ l p]	[h e ɛ l p]
hat	[h ɑ t]	[h æ̞ t]	[h ʌ t]	[h ᵊ æ t]	[h æ ᵊ t]	[h æ ɪ t]

PROCEED TO: Clinical Phonetics Tape 2A: Vowels and Diphthongs Module #5: Multiple Element Changes

MODULE TIME	
TOTAL	4:09
ELAPSED	13:51–18:00

Clinical Phonetics Tape 2A Vowels and Diphthongs Module #5: Multiple Element Changes

TRANSCRIPTION KEY

	STIMULUS WORD	INTENDED	CONSENSUS	ALTERNATIVES	COMMENTS
1	dog	[ɔ]	[a͡ʊ]	[ʌʊ], [a͡ʊ]	
2	swing	[ɪ]	[ɪ]	[ɪ̞], [ɛ̝]	
3	hat	[æ]	[æ ᵊ]		[h æ ᵊ t]!
4	shoe	[u]	[u ᶦ]	[u ᵊ]	Breathy offglide
5	bell	[ɛ]	[ɛ]		
6	toothbrush	[u]	[u ᶦ]		
7	smooth	[u]	[u ᵊ]		Hoarse voice; breathy offglide
8	key	[i]	[i ː ᵊ]	[i ː ᶦ]	
9	hat	[æ]	[e ᶦ]	[æ̝ ᶦ], [ɛ̞ ᶦ]	
10	saw	[ɔ]	[a͡ʊ]	[ɑ°], [ɔ°]	
11	keys	[i]	[i]		
12	box	[ɑ]	[ɑ ᶷ]	[ɑ ᵊ], [ɑ ᵓ]	
13	man	[æ]	[ẽ ᵊ]	[æ̃ ᵊ]	
14	shoe	[u]	[u ᵊ]	[u ː ᵊ]	
15	house	[a͡ʊ]	[a͡ʊ ᵊ]		
16	tree	[i]	[i]	[ᵊ i]	Slight onglide?
17	gun	[ʌ]	[ʌ]		
18	saw	[ɔ]	[ɔ ᵊ]		
19	on	[ɔ]	[ʊ ᵊ]	[ɔ ᵊ]	
20	tree	[i]	[i ᵊ]		

Notes: For all but the most detailed phonological inquiry, the distinction between an on-/offglide and diphthongization is unimportant. However, most of the multiple elements here (the addition of a vowel) should be readily discriminable. Practice of the type suggested in the text, making diphthongs from monophthongs, should be helpful if you are having difficulty hearing the intrusive vowels.

MODULE TIME	
TOTAL	4:09
ELAPSED	13:51–18:00

Clinical Phonetics Tape 2A
Vowels and Diphthongs Module #5: Multiple Element Changes

TRANSCRIPTION SHEET

	STIMULUS WORD	INTENDED	PERCEIVED	ALTERNATIVES	COMMENTS
1	dog	[ɔ]	[ ]		
2	swing	[ɪ]	[ ]		
3	hat	[æ]	[ ]		
4	shoe	[u]	[ ]		
5	bell	[ɛ]	[ ]		
6	toothbrush	[u]	[ ]		
7	smooth	[u]	[ ]		
8	key	[i]	[ ]		
9	hat	[æ]	[ ]		
10	saw	[ɔ]	[ ]		
11	keys	[i]	[ ]		
12	box	[ɑ]	[ ]		
13	man	[æ]	[ ]		
14	shoe	[u]	[ ]		
15	house	[a͡ʊ]	[ ]		
16	tree	[i]	[ ]		
17	gun	[ʌ]	[ ]		
18	saw	[ɔ]	[ ]		
19	on	[ɔ]	[ ]		
20	tree	[i]	[ ]		

Vowels and Diphthongs Module #6: Vowel and Diphthong Lengthening

Vowel or diphthong **lengthening** is symbolized by [ː] immediately following the lengthened element. Use of this symbol often results from extremely subjective judgments. As discussed in Chapter 4, differences in vowel duration are measured in milliseconds. Yet, such differences *are* detectable, and we do have expectations of the relative duration of vowels in different phonetic environments. Such expectations are part of our phonological competence. Vowel length must be appropriate for a person to sound like a native speaker of a particular linguistic community. And for situations in which vowels may be the focus of management—such as with hearing-impaired individuals and individuals with severely impaired intelligibility due to structural or neuromotor deficits—vowel length is a feature that requires clinical attention.

One particular situation where vowel duration is important may occur when transcribing children with severely delayed speech. Some of these children delete the final consonants of words. This situation interacts with the fact that in English vowels are relatively longer before voiced obstruents than before voiceless obstruents. For example, the vowel /i/ is longer before voiced /d/ in *bead* than it is before voiceless /t/ in *beat*. The child with delayed speech who uses appropriate vowel duration preceding an omitted final consonant may be showing "knowledge" of this final sound, which he or she does not actually produce (Renfrew, 1966; Shriberg and Kwiatkowski, 1980; Ingram, 1989). If we listen closely to the child who deletes final /t/ and /d/ in the words *beat* and *bead*, for example, we may discover that the child actually makes the /i/ longer before /d/. We can thus give the child credit for observing this phonological regularity of English, which may also indicate knowledge of voicing distinctions in omitted final consonants (see Smit and Bernthal, 1983, for an extensive discussion).

One note before we begin transcription. Speech clinicians sometimes give exaggerated models of a sound within a stimulus word to make it more salient for the child. A problem with this technique is that children often will copy, faithfully, everything the clinician does, including exaggerated vowel duration. In addition, children may use a singsong pattern when reading or an overarticulated manner when "naming" objects, which may result in lengthened vowels.[3] These imitative behaviors are seldom of linguistic significance and should be differentiated in phonological analyses from behaviors that reflect a rule-governed aspect of the child's phonology.

[3]Many of the words on the training audio samples were edited from children's responses to articulation tests. Such responses sound different from candid samples of speech. Ladefoged (1993) refers to such speech as *citation forms,* nicely characterizing these isolated forms as "citing," in contrast to "talking," as in natural, continuous speech.

PROCEED TO: Clinical Phonetics Tape 2A: Vowels and Diphthongs Module #6: Vowel and Diphthong Lengthening

MODULE TIME	
TOTAL	3:28
ELAPSED	18:00–21:28

Clinical Phonetics Tape 2A
Vowels and Diphthongs Module #6: Vowel and Diphthong Lengthening

TRANSCRIPTION KEY

	STIMULUS WORD	INTENDED	CONSENSUS	ALTERNATIVES	COMMENTS
1	he's running in a pile of dirt	[i]	[iː]		
2	chicken	[ɪ]	[ɪ]		
3	zipper	[ɚ]	[ɝ]	[ɝᵊ]	Change in stress
4	ladder	[æ]	[aː]	[æː]	
5	car	[ɑ]	[ɑː]		
6	elephant	[ɛ]	[aː]	[ɛ̞ː], [æ̝]	Almost sounds like "Alan Funt"!
7	finger	[ɪ]	[ɪ]		
8	bathe	[e͡ɪ]	[e͡ɪː]		
9	shoe	[u]	[uː]		
10	bell	[ɛ]	[ɛː]	[ɛ̞ː]	
11	blocks	[ɑ]	[ɑː]		
12	balloons	[u]	[uː]		The /n/ is slightly lengthened also.
13	top	[ɔ]	[ɔ]		
14	saw	[ɔ]	[ɑːᵊ]	[ɑːᶷᵊ], [ɔːᶷᵊ]	The vowel changes.
15	potato	[e͡ɪ]	[e͡ɪː]		

Notes: Your response should be in fairly high agreement with the key for this module. Notice that use of the lengthening diacritic is a dichotomous matter: You either perceived the target sound as lengthened or you did not. Did you use this diacritic more or less often than the key? Keep in mind that the consensus entry represents a conservative use of this diacritic. That is, the diacritic is used only when the vowel is readily perceived as lengthened. This is a conservative response definition, as illustrated in Chapter 7—"innocent until proven guilty."

MODULE TIME	
TOTAL	3:28
ELAPSED	18:00–21:28

Clinical Phonetics Tape 2A Vowels and Diphthongs Module #6: Vowel and Diphthong Lengthening

TRANSCRIPTION SHEET

	STIMULUS WORD	INTENDED	PERCEIVED	ALTERNATIVES	COMMENTS
1	he's running in a pile of dirt	[i]	[ ]		
2	chicken	[ɪ]	[ ]		
3	zipper	[ɚ]	[ ]		
4	ladder	[æ]	[ ]		
5	car	[ɑ]	[ ]		
6	elephant	[ɛ]	[ ]		
7	finger	[ɪ]	[ ]		
8	bathe	[e͞ɪ]	[ ]		
9	shoe	[u]	[ ]		
10	bell	[ɛ]	[ ]		
11	blocks	[ɑ]	[ ]		
12	balloons	[u]	[ ]		
13	top	[ɔ]	[ ]		
14	saw	[ɔ]	[ ]		
15	potato	[e͞ɪ]	[ ]		

Vowels and Diphthongs Module #7: Vowel and Diphthong Nasalization

A second change in vowel and diphthong manner occurs when nasal resonance is added to a vowel. **Nasalization** of vowels and diphthongs can be important for diagnostic purposes. The reasons are similar to those that we presented for transcribing on-/offglides, diphthongization, and duration. Nasalization may tell us something about the structural integrity of the speech mechanism and the regulation of articulatory timing. Nasality is an index of how well the velopharynx is functioning in speakers who have had a cleft palate or have a neuromotor problem. Some nasality on vowels will occur normally in conversational speech, especially when the vowels precede nasal consonants. In the word *man,* for example, the velum must be open for the two nasals but may be only partially closed for the vowel in between. This type of assimilation is termed **assimilative nasality.**

Transcription of nasalization can also yield information about the child with delayed speech development. The child who omits final /n/ and final /t/ will say [pæ] for both *pan* and *pat.* If we listen closely, however, we may hear a nasalized vowel [pæ̃] only in *pan.* What does this indicate? As with rule-governed vowel duration changes, it could indicate the child's awareness of the final nasal sound, even though he or she does not actually lift the tongue tip to say /n/ or /t/.

Problems in transcribing nasality are well known to speech clinicians. Researchers have attempted to develop objective ways of assessing relative nasality, although instrumental measures of nasality are validated ultimately by listeners' judgments. Clinicians must be alert to possible listener bias when transcribing nasality. For example, Ramig (1975) found that children were rated as more nasal when judges were aware of the children's cleft palate history. Such case-history information is not provided in the following module, although some of the samples are from people with repaired palatal clefts.

PROCEED TO: Clinical Phonetics Tape 2A: Vowels and Diphthongs Module #7: Vowel and Diphthong Nasalization

MODULE TIME	
TOTAL	3:37
ELAPSED	21:28–25:05

Clinical Phonetics Tape 2A
Vowels and Diphthongs Module #7:
Vowel and Diphthong Nasalization

TRANSCRIPTION KEY

	STIMULUS WORD	INTENDED	CONSENSUS	ALTERNATIVES	COMMENTS
1	kiss	[ɪ]	[ɪ̃]		
2	a knife	[a͡ɪ]	[ã͡ɪ]		Slight
3	bicycle	[a͡ɪ]	[a͡ɪ]		
4	a window	[ɪ], [o͡ʊ]	[ɪ̃], [õ͡ʊ]		
5	sky	[a͡ɪ]	[a͡ɪ]		
6	a bunny rabbit	[ʌ], [æ], [ɪ]	[ʌ̃], [æ̃], [ɪ̃]		
7	I like ice cream	[a͡ɪ], [a͡ɪ], [a͡ɪ], [i]	[ɑ̃], [ã͡ɪ], [ã͡ɪ], [ĩ]		All nasalized
8	baby	[e͡ɪ], [ɪ]	[e͡ɪ], [ɪ]	[ẽ͡ɪ]	
9	wagon	[æ]	[æ̃]		
10	soap	[o͡ʊ]	[õ͡ʊ]		
11	grass	[æ]	[æ̃]		
12	cracker	[æ], [ɚ]	[æ̃], [ɚ̃]		[æ̃] is only slight.
13	orange	[ɔ], [ɪ]	[ɔ̃], [ɪ̃]	[ɔ̃͡ɪ]	Sounds like a diphthong
14	banana	[æ]	[æ̃]	[æ̞̃ː], [ɑ̃]	
15	lamp	[æ]	[ɑ̃]		[j ɑ̃ ᵐ p]
16	balloon	[u]	[ũ]		[b ɪ j ũː]

Notes: Most of these items keyed for nasality were quite obviously nasalized. You should readily be able to produce nasalized vowels throughout the entire vowel quadrilateral. Practice in minimal pairs too, *man–pat,* should sharpen your discrimination skills for assimilative nasality.

MODULE TIME	
TOTAL	3:37
ELAPSED	21:28–25:05

Clinical Phonetics Tape 2A
Vowels and Diphthongs Module #7: Vowel and Diphthong Nasalization

TRANSCRIPTION SHEET

	STIMULUS WORD	INTENDED	PERCEIVED	ALTERNATIVES	COMMENTS
1	kiss	[ɪ]	[ ]		
2	a knife	[a͡ɪ]	[ ]		
3	bicycle	[a͡ɪ]	[ ]		
4	a window	[ɪ], [o͡ʊ]	[ ], [ ]		
5	sky	[a͡ɪ]	[ ]		
6	a bunny rabbit	[ʌ], [æ], [ɪ]	[ ], [ ], [ ]		
7	I like ice cream	[a͡ɪ], [a͡ɪ], [a͡ɪ], [i]	[ ], [ ], [ ], [ ]		
8	baby	[e͡ɪ], [ɪ]	[ ], [ ]		
9	wagon	[æ]	[ ]		
10	soap	[o͡ʊ]	[ ]		
11	grass	[æ]	[ ]		
12	cracker	[æ], [ɚ]	[ ], [ ]		
13	orange	[ɔ], [ɪ]	[ ], [ ]		
14	banana	[æ]	[ ]		
15	lamp	[æ]	[ ]		
16	balloon	[u]	[ ]		

Vowels and Diphthongs Module #8: Summary Quiz

Here's a chance to test your learning of all five types of sound changes that occur clinically on vowels and diphthongs. You may want to review each of the previous modules first—or perhaps spend more time on particular modules that were most difficult.

PROCEED TO: Clinical Phonetics Tape 2A: Vowels and Diphthongs Module #8: Summary Quiz

MODULE TIME	
TOTAL	4:18
ELAPSED	25:05–29:23

Clinical Phonetics Tape 2A
Vowels and Diphthongs Module #8: Summary Quiz

TRANSCRIPTION KEY

	STIMULUS WORD	INTENDED	CONSENSUS	ALTERNATIVES	COMMENTS
1	spider web	[ɛ]	[ʌ]		[w ʌ b̥]
2	baby	[e͡ɪ]	[e̞]	[e̞ᶦ]	
3	cat	[æ]	[æᵊ]	[æː]	
4	skates	[e͡ɪ]	[e͡ɪ]		
5	saw	[ɔ]	[ɑᶷ]	[ɑ°], [ɔ°]	
6	jars	[ɑ]	[ɑː]		
7	yes	[ɛ]	[ɛ]		
8	bed	[ɛ]	[ʌ]		
9	scissors	[ɪ]	[i]		
10	feather	[ɛ]	[ɛ̞]	[ɛ]	
11	hat	[æ]	[æᶦ]		
12	dog	[ɔ]	[ɔː]		
13	blue	[u]	[u̝]	[ᵊu], [uᵓ], [ʊᶷ]	Really difficult!
14	balloons	[u]	[ũ]		[b l ũ n z̥]
15	boat	[o͡ʊ]	[o͡ʊ̞]	[ʊᶷ], [ᶷu]	
16	garage	[ɑ]	[ɑː]		
17	matches	[ə]	[ʌ]		
18	fork	[ɔ]	[ɔ]	[oᵊ]	
19	cracker	[æ]	[æ̃]		
20	tongue	[ʌ]	[ʌ]		
21	he's so funny	[i], [o͡ʊ], [ʌ], [ɪ]	[ɪ], [o͡ʊ], [ʌ], [ɪ]		

Notes: If you agree with the "consensus" or "alternative" key somewhere above 75 percent on these 24 vowels/diphthongs, you are doing very nicely. After this quiz, you should be able to analyze quite closely where you should concentrate your efforts for additional practice. Keep in mind that you would undoubtedly do better with a *live* child in front of you.

MODULE TIME	
TOTAL	4:18
ELAPSED	25:05–29:23

Clinical Phonetics Tape 2A
Vowels and Diphthongs Module #8: Summary Quiz

TRANSCRIPTION SHEET

	STIMULUS WORD	INTENDED	PERCEIVED	ALTERNATIVES	COMMENTS
1	spider web	[ɛ]	[ ]		
2	baby	[e͡ɪ]	[ ]		
3	cat	[æ]	[ ]		
4	skates	[e͡ɪ]	[ ]		
5	saw	[ɔ]	[ ]		
6	jars	[ɑ]	[ ]		
7	yes	[ɛ]	[ ]		
8	bed	[ɛ]	[ ]		
9	scissors	[ɪ]	[ ]		
10	feather	[ɛ]	[ ]		
11	hat	[æ]	[ ]		
12	dog	[ɔ]	[ ]		
13	blue	[u]	[ ]		
14	balloons	[u]	[ ]		
15	boat	[o͡ʊ]	[ ]		
16	garage	[ɑ]	[ ]		
17	matches	[ə]	[ ]		
18	fork	[ɔ]	[ ]		
19	cracker	[æ]	[ ]		
20	tongue	[ʌ]	[ ]		
21	he's so funny	[i], [o͡ʊ], [ʌ], [ɪ]	[ ], [ ], [ ], [ ]		

PART B: TRANSCRIPTION OF STOP SOUND CHANGES

As in "Part A: Transcription of Vowel and Diphthong Sound Changes," stop training is divided into two sections—background information and training modules. Background information underscores facts about stop production and perception that should prove useful both for transcription and for clinical assessment and management. Modules for stop sound changes consist of six transcription training modules: (1) stop substitutions, (2) voicing of voiceless stops, (3) devoicing of voiced stops, (4) glottal stop substitutions, (5) stop deletions, and (6) frictionalized stops. Additionally, a seventh module provides a summary quiz of all stop sound changes. These transcription modules are recorded on Clinical Phonetics Tape 2.

You may be happy to hear that transcription of stop changes generally is less taxing than vowel and diphthong transcription!

BACKGROUND INFORMATION

Description of Stops

As introduced in Chapter 5, page 64, stops are formed by ". . . a complete closure of the vocal tract, so that airflow ceases temporarily and air pressure builds up behind the point of closure." To review, the three cognate pairs, /p b /, /t d /, and /k g /, are made along the vocal tract by the lips, tongue tip, and tongue dorsum, respectively. In addition to these six phonemes, American English speakers also have an allophone of /t/ and /d/, the flap [ɾ], and the glottal stop [ʔ]. The flap is used by most speakers of English in place of /t/ when it occurs between a preceding stressed vowel and a following unstressed vowel within a word (e.g., *letter* [l ɛ ɾ ɚ]) or between words (e.g., *quit it* [k w ɪ ɾ ɪ t]). The glottal stop sometimes occurs as an allophone of /t/ before syllabic nasals, such as *button* [b ʌ ʔ n̩] and in certain American dialectal forms, such as *bottle* [ˈb ɑ ʔ l̩]. Glottal stops can also occur between two vowels and serve to separate them, such as *uh-oh* [ɔ ʔ o͡ʊ]. Although [ɾ] and [ʔ] are allophones that occur frequently in both normal and delayed speech, only the glottal stop [ʔ] will be considered in the training modules to follow.

Distribution and Frequency of Occurrence of Stops

Tables B-1 and B-2 in Appendix B present information on the distribution of stops in adult English in singletons and in clusters, respectively. Unlike vowels, which are distributed only in certain syllables, the six phonemic stop consonants occur in all word positions regardless of syllable stress. Stops also occur frequently in clusters, as indicated in Tables B-2 and B-11. Note that we can expect /t/ and /d/, the two alveolar stops, to occur most frequently in children's speech (Table B-10).

TABLE 8-2

Allophone Description		Symbol[a]	Word
Unaspirated	/t/	[t⁼]	s*t*op
Aspirated	/t/	[tʰ]	*t*op
Unreleased	/t/	[t -]	bough*t* two
Flapped	/t/	[ɾ]	bu*tt*er
Nasally released	/t/	[t̃]	bu*tt*on
Laterally released	/t/	[tᴸ]	li*tt*le
Dental	/t/	[t̪]	both *T*om and I
Back (alveopalatal)	/t/	[t̠]	mea*t* shop

[a]MacKay's diacritics.

The broad distribution of stops in our language, together with the nature of stop production, yields a wide variety of stop allophones in spoken English. Thus, to sound like "native" speakers, children learning English, as well as adults learning English as a second language, must learn to produce these allophones under the appropriate conditions. For example, MacKay (1978) lists the allophones for /t/, as shown in Table 8-2.

Notice that from a management perspective, stimuli for a stop production program must account for these differing allophones. To promote *carryover* (generalization to free speech), the clinician should have the child practice making the target stop in diverse allophone contexts. Accordingly, clinicians must maintain consistent scoring or transcription skills across the wide variety of stop allophones.

TRAINING MODULES

Articulation errors on stops are rarely seen in school-aged children. Preschool children and people with structural and neuromotor problems, however, often have stop errors. Particularly for people with motor speech deficits, reduced intelligibility may be associated with imprecise stop articulation.

Our work with young children with moderate to severely delayed speech indicates that the majority of stop misarticulations can be divided into six clinical types: (1) stop substitutions, (2) voicing of voiceless stops, (3) devoicing of voiced stops, (4) glottal stop substitutions, (5) stop deletions, and (6) frictionalized stops.

Stops Module #1: Stop Substitutions

Stop substitutions made by a young child usually involve changes among the three primary stop positions of English.

If stops are to be replaced by another phoneme (other than the voiced/voiceless cognate to be covered in the following module), they are almost invariably replaced by another stop. It is rare to see a stop replaced, for example, by a liquid, a glide, or a true fricative. Hence, we normally (abnormally!) get [t/k] or [d/g] (see Ingram's 1989 discussion of "fronting" phenomena), or sometimes sounds are "backed"—[k/t], [g/d]. Among the six stops, /p/ and /b/ are the most stable: They seldom are the "victims" in developmental substitutions. When they are replaced, it generally is due to assimilation influences (see Ingram, 1989, and Bernthal and Bankson, 1993, for discussions of assimilation processes).

For this training module, we need concentrate only on stop substitutions *within* the voiceless series /p t k / or within the voiced series /b d g /. We will hold voicing constant in the practice that follows next and reserve cognate substitution discrimination for separate practice.

Discriminating stop substitutions is usually a straightforward task, provided that the stop is loud enough. Be alert for one situation, however—the tendency to perceive /t/ for /k/ or /d/ for /g/ in clusters involving /l/ and /r/. For example, we tend to hear [t/k] in words like *clean* or [d/g] in words like *glee*. In these phonetic contexts, the /k/ and /g/ sounds may be made more forward in the mouth in anticipation of the more anterior /l/.

PROCEED TO: Clinical Phonetics Tape 2B: Stops Module #1: Stop Substitutions

MODULE TIME	
TOTAL	2:54
ELAPSED	00:00–02:54

Clinical Phonetics Tape 2B
Stops Module #1:
Stop Substitutions

TRANSCRIPTION KEY

	STIMULUS WORD	INTENDED	CONSENSUS	ALTERNATIVES	COMMENTS
1	table	[b]	[d]		
2	crackers	[k]	[t]		
3	cake	[k]	[t]		
4	gun	[g]	[d]		
5	dog	[d]	[d]		
6	apple	[p]	[p]		
7	bus	[b]	[d]		
8	pin	[p]	[p]		
9	dog	[d]	[d]		
10	can	[k]	[p]	[t]	Judges were split evenly on this one.
11	carrot	[k]	[t]		
12	wagon	[g]	[d]		
13	clock	[k]	[t]		
14	boat	[b], [t]	[b], [t]		
15	book	[b], [k]	[p], [k]	[t]	
16	pocket	[p], [k], [t]	[p], [p], [t]		

Note: This array of stop substitutions should be fairly easy to discriminate.

MODULE TIME	
TOTAL	2:54
ELAPSED	00:00–02:54

Clinical Phonetics Tape 2B
Stops Module #1:
Stop Substitutions

TRANSCRIPTION SHEET

	STIMULUS WORD	INTENDED	PERCEIVED	ALTERNATIVES	COMMENTS
1	table	[b]	[ ]		
2	crackers	[k]	[ ]		
3	cake	[k]	[ ]		
4	gun	[g]	[ ]		
5	dog	[d]	[ ]		
6	apple	[p]	[ ]		
7	bus	[b]	[ ]		
8	pin	[p]	[ ]		
9	dog	[d]	[ ]		
10	can	[k]	[ ]		
11	carrot	[k]	[ ]		
12	wagon	[g]	[ ]		
13	clock	[k]	[ ]		
14	boat	[b], [t]	[ ], [ ]		
15	book	[b], [k]	[ ], [ ]		
16	pocket	[p], [k], [t]	[ ], [ ], [ ]		

Stops Module #2: Voicing of Voiceless Stops

Discriminating voicing characteristics can be difficult. For example, deciding whether [p/b] or [b/p] substitutions have occurred are among the most troublesome of transcription tasks. You may have perceived voicing changes in some of the items in the previous module on stop substitutions. Given the complexity of the speech production and speech perception processes involved, it is not surprising that we have difficulty judging voicing changes. Before proceeding with the transcription training on voicing characteristics in this and the following module, review the discussion of stop production beginning on page 64. After you have reacquainted yourself with how voiced and voiceless consonants differ in word-initial and word-final position, continue with the following discussion.

In the word-initial position, the most common voicing error in young children is either to fully voice a voiceless stop (to substitute [d/t]; *two* [d u]) or to partially voice a voiceless stop ([t̬/t]; *two* [t̬ u]). Strictly speaking, the "error" in each case may be related to voice onset time—voicing for the vowel starts too early for a "voiceless" stop to be made or heard. As developed earlier, differences in voice onset time of only 10 to 30 milliseconds can be very hard to discriminate. Normal children usually take many years before they can reliably coordinate voice onset time (Kent, 1976). Therefore, because voicing changes are the rule with many preschool children, they should not automatically be considered as "errors." Generally, we recognize cognate substitutions in the initial position—[b/p], [d/t], [g/k]. But how does the transcriber accurately perceive voice onset times that are just slightly advanced, that is, partially voiced?

Initial voiceless stops that sound partially voiced frequently should be transcribed as unaspirated. Thus, whenever initial /p/, /t/, or /k/ is perceived as partially voiced, it would be transcribed as [p˭], [t˭], and [k˭], respectively. Two considerations justify the use of this convention.

First, by using the aspiration symbol, we more accurately describe the factor that influences our perception of voicing in English. That is, the lack of aspiration of the initial voiceless sound makes it appear to be partially voiced. Therefore, [p˭], [t˭], and [k˭] are more appropriate than [p̬], [t̬], [k̬]. Second, by retaining the symbol of the target sound (such as [p˭]), rather than using a modified version of its cognate (such as [b̥]), a less severe claim is made about the child's phonological system. As discussed previously, it is more conservative to say that a child is modifying a certain phoneme than it is to say that he or she is *replacing* that phoneme with another phoneme or another modified phoneme. In general, we believe that substitution errors are more serious than some other error types; therefore, they should not be attributed to the child unless the evidence is clear-cut.

To sum up, the most common voicing "errors" in young children are to fully voice or partially voice an initial voiceless stop. On their way to adult speech, children require a lengthy period in which to acquire the motor control necessary for appropriate voice onset time values. Recall too that because voiceless sounds require more oral air pressure than voiced sounds, voiceless stops may be more difficult for the child or adult with a structural or neuromotor deficit. Initial voiceless sounds that are made weakly will also sound fully or partially voiced. We suggest that attention to the aspiration feature is the best approach for all such transcription situations. If initial voiceless stops /p/, /t/, or /k/ do not sound fully voiceless or fully aspirated, transcribe them as [p˭], [t˭], or [k˭].

PROCEED TO: Clinical Phonetics Tape 2B: Stops Module #2: Voicing of Voiceless Stops

Clinical Phonetics Tape 2B
Stops Module #2:
Voicing of Voiceless Stops

TRANSCRIPTION KEY

MODULE TIME	
TOTAL	1:57
ELAPSED	02:54–04:51

EXAMPLES			
ASPIRATED	[pʰɑ]	UNASPIRATED	[p˭ɑ]
	[tʰu]		[t˭u]

	STIMULUS WORD	INTENDED	CONSENSUS	ALTERNATIVES	COMMENTS
1	potato	[pʰ]	[pʰ]	[p˭], [b]	
2	potato	[pʰ]	[p˭]	[b]	
3	cat	[kʰ]	[kʰ]		
4	potatoes	[pʰ]	[p˭]		Change of stress [bəˈte͡ɪtoz]?
5	spoon	[p˭]	[pʰ]		This is not an example of devoicing.
6	star	[t˭]	[t˭]		
7	skates	[k˭]	[k˭]		
8	spoon	[p˭]	[p˭]		

Notes: Another way to practice making this sound change is to contrast voiceless stop contrasts as they occur initially as singletons and as the second member of a cluster. In item 6, for example, practice saying /t/ in the word *star* [t˭] versus /t/ in *tar* [tʰ].

Clinical Phonetics Tape 2B
Stops Module #2:
Voicing of Voiceless Stops

TRANSCRIPTION SHEET

MODULE TIME	
TOTAL	1:57
ELAPSED	02:54–04:51

EXAMPLES			
ASPIRATED	[p^{h}ɑ]	UNASPIRATED	[$p^{=}$ɑ]
	[t^{h}u]		[$t^{=}$u]

	STIMULUS WORD	INTENDED	PERCEIVED	ALTERNATIVES	COMMENTS
1	potato	[p^{h}]	[ ]		
2	potato	[p^{h}]	[ ]		
3	cat	[k^{h}]	[ ]		
4	potatoes	[p^{h}]	[ ]		
5	spoon	[$p^{=}$]	[ ]		
6	star	[$t^{=}$]	[ ]		
7	skates	[$k^{=}$]	[ ]		
8	spoon	[$p^{=}$]	[ ]		

Stops Module #3: Devoicing of Voiced Stops

The tendency toward partial devoicing of final voiced stops, particularly if they are unreleased, is common in casual or fast adult speech. In children, too, voicing of final voiced stops will often cease before articulation of the stop is completed. The symbol for partial devoicing is [̥].

Our strategy for discriminating *partially* devoiced final stops from those that are *fully* devoiced is to listen to the duration of the preceding vowel. If the length of the vowel seems appropriately long for a final voiced sound (relatively longer than before a final voiceless sound), the normally occurring partial devoicing is an appropriate allophone, such as [b̥], [d̥], and [ɡ̊]. However, if you hear what appears to be a cognate substitution, such as [p/b], [t/d], or [k/g], and the length of the preceding vowel is too short for a final voiced stop, it is appropriate to use the symbol for the substituted cognate.

PROCEED TO: Clinical Phonetics Tape 2B: Stops Module #3: Devoicing of Voiced Stops

MODULE TIME	
TOTAL	3:19
ELAPSED	04:51–08:10

Clinical Phonetics Tape 2B
Stops Module #3:
Devoicing of Voiced Stops

TRANSCRIPTION KEY

	STIMULUS WORD	INTENDED	CONSENSUS	ALTERNATIVES	COMMENTS
1	egg	[g]	[kʰ]		
2	bathtub	[b]	[pʰ]		
3	the bird	[d]	[d̥]		"Almost" [t]
4	dog	[g]	[g̊]		
5	egg	[g]	[g̊ʰ]		Compare to No. 1.
6	bathtub	[b]	[b]		Slight devoicing at end
7	bed	[d]	[d̥ʰ]		
8	spider web	[b]	[p]		
9	bib	[b]	[b̥ʰ]		Close to [p]
10	pig	[g]	[k]		Short vowel
11	bed	[d]	[tʰ]		Long vowel
12	bed	[d]	[d]		Compare to Nos. 7, 11.
13	wagon	[g]	[g̊]		
14	window	[d]	[d]		
15	blue	[b]	[b̥]	[b]	
16	brush	[b]	[b̥]	[b]	
17	doggie, a big dog	[g], [b], [g]	[g], [p], [g̊ʰ]	[g]	

Note: Judges agreed quite well on almost all items.

MODULE TIME	
TOTAL	3:19
ELAPSED	04:51–08:10

Clinical Phonetics Tape 2B
Stops Module #3:
Devoicing of Voiced Stops

TRANSCRIPTION SHEET

	STIMULUS WORD	INTENDED	PERCEIVED	ALTERNATIVES	COMMENTS
1	egg	[g]	[ ]		
2	bathtub	[b]	[ ]		
3	the bird	[d]	[ ]		
4	dog	[g]	[ ]		
5	egg	[g]	[ ]		
6	bathtub	[b]	[ ]		
7	bed	[d]	[ ]		
8	spider web	[b]	[ ]		
9	bib	[b]	[ ]		
10	pig	[g]	[ ]		
11	bed	[d]	[ ]		
12	bed	[d]	[ ]		
13	wagon	[g]	[ ]		
14	window	[d]	[ ]		
15	blue	[b]	[ ]		
16	brush	[b]	[ ]		
17	doggie, a big dog	[g], [b], [g]	[ ], [ ], [ ]		

Stops Module #4: Glottal Stop Substitutions

As described in the first part of this text, a glottal stop is a stop made by a quick opening or closing, or both, of the vocal folds. It is heard as an abrupt onset of the vowel or an abrupt offset of the vowel. If you say the following two series of words rapidly, you should hear the similarity between the glottal stop and the other three voiceless stops: [p ɑ], [t ɑ], [k ɑ], [ʔ ɑ]; [ɑ p], [ɑ t], [ɑ k], [ɑ ʔ].

Part of the difficulty in perceiving glottal stops is due to the fact that the articulators involved in their production are the vocal folds. The "catch" glottal stop made by the vocal folds is not always easily distinguished from the normal onset or offset of phonation. Difficulty depends also, as with other discrimination tasks, on how forcefully the glottal stop is articulated. A forcefully produced glottal stop is much easier to identify than a lightly articulated glottal stop. In the latter case, it is very difficult to discriminate the glottal stop from normal voice onset or offset. For a prevocalic glottal stop, the basic cue is an abrupt onset often followed by an aspirated vowel (such as [ʔ ʰɑ]). For a postvocalic glottal stop, the cue is an abrupt offset (such as [ɑ ʔ]). Children with delayed speech generally use glottal stops as substitutions for final consonants. Children with repaired cleft palates may use glottal stops in all positions.

To summarize, listening for a glottal stop addition or substitution is difficult. In the initial position, the cue is an abrupt onset of the following vowel. In postvocalic or final position, the cue is an abrupt offset of the preceding vowel. In the final position, we also may hear a release of air comparable to released final /t/, /k/, or /p/ (such as *pet* [p ɛ ʔ ʰ]).

PROCEED TO: Clinical Phonetics Tape 2B: Stops Module #4: Glottal Stop Substitutions

MODULE TIME	
TOTAL	1:49
ELAPSED	08:10–09:59

Clinical Phonetics Tape 2B
Stops Module #4:
Glottal Stop Substitutions

TRANSCRIPTION KEY

	STIMULUS WORD	INTENDED	CONSENSUS	ALTERNATIVES	COMMENTS
1	sheep	[p]	[ʔ]		Shortened vowel
2	monkey	[k]	[ʔ]		
3	table	[b]	[ʔ]		
4	apple	[p]	[ʔ]		
5	monkey	[k]	[k]		
6	matches	[tʃ]	[ʔ]		
7	dishes	[ʃ]	[ʔ]		The "click" after the word is from a counter used in management.
8	ladder	[d]	[ʔ]		

Notes: Items that clearly demonstrate glottal stop substitutions were difficult to isolate from our audiotapes of children with delayed speech. Particularly in postvocalic, word-final position, glottal stops are difficult to discriminate by perceptual phonetics, such as item 1 above.

MODULE TIME	
TOTAL	1:49
ELAPSED	08:10–09:59

Clinical Phonetics Tape 2B
Stops Module #4:
Glottal Stop Substitutions

TRANSCRIPTION SHEET

	STIMULUS WORD	INTENDED	PERCEIVED	ALTERNATIVES	COMMENTS
1	sheep	[p]	[ ]		
2	monkey	[k]	[ ]		
3	table	[b]	[ ]		
4	apple	[p]	[ ]		
5	monkey	[k]	[ ]		
6	matches	[tʃ]	[ ]		
7	dishes	[ʃ]	[ ]		
8	ladder	[d]	[ ]		

Stops Module #5: Stop Deletions

Stop deletions occur frequently enough in children with both normal and delayed speech to warrant attention in this series.

Two types of situations arise. First, unreleased stop allophones occur in several phonetic contexts. In the following contexts, stops are likely to be perceived as having been deleted:

1. When followed by another stop (*cupcake* [k ʌ p˺ k e k]).
2. When between two consonants (*printshop* [p r ɪ n t˺ ʃ ɑ p]).
3. When in a final homorganic cluster (*bank* [b æ ŋ k˺]).

In each of these three phonetic contexts, stops generally are unreleased in adult speech as well as in children's speech. In such contexts, they may be perceived as deleted.

Second, there is one context in which stops actually are deleted that occurs uniquely in children with delayed speech—word-final stops. Final consonant deletion, including deletion of final stops, is a frequent error type in children with delayed speech. Knowing whether a child articulated a final stop can be important diagnostically, particularly because final /t/ and /d/ can mark past tense (*play* [p l e͡ɪ]; *played* [p l e͡ɪ d]).

Two strategies aid in discriminating stop deletions if the stop is only weakly articulated or unreleased. First, visual information is needed. Lip closure for /p/ and /b/ targets is most easily seen, whether live or from video recording. "Seeing" tongue activity for /t/, /d/, /k/, and /g/, however, depends on the size of the child's mouth, the angle of view, and so forth. If transcription of any of the six stops is important, as suggested in Chapter 7, try to make the necessary observations live while testing or later from a video recording.

The second strategy for transcribing stops in final position is to listen to the preceding vowel. As discussed earlier in the training for vowels, the child who deletes final stops may *mark* the preceding vowel in some way. Some possible situations, for example, are:

Stimulus Word	*Child's Production*
dog	[d ɔ ː]
dot	[d ɔ]
pin	[p ɪ̃]
pick	[p ɪ]
bike	[b ɑ͡ɪ ᵊ]
bye	[b ɑ͡ɪ]

The missing target phoneme in the stimulus words *dog, pin,* and *bike* is marked by the preceding vowel—by lengthening, by nasalization, and by an offglide, respectively. Compare these marked vowels to those said in response to the stimulus words *dot, pick,* and *bye.* Such subtle changes are important to transcribe when they affect our analysis of a child's speech development.

We use the "circle" convention and the question mark symbol quite often when we are unsure whether a final stop is present, such as *pat* [p æ ⓣ], [p æ ⓘ?]. Rather than call a stop deleted or simply guess, we circle the questionable segment. Quite often, such difficult decisions involve possibly unreleased final stops, such as [d ɔ (g˺)].

In summary, transcription of children with both normal and delayed speech will require careful attention to stop deletions, particularly final stop deletions. Visual verification of a stop gesture may be necessary to discriminate stops that are weakly articulated or not audibly released. Because articulation of vowels preceding final stops can be important for phonological analysis, the use of vowel diacritics to mark vowel characteristics is useful. Of course, the same types of agreement problems for vowel transcription are evident in such situations as those discussed in the vowel section. Specifically, you will need to use reliable symbols for duration, nasality, place modifications, and multiple element changes. Finally, use of the circle convention shown in Figure 6-6 ([t ɔ ⓟ]) or a question mark [p æ (?)]) should reflect the amount of confidence you place in your transcription.

PROCEED TO: Clinical Phonetics Tape 2B: Stops Module #5: Stop Deletions

MODULE TIME	
TOTAL	4:12
ELAPSED	09:59–14:11

Clinical Phonetics Tape 2B
Stops Module #5:
Stop Deletions

TRANSCRIPTION KEY

	STIMULUS WORD	INTENDED	CONSENSUS	ALTERNATIVES	COMMENTS
1	some might not	[t]	[Ø]		Because /t/ is homorganic with /n/, a deletion here is not unusual.
2	cup	[p]	[p^h]		"Popping" release
3	glasses	[g]	[Ø]		Something here?
4	black	[k]	[Ø]	[k˺]	No voicing at release
5	hat	[t]	[t^h]		Breathy voice
6	book	[k]	[k˺]	[t˺], [ʔ]	Note vowel [a].
7	lamp	[p]	[p^h]		
8	cake	[k]	[k^h]		
9	thank you	[k]	[Ø]		
10	dog	[g]	[Ø]		
11	soft	[t]	[Ø]		
12	bird	[d]	[Ø]		
13	top	[p]	[p^h]		
14	ladder	[d]	[Ø]		
15	radio	[d]	[Ø]	[ʔ]	/d/ replaced by a voiceless segment
16	bed	[d]	[Ø]		[b ɛ ^{ə}Ø]
17	jump	[p]	[p^h]		
18	that	[t]	[Ø]		
19	that bite	[t], [t]	[Ø], [Ø]		
20	kitty cat	[t], [t]	[Ø], [Ø]		

MODULE TIME	
TOTAL	4:12
ELAPSED	09:59–14:11

Clinical Phonetics Tape 2B
Stops Module #5:
Stop Deletions

TRANSCRIPTION SHEET

	STIMULUS WORD	INTENDED	PERCEIVED	ALTERNATIVES	COMMENTS
1	some might no<u>t</u>	[t]	[ ]		
2	cu<u>p</u>	[p]	[ ]		
3	<u>g</u>lasses	[g]	[ ]		
4	bla<u>ck</u>	[k]	[ ]		
5	ha<u>t</u>	[t]	[ ]		
6	boo<u>k</u>	[k]	[ ]		
7	lam<u>p</u>	[p]	[ ]		
8	ca<u>k</u>e	[k]	[ ]		
9	than<u>k</u> you	[k]	[ ]		
10	do<u>g</u>	[g]	[ ]		
11	sof<u>t</u>	[t]	[ ]		
12	bir<u>d</u>	[d]	[ ]		
13	to<u>p</u>	[p]	[ ]		
14	la<u>dd</u>er	[d]	[ ]		
15	ra<u>d</u>io	[d]	[ ]		
16	be<u>d</u>	[d]	[ ]		
17	jum<u>p</u>	[p]	[ ]		
18	tha<u>t</u>	[t]	[ ]		
19	tha<u>t</u> bi<u>t</u>e	[t], [t]	[ ], [ ]		
20	ki<u>tt</u>y ca<u>t</u>	[t], [t]	[ ], [ ]		

Stops Module #6: Frictionalized Stops

One type of stop modification that occurs with some frequency in clinical populations is the **frictionalized stop** (also called a **spirantized stop**). Frictionalized stops, usually considered "distortions," do not have a crisp stop release; they have a gradual, rather than a sudden, movement away from the closure. Consequently, the resulting sound is less abrupt than the usual plosive burst of a stop release, sounding spirantized or more "drawn out." Frictionalized stops sound in between a stop and a fricative. You can simulate a frictionalized stop quite easily by making a /t/ and, while keeping oral pressure high, taking your tongue tip away from the alveolar ridge slowly rather than rapidly—[t͓].

We find occasion to use the frictionalized symbol [͓] often with young children and also with people who have neuromotor disorders. For young children with delayed speech, the frictionalized stop may indicate the beginning development of a new class of sounds, the fricatives—which initially appear at the same places of articulation (are homorganic to) as the previously acquired stops. A frictionalized /t/ ([t͓]) sound may be a transitional behavior before a child begins to make a good /s/. For children with neuromotor disorders, frictionalized stops may reflect difficulties in timing and other motor control domains, for stops require a rapid release.

It should be noted that we and others have also used "weakly released" to refer to stops that are not sharply released (the [̬] diacritic has been used to indicate "weak"). For example, Campbell and Dollaghan's (1995) description of the speech of a group of children and adolescents following traumatic brain injury includes the term "weak articulation of stop consonants" for four of the nine subjects.

PROCEED TO: Clinical Phonetics Tape 2B: Stops Module #6: Frictionalized Stops

Clinical Phonetics Tape 2B
Stops Module #6:
Frictionalized Stops

TRANSCRIPTION KEY

MODULE TIME	
TOTAL	1:36
ELAPSED	14:11–15:47

EXAMPLES			
NORMAL	[ki]	FRICTIONALIZED	[k͓i]
	[s t e͡ɪ]		[s t͓ e͡ɪ]

	STIMULUS WORD	INTENDED	CONSENSUS	ALTERNATIVES	COMMENTS
1	train	[t]	[t͓]		
2	soap	[p]	[pʰ]		
3	truck	[t]	[t͓]		
4	comb	[k]	[k͓]	[t͡s]	
5	car	[k]	[kʰ]		Note that even a normally released /k/ sounds "noisy."
6	with its path	[p]	[p͓]		Not stop closure

Notes: Clear examples of frictionalized stops are difficult to isolate. Keep in mind that this diacritic symbolizes a range of sound changes, from almost /s/-like to barely any closure for the stop. The speaker in item 6, for example, was a dysarthric individual whose articulation of stops was consistently imprecise.

Clinical Phonetics Tape 2B
Stops Module #6:
Frictionalized Stops

TRANSCRIPTION SHEET

MODULE TIME	
TOTAL	1:36
ELAPSED	14:11–15:47

EXAMPLES			
NORMAL	[k i]	FRICTIONALIZED	[k͓i]
	[s t e͡ɪ]		[s t͓ e͡ɪ]

	STIMULUS WORD	INTENDED	PERCEIVED	ALTERNATIVES	COMMENTS
1	train	[t]	[ ]		
2	soap	[p]	[ ]		
3	truck	[t]	[ ]		
4	comb	[k]	[ ]		
5	car	[k]	[ ]		
6	with its path	[p]	[ ]		

Stops Module #7: Summary Quiz

Here is an opportunity to test your discrimination skills for all stop errors. Good luck!

PROCEED TO: Clinical Phonetics Tape 2B: Stops Module #7: Summary Quiz

MODULE TIME	
TOTAL	5:02
ELAPSED	15:47–20:49

Clinical Phonetics Tape 2B
Stops Module #7:
Summary Quiz

TRANSCRIPTION KEY

	STIMULUS WORD	INTENDED	CONSENSUS	ALTERNATIVES	COMMENTS
1	bed	[b], [d]	[b], [d]		
2	bib	[b], [b]	[b], [bʰ]		
3	bread	[b], [d]	[Ø], [d̥]		
4	gun	[g]	[d]		
5	kitty cat	[k], [t], [k], [t]	[k], [t], [t], [t]		
6	toothbrush	[t], [b]	[t͓ʰ]*, [b]		*Aspirated and frictionalized release
7	frog	[g]	[g̥]		
8	bird	[b], [d]	[b], [d̥]		
9	dishes	[d]	[d]		[dɪʔɪ]
10	a ladder	[d]	[tʰ]		
11	paper	[p], [p]	[pʰ], [p]		
12	monkey	[k]	[b̥]	[pᵇ]	[mʌpᵇi]; [mʌ>bi]
13	bird	[b], [d]	[b], [d̥]		
14	radio	[d]	[Ø]		
15	carrot	[k], [t]	[t⁼], [t]		
16	bed	[b], [d]	[b], [t]		[bæːt]
17	cup	[k], [p]	[t], [p̚]		[tʌp̚]
18	book	[b], [k]	[p], [p]	[k], [ʔ]	Not enough to tell which
19	dog	[d], [g]	[d], [g̥]		
20	pig	[p], [g]	[p], [k]		
21	baby	[b], [b]	[b], [b]		
22	bed	[b], [d]	[b], [Ø]		
23	tail	[t]	[t]		
24	TV	[t]	[p]		[pifi]!
25	dog	[d], [g]	[d], [Ø]		

Notes: There are 44 stops to discriminate; each agreement is worth approximately 2.3 points. Which error types do you consistently discriminate correctly? Which need more practice? Which diacritics do you tend to overuse? underuse?

MODULE TIME	
TOTAL	5:02
ELAPSED	15:47–20:49

Clinical Phonetics Tape 2B
Stops Module #7:
Summary Quiz

TRANSCRIPTION SHEET

	STIMULUS WORD	INTENDED	PERCEIVED	ALTERNATIVES	COMMENTS
1	bed	[b], [d]	[ ], [ ]		
2	bib	[b], [b]	[ ], [ ]		
3	bread	[b], [d]	[ ], [ ]		
4	gun	[g]	[ ]		
5	kitty cat	[k], [t], [k], [t]	[ ], [ ], [ ], [ ]		
6	toothbrush	[t], [b]	[ ], [ ]		
7	frog	[g]	[ ]		
8	bird	[b], [d]	[ ], [ ]		
9	dishes	[d]	[ ]		
10	a ladder	[d]	[ ]		
11	paper	[p], [p]	[ ], [ ]		
12	monkey	[k]	[ ]		
13	bird	[b], [d]	[ ], [ ]		
14	radio	[d]	[ ]		
15	carrot	[k], [t]	[ ], [ ]		
16	bed	[b], [d]	[ ], [ ]		
17	cup	[k], [p]	[ ], [ ]		
18	book	[b], [k]	[ ], [ ]		
19	dog	[d], [g]	[ ], [ ]		
20	pig	[p], [g]	[ ], [ ]		
21	baby	[b], [b]	[ ], [ ]		
22	bed	[b], [d]	[ ], [ ]		
23	tail	[t]	[ ]		
24	TV	[t]	[ ]		
25	dog	[d], [g]	[ ], [ ]		

PART C: TRANSCRIPTION OF FRICATIVES AND AFFRICATE SOUND CHANGES

The popular media tend to use the term *lisp* to refer to the use of any incorrect speech sound. Technically, however, a lisp refers only to substitution and distortion errors on fricatives and affricates, sounds we are concerned with in the modules to follow. Such errors are the most prevalent type of residual articulation error. Because of the high prevalence of fricative/affricate errors in school-aged children, some clinicians may find this training unit to be the most useful part of this chapter. We will need first to develop a clear understanding of the salient articulatory, acoustic, and linguistic differences among fricative and affricate sounds.

BACKGROUND INFORMATION

Description of Fricatives

The terms **continuant, fricative,** and **sibilant** tend to be confused with one another. In the following list, note how these terms are superordinate to one another (see Appendix A, Table A-5 for a detailed review of relevant considerations).

Continuants: /θ ð f v s z ʃ ʒ h l r w m n ŋ /
Fricatives: /θ ð f v s z ʃ ʒ h /
Sibilants: /s z ʃ ʒ /

Among the 15 continuant consonants, only 9 are fricatives. And among these 9 fricatives, only 4 are sibilants. Production of the English fricatives and affricates was described in Chapter 5. Here, four characteristics of fricative and affricate sounds are important to underscore for the purpose of clinical transcription.

Duration and Intensity Differences. The voiceless fricatives /θ/, /f/, /s/, /ʃ/ are often longer in duration and are more intense than their respective voiced cognates /ð/, /v/, /z/, /ʒ/. Increased duration and intensity of the noise segment were previously noted also for the voiceless stops /p/, /t/, /k/, as compared with their voiced cognates /b/, /d/, /g/. The clinical implication of this fact is that errors on voiceless sounds will be more noticeable than errors on voiced sounds. Because voiceless sounds normally are articulated longer and louder, errors on them are more obvious to a listener. For this reason, voiceless sounds are given priority in speech management programs.

Frequency (Pitch) Differences. As a general rule, as the place of articulation moves toward the back of the oral cavity, the pitch of the fricative noise gets lower. Try saying the following sounds in sequence, listening for the perception of a successively lowering noise pitch: /s/, /ʃ/, /h/. The noise pitch of fricatives is an important identifying characteristic, one that we will be using as a discrimination cue in an upcoming training module.

Tongue Configuration (Placement-Grooving) Differences. In production of /θ/, /ð/, /s/, /z/, /ʃ/, and /ʒ/, the sides of the tongue from front to back are in firm contact with the inner surface of the upper teeth or with the lateral portions of the alveolar ridge up to the canine teeth. The positioning for the tip of the tongue and the middle of the tongue changes most among these six sounds. For /θ/ and /ð/, there is no grooving of the tongue; it is flat. For /s/ and /z/, a narrow groove along the midline of the tongue is needed, with air funneled up to and out over the apex (not the very tip) of the tongue. The tongue tip, in fact, can be placed either somewhere just behind the upper teeth or somewhere behind the lower teeth. We tend to think that only the tip of the tongue is involved in /s/ production when, in fact, the whole apex usually is involved. Finally, for /ʃ/ and /ʒ/, grooving is not as narrow as for /s/ and /z/. The wider groove for /ʃ/ and /ʒ/ makes the friction noise much more diffuse than that for /s/ and /z/.

By sucking air inwards as you put your tongue in position for each sound, /θ/, /s/, /ʃ/, you should feel cool air passing over the point of the fricative source. Try it. Also, to feel the central emission of the airstream, for /s/ and /z/ in particular, make a sustained /s/ and run your finger from one side to the other directly along your teeth. The airstream will be partially interrupted as your finger passes by the central incisors.

Lip Position Differences. Lip position for all fricatives and affricates (excepting /f/ and /v/) is neutral or flat and spread. Some people round lips slightly for /ʃ/, /ʒ/, and /tʃ/, /ʤ/, however. The /h/ sound is entirely free of specifications for lip and tongue postures (as long as the vocal tract is open). Hence, lip and tongue positions for any given /h/ are determined by the shape of the vowel to follow. Consider the alternative lip and tongue positions for /h/ in the following words: *he, hot,* and *hoot.* Because it is free to assume the position of the following vowel (but, unlike the vowel, remains unvoiced), /h/ is sometimes called a "voiceless vowel" or "voiceless glide."

Distribution and Frequency of Occurrence of Fricatives

The distributional and frequency of occurrence data for fricatives and affricates are presented in Appendix B. With the exception of /ʒ/ and /h/, which do not occur in word-initial and word-final positions, respectively, these 11 sounds occur in all word positions. The cluster data are particularly relevant for such clinical tasks as the choice of management stimuli. In initial position, voiceless fricative clusters are more prevalent than voiced, with /s/ clusters by far the most widespread. Notice, too, that /s/ is the premier fricative, with /tʃ/ and especially /ʒ/ occurring much less frequently.

In summary, in consideration of all the characteristics reviewed here—intensity, duration, distribution, and frequency of occurrence—the sibilants /s/, /z/ (in word-final position as a grammatical morpheme), and /ʃ/ are the most important fricatives. Errors on these sounds are most "costly" to a child or adult, when we calculate their effects on intelligibility of speech or as a speech disability. Consequently, in the training modules to follow, a greater proportion of the training stimuli will be concerned with the transcription of /s/, /z/, and /ʃ/ errors.

TRAINING MODULES

Overview

Learning to transcribe errors on the nine fricatives and two affricates is going to be a large task. Before we subdivide them into modules on the basis of common discrimination problems, we will discuss errors that are common to all the fricatives and affricates, except /h/. Four errors are most frequent in the fricative and affricate production of young children with delayed speech, as follows.

Deletions. A major decision in transcribing fricatives of preschool children whose speech is delayed is whether any fricative noise is present. We can easily see why this is such a problem. Recall that fricatives, especially /θ/, /ð/, /f/, and /v/, are low-intensity sounds. These sounds may not be audible at all on audio recordings if a child makes them softly. And if the sibilants /s/, /z/, /ʃ/, and /ʒ/ are made weakly, they can be confused with audio hiss. We will need to practice hearing the presence or absence of any fricative-like sound for all of the fricatives.

Stopping. We find somewhat older (beyond preschool) children with delayed speech who very commonly replace fricatives with stops (**stopping**). Fricatives can be replaced by a stop that is made at the same place of articulation—for example, [b/v], [p/f], [d/z], [t/s]—or by a stop made at a different place.

Voicing Changes. As with stops, a number of factors related to stress may influence voicing changes in fricative production. Although our position has been to deemphasize the clinical importance of voicing "errors" in young children, some practice in discriminating voicing errors is provided.

Distortions. The last stage of fricative development begins when fricatives are distorted (approximated) in some manner. We will be using several diacritics for tongue changes involved in sibilant distortions in later training modules.

In summary, children with delayed speech may: (1) delete, (2) stop, (3) voice/devoice, and/or (4) distort the 11 fricative and affricate sounds. The likelihood of each of these error types varies with the specific target sound involved. Accordingly, the training modules to follow are organized by target sound groups, with proportionately more practice on errors that occur more frequently in children with delayed speech.

Fricatives and Affricates Module #1: /f/ and /v/ Changes

Frequently occurring clinical problems with /f/ and /v/ fall into three types: (1) *deletions*—deciding whether the sound was present at all; (2) stop *substitutions*—deciding whether /f/ or /v/ was replaced by a stop (nearly always /p/ or /b/); or (3) *voicing* changes—deciding whether these sounds were correctly voiced. The practice module that follows provides examples of each of these sound changes.

PROCEED TO: Clinical Phonetics Tape 2B: Fricatives and Affricates Module #1: /f/ and /v/ Changes

MODULE TIME	
TOTAL	5:35
ELAPSED	20:49–26:24

Clinical Phonetics Tape 2B
Fricatives and Affricates Module #1:
/f/ and /v/ Changes

TRANSCRIPTION KEY

	STIMULUS WORD	INTENDED	CONSENSUS	ALTERNATIVES	COMMENTS
1	leaf	[f]	[Ø]		
2	knife	[f]	[f]		
3	telephone	[f]	[f]		
4	fork	[f]	[Ø]		
5	vacuum	[v]	[v]		
6	vacuum	[v]	[Ø]		
7	TV	[v]	[t]		Noisy
8	knife	[f]	[s]		
9	fork	[f]	[p˭]		
10	vacuum	[v]	[b]		
11	knife	[f]	[f]		
12	stove	[v]	[b̥]		
13	a leaf	[f]	[f]		
14	TV	[v]	[f]		
15	five	[v]	[v̥]		
16	vacuum	[v]	[v̥]		
17	stove	[v]	[v̥]		
18	leaf	[f]	[v]		
19	TV	[v]	[v̥]	[b v̥]	
20	stove	[v]	[v̥]		
21	elephant	[f]	[f]		
22	vacuum	[v]	[w]		
23	knife	[f]	[t]		
24	a feather	[f]	[f]		
25	TV	[v]	[v̥]		

MODULE TIME	
TOTAL	5:35
ELAPSED	20:49–26:24

Clinical Phonetics Tape 2B Fricatives and Affricates Module #1: /f/ and /v/ Changes

TRANSCRIPTION SHEET

	STIMULUS WORD	INTENDED	PERCEIVED	ALTERNATIVES	COMMENTS
1	lea<u>f</u>	[f]	[ ]		
2	kni<u>f</u>e	[f]	[ ]		
3	tele<u>ph</u>one	[f]	[ ]		
4	<u>f</u>ork	[f]	[ ]		
5	<u>v</u>acuum	[v]	[ ]		
6	<u>v</u>acuum	[v]	[ ]		
7	T<u>V</u>	[v]	[ ]		
8	kni<u>f</u>e	[f]	[ ]		
9	<u>f</u>ork	[f]	[ ]		
10	<u>v</u>acuum	[v]	[ ]		
11	kni<u>f</u>e	[f]	[ ]		
12	sto<u>v</u>e	[v]	[ ]		
13	a lea<u>f</u>	[f]	[ ]		
14	T<u>V</u>	[v]	[ ]		
15	fi<u>v</u>e	[v]	[ ]		
16	<u>v</u>acuum	[v]	[ ]		
17	sto<u>v</u>e	[v]	[ ]		
18	lea<u>f</u>	[f]	[ ]		
19	T<u>V</u>	[v]	[ ]		
20	sto<u>v</u>e	[v]	[ ]		
21	ele<u>ph</u>ant	[f]	[ ]		
22	<u>v</u>acuum	[v]	[ ]		
23	kni<u>f</u>e	[f]	[ ]		
24	a <u>f</u>eather	[f]	[ ]		
25	T<u>V</u>	[v]	[ ]		

Fricatives and Affricates Module #2: /h/ Deletions

The only type of /h/ error that occurs with any frequency in delayed speech is /h/ deletion. Pronouns such as *him, her, his,* and *he* and auxiliary verbs such as *had* and *has* are likely to be said with /h/ deletions when they occur in an unstressed position in a sentence (*He put his hat on his head* [hi pʊt ɪz hæt ɔn ɪz hɛd]). This is a casual speech phenomenon; we all "drop h's" when speaking casually or rapidly. Because /h/ deletions in such contexts are normal, only /h/ deletions in stressed positions (for example, the words *hat* and *head* in the previous sentence) might be of interest clinically. Nevertheless, clinicians should be able to transcribe /h/ deletions reliably whenever they occur.

PROCEED TO: Clinical Phonetics Tape 2B: Fricatives and Affricates Module #2: /h/ Deletions

MODULE TIME	
TOTAL	1:48
ELAPSED	26:24–28:12

Clinical Phonetics Tape 2B
Fricatives and Affricates Module #2:
/h/ Deletions

TRANSCRIPTION KEY

	STIMULUS WORD	INTENDED	CONSENSUS	ALTERNATIVES	COMMENTS
1	house	[h]	[Ø]		Ø/s also
2	dog house	[h]	[Ø]		
3	he's this high	[h], [h]	[h], [h]		
4	and he's a poodle	[h]	[Ø]		Normal in this context
5	house	[h]	[h]		
6	they were voting for him	[h]	[Ø]		Same as No. 4
7	hanger	[h]	[h]		
8	hammer	[h]	[Ø]		

MODULE TIME	
TOTAL	1:48
ELAPSED	26:24–28:12

Clinical Phonetics Tape 2B
Fricatives and Affricates Module #2:
/h/ Deletions

TRANSCRIPTION SHEET

	STIMULUS WORD	INTENDED	PERCEIVED	ALTERNATIVES	COMMENTS
1	house	[h]	[ ]		
2	dog house	[h]	[ ]		
3	he's this high	[h], [h]	[ ], [ ]		
4	and he's a poodle	[h]	[ ]		
5	house	[h]	[ ]		
6	they were voting for him	[h]	[ ]		
7	hanger	[h]	[ ]		
8	hammer	[h]	[ ]		

Fricatives and Affricates Module #3: Voiceless and Voiced *th* Changes

Studies of the prevalence of articulation errors have consistently found /θ/ and /ð/ to be among the last consonants articulated correctly in normal phonetic development. The usual "tongue between teeth" description of these sounds is not necessarily true of conversational speech. A wide range of placement of the tongue tip will produce /θ/ and /ð/, *as long as the tongue is in firm contact with the upper side teeth from front to back.* The tongue tip may be in light contact with the inner surface of the upper teeth or be placed between the upper and lower incisors. Because children evidently take longer to articulate these sounds correctly, we provide considerable practice on discrimination of errors in these sounds. This module will include the three types of errors found in children—deletions, substitutions, and distortions.

Deletions. In adult speech, /θ/ and /ð/ tend to be omitted in rapid speech (*Who's that* [h u z æ t]) and in clusters (*fifths* [f ɪ f s]). Because they are low in intensity, /θ/ and /ð/ are hard to identify auditorily.

Substitutions. The most likely substitution for /θ/ is /f/ or /t/; for /ð/, the most likely substitution is /v/ or /d/. Confirming /f/ or /v/ as the substituted sound, however, often requires visual evidence—seeing the teeth–lip closure. Again, the low intensity of these sounds makes them difficult to discriminate either live or from audio.

Distortions. The most common distortion for /θ/ and /ð/ are dentalized stops [t̪], [d̪]. By practicing making the following contrasts you can reacquaint yourself with dentalization of stops and fricatives. The tongue tip should be adjacent to or actually touching the inner margin of the teeth. Practice making the following contrasts.

1 Fricatives	2 Stops	3 Dentalized Stops	4 Dentalized Fricatives
those [ðo͡ʊz]	[do͡ʊz]	[d̪o͡ʊz]	[z̪o͡ʊz]
these [ðiz]	[diz]	[d̪iz]	[z̪iz]
thin [θɪn]	[tɪn]	[t̪ɪn]	[s̪ɪn]

Notice that the distortions in columns 3 and 4 are neither pure stops nor pure fricatives, respectively.

PROCEED TO: Clinical Phonetics Tape 3A: Fricatives and Affricates Module #3: Voiceless and Voiced *th* Changes

MODULE TIME	
TOTAL	6:32
ELAPSED	00:00–06:32

Clinical Phonetics Tape 3A
Fricatives and Affricates Module #3: *th* Changes

TRANSCRIPTION KEY

	STIMULUS WORD	INTENDED	CONSENSUS	ALTERNATIVES	COMMENTS
	DELETIONS				
1	ba<u>th</u>e	[ð]	[Ø]		[θ]?
2	too<u>th</u>brush	[θ]	[Ø]		
3	bro<u>th</u>er	[ð]	[ð]		
4	<u>th</u>at apple	[ð]	[ð]		
5	fea<u>th</u>er	[ð]	[Ø]	[ʔ]	Abrupt onset of second syllable
6	ba<u>th</u>	[θ]	[Ø]		[θ]?
7	tee<u>th</u>	[θ]	[θ]		
	SUBSTITUTIONS				
8	fea<u>th</u>er	[ð]	[l]		
9	<u>th</u>at	[ð]	[d]		
10	ba<u>th</u>tub	[θ]	[s]		
11	fea<u>th</u>er	[ð]	[d]		
12	tee<u>th</u>	[θ]	[f]		
13	smoo<u>th</u>	[ð]	[ð]	[ð̥]	
14	<u>th</u>is	[ð]	[d]		
15	ba<u>th</u>e	[ð]	[v]	[v̥]	
	DISTORTIONS				
16	<u>th</u>at	[ð]	[z̪]	[z̪̥]	
17	<u>th</u>ree	[θ]	[s̪]		
18	fea<u>th</u>er	[ð]	[ð̽]		
19	<u>th</u>is	[ð]	[t͓]		
20	ba<u>th</u>	[θ]	[θ]	[ᵗð̥̽], [t̪͓]	
21	tee<u>th</u>	[θ]	[θt]		
22	<u>th</u>at	[ð]	[ð̯̽]		Lateralized?
	ANY ERROR				
23	too<u>th</u>ache	[θ]	[θ]		
24	<u>th</u>umb	[θ]	[s]		
25	<u>th</u>is	[ð]	[z̪]		One judge heard as a palatalized /z/, [z̡].
26	<u>th</u>is apple	[ð]	[d]		
27	<u>th</u>ank you	[θ]	[s]		
28	ba<u>th</u>tub	[θ]	[Ø]		
29	<u>th</u>ank you	[θ]	[θ̯]		
30	a <u>th</u>umb	[θ]	[f]		

MODULE TIME	
TOTAL	6:32
ELAPSED	00:00–06:32

Clinical Phonetics Tape 3A
Fricatives and Affricates Module #3: *th* Changes

TRANSCRIPTION SHEET

	STIMULUS WORD	INTENDED	PERCEIVED	ALTERNATIVES	COMMENTS
	DELETIONS				
1	bathe	[ð]	[ ]		
2	toothbrush	[θ]	[ ]		
3	brother	[ð]	[ ]		
4	that apple	[ð]	[ ]		
5	feather	[ð]	[ ]		
6	bath	[θ]	[ ]		
7	teeth	[θ]	[ ]		
	SUBSTITUTIONS				
8	feather	[ð]	[ ]		
9	that	[ð]	[ ]		
10	bathtub	[θ]	[ ]		
11	feather	[ð]	[ ]		
12	teeth	[θ]	[ ]		
13	smooth	[ð]	[ ]		
14	this	[ð]	[ ]		
15	bathe	[ð]	[ ]		
	DISTORTIONS				
16	that	[ð]	[ ]		
17	three	[θ]	[ ]		
18	feather	[ð]	[ ]		
19	this	[ð]	[ ]		
20	bath	[θ]	[ ]		
21	teeth	[θ]	[ ]		
22	that	[ð]	[ ]		
	ANY ERROR				
23	toothache	[θ]	[ ]		
24	thumb	[θ]	[ ]		
25	this	[ð]	[ ]		
26	this apple	[ð]	[ ]		
27	thank you	[θ]	[ ]		
28	bathtub	[θ]	[ ]		
29	thank you	[θ]	[ ]		
30	a thumb	[θ]	[ ]		

Fricatives and Affricates Module #4: Fricative and Affricate Voicing Changes

Voicing changes of fricatives and affricates follow the same pattern as the voicing changes seen in the stops. Word-initial voiceless fricatives/affricates tend to be voiced; word-final fricative/affricates tend to be devoiced. Furthermore, the phonological rules for voicing assimilations in different phonetic contexts are essentially similar to those discussed for stops: fricatives and affricates tend to take on the voicing characteristics of adjacent consonants. The following module provides practice in discriminating voicing changes in certain fricatives and affricates.

PROCEED TO: Clinical Phonetics Tape 3A: Fricatives and Affricates Module #4: Fricative and Affricate Voicing Changes

Clinical Phonetics Tape 3A
Fricatives and Affricates Module #4: Fricative and Affricate Voicing Changes
TRANSCRIPTION KEY

MODULE TIME	
TOTAL	5:53
ELAPSED	06:32–12:25

EXAMPLES			
NORMAL	[zu]	DEVOICED	[z̥u]
	[ɪz]		[ɪz̥]

	STIMULUS WORD	INTENDED	CONSENSUS	ALTERNATIVES	COMMENTS
	PREVOCALIC POSITION				
1	<u>v</u>acuum	[v]	[v]		
2	<u>z</u>ebra	[z]	[z̥͎]		Whistled
3	<u>z</u>ipper	[z]	[z̥]		
4	<u>v</u>acuum	[v]	[v̥]		Slightly devoiced
5	<u>j</u>umping	[ʤ]	[ʤ]		Slightly devoiced
6	<u>j</u>ars	[ʤ]	[ʤ̥]		
	INTERVOCALIC POSITION				
7	T<u>V</u>	[v]	[v]		Noisy
8	fea<u>th</u>er	[ð]	[ð]		
9	pa<u>g</u>es	[ʤ]	[ʤ̥]		Second syllable is breathy.
10	sci<u>ss</u>ors	[z]	[z]		
11	se<u>v</u>en	[v]	[v]		
12	fea<u>th</u>er	[ð]	[ð̥]		
13	sci<u>ss</u>ors	[z]	[z̥]		Almost [s]
	POSTVOCALIC POSITION				
14	fi<u>v</u>e	[v]	[v̥]		
15	sto<u>v</u>e	[v]	[v̥]		
16	smoo<u>th</u>	[ð]	[ð̥]	[θ]	
17	glasse<u>s</u>	[z]	[z̥]	[z]	Devoiced only at the very end
18	feather<u>s</u>	[z]	[s͎]	[z̥͎]	
19	toe<u>s</u>	[z]	[z̥]	[z̞̥]	
20	smoo<u>th</u>	[ð]	[ð̥]		
21	dishe<u>s</u>	[z]	[z̥]		
	ASSORTED POSITIONS				
22	tele<u>ph</u>one	[f]	[f]		
23	T<u>V</u>	[v]	[v̥]		Noise
24	ca<u>g</u>e	[ʤ]	[ʤ̥]		
25	matche<u>s</u>	[z]	[z]		
26	toe<u>s</u>	[z]	[z̥]		
27	gara<u>g</u>e	[ʤ]	[ʤ̥]		
28	<u>z</u>ebra	[z]	[z̥]	[s]	

Note: One of the best comparisons is between the final /z/ in No. 25 *matches* versus No. 26 *toes.*

Clinical Phonetics Tape 3A
Fricatives and Affricates Module #4: Fricative and Affricate Voicing Changes
TRANSCRIPTION SHEET

MODULE TIME	
TOTAL	5:53
ELAPSED	06:32–12:25

EXAMPLES			
NORMAL	[zu]	DEVOICED	[z̥u]
	[ɪz]		[ɪz̥]

	STIMULUS WORD	INTENDED	PERCEIVED	ALTERNATIVES	COMMENTS
	PREVOCALIC POSITION				
1	vacuum	[v]	[ ]		
2	zebra	[z]	[ ]		
3	zipper	[z]	[ ]		
4	vacuum	[v]	[ ]		
5	jumping	[ʤ]	[ ]		
6	jars	[ʤ]	[ ]		
	INTERVOCALIC POSITION				
7	TV	[v]	[ ]		
8	feather	[ð]	[ ]		
9	pages	[ʤ]	[ ]		
10	scissors	[z]	[ ]		
11	seven	[v]	[ ]		
12	feather	[ð]	[ ]		
13	scissors	[z]	[ ]		
	POSTVOCALIC POSITION				
14	five	[v]	[ ]		
15	stove	[v]	[ ]		
16	smooth	[ð]	[ ]		
17	glasses	[z]	[ ]		
18	feathers	[z]	[ ]		
19	toes	[z]	[ ]		
20	smooth	[ð]	[ ]		
21	dishes	[z]	[ ]		
	ASSORTED POSITIONS				
22	telephone	[f]	[ ]		
23	TV	[v]	[ ]		
24	cage	[ʤ]	[ ]		
25	matches	[z]	[ ]		
26	toes	[z]	[ ]		
27	garage	[ʤ]	[ ]		
28	zebra	[z]	[ ]		

Fricatives and Affricates Module #5: Fricative and Affricate Substitutions

Substitution errors for fricatives and affricates generally involve either other fricatives or a stop. Seldom are fricatives replaced by sounds outside the class of obstruents; that is, not by nasal, liquid, or glide sounds. Our suggestions for transcribing fricative and affricate substitutions parallel those given for apparently phonemic substitutions for vowels and stops. We suggest a conservative approach. Do not label an error a fricative *substitution* unless the perceived sound is said essentially as it would be when used appropriately. Hence, for example, a perceived [t͡s/ʃ] is not the same as [tʃ/s]. Recall that in five-way scoring, tallying an error as a phonemic *substitution* rather than as a *distortion* could lead to incorrect analysis of the error pattern (see Chapter 7). The following module provides practice discriminating substitutions for fricatives and affricates; sounds for which substitutions are most common are: /s/, /z/, /ʃ/, /ʒ/, /tʃ/, and /ʤ/.

PROCEED TO: Clinical Phonetics Tape 3A: Fricatives and Affricates Module #5: Fricative and Affricate Substitutions

MODULE TIME	
TOTAL	5:49
ELAPSED	12:25–18:14

Clinical Phonetics Tape 3A
Fricatives and Affricates Module #5: Fricative and Affricate Substitutions

TRANSCRIPTION KEY

	STIMULUS WORD	INTENDED	CONSENSUS	ALTERNATIVES	COMMENTS
	/s/				
1	saw	[s]	[θ]		
2	house	[s]	[t]		
3	saw	[s]	[t]		
4	whistle	[s]	[s]		
5	seal	[s]	[s]		
	/z/				
6	zipper	[z]	[d͡ʒ]	[ʤ]	
7	a zebra	[z]	[z]		
8	scissors	[z]	[d]		
9	toes	[z]	[z̥]		
10	zipper	[z]	[j]		
11	hose	[z]	[d]		
	/ʃ/				
12	brush	[ʃ]	[s]		
13	fish	[ʃ]	[t]		[tʰ]
14	shoe	[ʃ]	[ʃ]		
15	station	[ʃ]	[s]		
16	dishes	[ʃ]	[ʃ]		
17	shoe	[ʃ]	[s]		
	/ʒ/				
18	measuring cup	[ʒ]	[ʒ]		
19	television	[ʒ]	[z̥]	[z̺̥]	
20	beige	[ʒ]	[z]		
21	measure	[ʒ]	[n]		
	/ʧ/				
22	chair	[ʧ]	[ʃ]		
23	watch	[ʧ]	[ʧ]		
24	sandwich	[ʧ]	[k͡s]	[t͡s]	[s] distorted?
25	matches	[ʧ]	[ʧ]		Stress change
26	chicken	[ʧ]	[t]		
	/ʤ/				
27	jar	[ʤ]	[s]	[s̪]	
28	orange juice	[ʤ]	[d]		
29	GI Joe	[ʤ], [ʤ]	[ʤ], [ʤ]		!!

MODULE TIME	
TOTAL	5:49
ELAPSED	12:25–18:14

Clinical Phonetics Tape 3A Fricatives and Affricates Module #5: Fricative and Affricate Substitutions

TRANSCRIPTION SHEET

	STIMULUS WORD	INTENDED	PERCEIVED	ALTERNATIVES	COMMENTS
	/s/				
1	<u>s</u>aw	[s]	[ ]		
2	hou<u>s</u>e	[s]	[ ]		
3	<u>s</u>aw	[s]	[ ]		
4	whi<u>st</u>le	[s]	[ ]		
5	<u>s</u>eal	[s]	[ ]		
	/z/				
6	<u>z</u>ipper	[z]	[ ]		
7	a <u>z</u>ebra	[z]	[ ]		
8	sci<u>ss</u>ors	[z]	[ ]		
9	toe<u>s</u>	[z]	[ ]		
10	<u>z</u>ipper	[z]	[ ]		
11	ho<u>s</u>e	[z]	[ ]		
	/ʃ/				
12	bru<u>sh</u>	[ʃ]	[ ]		
13	fi<u>sh</u>	[ʃ]	[ ]		
14	<u>sh</u>oe	[ʃ]	[ ]		
15	sta<u>ti</u>on	[ʃ]	[ ]		
16	di<u>sh</u>es	[ʃ]	[ ]		
17	<u>sh</u>oe	[ʃ]	[ ]		
	/ʒ/				
18	mea<u>s</u>uring cup	[ʒ]	[ ]		
19	televi<u>s</u>ion	[ʒ]	[ ]		
20	beige	[ʒ]	[ ]		
21	mea<u>s</u>ure	[ʒ]	[ ]		
	/tʃ/				
22	<u>ch</u>air	[tʃ]	[ ]		
23	wat<u>ch</u>	[tʃ]	[ ]		
24	sandwi<u>ch</u>	[tʃ]	[ ]		
25	mat<u>ch</u>es	[tʃ]	[ ]		
26	<u>ch</u>icken	[tʃ]	[ ]		
	/ʤ/				
27	<u>j</u>ar	[ʤ]	[ ]		
28	orange <u>j</u>uice	[ʤ]	[ ]		
29	<u>G</u>I <u>J</u>oe	[ʤ], [ʤ]	[ ], [ ]		

Fricatives and Affricates Module #6: Dentalized Sibilants

This training module and the two following training modules focus on distortion errors on the sibilant sounds /s/, /z/, /ʃ/, and /ʒ/. The audio examples will focus primarily on the distortions of these sounds that most often occur. The task in these modules is to learn to discriminate among three possible distortion types. To aid in this difficult task, let us first review some information about the production and acoustics of sibilants (you may also wish to review the description of sibilant productions given on pages 64, 76, 84, and 202).

First, recall that tongue placement and tongue shape (grooving) play the principal role in our production of sibilants. The front sounds made at the alveolar ridge, /s/ and /z/, are less intense (perceptually, they are softer) than the palatals /ʃ/ and /ʒ/. Recall also that the frequency (perceptually, the noise pitch) of lingual fricatives generally goes down as the point of articulation progresses from the front to the back of the oral cavity. That is, /s/ sounds higher pitched than /ʃ/. Both intensity and frequency factors, which result from the positioning of the tongue, will figure in our discussion of differences among distortion errors.

Finally, recall that although the tongue is the primary agent for sibilant production, both the teeth and the lips play important secondary roles. If you grasp your bottom lip between your fingers and alternately pull it down and back up while making a sustained fricative /s/, you will hear /s/ change in pitch. And if you slowly protrude your lower teeth forward while making /s/, you will hear /s/ change in pitch. Further, if you say /s/ with neutral or slightly rounded lips, then say it with lips fully rounded, you will hear /s/ change in pitch. The point is that although tongue shape and placement play the primary role in sibilant production, the teeth and the lips (particularly the bottom lip) do play an important secondary role. As clinicians are well aware, slight-to-severe sibilant distortions may be caused by structural abnormalities in a client's oral mechanism.

With these overall descriptive facts in mind, let us now consider the most frequent of all articulation errors, the dentalized /s/ [s̪]. Any distortion of /s/ or /z/ wherein the tongue gets too close to or actually abuts the alveolar ridge or teeth may be transcribed as [s̪] or [z̪]. A host of symbols has been proposed to capture subtle differences among /s/ distortions in this area. Trim (1953), for example, proposed 18 symbols to represent /s/ distortions. Although highly trained phoneticians can become skilled in using many of these symbols reliably, such discriminations are difficult, if not impossible, to teach on audio sample. Moreover, the clinical need for and benefits to be derived from such close transcription have yet to be demonstrated. In any case, we encompass the many possible frontal variants of /s/ sounds with the single symbol [s̪].

The ability to discriminate the varieties of dentalized /s/ [s̪] sounds from "normal" /s/ is markedly facilitated when the student-clinician can produce these distortion errors. Try pushing your tongue tip just millimeters forward and reducing the narrow groove along the middle of the tongue while making /s/. You should be able to make a variety of sounds, each of which is neither a correct /s/ nor a correct /θ/. These sounds should be somewhere in between /s/ and /θ/. The key perceptual feature of dentalized /s/ [s̪] is that in some way the fricative sound is "flattened." The high-pitched "sharpness" of /s/ is lost; instead it sounds anywhere from almost completely stopped to "flat." Also, because it is more forward and less sibilant, dentalized /s/ should seem less loud than correct /s/.

Be sure you can make the many varieties of dentalized /s/ and /z/ readily before proceeding to the following training module. Practice making the many varieties of dentalized /s̪/ by yourself and with a colleague. See if your friend can discriminate your intended distortions from your intended correct /s/. Pulling down your bottom lip during [s] and [s̪] production will allow you to more clearly hear the difference.

PROCEED TO: Clinical Phonetics Tape 3A: Fricatives and Affricates Module #6: Dentalized Sibilants

Clinical Phonetics Tape 3A
Fricatives and Affricates Module #6: Dentalized Sibilants

TRANSCRIPTION KEY

MODULE TIME	
TOTAL	5:16
ELAPSED	18:14–23:30

EXAMPLES			
NORMAL	[si]	DENTALIZED	[s̪i]
	[a͡ɪs]		[a͡ɪs̪]

	STIMULUS WORD	INTENDED	CONSENSUS	ALTERNATIVES	COMMENTS
	FINAL POSITION				
1	crayons	[z]	[z̥]	[t͡s̪]	Intrusive [t]?
2	doghouse	[s]	[s]		
3	fingers	[z]	[z̪̥]		
4	potatoes	[z]	[z̪]		
5	stories	[z]	[z]	[z̥]	
6	glasses	[z]	[z]		The intervocalic /s/ may be dentalized.
7	nose	[z]	[z̪]		
8	bus	[s]	[s]		Slightly dentalized
9	matches	[z]	[z]		
10	house	[s]	[s̪]	[s̡]	One judge heard as palatalized /s/.
	INITIAL POSITION				
11	saw	[s]	[s̪]		
12	a zebra	[z]	[z̪]		Slightly
13	smooth	[s]	[s̪]	[θ͡s̪]	Close to [θ/s]
14	spoon	[s]	[s]		
15	said	[s]	[s̪]	[s̡]	Palatalized?
16	stars	[s]	[s̪]		
17	soft	[s]	[s]		
18	sun	[s]	[s̪]		
	ASSORTED POSITIONS				
19	school bus	[s], [s]	[s], [s]		
20	grass	[s]	[s̪]		
21	six	[s], [s]	[s̪], [s̪]	[s]	
22	toothpaste	[s]	[s̪]		
23	smooth	[s]	[s]		
24	a zebra	[z]	[z̪]		
25	dishes	[z]	[z̪]	[z̪̥]	
26	/s/ (isolation)	[s]	[s]		Hard to tell, isn't it!

Notes: Good examples of dentalized /s/ and /z/ are No. 15, No. 20, and No. 24. Be sure you can make the range of dentalized /s/ and /z/, from slight dentalization to almost [θ], [ð].

Clinical Phonetics Tape 3A
Fricatives and Affricates Module #6: Dentalized Sibilants

TRANSCRIPTION SHEET

MODULE TIME	
TOTAL	5:16
ELAPSED	18:14–23:30

EXAMPLES			
NORMAL	[si]	DENTALIZED	[s̪i]
	[a͡ɪs]		[a͡ɪs̪]

	STIMULUS WORD	INTENDED	PERCEIVED	ALTERNATIVES	COMMENTS
	FINAL POSITION				
1	crayons	[z]	[ ]		
2	doghouse	[s]	[ ]		
3	fingers	[z]	[ ]		
4	potatoes	[z]	[ ]		
5	stories	[z]	[ ]		
6	glasses	[z]	[ ]		
7	nose	[z]	[ ]		
8	bus	[s]	[ ]		
9	matches	[z]	[ ]		
10	house	[s]	[ ]		
	INITIAL POSITION				
11	saw	[s]	[ ]		
12	a zebra	[z]	[ ]		
13	smooth	[s]	[ ]		
14	spoon	[s]	[ ]		
15	said	[s]	[ ]		
16	stars	[s]	[ ]		
17	soft	[s]	[ ]		
18	sun	[s]	[ ]		
	ASSORTED POSITIONS				
19	school bus	[s], [s]	[ ], [ ]		
20	grass	[s]	[ ]		
21	six	[s], [s]	[ ], [ ]		
22	toothpaste	[s]	[ ]		
23	smooth	[s]	[ ]		
24	a zebra	[z]	[ ]		
25	dishes	[z]	[ ]		
26	/s/ (isolation)	[s]	[ ]		

Fricatives and Affricates Module #7: Lateralized Sibilants

Lateral "lisps" ([s], [z], [ʃ] [ʒ]) have been referred to as sounding "wet" or "slurpy." These terms do, in fact, capture a perceptual aspect of the lateralized sibilant. Once this percept is learned, lateralization of /s/ and other sounds is readily recognized.

Here is how to teach yourself to make a lateral lisp. Place your tongue in the position that you would to say /l/ as in *look.* Now, keep your tongue tip *firmly* anchored on your alveolar ridge and try to say /s/. What you should generate is air turbulence over the *sides* of the tongue. Hence, the term *lateral* /s/. You can confirm the lateral air emission by tapping your cheek as you sustain the lateralized /s/ [s]. The sound will change in its quality as you divert the airstream by tapping your cheeks. In fact, you can shunt the air from one side to the other with your tongue, creating either a unilateral lisp or, if directed around both sides at once, a bilateral lisp. In our experience, most children with lateral lisps will have air coming out both sides.

Be sure you can make a "respectable" [s], [z], [ʃ], and [ʒ] before proceeding to the audio sample training on discrimination of lateralization. You should not hear or feel air coming across the central incisors. You can check for this by placing a single strip of tissue in front of your incisors, with or without your bottom lip pulled down. The tissue should not flutter; it should flutter only as you bring the tissue to the side(s) of the lips to which the airstream has been diverted. Again, practice with a colleague should be helpful.

PROCEED TO: Clinical Phonetics Tape 3A: Fricatives and Affricates Module #7: Lateralized Sibilants

Clinical Phonetics Tape 3A
Fricatives and Affricates Module #7: Lateralized Sibilants

TRANSCRIPTION KEY

MODULE TIME	
TOTAL	2:39
ELAPSED	23:30–26:09

EXAMPLES			
NORMAL	[si]	LATERALIZED	[s̯i]
	[a͡ɪs]		[a͡ɪs̯]

	STIMULUS WORD	INTENDED	CONSENSUS	ALTERNATIVES	COMMENTS
1	keys	[z]	[z̥̯]		Slightly
2	glasses	[s], [z]	[s̯], [z̯]		
3	star	[s]	[s]		
4	/s/	[s]	[s̯]		Very difficult in isolation on audio sample
5	scissors	[s], [z], [z]	[s̯], [z̯], [z̥̯]		
6	saddle	[s]	[s̯]		
7	sack	[s]	[s̯]		
8	pencil	[s]	[s̯]		
9	fish	[ʃ]	[s̯]		
10	gates	[s]	[s]		
11	this is fireworks	[s], [z], [s]	[s̯], [z̯], [s̯]		

Note: Judges each had a "favorite" best example; item 11 appears to contain good examples of lateralized sibilants.

Clinical Phonetics Tape 3A
Fricatives and Affricates Module #7:
Lateralized Sibilants

TRANSCRIPTION SHEET

MODULE TIME	
TOTAL	2:39
ELAPSED	23:30–26:09

EXAMPLES			
NORMAL	[si]	LATERALIZED	[si̯]
	[a͡ɪs]		[a͡ɪs̯]

	STIMULUS WORD	INTENDED	PERCEIVED	ALTERNATIVES	COMMENTS
1	keys	[z]	[ ]		
2	glasses	[s], [z]	[ ], [ ]		
3	star	[s]	[ ]		
4	/s/	[s]	[ ]		
5	scissors	[s], [z], [z]	[ ], [ ], [ ]		
6	saddle	[s]	[ ]		
7	sack	[s]	[ ]		
8	pencil	[s]	[ ]		
9	fish	[ʃ]	[ ]		
10	gates	[s]	[ ]		
11	this is fireworks	[s], [z], [s]	[ ], [ ], [ ]		

Fricatives and Affricates Module #8: Retroflexed Sibilants

The last type of sibilant distortion, retroflexed [s̫], [z̫], [ʃ̫], [ʒ̫], occurs only infrequently in children.[4] Retroflexed /s/, [s̫], with or without a whistling component, [s̫̑], is a common /s/ variant in certain Southern and rural communities. Also, Rousey and Moriarity (1965) present some evidence that a form of a whistling, retroflexed /s/ may occur temporarily when a person is nervous.

To make [s̫], first put your tongue in the position you normally would for /r/ or /ɝ/ as in *run* or *earn.* Now, keep your tongue poised in this retroflex position and try making /s/—try to generate a friction sound while your tongue is in the retroflex position. As you tense your tongue and experiment with different approximations of your tongue tip to the roof of your mouth, you should be able to make a retroflexed /s/, including a whistle component [s̫̑]. The trick is to make a very narrow groove in the center of the tongue and to tighten up the tongue as it curls backwards. Because the sound is made so far back in the oral cavity, its pitch should be lower than the dentalized /s/ [s̪] or the lateralized /s/ [s̯]. Try saying *bursar* [b ɝ s̫ ɚ], *purse* [p ɝ s̫], *mercy* [m ɝ s̫ ɪ]. Now try making retroflexed /s/ in words like *see, say,* and *Mississippi.* If your tongue is properly rolled back, your retroflexed /s/'s will sound like Humphrey Bogart's ("play it again, Sam").

[4]Another type of /s/ distortion, palatalized /s/ [sʲ], is perceptually quite similar to retroflexed /s/. Palatalized /s/ has a flattened tongue in the region of the turbulence. If you say the words "gas shortage" and freeze on the underlined continuant, you should be making [sʲ]. The [s] sounds like a sibilant midway between /s/ and /ʃ/. Palatalized /s/'s occur often in children. Unfortunately, however, we have not been able to teach reliable discrimination of this sound by audio recordings.

PROCEED TO: Clinical Phonetics Tape 3A: Fricatives and Affricates Module #8: Retroflexed Sibilants

Clinical Phonetics Tape 3A
Fricatives and Affricates Module #8:
Retroflexed Sibilants

TRANSCRIPTION KEY

MODULE TIME	
TOTAL	2:51
ELAPSED	26:09–29:00

EXAMPLES			
NORMAL	[si]	RETROFLEXED	[s̢i]
	[a͡ɪs]		[a͡ɪs̢]

	STIMULUS WORD	INTENDED	CONSENSUS	ALTERNATIVES	COMMENTS
1	whistle	[s]	[s̢]		Slight
2	walking in the bus	[s]	[s̢]		
3	scissors	[s], [z], [z]	[s̢͎], [z̢͎], [z̢͎]		
4	zebra	[z]	[z̢̥͎]		Devoiced, retroflexed, and whistled!
5	Christmas tree	[s], [s]	[s], [s]		
6	ice	[s]	[s̢]		
7	base	[s]	[s̢]		
8	gas	[s]	[s̢]		
9	carrots	[s]	[s̢]	[s̪]	
10	bus	[s]	[s̢]		
11	mice	[s]	[s̢]		
12	choice	[s]	[s̢]		

Notes: These are difficult discriminations to make from audio recordings. Practice in *making* the three types of sibilant distortions—dentalized, lateralized, and retroflexed—will allow you to compare the three. Try saying the same word with a correct /s/ or /z/, then with each of the distortion types. Can someone else label correctly what you intended? How do your recorded distortions sound? Can you discriminate your own distortion types when you hear them played back on audiotape or CD?

Clinical Phonetics Tape 3A
Fricatives and Affricates Module #8: Retroflexed Sibilants

TRANSCRIPTION SHEET

MODULE TIME	
TOTAL	2:51
ELAPSED	26:09–29:00

EXAMPLES			
NORMAL	[si]	RETROFLEXED	[s̢i]
	[a͡ɪs]		[a͡ɪs̢]

	STIMULUS WORD	INTENDED	PERCEIVED	ALTERNATIVES	COMMENTS
1	whistle	[s]	[ ]		
2	walking in the bus	[s]	[ ]		
3	scissors	[s], [z], [z]	[ ], [ ], [ ]		
4	zebra	[z]	[ ]		
5	Christmas tree	[s], [s]	[ ], [ ]		
6	ice	[s]	[ ]		
7	base	[s]	[ ]		
8	gas	[s]	[ ]		
9	carrots	[s]	[ ]		
10	bus	[s]	[ ]		
11	mice	[s]	[ ]		
12	choice	[s]	[ ]		

Fricatives and Affricates Module #9: Sibilants Quiz

Here is an opportunity to test your skill in discriminating sibilant distortions. The following module contains a variety of the sibilant distortions practiced up to this point—the emphasis will be on /s/ and /z/ distortions.

PROCEED TO: Clinical Phonetics Tape 3B: Fricatives and Affricates Module #9: Sibilants Quiz

MODULE TIME	
TOTAL	2:54
ELAPSED	00:00–02:54

Clinical Phonetics Tape 3B
Fricatives and Affricates Module #9:
Sibilants Quiz

TRANSCRIPTION KEY

	STIMULUS WORD	INTENDED	CONSENSUS	ALTERNATIVES	COMMENTS
1	I lost my red socks	[s], [s], [s]	[s̪], [s̪], [s̪]		Slight; the first /s/ in *socks* is most dentalized.
2	icy	[s]	[s̭]		
3	glasses	[s], [z]	[s̪], [z̪]		
4	lacing	[s]	[s̭]		
5	house	[s]	[s̢]		
6	this Christmas	[s], [s], [s]	[s], [s], [s]		
7	placemat	[s]	[s̪]		
8	whistle	[s]	[s̢]		
9	1977	[s], [s]	[s̭], [s̭]		
10	juicy	[s]	[s]		Noise
11	bus	[s]	[s̪]		
12	scissors	[s], [z], [z]	[s], [z], [z]		
13	balloons	[z]	[z̪̥]		
14	minus	[s]	[s̢]	[s̭]	One judge thought it sounded both retroflexed and lateralized!

Notes: One of the most difficult modules in this series. Keep in mind that in five-way scoring, all "distortions" are tallied as incorrect. If you are correctly discriminating normal from distorted but not getting the distortion category correct, you would be "reliable" in both five-way scoring and two-way scoring.

MODULE TIME	
TOTAL	2:54
ELAPSED	00:00–02:54

Clinical Phonetics Tape 3B Fricatives and Affricates Module #9: Sibilants Quiz

TRANSCRIPTION SHEET

	STIMULUS WORD	INTENDED	PERCEIVED	ALTERNATIVES	COMMENTS
1	I lo<u>s</u>t my red <u>s</u>ock<u>s</u>	[s], [s], [s]	[ ], [ ], [ ]		
2	i<u>c</u>y	[s]	[ ]		
3	gla<u>ss</u>e<u>s</u>	[s], [z]	[ ], [ ]		
4	la<u>c</u>ing	[s]	[ ]		
5	hou<u>s</u>e	[s]	[ ]		
6	thi<u>s</u> Chri<u>s</u>tma<u>s</u>	[s], [s], [s]	[ ], [ ], [ ]		
7	pla<u>c</u>emat	[s]	[ ]		
8	whi<u>s</u>tle	[s]	[ ]		
9	19<u>77</u>	[s], [s]	[ ], [ ]		
10	jui<u>c</u>y	[s]	[ ]		
11	bu<u>s</u>	[s]	[ ]		
12	<u>s</u>ci<u>ss</u>or<u>s</u>	[s], [z], [z]	[ ], [ ], [ ]		
13	balloon<u>s</u>	[z]	[ ]		
14	minu<u>s</u>	[s]	[ ]		

Fricatives and Affricates Module #10: Summary Quiz

Summary Quiz time once more! As in Part A for vowels and Part B for stops, this final quiz in Part C provides a good chance for you to review all the fricative and affricate errors taught to this point. You may want to review your work on the previous modules before beginning here. *Bonne chance!*

PROCEED TO: Clinical Phonetics Tape 3B: Fricatives and Affricates Module #10: Summary Quiz

MODULE TIME	
TOTAL	5:31
ELAPSED	02:54–08:25

Clinical Phonetics Tape 3B
Fricatives and Affricates Module #10: Summary Quiz

TRANSCRIPTION KEY

	STIMULUS WORD	INTENDED	CONSENSUS	ALTERNATIVES	COMMENTS
1	mi<u>ss</u>ing	[s]	[θ]		
2	i<u>c</u>e cream cone	[s]	[s̯]		
3	no<u>s</u>e	[z]	[z̥]		
4	<u>z</u>ebra	[z]	[ð̌]	[ð̥̌]	
5	<u>sc</u>i<u>ss</u>or<u>s</u>	[s], [z], [z]	[s̪], [ð̌], [ð̌]	[d]	
6	thi<u>s</u> boy ha<u>s</u> a too<u>th</u>ache	[s], [z], [θ]	[s̪], [z̪], [θ]	[θ]	
7	fea<u>th</u>er	[ð]	[d]		
8	the dog <u>s</u>it<u>s</u> up	[s], [s]	[s̪], [s̪]		Second /s/ is better.
9	<u>z</u>ipper	[z]	[z̥]	[z̥]	
10	<u>sh</u>oe	[ʃ]	[s]		
11	di<u>sh</u>e<u>s</u>	[ʃ], [z]	[ʃ], [z]	[z̪]	
12	<u>z</u>ipper	[z]	[d]		
13	fi<u>sh</u>	[ʃ]	[t͡s]		
14	<u>s</u>tar	[s]	[s̪]		
15	carrot<u>s</u>	[s]	[s̪]		Possibly [θ]
16	carrot<u>s</u>	[s]	[θ]		Contrast with No. 15
17	hou<u>s</u>e	[s]	[ø]		Dubbing noise but /s/ is deleted
18	<u>s</u>poon	[s]	[ø]		[p⁼ũ]
19	<u>s</u>kate<u>s</u>	[s], [s]	[ø], [s]		[k⁼e͞ɪts]
20	<u>s</u>tar<u>s</u>	[s], [z]	[s̢], [z̢̥]		
21	fi<u>sh</u>	[ʃ]	[p]		Noisy
22	fi<u>v</u>e toe<u>s</u>	[f], [v], [z]	[f], [v], [z̥̭]		[v] is barely audible.
23	T<u>V</u>	[v]	[f]	[v̥]	
24	mea<u>s</u>ure	[ʒ]	[z̪]	[ð]	Judges split on these two transcriptions.
25	<u>sh</u>oe	[ʃ]	[ʃ̯]		
26	<u>s</u>ta<u>t</u>ion	[s], [ʃ]	[s], [s]	[s̪]	Second /s/ may be slightly dentalized.
27	<u>ch</u>air	[tʃ]	[t͓ʰ]		
28	pla<u>c</u>emat	[s]	[s]	[s̪]	
29	mat<u>ch</u>e<u>s</u>	[tʃ], [z]	[tʃ], [z̪]		
30	a<u>s</u>leep	[s]	[s]		This speaker *can* say /s/ without lateralization.

MODULE TIME	
TOTAL	5:31
ELAPSED	02:54–08:25

Clinical Phonetics Tape 3B
Fricatives and Affricates Module #10: Summary Quiz

TRANSCRIPTION SHEET

	STIMULUS WORD	INTENDED	PERCEIVED	ALTERNATIVES	COMMENTS
1	missing	[s]	[ ]		
2	ice cream cone	[s]	[ ]		
3	nose	[z]	[ ]		
4	zebra	[z]	[ ]		
5	scissors	[s], [z], [z]	[ ], [ ], [ ]		
6	this boy has a toothache	[s], [z], [θ]	[ ], [ ], [ ]		
7	feather	[ð]	[ ]		
8	the dog sits up	[s], [s]	[ ], [ ]		
9	zipper	[z]	[ ]		
10	shoe	[ʃ]	[ ]		
11	dishes	[ʃ], [z]	[ ], [ ]		
12	zipper	[z]	[ ]		
13	fish	[ʃ]	[ ]		
14	star	[s]	[ ]		
15	carrots	[s]	[ ]		
16	carrots	[s]	[ ]		
17	house	[s]	[ ]		
18	spoon	[s]	[ ]		
19	skates	[s], [s]	[ ], [ ]		
20	stars	[s], [z]	[ ], [ ]		
21	fish	[ʃ]	[ ]		
22	five toes	[f], [v], [z]	[ ], [ ], [ ]		
23	TV	[v]	[ ]		
24	measure	[ʒ]	[ ]		
25	shoe	[ʃ]	[ ]		
26	station	[s], [ʃ]	[ ], [ ]		
27	chair	[tʃ]	[ ]		
28	placemat	[s]	[ ]		
29	matches	[tʃ], [z]	[ ], [ ]		
30	asleep	[s]	[ ]		

PART D: TRANSCRIPTION OF GLIDE AND LIQUID SOUND CHANGES

BACKGROUND INFORMATION

Description of Glides and Liquids

Glides and liquids are grouped together for this next series of training modules. The reason for this is that these two sound classes have much in common, as the following outline of their phonetic relationships clearly shows (see also Appendix A, Table A-5).

Sonorants (versus the **obstruents,** which are **stops, fricatives,** and **affricates**)

- **Nasals**
- **Vowels** and **diphthongs**
- **Glides**—/w/, /j/
- **Liquids**—/l/, /r/

Thus, the two glide sounds /w/, /j/ and the two liquid sounds /l/, /r/ all share a family tie to the class of sonorants. As noted for stop errors in Part B, children's errors on /w/, /j/, /l/, and /r/ are most likely to remain within class. That is, these four sonorant sounds are not likely to be replaced by obstruents when a substitution error occurs; they most likely will be replaced by another sonorant.

Distribution

The frequency of occurrence of each of the two glides and the two liquids differs markedly, as indicated in Appendix B. The consonant /r/, for example, ranks among the most frequent sounds, whereas /j/ is a very infrequent sound. The fact that many languages have only one liquid or none at all suggests that liquids are difficult to discriminate and to produce. English-speaking children must learn to differentiate among four glides and liquids. As we will discuss, they generally have little or no trouble with glides, but they have a great deal of difficulty with the two liquids.

Appendix B, Table B-1, includes a summary of the distributional rules for the occurrence of liquids and glides. Note that /w/ and /j/, which require a tense onset followed by a gliding movement, do not occur in word-final position. Because our orthography uses the letters "w" and "y" to end words (*tomorrow* and *buy*), we tend to forget this distributional characteristic of the glides /w/ and /j/. Note also (Table B-2) that glides and liquids are the only sounds permitted in the third position in an initial three-consonant cluster, such as [s k w] or [s p l], and that clusters containing glides and liquids occur frequently (Table B-11).

TRAINING MODULES

The glides /w/ and /j/ are among the first consonants that children articulate correctly. Therefore, children who have significant errors on /w/ and /j/ generally have extremely delayed speech. Substitutions for glides occur frequently enough to warrant the discrimination training presented in the following module.[5]

Glides and Liquids Module #1: Glide Changes

The task in this brief training module is straightforward. Here is an opportunity to transcribe changes for the glides /w/ and /j/.

[5]The distinction between /w/ ([w]) and /hw/ ([ʍ]) (*witch–which; wail–whale*) is not preserved in many American English dialects. For convenience, we use [w] for all training stimuli.

PROCEED TO: Clinical Phonetics Tape 3B: Glides and Liquids Module #1: Glide Changes

MODULE TIME	
TOTAL	2:05
ELAPSED	08:25–10:30

Clinical Phonetics Tape 3B
Glides and Liquids Module #1:
Glide Changes

TRANSCRIPTION KEY

	STIMULUS WORD	INTENDED	CONSENSUS	ALTERNATIVES	COMMENTS
1	onion	[j]	[w]		
2	flower	[w]	[w]		[w] does not always occur; i.e., [f l a͡ʊ ɚ].
3	sweeping	[w]	[l]		
4	swing	[w]	[r̮]		Derhotacized /r/ See Module #4.
5	yes	[j]	[j]		
6	sandwich	[w]	[w]		
7	flower	[w]	[l]		See comment for item 2.
8	thank you	[j]	[l]		[θ̯]
9	whistle	[w]	[w]		
10	yes	[j]	[w]		[s]

MODULE TIME	
TOTAL	2:05
ELAPSED	08:25–10:30

Clinical Phonetics Tape 3B
Glides and Liquids Module #1:
Glide Changes

TRANSCRIPTION SHEET

	STIMULUS WORD	INTENDED	PERCEIVED	ALTERNATIVES	COMMENTS
1	onion	[j]	[ ]		
2	flower	[w]	[ ]		
3	sweeping	[w]	[ ]		
4	swing	[w]	[ ]		
5	yes	[j]	[ ]		
6	sandwich	[w]	[ ]		
7	flower	[w]	[ ]		
8	thank you	[j]	[ ]		
9	whistle	[w]	[ ]		
10	yes	[j]	[ ]		

Glides and Liquids Module #2: /l/ Substitutions

The liquids /l/ and /r/ generally are conceded to be among the most difficult sounds in a language to articulate. Among the 24 English consonants, only /l/ requires the airstream to be emitted laterally—over the sides of the tongue. In the first of two /l/ sound change training modules, we are concerned with substitutions of other phonemes for /l/. As noted earlier, substitutions for /l/ generally will be one of the other sonorants—either a glide, a liquid, or a vowel-like sound. Clinicians typically have difficulty discriminating whether a child said final /l/ correctly or whether there was a vowel substitution (for example, *tail* [te͡ɪo]). Clinicians may be unaware that /l/ in this position is normally velarized, making it more similar acoustically to back vowels, and that tongue tip contact is not always made for postvocalic /l/. In the training module immediately following this one, a more detailed description of velarized /l/ will be provided. Here, it is sufficient to note that a velarized /l/ allophone occurs in the postvocalic position.

PROCEED TO: Clinical Phonetics Tape 3B: Glides and Liquids Module #2: /l/ Substitutions

MODULE TIME	
TOTAL	3:22
ELAPSED	10:30–13:52

Clinical Phonetics Tape 3B Glides and Liquids Module #2: /l/ Substitutions

TRANSCRIPTION KEY

	STIMULUS WORD	INTENDED	CONSENSUS	ALTERNATIVES	COMMENTS
1	ladder	[l]	[j]		
2	bell	[l]	[l]		
3	nail	[l]	[ne͡ɪoᶻ̪̥]	[ne͡ɪʊᶻ̪̥]	
4	lion	[l]	[l]		
5	football	[l]	[fʊʔbaʊ]	[fʊbal]	
6	blocks	[l]	[w]		
7	seal	[l]	[siᵊ]		
8	that apple	[l]	[æpʊ]	[æ p o]	
9	whistle	[l]	[w ɪ s o]	[w ɪ s ʊ]	
10	leaf	[l]	[l]		Lengthened
11	lamp	[l]	[r]	[r̮]	
12	baseball	[l]	[be͡ɪsbɔʊ]		
13	tail	[l]	[te͡ɪo̤]		Note symbol for breathy or murmured
14	we saw a puppet lady	[l]	[j]		
15	wheel	[l]	[w i o]		
16	ladder	[l]	[w]		
17	seal	[l]	[siowə]	[sɪʊwə]	Unusual

Note: Differences between [o] and [ʊ] as replacements for final [l] are unimportant.

MODULE TIME	
TOTAL	3:22
ELAPSED	10:30–13:52

Clinical Phonetics Tape 3B
Glides and Liquids Module #2:
/l/ Substitutions

TRANSCRIPTION SHEET

	STIMULUS WORD	INTENDED	PERCEIVED	ALTERNATIVES	COMMENTS
1	ladder	[l]	[ ]		
2	bell	[l]	[ ]		
3	nail	[l]	[ ]		
4	lion	[l]	[ ]		
5	football	[l]	[ ]		
6	blocks	[l]	[ ]		
7	seal	[l]	[ ]		
8	that apple	[l]	[ ]		
9	whistle	[l]	[ ]		
10	leaf	[l]	[ ]		
11	lamp	[l]	[ ]		
12	baseball	[l]	[ ]		
13	tail	[l]	[ ]		
14	we saw a puppet lady	[l]	[ ]		
15	wheel	[l]	[ ]		
16	ladder	[l]	[ ]		
17	seal	[l]	[ ]		

Glides and Liquids Module #3: Velarized /l/

As introduced in the previous module, velarized /l/ [l̰] is an allophone of /l/ that occurs primarily after a vowel at the ends of words. For the purposes of clinical phonetics, a velarized or "dark" /l/ can be differentiated from a "clear" /l/ by the activity of the back of the tongue during the articulation of this lateral sound (recall the discussion of the use of these terms beginning on page 70). For normal or "clear" /l/, the back of the tongue is positioned low in the oral cavity, and the high point of the tongue is at the alveolar ridge. Consider the position of the front and back of the tongue for [l] in the word *leap.*

For a "dark" or velarized /l/ [l̰], the back of the tongue is close to the velum. Our perception of a "darker" quality to the /l/ is associated with this secondary articulation within the oral cavity. The tongue tip may not even touch the alveolar ridge during velarized /l/ production. Consider the position of the front and back of the tongue for /l/ in the word *peal.* Now compare *leap* [l i p] and *peal* [pil̰] to appreciate the different qualities.

Whereas velarized /l/ [l̰] is a predictable allophone in postvocalic, word-final position, some individuals use a dark /l/ habitually in all phonetic positions. Such errors in adults generally go unnoticed by most people. Occasionally, however, the velarization is so pronounced that it draws attention to itself. The following module provides practice in hearing clear and dark /l/'s in an adult who could produce either at will after a program of speech management to correct velarized /l/.

PROCEED TO: Clinical Phonetics Tape 3B: Glides and Liquids Module #3: Velarized /l/

Clinical Phonetics Tape 3B
Glides and Liquids Module #3:
Velarized /l/

TRANSCRIPTION KEY

MODULE TIME	
TOTAL	3:10
ELAPSED	13:52–17:02

EXAMPLES			
NORMAL	[lɔ]	VELARIZED	[l̰ɔ]
	[ɔl]		[ɔl̰]

	STIMULUS WORD	INTENDED	CONSENSUS	ALTERNATIVES	COMMENTS
1	land	[l]	[l̰]		
2	ability	[l]	[l̰]		
3	asleep	[l]	[l̰]		Slightly
4	frolic	[l]	[l]		
5	alarm	[l]	[l̰]		Slightly
6	follow	[l]	[l̰]		Slightly
7	belong	[l]	[l̰]		
8	limb	[l]	[l̰]		
9	please	[l]	[l]		
10	black	[l]	[l̰]		[b ə l̰ æ k]
11	class	[l]	[l]		
12	glad	[l]	[l̰]		
13	I believe I belong in this village	[l], [l], [l]	[l̰], [l̰], [l̰]	[l], [l]	Slight velarization on first and last /l/
14	The lake is so still it is almost like glass	[l], [l], [l], [l], [l]	[l̰], [l̰], [l̰], [l̰], [l̰]	[l], [l]	

Notes: Comparison of No. 11 and No. 12, essentially the same phonetic context for the /l/, demonstrates a normal and a velarized /l/, respectively. Items 13 and 14 are extremely difficult to transcribe. They are included here to demonstrate the effect of velarized /l/ in continuous speech.

Clinical Phonetics Tape 3B Glides and Liquids Module #3: Velarized /l/

TRANSCRIPTION SHEET

MODULE TIME	
TOTAL	3:10
ELAPSED	13:52–17:02

EXAMPLES			
NORMAL	[lɔ]	VELARIZED	[l̴ɔ]
	[ɔl]		[ɔl̴]

	STIMULUS WORD	INTENDED	PERCEIVED	ALTERNATIVES	COMMENTS
1	land	[l]	[ ]		
2	ability	[l]	[ ]		
3	asleep	[l]	[ ]		
4	frolic	[l]	[ ]		
5	alarm	[l]	[ ]		
6	follow	[l]	[ ]		
7	belong	[l]	[ ]		
8	limb	[l]	[ ]		
9	please	[l]	[ ]		
10	black	[l]	[ ]		
11	class	[l]	[ ]		
12	glad	[l]	[ ]		
13	I believe I belong in this village	[l], [l], [l]	[ ], [ ], [ ]		
14	The lake is so still it is almost like glass	[l], [l], [l], [l], [l]	[ ], [ ], [ ], [ ], [ ]		

Glides and Liquids Module #4: Derhotacized /r/, /ɝ/, /ɚ/

Whether due to their perceptual characteristics, their articulatory demands, or some combination of both, /r/ and /ɝ/ seem to be hard for children to acquire. Children who make errors on one of these sounds (including also the unstressed vowel [ɚ]) usually make errors on the other (Shriberg, 1975, 1980b). Notice that the onset position for the consonant /r/ is the vowel /ɝ/, just as the consonants /w/ and /j/ have onsets similar to /u/ and /i/, respectively. In addition to the derhotacized /r/ [r̮] that we will learn to discriminate in this module, two other types of errors on /r/, /ɝ/, and /ɚ/ will require discrimination training: w/r and velarized /r/ [r̰].

Derhotacized /r/ [r̮] is the most common error type for /r/ in school-aged children and in adults. In overall prevalence of articulation error types, it ranks second only to dentalized /s/ [s̪].

To make a derhotacized /r/, put your tongue in the position you would to say /ʃ/—as though you were going to say *shoe.* Now glide away from this position as you say . . . *rue.* Try beginning in the /ʃ/ position as you say *read, ride, road.* You should hear a slightly lengthened derhotacized /r/ [r̮] that may vary with the height of the following vowel. Derhotacized /r/ sounds cover a wide range of "*r*-ness," from just a trace of *r* coloring to almost [r]. As you attempt to make derhotacized /r/ sounds, [r̮], be sure to focus on tongue postures, not lip gestures such as rounding or protrusion. Lip rounding of /r/ is determined partly by the following vowel, not only by the "*r*-ness" of the consonant itself (contrast the amount of lip rounding in *read* versus that in *rude*).

Here are some examples that should reacquaint you with the proper use of the symbols for derhotacized /r/ introduced earlier in this text.

Item	*If Correct*	*If Derhotacized*
read	[r i d]	[r̮ i d]
early	[ɝ l ɪ]	[ɝ̮ l ɪ]
crayon	[k r e͡ɪ ɑ n]	[k r̮ e͡ɪ ɑ n]
acre	[e͡ɪ k ɚ]	[e͡ɪ k ɚ̮]
Brewers	[b r u ɚ z]	[b r̮ u ɚ̮ z]

PROCEED TO: Clinical Phonetics Tape 3B: Glides and Liquids Module #4: Derhotacized /r/, /ɝ/, /ɚ/

Clinical Phonetics Tape 3B
Glides and Liquids Module #4: Derhotacized /r/, /ɝ/, /ɚ/

TRANSCRIPTION KEY

MODULE TIME	
TOTAL	5:57
ELAPSED	17:02–22:59

EXAMPLES			
NORMAL	[ri]	DERHOTACIZED	[r̮i]
	[ir]		[ir̮]

	STIMULUS WORD	INTENDED	CONSENSUS	ALTERNATIVES	COMMENTS
1	car	[r]	[r]		Slightly devoiced
2	a zebra	[r]	[r̮]	[w]	Also labialized, i.e., [r̮ʷ]
3	/ɝ/	[ɝ]	[ɝ]		
4	they having a fire	[r]	[ʊ]	[ə]	[f ɑ͡ɪ ʊ] or [f ɑ͡ɪ ə]
5	/ɝ/	[ɝ]	[ʌːᵊ]	[ɛːᵊ], [ʊᵒᵊ]	Other transcriptions too!
6	chair	[r]	[ɛ̠ə]	[ɛ ɪ ə], [ɛ ɔ]	
7	raining	[r]	[r̮]		Labialized [r̮ʷ]
8	/ɝ/	[ɝ]	[ʌ˞]	[ɔ˞], [ɔ˞ᶷ]	
9	car	[r]	[r]		
10	finger	[ɚ]	[ə]	[ɚ̮], [ʊ]	Perhaps some slight *r* coloring
11	garage	[r]	[r]	[rʷ]	
12	Is the cake ready	[r]	[r̮]	[rʷ]	Slightly
13	feather	[ɚ]	[ɚ]	[ɚ̮]	Ends abruptly
14	chair	[r]	[r̮]		Almost normal
15	big brother	[r], [ɚ]	[r̮], [ɚ̮]		
16	/ɝ/	[ɝ]	[ɝ̮]		
17	orbit	[r]	[r̮]		
18	sit right here	[r], [r]	[r̮], [r]		Second /r/ slightly derhotacized?
19	read	[r]	[r]		
20	He was running to school	[r]	[r]		
21	scissors	[ɚ]	[ɚ̮]	[ə]	
22	camper	[ɚ]	[ʊ]		[k æ m p ᶷ]
23	three, four, five	[r], [r]	[r̮], [ə]		[f ɔ ə]
24	cricket	[r]	[r]		
25	brush	[r]	[r̮]		
26	chair	[r]	[r]		
27	sit right here	[r], [r]	[r̮], [r̮]		Last /r/ is only slightly derhotacized.

Notes: Items 16 and 17 provide good examples of derhotacized /ɝ/ and /r/, respectively. If you are hearing *w*-like sounds in place of /r/, recall that use of this symbol indicates a phonemic substitution. The number of alternative transcriptions for the incorrect /r/ sounds brings to mind similar problems with vowel-diphthong sound modifications. These judgments are extremely demanding; specification of the central or back vowel that replaced /r/, /ɝ/, or /ɚ/ generally is not critical. The derhotacized symbols [r̮], [ɝ̮], or [ɚ̮] can be used to cover the variety of sounds that replace [r], [ɝ], or [ɚ] with only *partial r* coloring.

Clinical Phonetics Tape 3B
Glides and Liquids Module #4: Derhotacized /r/, /ɝ/, /ɚ/

TRANSCRIPTION SHEET

MODULE TIME	
TOTAL	5:57
ELAPSED	17:02–22:59

EXAMPLES			
NORMAL	[ri]	DERHOTACIZED	[r̮i]
	[ir]		[ir̮]

	STIMULUS WORD	INTENDED	PERCEIVED	ALTERNATIVES	COMMENTS
1	car	[r]	[ ]		
2	a zebra	[r]	[ ]		
3	/ɝ/	[ɝ]	[ ]		
4	they having a fire	[r]	[ ]		
5	/ɝ/	[ɝ]	[ ]		
6	chair	[r]	[ ]		
7	raining	[r]	[ ]		
8	/ɝ/	[ɝ]	[ ]		
9	car	[r]	[ ]		
10	finger	[ɚ]	[ ]		
11	garage	[r]	[ ]		
12	Is the cake ready	[r]	[ ]		
13	feather	[ɚ]	[ ]		
14	chair	[r]	[ ]		
15	big brother	[r], [ɚ]	[ ], [ ]		
16	/ɝ/	[ɝ]	[ ]		
17	orbit	[r]	[ ]		
18	sit right here	[r], [r]	[ ], [ ]		
19	read	[r]	[ ]		
20	He was running to school	[r]	[ ]		
21	scissors	[ɚ]	[ ]		
22	camper	[ɚ]	[ ]		
23	three, four, five	[r], [r]	[ ], [ ]		
24	cricket	[r]	[ ]		
25	brush	[r]	[ ]		
26	chair	[r]	[ ]		
27	sit right here	[r], [r]	[ ], [ ]		

Glides and Liquids Module #5: /r/ Quiz

The previous training module provided practice in transcribing derhotacized /r/ sounds. The following module provides practice in contrasting correct /r/, derhotacized /r/ [r̮], and w/r substitutions. Our suggestion for transcribing what appears to be w/r is consistent with all previous cautions about use of substitutions—be sure you really hear [w] (Chaney, 1988). Derhotacized /r/ [r̮] is much more prevalent than w/r in school-aged children and adults, while w/r is heard in very young children. This /r/ quiz provides an excellent opportunity to practice an important discrimination, one that clinicians often report difficulty in making in the course of their work with school-aged children with /r/ problems.

PROCEED TO: Clinical Phonetics Tape 3B: Glides and Liquids Module #5: /r/ Quiz

MODULE TIME	
TOTAL	4:35
ELAPSED	22:59–27:34

Clinical Phonetics Tape 3B Glides and Liquids Module #5: /r/ Quiz

TRANSCRIPTION KEY

	STIMULUS WORD	INTENDED	CONSENSUS	ALTERNATIVES	COMMENTS
1	smooth rock	[r]	[w]		
2	read	[r]	[w]	[r̮]	
3	rain	[r]	[r]		Noisy onset
4	carrots	[r]	[w]		
5	sit on the bridge	[r]	[w]		Did he say *sit?*
6	he can't run very good	[r], [r]	[r̮], [r]		
7	barn	[r]	[ɑ ɔ]	[b ɑ o n], [b a͡ʊː n]	
8	ring	[r]	[r̮]		Close to [w]
9	He was running to school	[r]	[r̮]		Close to [w]
10	color the map red	[ɚ], [r]	[ɚ̮], [r̮]		
11	crackers	[r], [ɚ]	[w], [ʊ]	[ə], [ɔ]	
12	rabbit	[r]	[r]		
13	Christmas tree	[r], [r]	[w], [r̮]		
14	parking	[r]	[r]		
15	Did the bell ring	[r]	[w]		
16	broom	[r]	[r̮]		Almost [w]
17	ice water	[ɚ]	[ɚ̮]	[ʊ], [o]	
18	He can ride a bike	[r]	[r̮]		
19	fireman	[r]	[ʊ]	[f ɑ͡ɪ əʷ m æ n]	
20	doorway	[r]	[r]		
21	zipper	[ɚ]	[ɚ]		

Notes: Notice some clear examples of correct /r/ and /ɚ/ and some clear examples of w/r. What falls in between these two either has *some r* coloring (derhotacized) or is transcribed as a pure vowel—usually /ə/, /ʊ/, or /ɔ/.

MODULE TIME	
TOTAL	4:35
ELAPSED	22:59–27:34

Clinical Phonetics Tape 3B Glides and Liquids Module #5: /r/ Quiz

TRANSCRIPTION SHEET

	STIMULUS WORD	INTENDED	PERCEIVED	ALTERNATIVES	COMMENTS
1	smooth rock	[r]	[ ]		
2	read	[r]	[ ]		
3	rain	[r]	[ ]		
4	carrots	[r]	[ ]		
5	sit on the bridge	[r]	[ ]		
6	he can't run very good	[r], [r]	[ ], [ ]		
7	barn	[r]	[ ]		
8	ring	[r]	[ ]		
9	He was running to school	[r]	[ ]		
10	color the map red	[ɚ], [r]	[ ], [ ]		
11	crackers	[r], [ɚ]	[ ], [ ]		
12	rabbit	[r]	[ ]		
13	Christmas tree	[r], [r]	[ ], [ ]		
14	parking	[r]	[ ]		
15	Did the bell ring	[r]	[ ]		
16	broom	[r]	[ ]		
17	ice water	[ɚ]	[ ]		
18	He can ride a bike	[r]	[ ]		
19	fireman	[r]	[ ]		
20	doorway	[r]	[ ]		
21	zipper	[ɚ]	[ ]		

Glides and Liquids Module #6: Velarized /r/

Velarized /r/ [r̰] is an infrequent error in children. In one study of fifty children with /r/ errors, we found only one child with velarized /r/ (Shriberg, 1975). We include brief training on this error type.

A velarized /r/ [r̰] is essentially the same sound as a velarized /l/ [l̰]. Both are made by a gliding movement of the back of the tongue; they both are substitutes for liquids; hence, velarized /l/ and velarized /r/ sound essentially the same. Follow the same procedure to make a velarized /r/ [r̰] that was suggested for making a velarized /l/ [l̰]. Put the back of your tongue up toward /g/ or /k/ but do not allow the tongue to actually touch the velum. Now, with a gliding movement of the back of the tongue, say the words *red, run, room*. In practicing [r̰], you may notice that you are saying a fricative-like sound or even a stoplike sound. Neither of these is what you are aiming at. Rather, it should be a gliding movement away from the soft palate. The sound should be "dark"—as though it is coming from the very back of the oral cavity.

PROCEED TO: Clinical Phonetics Tape 4A: Glides and Liquids Module #6: Velarized /r/

MODULE TIME	
TOTAL	3:03
ELAPSED	00:00–03:03

Clinical Phonetics Tape 4A
Glides and Liquids Module #6: Velarized /r/

TRANSCRIPTION KEY

	STIMULUS WORD	INTENDED	CONSENSUS	ALTERNATIVES	COMMENTS
1	chair	[r]	[r]		
2	a zebra	[r]	[r̰]		Sounds almost like a stop, i.e., [z i b g ɑ]
3	play with Brett	[r]	[r̰]		
4	rain	[r]	[r̰]		Less far back than No. 2 and No. 3
5	brush	[r]	[r̰]		
6	garage	[r]	[r̰]		Slight
7	it's raining	[r]	[r]		
8	at a fire	[r]	[ʋ]		[fɑ͡ɪʋ]
9	brush	[r]	[r̰]		
10	parking	[r]	[r]		
11	garage	[r]	[r̰]		
12	chair	[r]	[ʌ]	[tʃe͡ɪɔ]	
13	running	[r]	[r̰]		
14	zebra	[r]	[r]		

Notes: Can you make velarized /r/ sounds easily and rapidly? Item 9 is a good model. Recall that velarized /r/ is made and sounds exactly like velarized /l/. For example, say velarized liquids in the word pairs *light* [l̰ ɑ͡ɪ t] and *right* [r̰ ɑ͡ɪ t]; *lead* [l̰ ɛ d] and *red* [r̰ ɛ d]; *load* [l̰ o͡ʊ d] and *road* [r̰ o͡ʊ d].

MODULE TIME	
TOTAL	3:03
ELAPSED	00:00–03:03

Clinical Phonetics Tape 4A
Glides and Liquids Module #6:
Velarized /r/

TRANSCRIPTION SHEET

	STIMULUS WORD	INTENDED	PERCEIVED	ALTERNATIVES	COMMENTS
1	chair	[r]	[ ]		
2	a zebra	[r]	[ ]		
3	play with Brett	[r]	[ ]		
4	rain	[r]	[ ]		
5	brush	[r]	[ ]		
6	garage	[r]	[ ]		
7	it's raining	[r]	[ ]		
8	at a fire	[r]	[ ]		
9	brush	[r]	[ ]		
10	parking	[r]	[ ]		
11	garage	[r]	[ ]		
12	chair	[r]	[ ]		
13	running	[r]	[ ]		
14	zebra	[r]	[ ]		

Glides and Liquids Module #7: Summary Quiz

It's that time again. . . . The following 25-item module should afford a good opportunity to test your clinical transcription skill on glides and liquids. In keeping with their clinical prevalence, /l/ and /r/ errors will receive the most emphasis. *¡Buena suerte!*

PROCEED TO: Clinical Phonetics Tape 4A: Glides and Liquids Module #7: Summary Quiz

MODULE TIME	
TOTAL	4:56
ELAPSED	03:03–07:59

Clinical Phonetics Tape 4A
Glides and Liquids Module #7:
Summary Quiz

TRANSCRIPTION KEY

	STIMULUS WORD	INTENDED	CONSENSUS	ALTERNATIVES	COMMENTS
1	play	[l]	[l̰]		
2	New York	[j], [r]	[j], [ɔᵊ]		
3	train	[r]	[w]		[tᵊwe͡ɪn]
4	brush	[r]	[l]		[bᵊlʌs]
5	balloons	[l]	[l]		
6	police car siren	[l], [r], [r]	[w], [Ø], [w]		[pᵊiˢkɑːsɑ͡ɪwən]
7	girl	[ɝ], [l]	[w], [ʊ]	[u]	[gʌwʊ]
8	ladder	[l], [ɚ]	[m], [ɝ]		Stress change [mædɝ]
9	carrot	[r]	[l]		?
10	chair	[r]	[r]		Noisy
11	apple	[l]	[ɝ]		[æpʰɝ]
12	yellow	[j], [l]	[j], [d]		[jɛdə̫] or [jɛdɔ]
13	sit right here	[r], [r]	[r̮], [r̮]		Second /r/ only slightly derhotacized
14	fireman	[r]	[r]		
15	yellow	[j], [l]	[ᵏj], [ð̌]		[ᵏjɛð̌oᵛ]
16	tail	[l]	[o]		[te͡ɪo]
17	measuring cup	[ɚ]	[ɚ]		
18	nail	[l]	[ːᵊ]	[ne͡ɪᵛ]	
19	broom	[r]	[Ø]		[bum]
20	feather	[ɚ]	[əᵓ]	[fɛð̌ɔː], [fɛð̌oᵊ]	
21	rain	[r]	[ᵊw]	[ᵛw]	
22	the drum	[r]	[r̰]		[dᵊr̰ʌm]
23	carrots	[r]	[w]		
24	a feather	[ɚ]	[ʊ]	[ɚ̮]	
25	finger	[ɚ]	[ɚ]		

MODULE TIME	
TOTAL	4:56
ELAPSED	03:03–07:59

Clinical Phonetics Tape 4A
Glides and Liquids Module #7:
Summary Quiz

TRANSCRIPTION SHEET

	STIMULUS WORD	INTENDED	PERCEIVED	ALTERNATIVES	COMMENTS
1	play	[l]	[ ]		
2	New York	[j], [r]	[ ], [ ]		
3	train	[r]	[ ]		
4	brush	[r]	[ ]		
5	balloons	[l]	[ ]		
6	police car siren	[l], [r], [r]	[ ], [ ], [ ]		
7	girl	[ɝ], [l]	[ ], [ ]		
8	ladder	[l], [ɚ]	[ ], [ ]		
9	carrot	[r]	[ ]		
10	chair	[r]	[ ]		
11	apple	[l]	[ ]		
12	yellow	[j], [l]	[ ], [ ]		
13	sit right here	[r], [r]	[ ], [ ]		
14	fireman	[r]	[ ]		
15	yellow	[j], [l]	[ ], [ ]		
16	tail	[l]	[ ]		
17	measuring cup	[ɚ]	[ ]		
18	nail	[l]	[ ]		
19	broom	[r]	[ ]		
20	feather	[ɚ]	[ ]		
21	rain	[r]	[ ]		
22	the drum	[r]	[ ]		
23	carrots	[r]	[ ]		
24	a feather	[ɚ]	[ ]		
25	finger	[ɚ]	[ ]		

PART E: TRANSCRIPTION OF NASAL SOUND CHANGES

BACKGROUND INFORMATION

Description and Distribution of Nasals

The three nasals, /m/, /n/, and /ŋ/, are among the easiest sounds to make. The lips [m], tongue apex or tip [n], and back of tongue [ŋ] only need to close off the oral cavity; the velum remains open. Notice also that it does not matter how tightly the lips are pressed for an acceptable /m/ or exactly where the tip of the tongue is for an acceptable /n/.

Appendix B contains a summary of the distributional and frequency of occurrence characteristics of /m/, /n/, and /ŋ/. /n/ is among the most frequent of the English consonants, with only /t/ occurring more frequently in some studies. /m/ and /n/ also occur frequently in clusters, particularly in word-final position. Only /ŋ/ is restricted in its position of occurrence—it cannot be used to begin a word.

TRAINING MODULES

Nasals are generally acquired early by normal-speaking children. Nasal errors and the problems associated with their transcription only occur, therefore, in very young, rather than older, children. And unless one considers n/ŋ in word-final position to be an error (which we generally do not when it occurs in an unstressed syllable), nasal errors are actually seen very seldom. The few errors that do occur may be divided into: (1) deletions and (2) an assortment of variations that we will present subsequently in the form of a summary quiz.

Nasals Module #1: Nasal Deletions

The most difficult problem you are likely to experience in transcribing /m/, /n/, and /ŋ/ is deciding whether or not a nasal was deleted. Consider a word such as *can.* The assimilative nasality that is normal on the preceding vowel [kæ̃n] may be sufficient to create the impression of the final /n/ without the final /n/ actually being articulated ([kæ̃]). Even in clusters, as in *bent,* assimilative vowel nasalization can suffice for a perception of /n/ ([bɛ̃]). Particularly in the speech of very young children, it can be difficult to decide whether /n/ and, to a lesser degree, /m/ and /ŋ/ were actually produced or whether we are responding only to assimilative nasality on the preceding vowel. In the training module that follows, keep in mind that you are lacking the visual information that will make this task somewhat easier in the live situation.

PROCEED TO: Clinical Phonetics Tape 4A: Nasals Module #1: Nasal Deletions

MODULE TIME	
TOTAL	03:09
ELAPSED	07:59–11:08

Clinical Phonetics Tape 4A
Nasals Module #1:
Nasal Deletions

TRANSCRIPTION KEY

	STIMULUS WORD	INTENDED	CONSENSUS	ALTERNATIVES	COMMENTS
1	ju<u>m</u>pi<u>ng</u>	[m], [ŋ]	[m], [ŋ]		
2	o<u>n</u>io<u>n</u>	[n], [n]	[Ø], [n]		[e͡ɪ jən]
3	s<u>m</u>ooth	[m]	[m]		
4	vale<u>n</u>ti<u>n</u>e	[n], [n]	[Ø], [n]	[ʔ]	
5	spoo<u>n</u>	[n]	[n]		
6	pla<u>n</u>ti<u>ng</u>	[n], [ŋ]	[Ø], [ŋ]		[plæ̃ː tɪŋ]
7	Joa<u>nn</u>e	[n]	[Ø]		[ʤ o͡ʊ æ̃ ᵊ]
8	ha<u>mm</u>er	[m]	[m]		Noisy
9	ca<u>n</u>	[n]	[ᵊ]		[k æ ː ᵊ]
10	gu<u>n</u>	[n]	[n]		
11	la<u>m</u>p	[m]	[m]	[Ø]	Reduced, i.e., [l æ̝̃ m pʰ]
12	thu<u>m</u>b	[m]	[m]		
13	parki<u>ng</u>	[ŋ]	[ŋ]		
14	ca<u>n</u>	[n]	[n]		
15	fire hydra<u>n</u>t	[n]	[Ø]		

MODULE TIME	
TOTAL	03:09
ELAPSED	07:59–11:08

Clinical Phonetics Tape 4A
Nasals Module #1:
Nasal Deletions

TRANSCRIPTION SHEET

	STIMULUS WORD	INTENDED	PERCEIVED	ALTERNATIVES	COMMENTS
1	jumping	[m], [ŋ]	[ ], [ ]		
2	onion	[n], [n]	[ ], [ ]		
3	smooth	[m]	[ ]		
4	valentine	[n], [n]	[ ], [ ]		
5	spoon	[n]	[ ]		
6	planting	[n], [ŋ]	[ ], [ ]		
7	Joanne	[n]	[ ]		
8	hammer	[m]	[ ]		
9	can	[n]	[ ]		
10	gun	[n]	[ ]		
11	lamp	[m]	[ ]		
12	thumb	[m]	[ ]		
13	parking	[ŋ]	[ ]		
14	can	[n]	[ ]		
15	fire hydrant	[n]	[ ]		

Nasals Module #2: Summary Quiz

This summary quiz contains a collection of errors on nasals taken from our clinical tape collection. These sound changes can be categorized into three types.

Denasalized. Denasalization occurs when a nasal is articulated as the homorganic stop, that is, [b/m], [d/n], and [g/ŋ]. Children with a common cold, sinusitus (inflammation of a sinus), a deviated septum, enlarged adenoids, or other nasal obstructions may consistently denasalize nasal consonants. The result may be perceived either as a complete substitution by the voiced homorganic stop (*Pam* [pæ͋b]) or as a nasal followed by an intrusive homorganic voiced stop (*Pam* [pæ͋ m^{b}]).

Devoiced Nasals. When children delete /s/ in an initial /sn/ or /sm/ cluster, the nasals may sound devoiced. For example, *Snoopy* [n̥͋upɪ], *smoke* [m̥͋oʊk]. Here we have used the nasal emission diacritic [͋] as well as the devoicing symbol [̥]; children often mark the missing fricative /s/ by voiceless emission of the nasal. Nasal emission also occurs frequently in the speech of children with repaired cleft palates.

Nasal Substitutions. Substitution of one nasal for another is generally restricted to certain lexical items (*balentime* for *valentine*). Less frequently, nasal confusions may be a consistent pattern in the child's phonological system. In the latter case, substitutions are almost invariably [m/n] or [n/m]. In word-final position, /ŋ/ may appear to be replaced by /n/(n/ŋ); but, more likely, the /ŋ/ was said as a syllabic, such as *walking* [wɔkŋ̍]. As noted before, these latter differences generally are not of clinical significance.

PROCEED TO: Clinical Phonetics Tape 4A: Nasals Module #2: Summary Quiz

MODULE TIME	
TOTAL	3:54
ELAPSED	11:08–15:02

Clinical Phonetics Tape 4A
Nasals Module #2:
Summary Quiz

TRANSCRIPTION KEY

	STIMULUS WORD	INTENDED	CONSENSUS	ALTERNATIVES	COMMENTS
1	angels	[n]	[n]		
2	jumping	[m], [ŋ]	[m], [ŋ]		
3	knife	[n]	[ᵈn]		[d n a͡ɪ͊ ə f]
4	a thumb	[m]	[m]		
5	window	[n]	[n]		
6	comb	[m]	[m͊]		[k o͡ʊ͊ m͊]
7	some	[m]	[m͊͡bᵊ]	[m͊ bᵊ]	[s ʌ m͊ bᵊ ʔ]
8	spoon	[n]	[n]	[n ᵗ]	
9	elephant	[n]	[n]	[n͊]	
10	gun	[n]	[n͊]		[g ʌ͊ n͊]
11	some	[m]	[m]	[mː]	
12	smoke	[m]	[m̥]		
13	snake	[n]	[n]		
14	hammer	[m]	[n]		
15	jumping	[m], [ŋ]	[m], [n]		
16	monkey	[m], [ŋ]	[m], [ŋ]		
17	nail	[n]	[m]		[m e͡ɪ͊ o]
18	snowman	[n], [m], [n]	[n], [m], [n]		Extra first syllable [s ɪ mᵊ n oᵊ m æ˕ n]
19	knife	[n]	[n]		
20	comb	[m]	[n͊]	[n]	

Note: Notice the variety of denasalization errors, including what sounds like an *epenthetic* (added) *stop,* such as No. 3 and No. 7.

MODULE TIME	
TOTAL	3:54
ELAPSED	11:08–15:02

Clinical Phonetics Tape 4A
Nasals Module #2:
Summary Quiz

TRANSCRIPTION SHEET

	STIMULUS WORD	INTENDED	PERCEIVED	ALTERNATIVES	COMMENTS
1	angels	[n]	[ ]		
2	jumping	[m], [ŋ]	[ ], [ ]		
3	knife	[n]	[ ]		
4	a thumb	[m]	[ ]		
5	window	[n]	[ ]		
6	comb	[m]	[ ]		
7	some	[m]	[ ]		
8	spoon	[n]	[ ]		
9	elephant	[n]	[ ]		
10	gun	[n]	[ ]		
11	some	[m]	[ ]		
12	smoke	[m]	[ ]		
13	snake	[n]	[ ]		
14	hammer	[m]	[ ]		
15	jumping	[m], [ŋ]	[ ], [ ]		
16	monkey	[m], [ŋ]	[ ], [ ]		
17	nail	[n]	[ ]		
18	snowman	[n], [m], [n]	[ ], [ ], [ ]		
19	knife	[n]	[ ]		
20	comb	[m]	[ ]		

GRAND QUIZ

You knew this was coming! This final module of Chapter 8 gives you a chance to transcribe 45 words completely. You will hear many "old friends" . . . sound changes of every type practiced in the preceding 34 training modules. Take time with each word. You may want to reread the discussion beginning on page 152 for suggestions on whole word transcription strategies. *Alles Gute!*

PROCEED TO: Clinical Phonetics Tape 4A: Grand Quiz

MODULE TIME	
TOTAL	8:36
ELAPSED	15:02–23:38

Clinical Phonetics Tape 4A
Grand Quiz

TRANSCRIPTION KEY

	STIMULUS WORD	CONSENSUS		STIMULUS WORD	CONSENSUS
1	a seal	[ə θ i l]	24	party	[pʰ ɑ r tʰ i̞]
2	scissors	[s ɪ z ɚ z̥]	25	feather	[f ɛ̠ ð ʊ]
3	shoe	[s u]	26	bus	[b ʌ s̪]
4	hammer	[h æ̝̃ m ᵇ ɚ]	27	a zebra	[ə z i b w ə]
5	lamp	[l ɑ̃ p]	28	yellow	[j ɛ̞ l o]
6	valentine	[v ɛ̞ w ə n t a͡ɪ m]	29	arrow	[æ̝ r o͡ʊ]
7	watch	[w ɔ t͡s̡] (palatal /s/)	30	crayons	[k r e͡ɪ ɑ̠̃ n t s̪]
8	soap	[s̪̯ o͡ʊ p]	31	roller skates	[r̮ o͡ʊ l ɚ̮ s k e͡ɪ t s̺]
9	bicycle	[b ã͡ɪ s ɪ̃ k ʊ̃]	32	wagon	(child was a young Republican) [ə r e͡ɪ g ə n]
10	chicken	[s̪ ɪ k ɪ n]	33	bathe	[b e͡ɪ̤ v̥]
11	pencils	[p ɛ̃ n s̪ o̠ z̪̊]	34	fall	[f ɔ l̰]
12	garage	[g w ɑ ᵊ d͡ʒ̊]	35	fish	[t͡ʃ ɪ f]
13	banana	[p⁼ ɪ k æ̝̃ n ɑ̃]	36	whistle	[b r ɪ ʔ ɪ]
14	spoon	[s p ũː n]	37	splash	[s̪ p l æ s̪]
15	dog	[d̪ ɔː g̊]	38	shoe	[tʰ u]
16	skates	[k⁼ e͡ɪ t s]	39	egg	[e͡ɪ g̊]
17	that apple	[d æ ɾ æ p o]	40	measure	[m æ ʔ ɪ]
18	zebra	[z̥ i b r ʌ]	41	blocks	[b w ɑ t s̺]
19	cat	[kʰ e ᵆ t]	42	string	[s̪ t r ɪ ŋ k]
20	teeth	[tʰ i f]	43	follow	[f ɑ l̰ o͡ʊ]
21	ladder	[w æ d̯ ɚ] (or flap [ɾ])	44	camper	[k æ̃ m p ʊ]
22	pipe	[p a͡ɪ ˃ p]	45	water	[w ɔ d ɚ̮]
23	doorway	[d ɔ w e͡ɪ]			

Note: You can calculate your agreement in many ways: Whole word agreement, agreement for all vowels, agreement for all consonants, agreement for all fricatives, and so forth.

MODULE TIME	
TOTAL	8:36
ELAPSED	15:02–23:38

Clinical Phonetics Tape 4A
Grand Quiz

TRANSCRIPTION SHEET

	STIMULUS WORD	PERCEIVED		STIMULUS WORD	PERCEIVED
1	a seal	[ ]	24	party	[ ]
2	scissors	[ ]	25	feather	[ ]
3	shoe	[ ]	26	bus	[ ]
4	hammer	[ ]	27	a zebra	[ ]
5	lamp	[ ]	28	yellow	[ ]
6	valentine	[ ]	29	arrow	[ ]
7	watch	[ ]	30	crayons	[ ]
8	soap	[ ]	31	roller skates	[ ]
9	bicycle	[ ]	32	wagon	[ ]
10	chicken	[ ]	33	bathe	[ ]
11	pencils	[ ]	34	fall	[ ]
12	garage	[ ]	35	fish	[ ]
13	banana	[ ]	36	whistle	[ ]
14	spoon	[ ]	37	splash	[ ]
15	dog	[ ]	38	shoe	[ ]
16	skates	[ ]	39	egg	[ ]
17	that apple	[ ]	40	measure	[ ]
18	zebra	[ ]	41	blocks	[ ]
19	cat	[ ]	42	string	[ ]
20	teeth	[ ]	43	follow	[ ]
21	ladder	[ ]	44	camper	[ ]
22	pipe	[ ]	45	water	[ ]
23	doorway	[ ]			

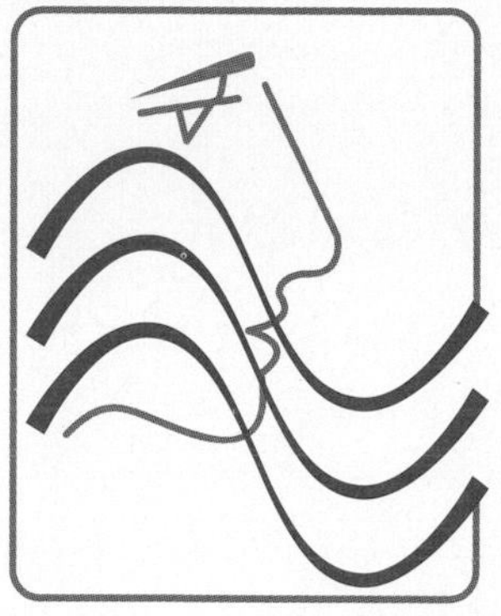

Transcription and Scoring Practice

9

To this point in the training series, you have learned:

1. How the sounds of English are made and how they are distributed in the language.
2. The most frequently occurring sound changes made by children with delayed speech and how to discriminate among them.
3. A set of symbols to represent both the normal sounds and a variety of sound changes.

This chapter will build upon these skills. The goal is to provide you with transcription practice on a variety of clinical tasks. Materials are presented that provide:

- Practice using two-way scoring, five-way scoring, and phonetic transcription.
- Practice in building transcription speed. Materials reflect the pace of transcription that occurs in the clinic (repetitions of items are *not* provided in these transcription modules).
- Exposure to some of the primary sampling procedures clinicians use to assess a child's speech, including several articulation tests and free speech samples.
- Further exposure to the variety of errors seen clinically.

This chapter, like the previous one, provides blank forms on the right-hand page and a completed key on the left-hand page. To allow for training in all three systems used by clinicians—two-way scoring, five-way scoring, and phonetic transcription—additional blank forms and keys are provided for certain modules. Feedback comments follow some of the modules.

PRACTICE MODULES

PRACTICE MODULE #1: SINGLE-SOUND ARTICULATION TEST

Speech-language clinicians commonly use forms of speech sampling that, for convenience, are termed **single-sound** articulation tests. These tests assess a target sound in three positions within a word—initial, medial, and final. As described in Chapter 7 (see also Figure 1-1), the **response complexity** for the clinician involves only one target sound per word. The clinician may ask a child to name a picture (elicitation) or to say a word after him or her (imitation). References and comparative discussion of some of the more widely used measures may be found in several textbooks on developmental phonological disorders, including Bernthal and Bankson (1993).

The single-sound articulation test used in this module is the Developmental Articulation Test (Hejna, 1955), administered by imitation to a seven-year-old girl with moderately to severely delayed speech. In this test, the girl attempts 17 of the consonant sounds as they occur in word-initial, word-medial, and word-final position (except /ŋ/, /w/, and /j/, which are tested only in the two positions in which they occur). For each word spoken by the child, score/transcribe *only* the target sound. Three blank test forms are presented, one each for two-way scoring, five-way scoring, and phonetic transcription, respectively. You may wish to gain practice using any or all of the three systems. For two-way scoring, use "plus" (+) and "zero" (0). For five-way scoring, use "plus" (+) for correct, "minus" (–) for deletion, "D" for distortion, and write in the symbol perceived for an addition and for a substitution; for example, [w] (for [w/r]), [t] (for [t/k]), and so forth. For phonetic transcription, use the symbols and diacritics that you have learned in previous chapters. Score or transcribe only the target sound in the space under each column. The first three columns for /m/ are completed to illustrate the procedure. Only the first 17 items have been dubbed for training.

PROCEED TO: Clinical Phonetics Tape 4A: Practice Module #1: Single-Sound Articulation Test

MODULE TIME	
TOTAL	4:42
ELAPSED	23:38–28:20

Clinical Phonetics Tape 4A
Practice Module #1:
Single-Sound Articulation Test

DEVELOPMENTAL ARTICULATION TEST—KEY

Name ____________________ Age____ Grade____ School___________ Date________

(Score as per the following examples. Substitution: b/p; Omission: -/p; Distortion: Dist/p.
***Note: Except where otherwise noted, Developmental Age Level signifies the chronological age by which approximately 90% or more children are using the sound correctly.**

Card	Dev. Age Level	Sound Tested	Check Words	1	2	3	Iso.	Comments
1	3	m	monkey, hammer, broom	+	+	O		
2	3	n	nails, penny, lion	+	+	+		
3	3	p	pig, puppy, cup	O	+	+		
4	3	h	house, dog-house, ----	+	+			
5	3	w	window, spider-web, ----	+	+			
6	4	b	boat, baby, (bib: 75%)	+	+	+		
7	4	k	cat, chicken, book	O	+	*O		*Indeterminant
8	4	g	girl, wagon, (pig: 75%)	+	O	O		
9	4	f	fork, telephone, knife	O	O	O		
10	5	y	yellow, onion, (thank-you; Alt.), --	O	O			
11	5	ng	----, fingers, ring		+	O		
12	5	d	dog, ladder, bed	+	O	+		
13	6	l	lamp, balloon, ball	O	O	O		
14	6	r	rabbit, barn, car	O	+	+		
15	6	t	table, potatoes, coat	+	O	*O		*Indeterminant
16	6	sh	shoe, dishes, fish	O	O	O		
17	6	ch	chair, matches, watch	O	O	O		
18	6	Blends	drum, clock, blocks, glasses, crayons					
19	7	v	vacuum, television, stove					
20	7	th	thumb, toothbrush, teeth					
21	7	j	jump-rope, orange-juice, orange					
22	7	s	sun, pencil, bus					
23	7	z	zebra, scissors, (rubbers: 75%)					
24	7	Blends	train, star, slide, swing, spoon					
25	8	~~th~~	this or that, feathers, ----					
26	8	Blends	scooter, snowman, desk, nest					

Notes: A strict response definition is used for this key. For example, initial unaspirated stops are scored incorrect; by a more liberal response definition, they would be correct.

MODULE TIME	
TOTAL	4:42
ELAPSED	23:38–28:20

Clinical Phonetics Tape 4A Practice Module #1: Single-Sound Articulation Test

DEVELOPMENTAL ARTICULATION TEST—SCORING BLANK

Name ____________ Age____ Grade____ School____________ Date__________

(Score as per the following examples. Substitution: b/p; Omission: -/p; Distortion: Dist/p.
*Note: Except where otherwise noted, Developmental Age Level signifies the chronological age by which approximately 90% or more children are using the sound correctly.

Card	Dev. Age Level	Sound Tested	Check Words	1	2	3	Iso.	Comments
1	3	m	monkey, hammer, broom	+	+	0		
2	3	n	nails, penny, lion					
3	3	p	pig, puppy, cup					
4	3	h	house, dog-house, ----					
5	3	w	window, spider-web, ----					
6	4	b	boat, baby, (bib: 75%)					
7	4	k	cat, chicken, book					
8	4	g	girl, wagon, (pig: 75%)					
9	4	f	fork, telephone, knife					
10	5	y	yellow, onion, (thank-you; Alt.), --					
11	5	ng	----, fingers, ring					
12	5	d	dog, ladder, bed					
13	6	l	lamp, balloon, ball					
14	6	r	rabbit, barn, car					
15	6	t	table, potatoes, coat					
16	6	sh	shoe, dishes, fish					
17	6	ch	chair, matches, watch					
18	6	Blends	drum, clock, blocks, glasses, crayons					
19	7	v	vacuum, television, stove					
20	7	th	thumb, toothbrush, teeth					
21	7	j	jump-rope, orange-juice, orange					
22	7	s	sun, pencil, bus					
23	7	z	zebra, scissors, (rubbers: 75%)					
24	7	Blends	train, star, slide, swing, spoon					
25	8	~~th~~	this or that, feathers, ----					
26	8	Blends	scooter, snowman, desk, nest					

Notes: Clinical Phonetics Tape 4A: Practice Module #1 is based on the Hejna Developmental Articulation Test Form reproduced with permission of Robert F. Hejna.

MODULE TIME	
TOTAL	4:42
ELAPSED	23:38–28:20

Clinical Phonetics Tape 4A Practice Module #1: Single-Sound Articulation Test

DEVELOPMENTAL ARTICULATION TEST—KEY

Name ______________ Age____ Grade____ School__________ Date__________

(Score as per the following examples. Substitution: b/p; Omission: -/p; Distortion: Dist/p.
*Note: Except where otherwise noted, Developmental Age Level signifies the chronological age by which approximately 90% or more children are using the sound correctly.

Card	Dev. Age Level	Sound Tested	Check Words	1	2	3	Iso.	Comments
1	3	m	monkey, hammer, broom	+	+	–		
2	3	n	nails, penny, lion	+	+	+		
3	3	p	pig, puppy, cup	D	+	+		
4	3	h	house, dog-house, ----	+	+			
5	3	w	window, spider-web, ----	+	+			
6	4	b	boat, baby, (bib: 75%)	+	+	+		
7	4	k	cat, chicken, book	D	+	(t/k)*		*Indeterminant
8	4	g	girl, wagon, (pig: 75%)	+	D	d/g		
9	4	f	fork, telephone, knife	p/f	w/f	A		A = Addition
10	5	y	yellow, onion, (thank-you; Alt.), --	–	–			
11	5	ng	----, fingers, ring		+	D		
12	5	d	dog, ladder, bed	+	D	+		
13	6	l	lamp, balloon, ball	D	b/l	–		
14	6	r	rabbit, barn, car	w/r	+	+		
15	6	t	table, potatoes, coat	+	D	?/t		
16	6	sh	shoe, dishes, fish	h/ʃ	t/ʃ	D		
17	6	ch	chair, matches, watch	D	t/tʃ	D		
18	6	Blends	drum, clock, blocks, glasses, crayons					
19	7	v	vacuum, television, stove					
20	7	th	thumb, toothbrush, teeth					
21	7	j	jump-rope, orange-juice, orange					
22	7	s	sun, pencil, bus					
23	7	z	zebra, scissors, (rubbers: 75%)					
24	7	Blends	train, star, slide, swing, spoon					
25	8	~~th~~	this or that, feathers, ----					
26	8	Blends	scooter, snowman, desk, nest					

Notes: A strict response definition is used for this key. For example, initial unaspirated stops are scored incorrect; by a more liberal response definition, they would be correct.

MODULE TIME	
TOTAL	4:42
ELAPSED	23:38–28:20

Clinical Phonetics Tape 4A
Practice Module #1:
Single-Sound Articulation Test

DEVELOPMENTAL ARTICULATION TEST—SCORING BLANK

Name __________ Age____ Grade____ School__________ Date________

(Score as per the following examples. Substitution: b/p; Omission: -/p; Distortion: Dist/p.
*Note: Except where otherwise noted, Developmental Age Level signifies the chronological age by which approximately 90% or more children are using the sound correctly.

Card	Dev. Age Level	Sound Tested	Check Words	1	2	3	Iso.	Comments
1	3	m	monkey, hammer, broom	+	+	−		
2	3	n	nails, penny, lion					
3	3	p	pig, puppy, cup					
4	3	h	house, dog-house, ----					
5	3	w	window, spider-web, ----					
6	4	b	boat, baby, (bib: 75%)					
7	4	k	cat, chicken, book					
8	4	g	girl, wagon, (pig: 75%)					
9	4	f	fork, telephone, knife					
10	5	y	yellow, onion, (thank-you; Alt.), --					
11	5	ng	----, fingers, ring					
12	5	d	dog, ladder, bed					
13	6	l	lamp, balloon, ball					
14	6	r	rabbit, barn, car					
15	6	t	table, potatoes, coat					
16	6	sh	shoe, dishes, fish					
17	6	ch	chair, matches, watch					
18	6	Blends	drum, clock, blocks, glasses, crayons					
19	7	v	vacuum, television, stove					
20	7	th	thumb, toothbrush, teeth					
21	7	j	jump-rope, orange-juice, orange					
22	7	s	sun, pencil, bus					
23	7	z	zebra, scissors, (rubbers: 75%)					
24	7	Blends	train, star, slide, swing, spoon					
25	8	~~th~~	this or that, feathers, ----					
26	8	Blends	scooter, snowman, desk, nest					

MODULE TIME	
TOTAL	4:42
ELAPSED	23:38–28:20

Clinical Phonetics Tape 4A
Practice Module #1:
Single-Sound Articulation Test

DEVELOPMENTAL ARTICULATION TEST—KEY

Name ______________________ **Age**____ **Grade**____ **School**____________ **Date**__________

(Score as per the following examples. Substitution: b/p; Omission: -/p; Distortion: Dist/p.
***Note: Except where otherwise noted, Developmental Age Level signifies the chronological age by which approximately 90% or more children are using the sound correctly.**

Card	Dev. Age Level	Sound Tested	Check Words	1	2	3	Iso.	Comments
1	3	m	monkey, hammer, broom	m	m	∅		
2	3	n	nails, penny, lion	n	n	n		
3	3	p	pig, puppy, cup	p=	p	p		
4	3	h	house, dog-house, ----	h	h			
5	3	w	window, spider-web, ----	w	ʸw			
6	4	b	boat, baby, (bib: 75%)	b	b	b		
7	4	k	cat, chicken, book	k=	k	(t̚)* (k̚)		*Indeterminant
8	4	g	girl, wagon, (pig: 75%)	g*	g̃ or ŋ	d		*Second time!!
9	4	f	fork, telephone, knife	p=	w̃	t͡f		
10	5	y	yellow, onion, (thank-you; Alt.), --	∅	(j̃ l)			*Indeterminant
11	5	ng	----, fingers, ring		ŋ	ŋᵏ		
12	5	d	dog, ladder, bed	d̥	d̽*	d		*Weak contact
13	6	l	lamp, balloon, ball	ɹ̡/*	b	∅		*Palatalized?
14	6	r	rabbit, barn, car	m̫	r	r		
15	6	t	table, potatoes, coat	t	t=	*ʔ		*Indeterminant: [ʔ] or [t̚] or [∅]
16	6	sh	shoe, dishes, fish	h	t̪	t͡s̡		
17	6	ch	chair, matches, watch	tθ̪	t̪	ts̪		
18	6	Blends	drum, clock, blocks, glasses, crayons					
19	7	v	vacuum, television, stove					
20	7	th	thumb, toothbrush, teeth					
21	7	j	jump-rope, orange-juice, orange					
22	7	s	sun, pencil, bus					
23	7	z	zebra, scissors, (rubbers: 75%)					
24	7	Blends	train, star, slide, swing, spoon					
25	8	~~th~~	this or that, feathers, ----					
26	8	Blends	scooter, snowman, desk, nest					

Notes: Note the problems this girl has in timing, particularly in velopharyngeal control.

MODULE TIME	
TOTAL	4:42
ELAPSED	23:38–28:20

Clinical Phonetics Tape 4A
Practice Module #1:
Single-Sound Articulation Test

DEVELOPMENTAL ARTICULATION TEST—SCORING BLANK

Name __________ Age____ Grade____ School__________ Date__________

(Score as per the following examples. Substitution: b/p; Omission: -/p; Distortion: Dist/p.
*Note: Except where otherwise noted, Developmental Age Level signifies the chronological age by which approximately 90% or more children are using the sound correctly.

Card	Dev. Age Level	Sound Tested	Check Words	1	2	3	Iso.	Comments
1	3	m	monkey, hammer, broom	m	m	ϕ		
2	3	n	nails, penny, lion					
3	3	p	pig, puppy, cup					
4	3	h	house, dog-house, ----					
5	3	w	window, spider-web, ----					
6	4	b	boat, baby, (bib: 75%)					
7	4	k	cat, chicken, book					
8	4	g	girl, wagon, (pig: 75%)					
9	4	f	fork, telephone, knife					
10	5	y	yellow, onion, (thank-you; Alt.), --					
11	5	ng	----, fingers, ring					
12	5	d	dog, ladder, bed					
13	6	l	lamp, balloon, ball					
14	6	r	rabbit, barn, car					
15	6	t	table, potatoes, coat					
16	6	sh	shoe, dishes, fish					
17	6	ch	chair, matches, watch					
18	6	Blends	drum, clock, blocks, glasses, crayons					
19	7	v	vacuum, television, stove					
20	7	th	thumb, toothbrush, teeth					
21	7	j	jump-rope, orange-juice, orange					
22	7	s	sun, pencil, bus					
23	7	z	zebra, scissors, (rubbers: 75%)					
24	7	Blends	train, star, slide, swing, spoon					
25	8	~~th~~	this or that, feathers, ----					
26	8	Blends	scooter, snowman, desk, nest					

Practice Module #2: Multiple-Sound Articulation Test

Multiple-sound articulation tests require the clinician to score or transcribe more than one target sound per item (see Figure 1-1). A wealth of technical issues has emerged from the comparison of the results of such tests to those obtained with single-sound measures. Such controversies are beyond the scope of this program, but discussions are available in many sources, including Bernthal and Bankson (1993) and Morrison and Shriberg (1992).

The multiple-sound articulation test selected for this module is the McDonald Screening Test, which follows from a view of speech production developed by McDonald (1964, 1968) that emphasizes the role of phonetic context on the articulation of target sounds. Because the McDonald Screening Test yields information on nine sounds, each tested ten times, it is a useful clinical measure; *however,* it is one of the more difficult tests to administer and to score or transcribe because clinicians must make decisions on as many as four sounds per word.

You will need to familiarize yourself with the format of the McDonald Screening Test before beginning practice (see page 271). Note that responses to each of the nine sounds are recorded in spaces within a column. Responses to the first item are completed to show how the test format is used. Only the first 21 items will be presented. Once again, your goal is to play each recorded stimulus only once. Try to minimize playbacks. Blanks are provided for two-way scoring, five-way scoring, and phonetic transcription. The child whose speech is being tested is five years old; his speech may be considered moderately delayed.

PROCEED TO: Clinical Phonetics Tape 4B: Practice Module #2: Multiple-Sound Articulation Test

MODULE TIME	
TOTAL	3:06
ELAPSED	00:00–03:06

Clinical Phonetics Tape 4B Practice Module #2: Multiple-Sound Articulation Test

INDIVIDUAL RECORD SHEET FOR A SCREENING DEEP TEST OF ARTICULATION

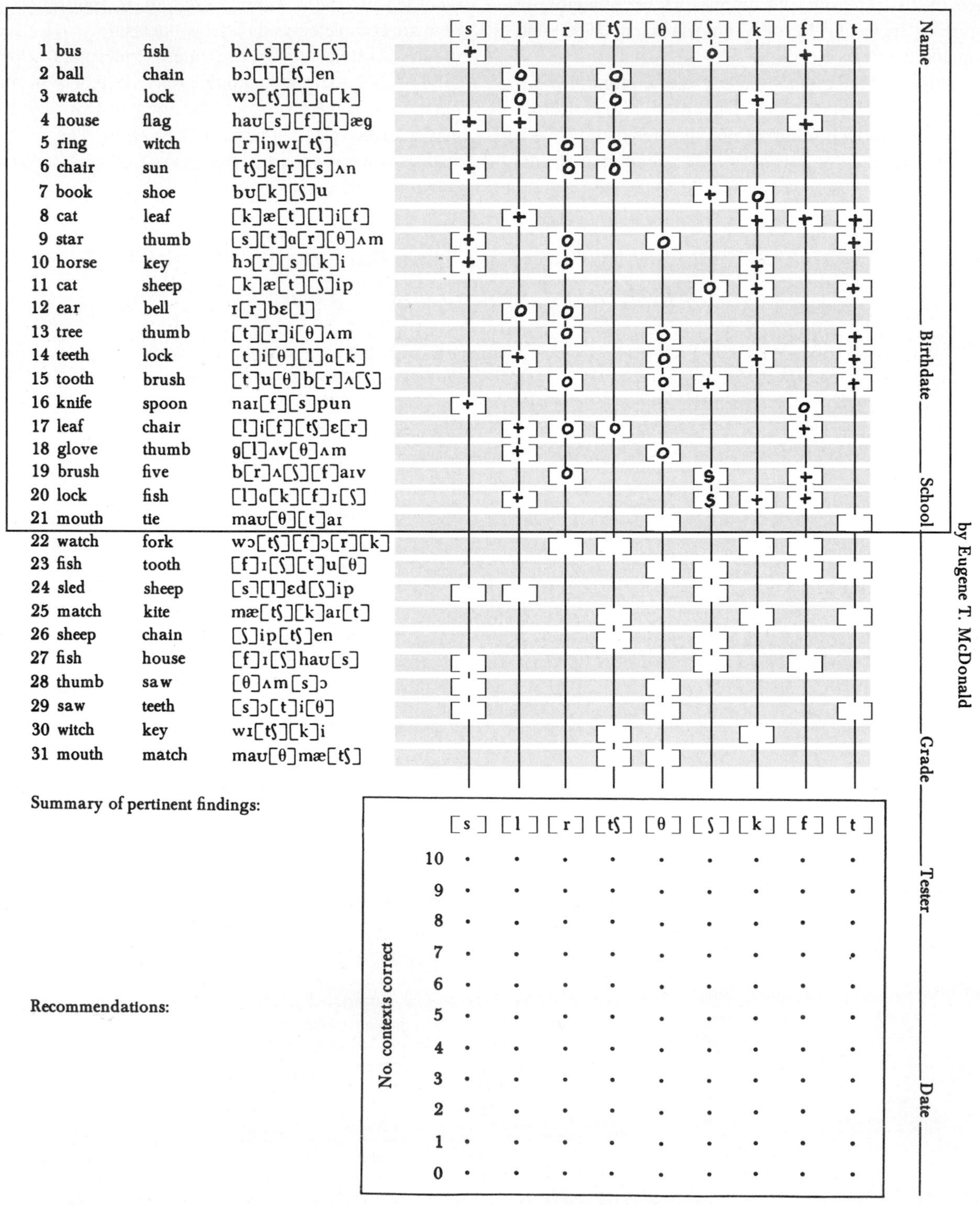

				[s]	[l]	[r]	[tʃ]	[θ]	[ʃ]	[k]	[f]	[t]
1	bus	fish	bʌ[s][f]ɪ[ʃ]	[+]					[o]		[+]	
2	ball	chain	bɔ[l][tʃ]en		[o]		[o]					
3	watch	lock	wɔ[tʃ][l]ɑ[k]		[o]		[o]			[+]		
4	house	flag	haʊ[s][f][l]æg	[+]	[+]						[+]	
5	ring	witch	[r]iŋwɪ[tʃ]			[o]	[o]					
6	chair	sun	[tʃ]ɛ[r][s]ʌn	[+]		[o]	[o]					
7	book	shoe	bʊ[k][ʃ]u						[+]	[o]		
8	cat	leaf	[k]æ[t][l]i[f]		[+]					[+]	[+]	[+]
9	star	thumb	[s][t]ɑ[r][θ]ʌm	[+]		[o]		[o]				[+]
10	horse	key	hɔ[r][s][k]i	[+]		[o]				[+]		
11	cat	sheep	[k]æ[t][ʃ]ip						[o]	[+]		[+]
12	ear	bell	ɪ[r]bɛ[l]		[o]	[o]						
13	tree	thumb	[t][r]i[θ]ʌm			[o]		[o]				[+]
14	teeth	lock	[t]i[θ][l]ɑ[k]		[+]			[o]		[+]		[+]
15	tooth	brush	[t]u[θ]b[r]ʌ[ʃ]			[o]		[o]	[+]			[+]
16	knife	spoon	naɪ[f][s]pun	[+]							[o]	
17	leaf	chair	[l]i[f][tʃ]ɛ[r]		[+]	[o]	[o]				[+]	
18	glove	thumb	g[l]ʌv[θ]ʌm		[+]			[o]				
19	brush	five	b[r]ʌ[ʃ][f]aɪv			[o]			[s]		[+]	
20	lock	fish	[l]ɑ[k][f]ɪ[ʃ]		[+]				[s]	[+]	[+]	
21	mouth	tie	maʊ[θ][t]aɪ					[ ]				[ ]
22	watch	fork	wɔ[tʃ][f]ɔ[r][k]			[ ]	[ ]			[ ]	[ ]	
23	fish	tooth	[f]ɪ[ʃ][t]u[θ]					[ ]	[ ]		[ ]	[ ]
24	sled	sheep	[s][l]ɛd[ʃ]ip	[ ]	[ ]				[ ]			
25	match	kite	mæ[tʃ][k]aɪ[t]				[ ]			[ ]		[ ]
26	sheep	chain	[ʃ]ip[tʃ]en				[ ]		[ ]			
27	fish	house	[f]ɪ[ʃ]haʊ[s]	[ ]					[ ]		[ ]	
28	thumb	saw	[θ]ʌm[s]ɔ	[ ]				[ ]				
29	saw	teeth	[s]ɔ[t]i[θ]	[ ]				[ ]				[ ]
30	witch	key	wɪ[tʃ][k]i				[ ]			[ ]		
31	mouth	match	maʊ[θ]mæ[tʃ]				[ ]	[ ]				

Name____ Birthdate____ School____ Grade____ Tester____ Date____

by Eugene T. McDonald

Summary of pertinent findings:

Recommendations:

No. contexts correct	[s]	[l]	[r]	[tʃ]	[θ]	[ʃ]	[k]	[f]	[t]
10	•	•	•	•	•	•	•	•	•
9	•	•	•	•	•	•	•	•	•
8	•	•	•	•	•	•	•	•	•
7	•	•	•	•	•	•	•	•	•
6	•	•	•	•	•	•	•	•	•
5	•	•	•	•	•	•	•	•	•
4	•	•	•	•	•	•	•	•	•
3	•	•	•	•	•	•	•	•	•
2	•	•	•	•	•	•	•	•	•
1	•	•	•	•	•	•	•	•	•
0	•	•	•	•	•	•	•	•	•

PHONETIC PROFILE

MODULE TIME	
TOTAL	3:06
ELAPSED	00:00–03:06

Clinical Phonetics Tape 4B
Practice Module #2:
Multiple-Sound Articulation Test

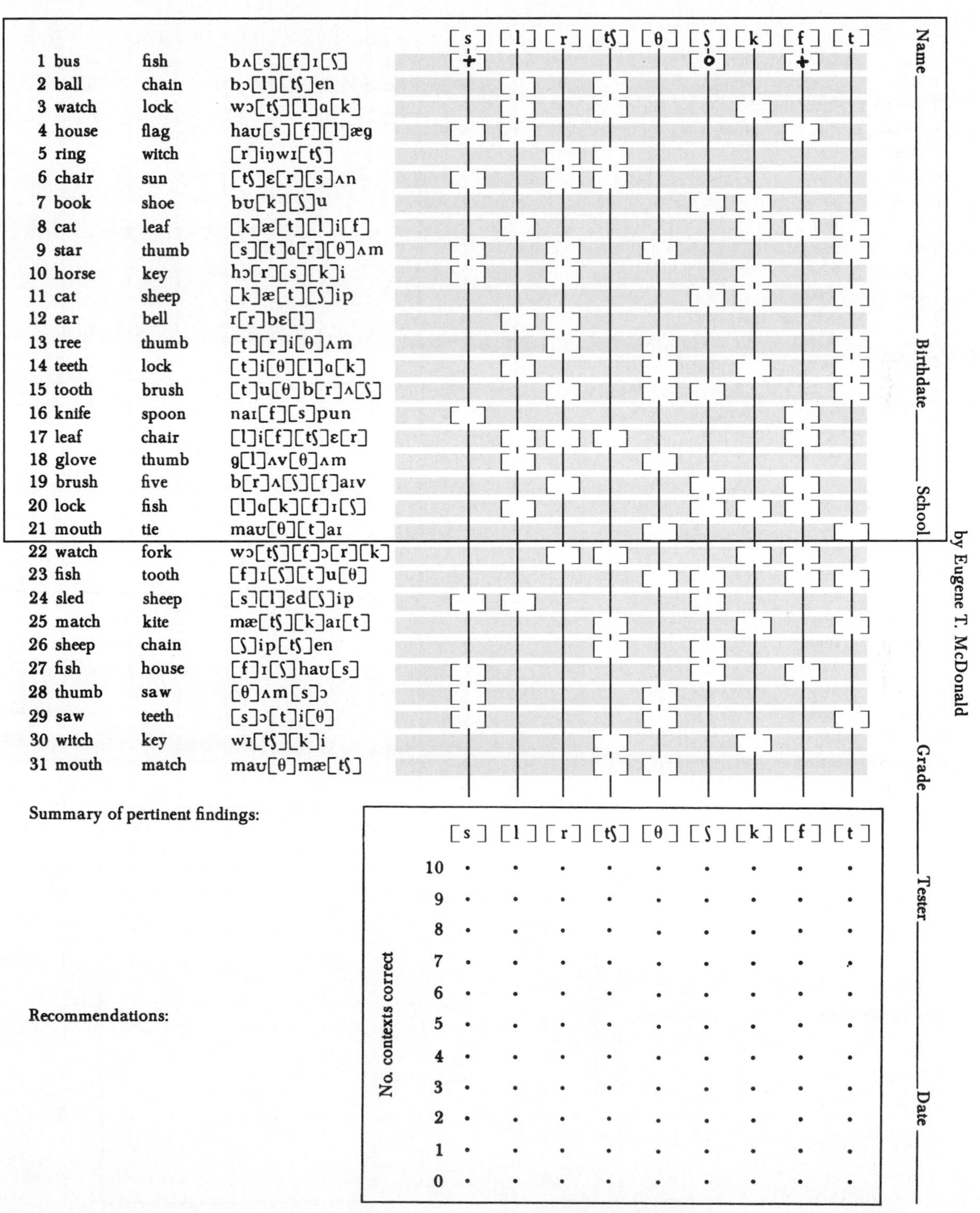

INDIVIDUAL RECORD SHEET FOR A SCREENING DEEP TEST OF ARTICULATION

				[s]	[l]	[r]	[tʃ]	[θ]	[ʃ]	[k]	[f]	[t]
1 bus	fish	bʌ[s][f]ɪ[ʃ]		+					o		+	
2 ball	chain	bɔ[l][tʃ]en										
3 watch	lock	wɔ[tʃ][l]ɑ[k]										
4 house	flag	haʊ[s][f][l]æg										
5 ring	witch	[r]iŋwɪ[tʃ]										
6 chair	sun	[tʃ]ɛ[r][s]ʌn										
7 book	shoe	bʊ[k][ʃ]u										
8 cat	leaf	[k]æ[t][l]i[f]										
9 star	thumb	[s][t]ɑ[r][θ]ʌm										
10 horse	key	hɔ[r][s][k]i										
11 cat	sheep	[k]æ[t][ʃ]ip										
12 ear	bell	ɪ[r]bɛ[l]										
13 tree	thumb	[t][r]i[θ]ʌm										
14 teeth	lock	[t]i[θ][l]ɑ[k]										
15 tooth	brush	[t]u[θ]b[r]ʌ[ʃ]										
16 knife	spoon	naɪ[f][s]pun										
17 leaf	chair	[l]i[f][tʃ]ɛ[r]										
18 glove	thumb	g[l]ʌv[θ]ʌm										
19 brush	five	b[r]ʌ[ʃ][f]aɪv										
20 lock	fish	[l]ɑ[k][f]ɪ[ʃ]										
21 mouth	tie	maʊ[θ][t]aɪ										
22 watch	fork	wɔ[tʃ][f]ɔ[r][k]										
23 fish	tooth	[f]ɪ[ʃ][t]u[θ]										
24 sled	sheep	[s][l]ɛd[ʃ]ip										
25 match	kite	mæ[tʃ][k]aɪ[t]										
26 sheep	chain	[ʃ]ip[tʃ]en										
27 fish	house	[f]ɪ[ʃ]haʊ[s]										
28 thumb	saw	[θ]ʌm[s]ɔ										
29 saw	teeth	[s]ɔ[t]i[θ]										
30 witch	key	wɪ[tʃ][k]i										
31 mouth	match	maʊ[θ]mæ[tʃ]										

Name______ Birthdate______ School______ Grade______ Tester______ Date______

by Eugene T. McDonald

Summary of pertinent findings:

Recommendations:

No. contexts correct	[s]	[l]	[r]	[tʃ]	[θ]	[ʃ]	[k]	[f]	[t]
10	•	•	•	•	•	•	•	•	•
9	•	•	•	•	•	•	•	•	•
8	•	•	•	•	•	•	•	•	•
7	•	•	•	•	•	•	•	•	•
6	•	•	•	•	•	•	•	•	•
5	•	•	•	•	•	•	•	•	•
4	•	•	•	•	•	•	•	•	•
3	•	•	•	•	•	•	•	•	•
2	•	•	•	•	•	•	•	•	•
1	•	•	•	•	•	•	•	•	•
0	•	•	•	•	•	•	•	•	•

PHONETIC PROFILE

MODULE TIME	
TOTAL	3:06
ELAPSED	00:00–03:06

Clinical Phonetics Tape 4B Practice Module #2: Multiple-Sound Articulation Test

INDIVIDUAL RECORD SHEET FOR A SCREENING DEEP TEST OF ARTICULATION

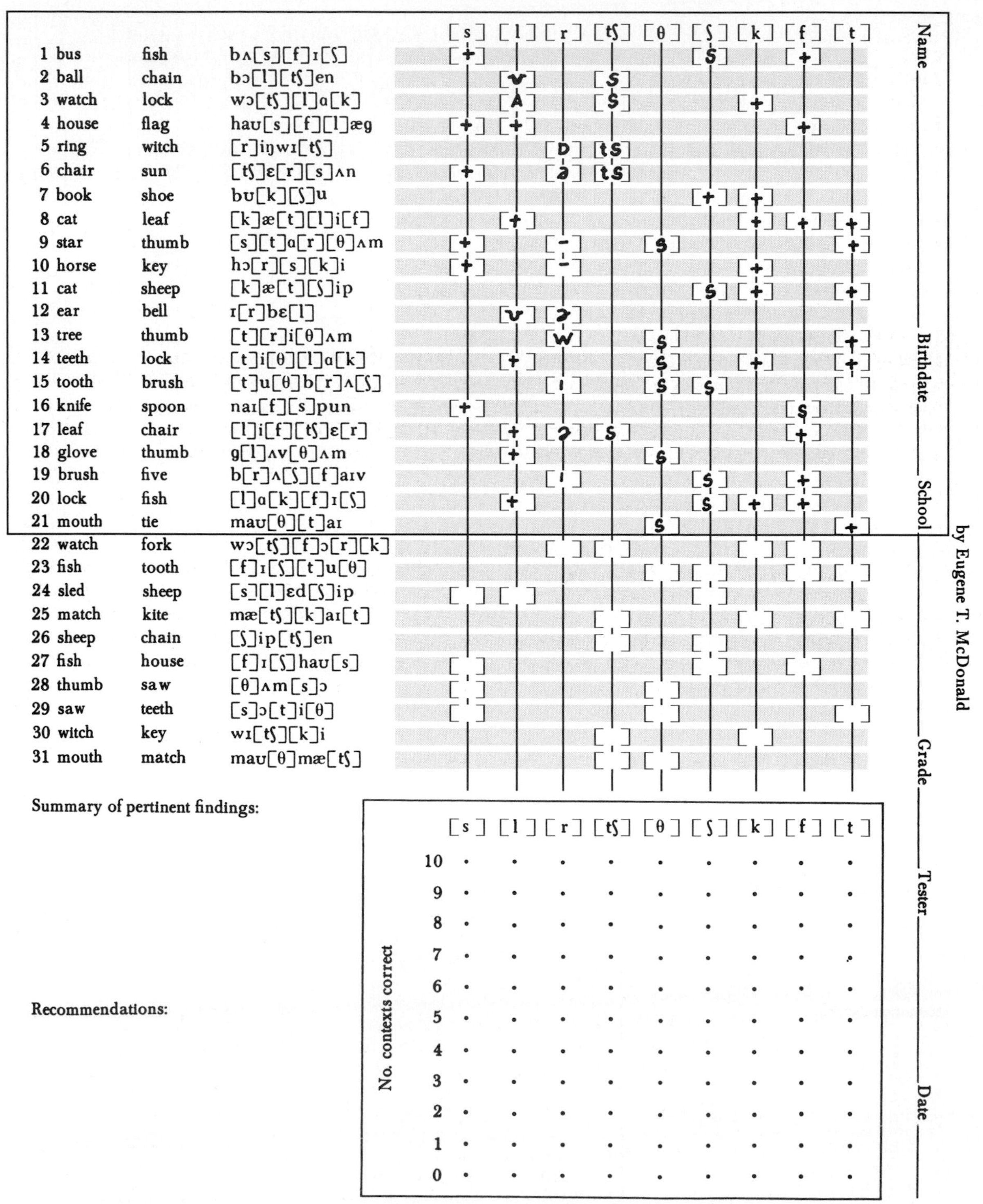

				[s]	[l]	[r]	[tʃ]	[θ]	[ʃ]	[k]	[f]	[t]
1	bus	fish	bʌ[s][f]ɪ[ʃ]	[+]					[s]		[+]	
2	ball	chain	bɔ[l][tʃ]en		[v]		[s]					
3	watch	lock	wɔ[tʃ][l]ɑ[k]		[A]		[s]			[+]		
4	house	flag	haʊ[s][f][l]æg	[+]	[+]						[+]	
5	ring	witch	[r]iŋwɪ[tʃ]			[D]	[ts]					
6	chair	sun	[tʃ]ɛ[r][s]ʌn	[+]		[ə]	[ts]					
7	book	shoe	bʊ[k][ʃ]u						[+]	[+]		
8	cat	leaf	[k]æ[t][l]i[f]		[+]					[+]	[+]	[+]
9	star	thumb	[s][t]ɑ[r][θ]ʌm	[+]		[-]		[s]				[+]
10	horse	key	hɔ[r][s][k]i	[+]		[-]				[+]		
11	cat	sheep	[k]æ[t][ʃ]ip						[s]	[+]		[+]
12	ear	bell	ɪ[r]bɛ[l]		[v]	[ɚ]						
13	tree	thumb	[t][r]i[θ]ʌm			[w]		[s]				[+]
14	teeth	lock	[t]i[θ][l]ɑ[k]		[+]			[s]		[+]		[+]
15	tooth	brush	[t]u[θ]b[r]ʌ[ʃ]			[ɪ]		[s]	[s]			[ ]
16	knife	spoon	naɪ[f][s]pun	[+]							[s]	
17	leaf	chair	[l]i[f][tʃ]ɛ[r]		[+]	[ɚ]	[s]				[+]	
18	glove	thumb	g[l]ʌv[θ]ʌm		[+]			[s]				
19	brush	five	b[r]ʌ[ʃ][f]aɪv			[ɪ]			[s]		[+]	
20	lock	fish	[l]ɑ[k][f]ɪ[ʃ]		[+]				[s]	[+]	[+]	
21	mouth	tie	maʊ[θ][t]aɪ					[s]				[+]
22	watch	fork	wɔ[tʃ][f]ɔ[r][k]			[ ]	[ ]			[ ]	[ ]	
23	fish	tooth	[f]ɪ[ʃ][t]u[θ]					[ ]	[ ]		[ ]	[ ]
24	sled	sheep	[s][l]ɛd[ʃ]ip	[ ]	[ ]				[ ]			
25	match	kite	mæ[tʃ][k]aɪ[t]				[ ]			[ ]		[ ]
26	sheep	chain	[ʃ]ip[tʃ]en				[ ]		[ ]			
27	fish	house	[f]ɪ[ʃ]haʊ[s]	[ ]					[ ]		[ ]	
28	thumb	saw	[θ]ʌm[s]ɔ	[ ]				[ ]				
29	saw	teeth	[s]ɔ[t]i[θ]	[ ]				[ ]				[ ]
30	witch	key	wɪ[tʃ][k]i				[ ]			[ ]		
31	mouth	match	maʊ[θ]mæ[tʃ]				[ ]	[ ]				

Name_____ Birthdate_____ School_____ Grade_____ Tester_____ Date_____

by Eugene T. McDonald

Summary of pertinent findings:

Recommendations:

No. contexts correct	[s]	[l]	[r]	[tʃ]	[θ]	[ʃ]	[k]	[f]	[t]
10	·	·	·	·	·	·	·	·	·
9	·	·	·	·	·	·	·	·	·
8	·	·	·	·	·	·	·	·	·
7	·	·	·	·	·	·	·	·	·
6	·	·	·	·	·	·	·	·	·
5	·	·	·	·	·	·	·	·	·
4	·	·	·	·	·	·	·	·	·
3	·	·	·	·	·	·	·	·	·
2	·	·	·	·	·	·	·	·	·
1	·	·	·	·	·	·	·	·	·
0	·	·	·	·	·	·	·	·	·

PHONETIC PROFILE

MODULE TIME	
TOTAL	3:06
ELAPSED	00:00–03:06

Clinical Phonetics Tape 4B
Practice Module #2:
Multiple-Sound Articulation Test

INDIVIDUAL RECORD SHEET FOR A SCREENING DEEP TEST OF ARTICULATION

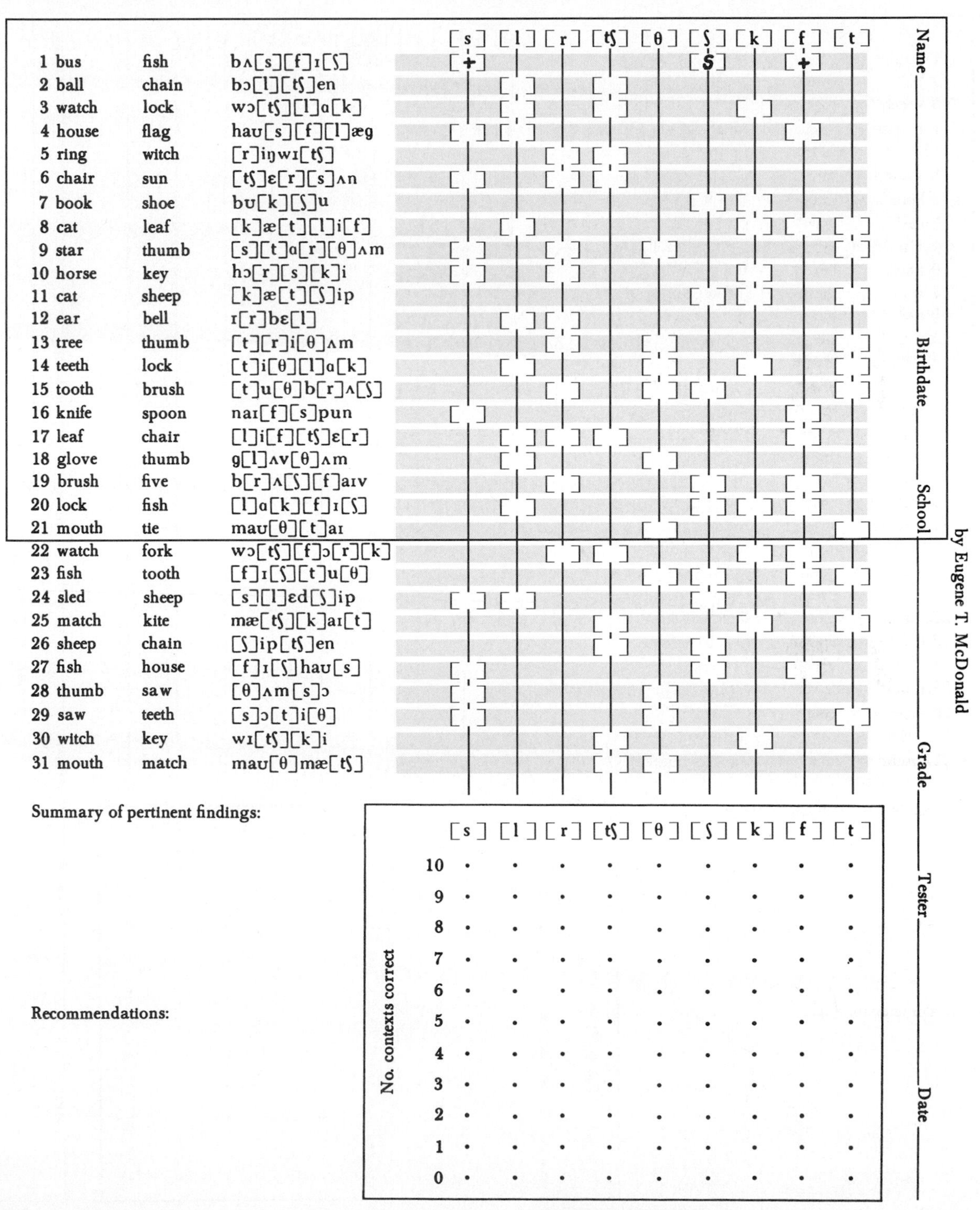

				[s]	[l]	[r]	[tʃ]	[θ]	[ʃ]	[k]	[f]	[t]
1	bus	fish	bʌ[s][f]ɪ[ʃ]	[+]					[ʃ]		[+]	
2	ball	chain	bɔ[l][tʃ]en									
3	watch	lock	wɔ[tʃ][l]ɑ[k]									
4	house	flag	haʊ[s][f][l]æg									
5	ring	witch	[r]ɪŋwɪ[tʃ]									
6	chair	sun	[tʃ]ɛ[r][s]ʌn									
7	book	shoe	bʊ[k][ʃ]u									
8	cat	leaf	[k]æ[t][l]i[f]									
9	star	thumb	[s][t]ɑ[r][θ]ʌm									
10	horse	key	hɔ[r][s][k]i									
11	cat	sheep	[k]æ[t][ʃ]ip									
12	ear	bell	ɪ[r]bɛ[l]									
13	tree	thumb	[t][r]i[θ]ʌm									
14	teeth	lock	[t]i[θ][l]ɑ[k]									
15	tooth	brush	[t]u[θ]b[r]ʌ[ʃ]									
16	knife	spoon	naɪ[f][s]pun									
17	leaf	chair	[l]i[f][tʃ]ɛ[r]									
18	glove	thumb	g[l]ʌv[θ]ʌm									
19	brush	five	b[r]ʌ[ʃ][f]aɪv									
20	lock	fish	[l]ɑ[k][f]ɪ[ʃ]									
21	mouth	tie	maʊ[θ][t]aɪ									
22	watch	fork	wɔ[tʃ][f]ɔ[r][k]									
23	fish	tooth	[f]ɪ[ʃ][t]u[θ]									
24	sled	sheep	[s][l]ɛd[ʃ]ip									
25	match	kite	mæ[tʃ][k]aɪ[t]									
26	sheep	chain	[ʃ]ip[tʃ]en									
27	fish	house	[f]ɪ[ʃ]haʊ[s]									
28	thumb	saw	[θ]ʌm[s]ɔ									
29	saw	teeth	[s]ɔ[t]i[θ]									
30	witch	key	wɪ[tʃ][k]i									
31	mouth	match	maʊ[θ]mæ[tʃ]									

Name _____ Birthdate _____ School _____ Grade _____ Tester _____ Date _____

by Eugene T. McDonald

Summary of pertinent findings:

Recommendations:

No. contexts correct	[s]	[l]	[r]	[tʃ]	[θ]	[ʃ]	[k]	[f]	[t]
10	•	•	•	•	•	•	•	•	•
9	•	•	•	•	•	•	•	•	•
8	•	•	•	•	•	•	•	•	•
7	•	•	•	•	•	•	•	•	•
6	•	•	•	•	•	•	•	•	•
5	•	•	•	•	•	•	•	•	•
4	•	•	•	•	•	•	•	•	•
3	•	•	•	•	•	•	•	•	•
2	•	•	•	•	•	•	•	•	•
1	•	•	•	•	•	•	•	•	•
0	•	•	•	•	•	•	•	•	•

PHONETIC PROFILE

MODULE TIME	
TOTAL	3:06
ELAPSED	00:00–03:06

Clinical Phonetics Tape 4B
Practice Module #2:
Multiple-Sound Articulation Test

INDIVIDUAL RECORD SHEET FOR A SCREENING DEEP TEST OF ARTICULATION

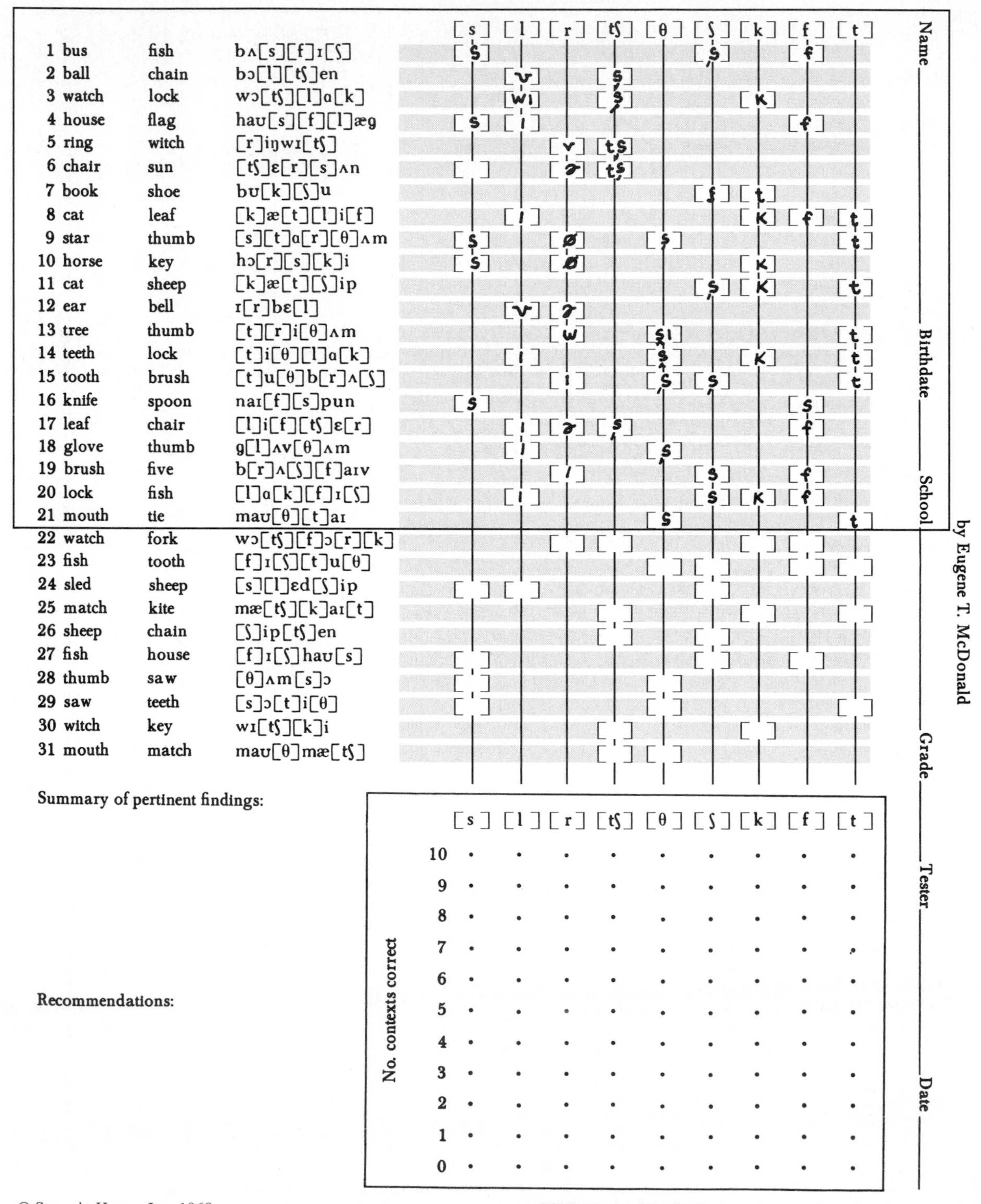

				[s]	[l]	[r]	[tʃ]	[θ]	[ʃ]	[k]	[f]	[t]
1 bus	fish	bʌ[s][f]ɪ[ʃ]		[s]					[s]		[f]	
2 ball	chain	bɔ[l][tʃ]en			[v]		[s]					
3 watch	lock	wɔ[tʃ][l]ɑ[k]			[wl]		[s]			[k]		
4 house	flag	haʊ[s][f][l]æg		[s]	[l]						[f]	
5 ring	witch	[r]iŋwɪ[tʃ]				[v]	[ts]					
6 chair	sun	[tʃ]ɛ[r][s]ʌn		[ ]		[ɚ]	[ts]					
7 book	shoe	bʊ[k][ʃ]u							[ʃ]	[t]		
8 cat	leaf	[k]æ[t][l]i[f]			[l]					[k]	[f]	[t]
9 star	thumb	[s][t]ɑ[r][θ]ʌm		[s]		[ø]		[s]				[t]
10 horse	key	hɔ[r][s][k]i		[s]		[ø]				[k]		
11 cat	sheep	[k]æ[t][ʃ]ip							[s]	[k]		[t]
12 ear	bell	ɪ[r]bɛ[l]			[v]	[ɚ]						
13 tree	thumb	[t][r]i[θ]ʌm				[w]		[sl]				[t]
14 teeth	lock	[t]i[θ][l]ɑ[k]			[l]			[s]		[k]		[t]
15 tooth	brush	[t]u[θ]b[r]ʌ[ʃ]				[l]		[s]	[s]			[t]
16 knife	spoon	naɪ[f][s]pun		[s]							[s]	
17 leaf	chair	[l]i[f][tʃ]ɛ[r]			[l]	[ɚ]	[s]				[f]	
18 glove	thumb	g[l]ʌv[θ]ʌm			[l]			[s]				
19 brush	five	b[r]ʌ[ʃ][f]aɪv				[l]			[s]		[f]	
20 lock	fish	[l]ɑ[k][f]ɪ[ʃ]			[l]				[s]	[k]	[f]	
21 mouth	tie	maʊ[θ][t]aɪ						[s]				[t]
22 watch	fork	wɔ[tʃ][f]ɔ[r][k]				[ ]	[ ]			[ ]	[ ]	
23 fish	tooth	[f]ɪ[ʃ][t]u[θ]						[ ]	[ ]		[ ]	[ ]
24 sled	sheep	[s][l]ɛd[ʃ]ip		[ ]	[ ]				[ ]			
25 match	kite	mæ[tʃ][k]aɪ[t]					[ ]			[ ]		[ ]
26 sheep	chain	[ʃ]ip[tʃ]en					[ ]		[ ]			
27 fish	house	[f]ɪ[ʃ]haʊ[s]		[ ]					[ ]		[ ]	
28 thumb	saw	[θ]ʌm[s]ɔ		[ ]				[ ]				
29 saw	teeth	[s]ɔ[t]i[θ]		[ ]				[ ]				[ ]
30 witch	key	wɪ[tʃ][k]i					[ ]			[ ]		
31 mouth	match	maʊ[θ]mæ[tʃ]					[ ]	[ ]				

Name ______ Birthdate ______ School ______ Grade ______ Tester ______ Date ______

by Eugene T. McDonald

Summary of pertinent findings:

Recommendations:

No. contexts correct	[s]	[l]	[r]	[tʃ]	[θ]	[ʃ]	[k]	[f]	[t]
10	•	•	•	•	•	•	•	•	•
9	•	•	•	•	•	•	•	•	•
8	•	•	•	•	•	•	•	•	•
7	•	•	•	•	•	•	•	•	•
6	•	•	•	•	•	•	•	•	•
5	•	•	•	•	•	•	•	•	•
4	•	•	•	•	•	•	•	•	•
3	•	•	•	•	•	•	•	•	•
2	•	•	•	•	•	•	•	•	•
1	•	•	•	•	•	•	•	•	•
0	•	•	•	•	•	•	•	•	•

PHONETIC PROFILE

Note: This boy makes both palatalized and lateralized sibilants and affricates.

MODULE TIME	
TOTAL	3:06
ELAPSED	00:00–03:06

Clinical Phonetics Tape 4B
Practice Module #2:
Multiple-Sound Articulation Test

INDIVIDUAL RECORD SHEET FOR A SCREENING DEEP TEST OF ARTICULATION

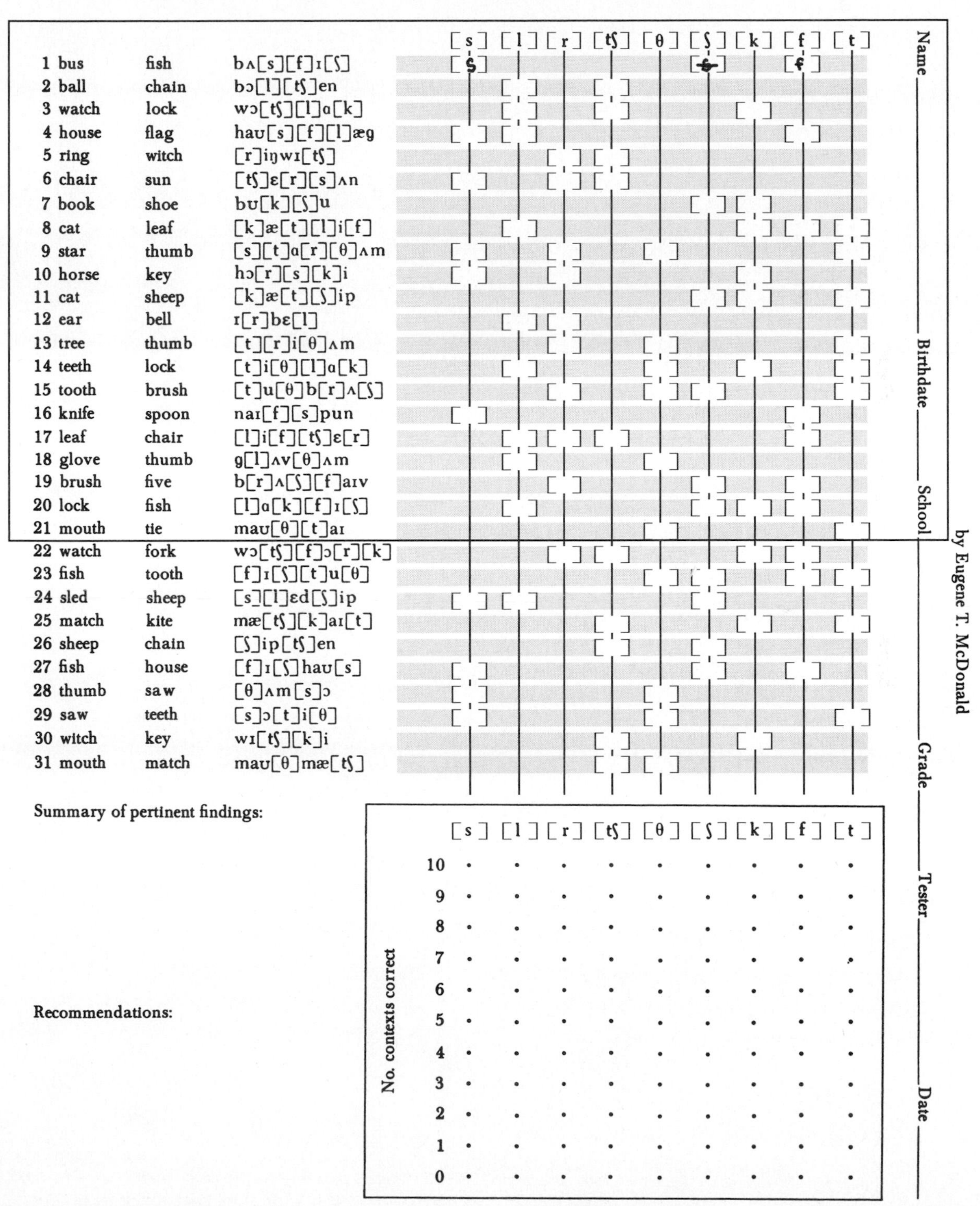

[s] [l] [r] [tʃ] [θ] [ʃ] [k] [f] [t]

1	bus	fish	bʌ[s][f]ɪ[ʃ]
2	ball	chain	bɔ[l][tʃ]en
3	watch	lock	wɔ[tʃ][l]ɑ[k]
4	house	flag	haʊ[s][f][l]æg
5	ring	witch	[r]iŋwɪ[tʃ]
6	chair	sun	[tʃ]ɛ[r][s]ʌn
7	book	shoe	bʊ[k][ʃ]u
8	cat	leaf	[k]æ[t][l]i[f]
9	star	thumb	[s][t]ɑ[r][θ]ʌm
10	horse	key	hɔ[r][s][k]i
11	cat	sheep	[k]æ[t][ʃ]ip
12	ear	bell	ɪ[r]bɛ[l]
13	tree	thumb	[t][r]i[θ]ʌm
14	teeth	lock	[t]i[θ][l]ɑ[k]
15	tooth	brush	[t]u[θ]b[r]ʌ[ʃ]
16	knife	spoon	naɪ[f][s]pun
17	leaf	chair	[l]i[f][tʃ]ɛ[r]
18	glove	thumb	g[l]ʌv[θ]ʌm
19	brush	five	b[r]ʌ[ʃ][f]aɪv
20	lock	fish	[l]ɑ[k][f]ɪ[ʃ]
21	mouth	tie	maʊ[θ][t]aɪ
22	watch	fork	wɔ[tʃ][f]ɔ[r][k]
23	fish	tooth	[f]ɪ[ʃ][t]u[θ]
24	sled	sheep	[s][l]ɛd[ʃ]ip
25	match	kite	mæ[tʃ][k]aɪ[t]
26	sheep	chain	[ʃ]ip[tʃ]en
27	fish	house	[f]ɪ[ʃ]haʊ[s]
28	thumb	saw	[θ]ʌm[s]ɔ
29	saw	teeth	[s]ɔ[t]i[θ]
30	witch	key	wɪ[tʃ][k]i
31	mouth	match	maʊ[θ]mæ[tʃ]

Name_____ Birthdate_____ School_____ Grade_____ Tester_____ Date_____

by Eugene T. McDonald

Summary of pertinent findings:

Recommendations:

No. contexts correct

[s] [l] [r] [tʃ] [θ] [ʃ] [k] [f] [t]

10
9
8
7
6
5
4
3
2
1
0

PHONETIC PROFILE

Practice Module #3: /s/ in Continuous Speech; Sample I

This transcription practice module and the two immediately following contain samples of continuous speech by children who have errors on /s/. As we discussed earlier, /s/ errors are the most prevalent type of residual articulation error. Clinicians commonly obtain continuous speech samples from children with /s/ errors to probe how well a child is generalizing and maintaining articulatory skills in a continuous speech situation. For such monitoring tasks, two-way scoring usually is sufficient. What the clinician generally needs is a statement of the percentage of items on which the child is correctly articulating the target sound. These data, in such forms as "percentage correct per minute" or "percentage correct per sample" are used in different phases of management programs.

We have found that a two-step approach for acquisition of this skill works well. First, students need to learn to *identify* a target sound each time it occurs in free speech. When accuracy in identifying target sounds as they occur in free speech is high enough, the next task is to *discriminate* correct production of target sounds from incorrect ones. The practice modules in this section follow this two-step approach.

Preliminary Practice—Identifying /s/ in Continuous Speech. Frequency of occurrence data (Appendix B) and research by Diedrich and Bangert (1981) indicate that /s/ occurs often in normal speech, approximately seven times per minute. When clinicians first try to *identify* each occurrence of /s/ in continuous speech, two types of errors are often made:

1. The most frequent error students make when counting /s/ in a speech sample is to include /z/. Try to disregard how words are spelled—think of how words sound (*pays* [peɪ͡z], *pads* [pædz], and so forth).
2. Another error is to miss /s/ sounds in words that have two or more /s/ sounds per word. Usually one or more of the /s/'s occur in a cluster (*stamps*).

Before listening to the continuous speech samples, see how often you can correctly identify the occurrence of /s/ in words. For each word in the following list—as rapidly as you can—say the word out loud and decide how many /s/ *sounds* it contains:

Item	*Number of /s/ Sounds*
1. stores	________
2. simplex	________
3. substantial	________
4. scissors	________
5. Mississippi	________
6. Missouri	________
7. transcribers	________
8. stencils	________
9. scratches	________
10. taxes	________

You can gain further practice by counting sounds in a number of ways. You can listen to the radio or television and count the number of /s/'s produced by a particular speaker. You can do the same while listening to a friend. Another excellent way to develop this skill is to record yourself reading or talking. The advantage here is that after listening and counting the /s/'s that occurred, you can replay the recording as often as needed to determine the actual count. Accuracy within 85 to 90 percent of the actual tally should be your objective before proceeding to the next stage.

Transcription Practice—Discriminating /s/ Errors in Continuous Speech. The following pages contain the transcripts (right-hand page) and the keys (left-hand page) for each of three speech samples. You can practice in either of two ways. First, you may wish to tally the correct and incorrect /s/'s without reference to the transcription. To do this, simply use a piece of scrap paper and tally each correct versus incorrect /s/ as you hear it on the recording. Alternately, you may wish to use the transcript to follow along and mark your decision over each /s/ that occurs as a phoneme on the transcript (watch those /z/'s). Keeping a tally without a transcript is what clinicians ordinarily do in the clinical situation. However, use of a transcript allows you to compare your answers item by item with the key. What you should be aiming for is a total percent correct figure that agrees with the key about 85 percent or more of the time.

Because the perceptual events in this task are fleeting, do not expect to agree exactly item by item with the key—our panel of listeners certainly did not agree with each other all the time.

The three children in these samples were either in kindergarten or first grade. They all are interviewed by the same clinician; the tapes have been edited only slightly. As you will hear, "kids say the darndest things."

PROCEED TO: Clinical Phonetics Tape 4B: Practice Module #3: /s/ in Continuous Speech; Sample I

MODULE TIME	
TOTAL	2:39
ELAPSED	03:06–05:45

Clinical Phonetics Tape 4B Practice Module #3: /s/ in Continuous Speech; Sample 1

TWO-WAY SCORING KEY

EXAMINER:	How old are you?
CHILD:	Five and a half.
E.:	Do you have any brothers or sisters?
C.:	A baby brother.
E.:	How old is he?
C.:	I don't know . . . I don't know how old he is. 'Bout four months̊ or maybe five.
E.:	Ahuh . . . he's pretty little. Can he sit up yet?
C.:	He can s̊tand up, but he, he can, you know, he can s̊tand up holding onto things.
E.:	Oh, then he's even more than five months. [Yeah] He's probably going on about ten months.
C.:	Yeah.
E.:	Do you know when his birthday is?
C.:	Ah, no.
E.:	Is it in summer? Was he born in summertime?
C.:	Yeah, in s̊ummer.
E.:	Who are your good friends that you like to play with?
C.:	At home or at s̊chool?
E.:	Either.
C.:	Ah, I'll jus⁺t s⁺ay at home. [OK] Ah, David, Mark, and Eric.
E.:	Oh, . . . what do you guys play when you get together?
C.:	Oh . . . all s̊orts̊ of things.
E.:	Like what?
C.:	Well, s̊(?)ometimes in the s̊(?)ummer we play football in the middle of the night.
E.:	Then you get to stay up late, huh?
C.: (school background noise)	Yeah, we play football when it's̊ (short) real dark and, ah . . . I don't know anything els̊e . . . all I know . . . we play football and baseball and hockey or . . .
E.:	Oh, that's what you play in winter is hockey, huh?
C.:	Yeah, we play hockey. We, you know, we go to a s̊kating rink and we bring our hockey s̊ticks̊ and pucks̊ and you know play hockey.
E.:	Great! . . . um . . . what are your favorite TV shows? What do you watch after school? Do you watch any TV after school?
C.:	No, . . . I . . . but I'll tell you what my bes⁺t TV programs are. [OK] Adam-12.
E.:	Adam-12? What's that?
C.:	It's̊ a polic⁺e show. [Oh] And, ah, the Rookies. That's̊ also a polic⁺e show too. [Oh] And, ah, the Mod S̊quad.
E.:	That's interesting. Do you watch any children's shows? Those are pretty grown-up shows.
C.:	Umm, no . . . I like grown-up shows better than children's shows!

Notes: As discussed in Chapter 7, it is difficult and, in some situations, unwarranted to score sibilants from an audio recording. The general goals of this task and the other five modules to follow are to help you develop your discrimination skills with this type of sample. While you may not be able to discriminate subtle distinctions among target consonants, you should be able to differentiate strident from nonstrident sibilants. You should be able to discriminate a clearly incorrect /s/ when it occurs in a stressed word, and so forth. Judges agreed on approximately 85 percent of target consonants in these modules. Your item-by-item agreement with the keys may not be this high, but your percentage of correct consonants for each child should be within ± 10 percentage points of the value calculated for the key. For example, the child in this module, Practice Module #3, was 80 percent correct on /s/ as calculated from this key. Your percentage of consonants correct should be between 70 and 90 percent.

MODULE TIME	
TOTAL	2:39
ELAPSED	03:06–05:45

Clinical Phonetics Tape 4B Practice Module #3: /s/ in Continuous Speech; Sample 1

TWO-WAY SCORING SHEET[a]

EXAMINER: How old are you?
CHILD: Five and a half.
E.: Do you have any brothers or sisters?
C.: A baby brother.
E.: How old is he?
C.: I don't know . . . I don't know how old he is. 'Bout four months or maybe five.
E.: Ahuh . . . he's pretty little. Can he sit up yet?
C.: He can stand up, but he, he can, you know, he can stand up holding onto things.
E.: Oh, then he's even more than five months. [Yeah] He's probably going on about ten months.
C.: Yeah.
E.: Do you know when his birthday is?
C.: Ah, no.
E.: Is it in summer? Was he born in summertime?
C.: Yeah, in summer.
E.: Who are your good friends that you like to play with?
C.: At home or at school?
E.: Either.
C.: Ah, I'll just say at home. [OK] Ah, David, Mark, and Eric.
E.: Oh, . . . what do you guys play when you get together?
C.: Oh . . . all sorts of things.
E.: Like what?
C.: Well, sometimes in the summer we play football in the middle of the night.
E.: Then you get to stay up late, huh?
C.: (school background noise) Yeah, we play football when it's real dark and, ah . . . I don't know anything else . . . all I know . . . we play football and baseball and hockey or . . .
E.: Oh, that's what you play in winter is hockey, huh?
C.: Yeah, we play hockey. We, you know, we go to a skating rink and we bring our hockey sticks and pucks and you know play hockey.
E.: Great! . . . um . . . what are your favorite TV shows? What do you watch after school? Do you watch any TV after school?
C.: No, . . . I . . . but I'll tell you what my best TV programs are. [OK] Adam-12.
E.: Adam-12? What's that?
C.: It's a police show. [Oh] And, ah, the Rookies. That's also a police show too. [Oh] And, ah, the Mod Squad.
E.: That's interesting. Do you watch any children's shows? Those are pretty grown-up shows.
C.: Umm, no . . . I like grown-up shows better than children's shows!

[a]Above each underlined sound, indicate if it is correct (+) or incorrect (0).

Practice Module #4: /s/ in Continuous Speech; Sample 2

PROCEED TO: Clinical Phonetics Tape 4B: Practice Module #4: /s/ in Continuous Speech; Sample 2

MODULE TIME	
TOTAL	3:37
ELAPSED	05:45–09:22

Clinical Phonetics Tape 4B
Practice Module #4:
/s/ in Continuous Speech; Sample 2

TWO-WAY SCORING KEY

E.: Did you tell me how old you are?
C.: Yeah, six. (difficult)
E.: OK. How many brothers and sisters do you have?
C.: I have one brother and one sister.
E.: What's your sister's name?
C.: Karen.
E.: Karen . . . How old is your brother?
C.: Seven. I mean eight.
E.: He's eight. Do you and he play a lot together?
C.: Yeah.
E.: What do you do?
C.: Most of the time we play basketball.
E.: Do ya?
C.: Yeah.
E.: You both good players?
C.: He (said) alotta time he (says) I'm better'n him.
E.: How many points dya usually get?
C.: My average is about . . . 20.0
E.: Hmm . . . pretty good, pretty good. Who are your other friends that you play with?
C.: Gary.
E.: And who else . . . ?
C.: At home or at school?
E.: Both.
C.: Teddy and Mark. [Uhuh] . . . and I used to play with Chad, and I play with Doug. [Uhuh] . . . and Jim and Rich.
E.: What do you like to play besides basketball?
C.: Baseball.
E.: You like sports, huh?
C.: Yeah.
E.: Do you . . . like to play any indoor games?
C.: Yeah.
E.: Like what?
C.: Trouble.
E.: Trouble . . . explain that to me.
C.: Well . . . you know, d'you know how to play Aggravation?
E.: No, I don't know how to play that either . . . so you'll have to start from the beginning.
C.: There's this little thing up here that's got a die an if that comes off . . . you just need a (?) . . . and you each have four men.

MODULE TIME	
TOTAL	3:37
ELAPSED	05:45–09:22

Clinical Phonetics Tape 4B
Practice Module #4:
/s/ in Continuous Speech; Sample 2

TWO-WAY SCORING SHEET

E.: Did you tell me how old you are?
C.: Yeah, six.
E.: OK. How many brothers and sisters do you have?
C.: I have one brother and one sister.
E.: What's your sister's name?
C.: Karen.
E.: Karen . . . How old is your brother?
C.: Seven. I mean eight.
E.: He's eight. Do you and he play a lot together?
C.: Yeah.
E.: What do you do?
C.: Most of the time we play basketball.
E.: Do ya?
C.: Yeah.
E.: You both good players?
C.: He (said) alotta time he (says) I'm better'n him.
E.: How many points dya usually get?
C.: My average is about . . . 20.0
E.: Hmm . . . pretty good, pretty good. Who are your other friends that you play with?
C.: Gary.
E.: And who else . . . ?
C.: At home or at school?
E.: Both.
C.: Teddy and Mark. [Uhuh] . . . and I used to play with Chad, and I play with Doug. [Uhuh] . . . and Jim and Rich.
E.: What do you like to play besides basketball?
C.: Baseball.
E.: You like sports, huh?
C.: Yeah.
E.: Do you . . . like to play any indoor games?
C.: Yeah.
E.: Like what?
C.: Trouble.
E.: Trouble . . . explain that to me.
C.: Well . . . you know, d'you know how to play Aggravation?
E.: No, I don't know how to play that either . . . so you'll have to start from the beginning.
C.: There's this little thing up here that's got a die an if that comes off . . . you just need a (?) . . . and you each have four men.

MODULE TIME	
TOTAL	3:37
ELAPSED	05:45–09:22

Clinical Phonetics Tape 4B
Practice Module #4:
/s/ in Continuous Speech; Sample 2, Continued

TWO-WAY SCORING KEY

E.: Uhuh.

C.: An ya try to . . . an there's a whole bunch of spaces, an ya try to go around the board an then it's got a ladder.

E.: Uhuh.

C.: Which is four spa (space) [not clear] an ya get each one up the ladder . . . first one to fill up their ladder wins.

E.: Aahhh . . .

C.: An then Aggravation . . . it's the same except there's, except you need a six or a one to get out in Aggravation . . . and also there's a shortcut. So (just) a little hole in the middle.

E.: Uhuh . . . who is the winner? The one who has . . .

C.: The one who gets 'em (?) . . .

E.: Who gets 'em all up the ladder?

C.: Yeah . . . I think there's six in Aggravation.

E.: Uhuh. That's interesting. How 'bout any other indoor games? Are there any other ones you like to play . . . any card games?

C.: Yeah.

E.: What?

C.: War.

E.: War . . . OK, I know how to play War, but I'd like you to explain it to me.

C.: Each person has half a deck of cards. [Mhmmm] An you take 'em and turn 'em over an' the highest one wins . . . (?)

E.: The one . . . what do you mean the highest . . . the highest . . . card?

C.: Yeah.

E.: OK. Person who has the highest card takes the two that are put out [Yeah], right?

C.: And if they're both the same then puts three down an then turn one over.

E.: Oh, . . . then that's called . . .

C.: War!

Notes: What type of distortion error on /s/ does this child have? (Hint: See "Fricatives and Affricates Module #7") Calculate his percentage of consonants correct by your two-way scoring and compare to the value derived from the key. Does your score agree within ± 10 percentage points? Notice this child's denasal and hoarse voice quality; as discussed in Chapter 7, voice quality can bias our perceptions of articulation.

MODULE TIME	
TOTAL	3:37
ELAPSED	05:45–09:22

Clinical Phonetics Tape 4B
Practice Module #4:
/s/ in Continuous Speech; Sample 2, Continued

TWO-WAY SCORING SHEET

E.: Uhuh.
C.: An ya try to . . . an there's a whole bunch of spaces, an ya try to go around the board an then it's got a ladder.
E.: Uhuh.
C.: Which is four spa (space) [not clear] an ya get each one up the ladder . . . first one to fill up their ladder wins.
E.: Aahhh . . .
C.: An then Aggravation . . . it's the same except there's, except you need a six or a one to get out in Aggravation . . . and also there's a shortcut. So (just) a little hole in the middle.
E.: Uhuh . . . who is the winner? The one who has . . .
C.: The one who gets 'em (?) . . .
E.: Who gets 'em all up the ladder?
C.: Yeah . . . I think there's six in Aggravation.
E.: Uhuh. That's interesting. How 'bout any other indoor games? Are there any other ones you like to play . . . any card games?
C.: Yeah.
E.: What?
C.: War.
E.: War . . . OK, I know how to play War, but I'd like you to explain it to me.
C.: Each person has half a deck of cards. [Mhmmm] An you take 'em and turn 'em over an' the highest one wins . . . (?)
E.: The one . . . what do you mean the highest . . . the highest . . . card?
C.: Yeah.
E.: OK. Person who has the highest card takes the two that are put out [Yeah], right?
C.: And if they're both the same then puts three down an then turn one over.
E.: Oh, . . . then that's called . . .
C.: War!

Practice Module #5: /s/ in Continuous Speech; Sample 3

PROCEED TO: Clinical Phonetics Tape 4B: Practice Module #5: /s/ in Continuous Speech; Sample 3

MODULE TIME	
TOTAL	3:54
ELAPSED	09:22–13:16

Clinical Phonetics Tape 4B
Practice Module #5:
/s/ in Continuous Speech; Sample 3

TWO-WAY SCORING KEY

E.: What were you doing in the classroom when I took you out?
C.: I was, um, putting some decorations on my box.
E.: Wow, very good. What kind of box were you making?
C.: A valentine box.
E.: That's nice. What are you gonna do with the valentine box?
C.: I'm going to put cards in it to send to people.
E.: Can you speak up a little bit?
C.: We're going to put valentine cards in it to send to people.
E.: Very nice. Did you write your valentines out yet?
C.: No.
E.: Did you buy them yet?
C.: Uh uh.
E.: When is Valentine's day?
C.: Seven more days.
E.: Seven, is that all?
C.: Yeah.
E.: Seven more school days, huh? That's great! . . . Who are your best friends? Who do you like to play with?
C.: My friend Jimmy that always socks me in the belly.(!!)
E.: He socks you in the belly . . . hope he doesn't do it very hard!
C.: He does.
E.: He does? [He does] What do you and Jimmy do?
C.: We play together and we spy on girls.
E.: You spy on them. Why do you spy on them?
C.: We like to. Today my friend was running away because he didn't like me.
E.: He didn't like you today?
C.: No. So then I told him something. Then he walked with me.
E.: Ah . . . sometimes friends are like that. They're changeable. One day they're real friendly and the next day they're not too friendly. . . . How many brothers and sisters do you have?
C.: Just one sister.
E.: Just one sister. And how old is she?
C.: Four.
E.: Do you play with her very much?
C.: No.
E.: No . . . I have a . . . couple of pictures here I'd like you to look at. What happened to all the snow?
C.: It melted.

MODULE TIME	
TOTAL	3:54
ELAPSED	09:22–13:16

Clinical Phonetics Tape 4B Practice Module #5: /s/ in Continuous Speech; Sample 3

TWO-WAY SCORING SHEET

E.: What were you doing in the classroom when I took you out?
C.: I was, um, putting some decorations on my box.
E.: Wow, very good. What kind of box were you making?
C.: A valentine box.
E.: That's nice. What are you gonna do with the valentine box?
C.: I'm going to put cards in it to send to people.
E.: Can you speak up a little bit?
C.: We're going to put valentine cards in it to send to people.
E.: Very nice. Did you write your valentines out yet?
C.: No.
E.: Did you buy them yet?
C.: Uh uh.
E.: When is Valentine's day?
C.: Seven more days.
E.: Seven, is that all?
C.: Yeah.
E.: Seven more school days, huh? That's great! . . . Who are your best friends? Who do you like to play with?
C.: My friend Jimmy that always socks me in the belly.(!!)
E.: He socks you in the belly . . . hope he doesn't do it very hard!
C.: He does.
E.: He does? [He does] What do you and Jimmy do?
C.: We play together and we spy on girls.
E.: You spy on them. Why do you spy on them?
C.: We like to. Today my friend was running away because he didn't like me.
E.: He didn't like you today?
C.: No. So then I told him something. Then he walked with me.
E.: Ah . . . sometimes friends are like that. They're changeable. One day they're real friendly and the next day they're not too friendly. . . . How many brothers and sisters do you have?
C.: Just one sister.
E.: Just one sister. And how old is she?
C.: Four.
E.: Do you play with her very much?
C.: No.
E.: No . . . I have a . . . couple of pictures here I'd like you to look at. What happened to all the snow?
C.: It melted.

MODULE TIME	
TOTAL	3:54
ELAPSED	09:22–13:16

Clinical Phonetics Tape 4B
Practice Module #5:
/s/ in Continuous Speech; Sample 3, Continued

TWO-WAY SCORING KEY

E.: Doggone it. If we had some snow, what could we do outside?
C.: We can make a snowman.
E.: What else could we do?
C.: Make a snow fort.
E.: Yeah, what else?
C.: We could sled.
E.: Yeah, what else?
C.: Um, we could, can't think of anything.
E.: Maybe you don't have skates, but . . .
C.: Yeah, I have skates.
E.: Do you have skates? So, then what could you do?
C.: Skate.
E.: Go ice skating?
C.: Yeah.
E.: Right. This hasn't been a very good winter for ice skating, has it?
C.: Uh uh.
E.: Let's look at this little fellow here. He's lucky he's got snow outside. You tell me a little story about, I mean a sentence about each one of these pictures. By the time you're finished, we'll have a little story, OK?
C.: He's getting ready to go out and he's almost ready. He's almost ready, and he's out.
E.: What's he putting, what's he doing here?
C.: Putting on his mitten and his coat. And now he's ready to sled. He's sledded down and he's going back up now.
E.: Here's one about a girl. It looks like a different time of year. What's your favorite time of year?
C.: Spring.
E.: Spring?
C.: Yeah.
E.: Why do you like spring?
C.: So I can play football and get muscles.
E.: Ah . . . what's she doing here?
C.: She's getting up, she puts on her dress. She's eating her breakfast . . . (she catches) a school bus . . . she walks up to school and gets ready to do her math.
E.: Ah . . . she's going to do math.

MODULE TIME	
TOTAL	3:54
ELAPSED	09:22–13:16

Clinical Phonetics Tape 4B
Practice Module #5:
/s/ in Continuous Speech; Sample 3, Continued

TWO-WAY SCORING SHEET

E.: Doggone it. If we had some snow, what could we do outside?
C.: We can make a snowman.
E.: What else could we do?
C.: Make a snow fort.
E.: Yeah, what else?
C.: We could sled.
E.: Yeah, what else?
C.: Um, we could, can't think of anything.
E.: Maybe you don't have skates, but . . .
C.: Yeah, I have skates.
E.: Do you have skates? So, then what could you do?
C.: Skate.
E.: Go ice skating?
C.: Yeah.
E.: Right. This hasn't been a very good winter for ice skating, has it?
C.: Uh uh.
E.: Let's look at this little fellow here. He's lucky he's got snow outside. You tell me a little story about, I mean a sentence about each one of these pictures. By the time you're finished, we'll have a little story, OK?
C.: He's getting ready to go out and he's almost ready. He's almost ready, and he's out.
E.: What's he putting, what's he doing here?
C.: Putting on his mitten and his coat. And now he's ready to sled. He's sledded down and he's going back up now.
E.: Here's one about a girl. It looks like a different time of year. What's your favorite time of year?
C.: Spring.
E.: Spring?
C.: Yeah.
E.: Why do you like spring?
C.: So I can play football and get muscles.
E.: Ah . . . what's she doing here?
C.: She's getting up, she puts on her dress. She's eating her breakfast . . . (she catches) a school bus . . . she walks up to school and gets ready to do her math.
E.: Ah . . . she's going to do math.

Practice Module #6: /r/ in Continuous Speech; Sample I

A second group of target sounds that speech-language pathologists must learn to identify and discriminate in continuous speech is the /r/, /ɝ/, and /ɚ/ sounds. Errors on *r* sounds are second only to /s/ in terms of their prevalence as a residual speech sound error.

The two-step approach for learning to transcribe /s/ in continuous speech also is suggested for *r* errors. Clinicians may or may not wish to include the three *r* types in the same tally. For some clinical purposes, a combined tally may be sufficient; however, for more discriminating purposes, separate counts of errors on /r/, /ɝ/, and /ɚ/ may be useful. Because every orthographic *r* is said as either /r/, /ɝ/, or /ɚ/, the *s–z* confusion experienced on /s/ does not occur. Rather, the opposite problem of *underestimating* the occurrence of /r/, /ɝ/, and /ɚ/ crops up. When a word contains two or more *r* sounds (*brother* [b r ʌ ð ɚ]; *Barbara* [b ɑ r b ə r ə]), it becomes especially difficult to identify and transcribe each *r* sound. The task also is more difficult for speakers with inconsistent *r* errors.

Once again, before proceeding to the speech sample modules, first develop your skill in counting *r* sounds in continuous speech. Use the procedures suggested for /s/—by listening to the radio or television or by recording yourself, and so forth. Try to keep separate tallies for the occurrence of /r/, /ɝ/, and /ɚ/; /r/ will occur most frequently among the three sounds, by about a 3:1 ratio over the long term. Your counts should be reliable within 85 to 90 percent (see Appendix D) before proceeding to the speech samples for error discrimination training.

PROCEED TO: Clinical Phonetics Tape 4B: Practice Module #6: /r/ in Continuous Speech; Sample I

MODULE TIME	
TOTAL	4:39
ELAPSED	13:16–17:55

Clinical Phonetics Tape 4B
Practice Module #6:
/r/ in Continuous Speech; Sample 1

TWO-WAY SCORING KEY

E.: Do you have any brothers or sisters?
C.: Only br̲̊other̲̊s . . . two of 'em.
E.: You have two brothers?
C.: Mm hmm.
E.: What are their names?
C.: Danny and Dave.
E.: Ah . . . and what do you play with Danny and Dave?
C.: I play with, I play Old Maid . . . I play Cr̲̊azy Eights . . . I played, I play Snap . . . I play car̲̊s, and I play . . . hmm . . . jump on Dave's bed downstair̲̊s. He has a double bed. [Uhuh.] And um, in the summer̲̊ we play at the night, we play kick the can and then we play . . .
E.: That sounds like fun.
C.: Um . . . play kick the ball. Not kick the ball, but . . . mmm . . . soccer̲̊ baseball.
E.: Uh huh.
C.: And, I don't know anything else we play.
E.: Uh huh. What do you do with your friends in wintertime?
C.: Hm, we . . . we jump in the snow, and we make angels.
E.: Oh, that sounds like fun. What else?
C.: Oh, I go, I go to David's house, and pr̲̊obably sleep over̲̊ at his house Fr̲̊iday so I can watch car̲̟toons with him. And, then with Doug . . . I play at school with him a little bit.
E.: Uh huh . . . I've a few pictures here . . . Can you tell me about this picture?
C.: Hmm . . . the boy's dr̲̟opping the bat and he's taking a, I think it looks like a . . .
E.: It's a glove, I think.
C.: Un huh . . . took that boy's, that boy's glove. Now the police is coming.
E.: Why?
C.: Cause he took the boy's glove.
E.: What else happened?
C.: Hmmm . . . and the window br̲̊oke.
E.: How'd that happen?
C.: Pr̲̊obably a stone.
E.: Do you think it was a stone?
C.: Oh, a bat!
E.: Did the bat break it, or what happened?
C.: He went up and br̲̊oke it. Then he r̲̟an.
E.: That's a possibility. What else could he have done with the bat to break the window, besides hit it with the bat?
C.: Hmm . . . thr̲̊ow it at it.

MODULE TIME	
TOTAL	4:39
ELAPSED	13:16–17:55

Clinical Phonetics Tape 4B
Practice Module #6:
/r/ in Continuous Speech; Sample 1

TWO-WAY SCORING SHEET

E.: Do you have any brothers or sisters?
C.: Only brothers . . . two of 'em.
E.: You have two brothers?
C.: Mm hmm.
E.: What are their names?
C.: Danny and Dave.
E.: Ah . . . and what do you play with Danny and Dave?
C.: I play with, I play Old Maid . . . I play Crazy Eights . . . I played, I play Snap . . . I play cars, and I play . . . hmm . . . jump on Dave's bed downstairs. He has a double bed. [Uhuh.] And um, in the summer we play at the night, we play kick the can and then we play . . .
E.: That sounds like fun.
C.: Um . . . play kick the ball. Not kick the ball, but . . . mmm . . . soccer baseball.
E.: Uh huh.
C.: And, I don't know anything else we play.
E.: Uh huh. What do you do with your friends in wintertime?
C.: Hm, we . . . we jump in the snow, and we make angels.
E.: Oh, that sounds like fun. What else?
C.: Oh, I go, I go to David's house, and probably sleep over at his house Friday so I can watch cartoons with him. And, then with Doug . . . I play at school with him a little bit.
E.: Uh huh . . . I've a few pictures here . . . Can you tell me about this picture?
C.: Hmm . . . the boy's dropping the bat and he's taking a, I think it looks like a . . .
E.: It's a glove, I think.
C.: Un huh . . . took that boy's, that boy's glove. Now the police is coming.
E.: Why?
C.: Cause he took the boy's glove.
E.: What else happened?
C.: Hmmm . . . and the window broke.
E.: How'd that happen?
C.: Probably a stone.
E.: Do you think it was a stone?
C.: Oh, a bat!
E.: Did the bat break it, or what happened?
C.: He went up and broke it. Then he ran.
E.: That's a possibility. What else could he have done with the bat to break the window, besides hit it with the bat?
C.: Hmm . . . throw it at it.

MODULE TIME	
TOTAL	4:39
ELAPSED	13:16–17:55

Clinical Phonetics Tape 4B Practice Module #6: /r/ in Continuous Speech; Sample 1, Continued

TWO-WAY SCORING KEY

E.: Could have. . . . How do you think this lady feels? I think maybe . . .
C.: She feel(s) mad!
E.: Oh boy . . .
C.: . . . and tr̲̟ash cans, tr̲̟ash over̲̊ there̲̊ for̲̊(?) tr̲̊uck.
E.: What 'bout him?
C.: He could've br̲̊oke the window too.
E.: What's he doing?
C.: He's going ar̲̊ound the block.
E.: Yeah, he's getting out of there, isn't he . . .
C.: Uh huh. So is he.
E.: Yeah. What would you do in that situation if you'd broken a window while you were playing baseball?
C.: I'd go r̲̊unning . . .
E.: Would ya?
C.: Yeah . . . pr̲̊obably [go ahead] pr̲̊obably playin' baseball in the middle of the str̲̊eet.
E.: Yeah . . . if you had broken the window, do you think you should say something?
C.: . . . sor̲r̲̊y!!
E.: Yeah . . . what's this man doing over here?
C.: He's getting in his car̲̊.
E.: Looks that way.
C.: Or̲̊, he's scr̲̊atchin' paint off his car̲̟.
E.: Maybe a witness, huh? Watchin' it all.
C.: Yeah.

MODULE TIME	
TOTAL	4:39
ELAPSED	13:16–17:55

Clinical Phonetics Tape 4B Practice Module #6: /r/ in Continuous Speech; Sample 1, Continued

TWO-WAY SCORING SHEET

E.: Could have. . . . How do you think this lady feels? I think maybe . . .
C.: She feel(s) mad!
E.: Oh boy . . .
C.: . . . and trash cans, trash over there for truck.
E.: What 'bout him?
C.: He could've broke the window too.
E.: What's he doing?
C.: He's going around the block.
E.: Yeah, he's getting out of there, isn't he . . .
C.: Uh huh. So is he.
E.: Yeah. What would you do in that situation if you'd broken a window while you were playing baseball?
C.: I'd go running . . .
E.: Would ya?
C.: Yeah . . . probably [go ahead] probably playin' baseball in the middle of the street.
E.: Yeah . . . if you had broken the window, do you think you should say something?
C.: . . . sorry!!
E.: Yeah . . . what's this man doing over here?
C.: He's getting in his car.
E.: Looks that way.
C.: Or, he's scratchin' paint off his car.
E.: Maybe a witness, huh? Watchin' it all.
C.: Yeah.

Practice Module #7: /r/ in Continuous Speech; Sample 2

PROCEED TO: Clinical Phonetics Tape 4B: Practice Module #7: /r/ in Continuous Speech; Sample 2

MODULE TIME	
TOTAL	3:13
ELAPSED	17:55–21:08

Clinical Phonetics Tape 4B
Practice Module #7:
/r/ in Continuous Speech; Sample 2

TWO-WAY SCORING KEY

E.: What did you get for Christmas?
C.: A bike . . . a helmet . . . a . . . race car set . . .
E.: Hmm . . . tell me about that race car set.
C.: It's electric . . . you plug it into the wall . . . and ya gotta set it up anyway ya want it to [Mhmm] . . . you want it to, except ya gotta put the car on these one little things where the electricity comes into the car [Mhmm] . . . and it goes around the track.
E.: Hmm . . . sounds neat.
C.: And sometimes you can make a bridge.
E.: Hmm, out of what?
C.: Out of the, out of the things that go like that [Mhmm] . . . and . . . and it goes up ta one hundred and sixty.
E.: Oh my gosh . . . hundred and sixty?
C.: First it starts out with twenty . . . then it goes to forty, then eighty, then one hundred ta sixty.
E.: Oh my gosh, that goes pretty fast, doesn't it. Do you have any pets?
C.: No.
E.: Who are your best friends?
C.: Byron.
E.: Byron . . .
C.: . . . and Richie.
E.: Byron and Richie. What do you, what do the three of you do together?
C.: We ride bikes sometimes [Mhmm] . . . and we . . .
E.: What else do you do?
C.: . . . play guns [Uhuh] . . . and sometimes I push Byron in his wagon.
E.: Oh . . . Let's look at one of these pictures . . . tell me something about this picture.
C.: A fireman's carrying a hurt guy.
E.: How'd he get hurt?
C.: In the fire.
E.: Well how could he get his head hurt in the fire? . . . What do you 'spose happened to him?
C.: He fell through the floor.
E.: What do you think started the fire?
C.: . . . Gasoline.
E.: How could the gasoline get started?
C.: Some guys could sneak in and start it.
E.: Oh, you mean you think it happened on purpose, huh? What are the firemen doing here?
C.: Puttin' out the fire.
E.: And they're . . .
C.: Climbing the ladder.<too weak>
E.: Are there different kinds of fire trucks, or, do you know . . .
C.: They're all the same except for the chief's car.
E.: The chief's car . . . what is this?
C.: A fire hydrant . . .

MODULE TIME	
TOTAL	3:13
ELAPSED	17:55–21:08

Clinical Phonetics Tape 4B Practice Module #7: /ɾ/ in Continuous Speech; Sample 2

TWO-WAY SCORING SHEET

E.: What did you get for Christmas?
C.: A bike . . . a helmet . . . a . . . race car set . . .
E.: Hmm . . . tell me about that race car set.
C.: It's electric . . . you plug it into the wall . . . and ya gotta set it up anyway ya want it to [Mhmm] . . . you want it to, except ya gotta put the car on these one little things where the electricity comes into the car [Mhmm] . . . and it goes around the track.
E.: Hmm . . . sounds neat.
C.: And sometimes you can make a bridge.
E.: Hmm, out of what?
C.: Out of the, out of the things that go like that [Mhmm] . . . and . . . and it goes up ta one hundred and sixty.
E.: Oh my gosh . . . hundred and sixty?
C.: First it starts out with twenty . . . then it goes to forty, then eighty, then one hundred ta sixty.
E.: Oh my gosh, that goes pretty fast, doesn't it. Do you have any pets?
C.: No.
E.: Who are your best friends?
C.: Byron.
E.: Byron . . .
C.: . . . and Richie.
E.: Byron and Richie. What do you, what do the three of you do together?
C.: We ride bikes sometimes [Mhmm] . . . and we . . .
E.: What else do you do?
C.: . . . play guns [Uhuh] . . . and sometimes I push Byron in his wagon.
E.: Oh . . . Let's look at one of these pictures . . . tell me something about this picture.
C.: A fireman's carrying a hurt guy.
E.: How'd he get hurt?
C.: In the fire.
E.: Well how could he get his head hurt in the fire? . . . What do you 'spose happened to him?
C.: He fell through the floor.
E.: What do you think started the fire?
C.: . . . Gasoline.
E.: How could the gasoline get started?
C.: Some guys could sneak in and start it.
E.: Oh, you mean you think it happened on purpose, huh? What are the firemen doing here?
C.: Puttin' out the fire.
E.: And they're . . .
C.: Climbing the ladder.<too weak>
E.: Are there different kinds of fire trucks, or, do you know . . .
C.: They're all the same except for the chief's car.
E.: The chief's car . . . what is this?
C.: A fire hydrant . . .

Practice Module #8: /ɾ/ in Continuous Speech; Sample 3

PROCEED TO: Clinical Phonetics Tape 4B: Practice Module #8: /ɾ/ in Continuous Speech; Sample 3

MODULE TIME	
TOTAL	3:54
ELAPSED	21:08–25:02

Clinical Phonetics Tape 4B
Practice Module #8:
/ɾ/ in Continuous Speech; Sample 3

TWO-WAY SCORING KEY

E.: And who do you play with?
C.: Umm . . . my fr̲̊iend David.
E.: A friend named David. What do you and David play?
C.: Umm . . . basketball, football, baseball, and, uh, soccer̲̊.
E.: Hmm.
C.: . . . and, uh, and sometimes, ah, pool.
E.: You play pool. . . . What kind of game is it? I really don't know much about pool.
C.: You r̲̊ack 'em up on this one r̲̊ack and, and like ther̲̊e's ones with r̲̊ed, like this r̲̊ed and other̲̊s and the ones that has the str̲̊ipes, and then the one what don't haves the str̲̊ipes . . . that's the solids . . . and the other̲̊s ar̲̊e str̲̊ipes.
E.: Hmm.
C.: And then the last one who gets all the balls and shoots the eight ball in, and then they win.
E.: Mmhmm. Do you ever win?
C.: Yeah.
E.: Who do you beat?
C.: My fr̲̊iend David.
E.: Mmhmm.
C.: And then I got one mor̲̊e fr̲̊iend . . . ah . . . he always comes down and play with me and, ah . . . and then I got lots of other̲̊ fr̲̊iends like ah . . . my fr̲̊iend Edgar̲̊. He always comes down and play with me. And . . . that's all the fr̲̊iends I got.
E.: Sounds like you've got a lot of friends. What'd ya get for Christmas?
C.: Umm . . . I got a Big Jim camper̲̊, a Big Jim war̲̊m-up suit and . . . umm, Big Jim basketball suit.
E.: Umhmm.
C.: And . . . got a walkie-talkie . . . and . . . I got a br̲̊and new bike, and . . . that's all.
E.: Sounds like you had a pretty good Christmas (sounds like a good Christmas). Did you ever see this picture . . . have you seen that?
C.: Umm, no.
E.: Can you tell me something about it?
C.: Ther̲̊e's a fir̲̊e and the fir̲̊eman came and pour̲̊ed it out and a guy got hur̲̊t in the fir̲̊e.
E.: How do you suppose he got hurt?
C.: In the fir̲̊e.
E.: What could have happened?
C.: He could, umm, started up the stove when his mom and dad was gone and he just . . . and the place star̲̊ted on fire.
E.: Hmm, but how would he get a hurt head from the fire?
C.: Maybe he fell against something when it star̲̊ted to fir̲̊e and then cr̲̊acked his head open.
E.: That could be. . . . What are the firemen doing here?
C.: Ah, climbing up and get some mor̲̊e people what's in the fir̲̊e.
E.: Umhmm. They're going to rescue them, I imagine. What is this called, you know?
C.: A fir̲̊e hydr̲̊ant.
E.: Mhmm. What are they for?
C.: Ah, for̲̊ fir̲̊es.
E.: Have you ever seen one used?
C.: My fr̲̊iend called up a fir̲̊eman and, and he said, umm to r̲̊un that thing out in the str̲̊eet so we had get wet, so we did and we got wet. . . .

MODULE TIME	
TOTAL	3:54
ELAPSED	21:08–25:02

Clinical Phonetics Tape 4B
Practice Module #8:
/r/ in Continuous Speech; Sample 3

TWO-WAY SCORING SHEET

E.: And who do you play with?
C.: Umm . . . my friend David.
E.: A friend named David. What do you and David play?
C.: Umm . . . basketball, football, baseball, and, uh, soccer.
E.: Hmm.
C.: . . . and, uh, and sometimes, ah, pool.
E.: You play pool. . . . What kind of game is it? I really don't know much about pool.
C.: You rack 'em up on this one rack and, and like there's ones with red, like this red and others and the ones that has the stripes, and then the one what don't haves the stripes . . . that's the solids . . . and the others are stripes.
E.: Hmm.
C.: And then the last one who gets all the balls and shoots the eight ball in, and then they win.
E.: Mmhmm. Do you ever win?
C.: Yeah.
E.: Who do you beat?
C.: My friend David.
E.: Mmhmm.
C.: And then I got one more friend . . . ah . . . he always comes down and play with me and, ah . . . and then I got lots of other friends like ah . . . my friend Edgar. He always comes down and play with me. And . . . that's all the friends I got.
E.: Sounds like you've got a lot of friends. What'd ya get for Christmas?
C.: Umm . . . I got a Big Jim camper, a Big Jim warm-up suit and . . . umm, Big Jim basketball suit.
E.: Umhmm.
C.: And . . . got a walkie-talkie . . . and . . . I got a brand new bike, and . . . that's all.
E.: Sounds like you had a pretty good Christmas (sounds like a good Christmas). Did you ever see this picture . . . have you seen that?
C.: Umm, no.
E.: Can you tell me something about it?
C.: There's a fire and the fireman came and poured it out and a guy got hurt in the fire.
E.: How do you suppose he got hurt?
C.: In the fire.
E.: What could have happened?
C.: He could, umm, started up the stove when his mom and dad was gone and he just . . . and the place started on fire.
E.: Hmm, but how would he get a hurt head from the fire?
C.: Maybe he fell against something when it started to fire and then cracked his head open.
E.: That could be. . . . What are the firemen doing here?
C.: Ah, climbing up and get some more people what's in the fire.
E.: Umhmm. They're going to rescue them, I imagine. What is this called, you know?
C.: A fire hydrant.
E.: Mhmm. What are they for?
C.: Ah, for fires.
E.: Have you ever seen one used?
C.: My friend called up a fireman and, and he said, umm to run that thing out in the street so we had get wet, so we did and we got wet. . . .

Practice Module #9: All Sounds in Continuous Speech; Sample 1

Transcribing all sounds in continuous speech can be considered the "grand quiz" of this chapter. Your task in these two modules is to transcribe each word in a series of continuous speech samples using all the appropriate symbols and diacritics for phonetic transcription. If it has been some time since you have used all the phonetic and diacritic symbols, review Chapter 6 and the material in Chapter 8. Obviously, this task ranks as the most difficult in the realm of clinical transcription (Figure 1-1, cell 24). The gloss provided on the left-hand page is the *consensus* from our panel—you may not agree with each and every transcription. You may wish to transcribe each of the two samples once without reference to the gloss. As discussed in Chapter 7, having available a gloss of what the child intended to say can influence markedly our perception of speech.

PROCEED TO: Clinical Phonetics Tape 4B: Practice Module #9: All Sounds in Continuous Speech; Sample 1

MODULE TIME	
TOTAL	1:29
ELAPSED	25:02–26:31

Clinical Phonetics Tape 4B Practice Module #9: All Sounds in Continuous Speech; Sample 1

TRANSCRIPTION KEY

Clinician	*Child*	*Transcription*
What kind of things do you do?	Well, well, I don't have any more school, so . . .	[wɛl wɛl ɑ͡ɪ dõ æʌ ɛnɪ mɔr su so͡ʊ]
Now you don't have any more school so what . . .	I stay home all day.	[ɑ͡ɪ s̺ e͡ɪ hom ɔ dɑ͡ɪ]
You stay home all day.	Yeah, play.	[jɛɑ pʰɑeː]
(What do you) Oh, and play . . . that sounds good. What kinds of things do you play?	Well, sometimes I go to . . . over to my (??) house.	[wɛːʊ sʌmtɑ͡ɪmz ɑ͡ɪ go͡ʊ tu̟ hɑ̟rvɚ tə mɑ͡ɪ(hɑ͡ɪs̪ ɑ͡ɪ̃nz̥̟)hɑ͡ʊːs]
Sometimes you go over to your friend's house?	Yeah.	[jɛ̃ᵊ]
What do you do there?	Well, I just take my Big Wheels or something.	[wɛᵘ ɑ͡ɪ̰ əs tɛk mɑɑ̞ bɪg wiɚ sʌ̃mpɛn]
Oh, you always take your Big Wheels or something, I see.	And, um	[ɑẽn ʌːm]
What else do you do?	Well, that's about all.	[wɛ d̪ɪts̺ bɑɔːᵘ]
That's about all?	Mhmm	[mː]
Do you ever get to play with your baby brother?	Yeah . . .	[jɑːᴵ]
Yeah, what kinds of things do you do with him?	Oh, wrestle . . .	[ɑ͡ɪ̃ wɛ̟̃s̪õː]
Wrestle . . . oh.	I roll him over on my stomach.	[ɑ̟ wo͡ʊᴵm hɝ̠vɚ ɔn mɑ s̪ʌmək]
You roll him over on your stomach. Does he like that?	Yeah. He's believing it's (the) trick . . .	[jɛ hiz bɪivɪŋ hɪz̥ z̪ʌ twɪkʰ]
He what?	He's believing it's a trick.	[ɪːts bi̝ːvɪŋ ɪts̺ ə twɪk]
Oh, he's believing it's a trick. Yeah. Oh, so he thinks he's doing tricks with you, huh. Does he laugh a lot when you do that?	Yeah.	[jɪʌ]
Yeah, does he get real silly?	Goes like this ______	[ɪ go͡ʊz̥ lɑ͡ɪk dɪt k͓k͓k͓]
Oh . . .		

MODULE TIME	
TOTAL	1:29
ELAPSED	25:02–26:31

Clinical Phonetics Tape 4B
Practice Module #9:
All Sounds in Continuous Speech;
Sample 1

TRANSCRIPTION SHEET

Clinician	*Child*	*Transcription*
What kind of things do you do?	Well, well, I don't have any more school, so . . .	
Now you don't have any more school so what . . .	I stay home all day.	
You stay home all day.	Yeah, play.	
(What do you) Oh, and play . . . that sounds good. What kinds of things do you play?	Well, sometimes I go to . . . over to my (??) house.	
Sometimes you go over to your friend's house?	Yeah.	
What do you do there?	Well, I just take my Big Wheels or something.	
Oh, you always take your Big Wheels or something, I see.	And, um	
What else do you do?	Well, that's about all.	
That's about all?	Mhmm	
Do you ever get to play with your baby brother?	Yeah . . .	
Yeah, what kinds of things do you do with him?	Oh, wrestle . . .	
Wrestle . . . oh.	I roll him over on my stomach.	
You roll him over on your stomach. Does he like that?	Yeah. He's believing it's (the) trick . . .	
He what?	He's believing it's a trick.	
Oh, he's believing it's a trick. Yeah. Oh, so he thinks he's doing tricks with you, huh. Does he laugh a lot when you do that?	Yeah.	
Yeah, does he get real silly?	Goes like this ______	
Oh . . .		

Practice Module #10: All Sounds in Continuous Speech; Sample 2

PROCEED TO: Clinical Phonetics Tape 4B: Practice Module #10: All Sounds in Continuous Speech; Sample 2

MODULE TIME	
TOTAL	1:31
ELAPSED	26:31–28:02

Clinical Phonetics Tape 4B Practice Module #10: All Sounds in Continuous Speech; Sample 2

TRANSCRIPTION KEY[a]

Clinician	*Child*	*Transcription*
How do you ride home?	On the buses.	[ɑ̃n də bʌsɪs]
Oh, on the buses. Tell me about the things that you do in the morning. . . that are just like the little girl.	Get up and get dressed.	[gɛʔ ʌp æ ɪ̃n gɛʔ gwɛstʰ]
(Talkover)	(??)	
And then you eat and then the school bus?	Mm, I come home.	[m̩ ɑɪ kʌ̃m hoʊm]
And you come home. Do you go to school in the morning . . . or in the afternoon?	No, in the morning.	[noʊ ɪn ə mɔrnɪn]
In the morning. What do you do (repeat) after you come home from school then?	Play.	[pʰw̥eɪ]
What kinds of things do you play?	Toys and stuff.	[tʰɔɪz̥n̩ stʌf]
Toys and stuff? Do you ever have lunch . . . when you come home?	Yeah.	[jɛəʰ]
What kinds of things do you have for lunch?	Sandwiches (and stuff).	[s̪æ̃nwɪtʃɪz]
Stuff like that? Do you make your own sandwiches? Or does Mom make them?	Mom makes them . . . Sometimes I make them self.	[mɑ̃ meɪ̃ks əm sʌmtɑ̃ɪ̃mz ɑɪ meɪk ðəm sɛuf]
Sometimes you make them yourself . . . Mom makes them. Yeah. What kind of sandwiches do you make yourself when you make them yourself?	Cheese . . . cheese and pickles.	[tʃɪztʃizæn pɪkʊᵊz̥]
Ah, I'm not sure I know how to make a cheese sandwich. What would you do? How would you tell me how to make a cheese sandwich?	First put mustard on it—I mean that stuff on it and then put (ch . . .) meat and then put cheese and then close it up!	[fɜs pʰɪt mʌstɪd ɑ̃n ɪt ɛ̃ min ðɛt stʌf ɑ̃ɪʔ ɛnɛn pɪts̪ː mĩt ɛnɛn pʊt tʃi ənɛ̃n kwɔz̪ ɪɾ ʌp]

[a]Recall that questionable segments are circled.

MODULE TIME	
TOTAL	1:31
ELAPSED	26:31–28:02

Clinical Phonetics Tape 4B Practice Module #10: All Sounds in Continuous Speech; Sample 2

TRANSCRIPTION SHEET

Clinician	*Child*	*Transcription*
How do you ride home?	On the buses.	
Oh, on the buses. Tell me about the things that you do in the morning . . . that are just like the little girl.	Get up and get dressed.	
(Talkover)	(??)	
And then you eat and then the school bus?	Mm, I come home.	
And you come home. Do you go to school in the morning . . . or in the afternoon?	No, in the morning.	
In the morning. What do you do (repeat) after you come home from school then?	Play.	
What kinds of things do you play?	Toys and stuff.	
Toys and stuff? Do you ever have lunch . . . when you come home?	Yeah.	
What kinds of things do you have for lunch?	Sandwiches (and stuff).	
Stuff like that? Do you make your own sandwiches? Or does Mom make them?	Mom makes them . . . Sometimes I make them self.	
Sometimes you make them yourself . . . Mom makes them. Yeah. What kind of sandwiches do you make yourself when you make them yourself?	Cheese . . . cheese and pickles.	
Ah, I'm not sure I know how to make a cheese sandwich. What would you do? How would you tell me how to make a cheese sandwich?	First put mustard on it—I mean that stuff on it and then put (ch . . .) meat and then put cheese and then close it up!	

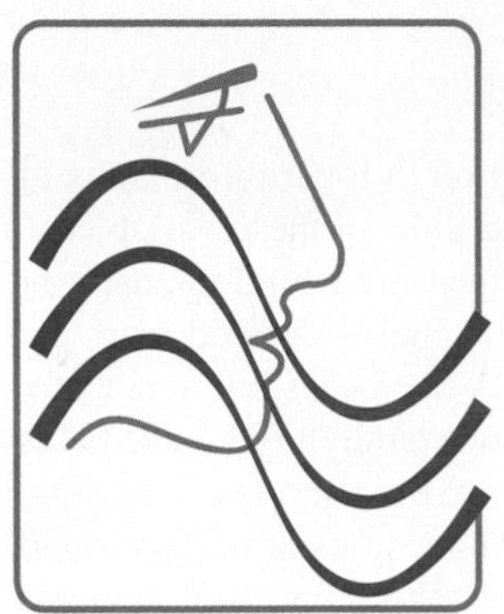

Acoustic Phonetics

10

When we hear speech, our ears sense acoustic vibrations of air molecules. Hence, the acoustic signal of speech, carried through the air, intervenes between the act of speech production in a speaker and the act of speech perception in a listener. For this reason, an understanding of the acoustics of speech is a central concern to a unified conception of communication processes and disorders. Acoustic descriptions of speech are useful for understanding both speech production and speech perception. Because changes in articulation cause changes in the acoustic output signal, we may use acoustic features to describe speech articulation, including disordered articulation. Because speech perception is based on the acoustic signals of speech, our scientific understanding of phonetic perception (including phonetic perception for the purpose of transcription) rests to a large degree on knowledge of speech acoustics.

Although acoustic analysis is not routinely used in most clinics that serve people with communication disorders, acoustic analyses can be very helpful in describing and diagnosing speech disorders and also can be used to document the effects of remediation. Acoustic analysis permits measurement or quantification of the physical signal of speech. Quantification is advantageous not only for the purposes of research but for clinical purposes as well. This chapter discusses the elements of speech acoustics. Because an understanding of basic concepts in acoustics is prerequisite to an understanding of the acoustics of speech, we begin with a brief introduction to the physics of sound.

BASIC CONCEPTS OF ACOUSTICS

Acoustics is the branch of physics that deals with the study of sound. In this chapter the interest is with sounds that can be produced by the human vocal tract and perceived by the human ear. Thus, the focus is on sounds that can be perceived and interpreted by the brain in relation to units of meaning. However, the discussion of this area is most conveniently introduced with a sound that probably is never produced by a human vocal tract and is rarely heard by the human ear except in laboratories. The sound is that produced by a simple tuning fork, as illustrated in Figure 10-1. The sound is called a **pure tone**.

The Basic Dimensions of Sound

When we strike a tuning fork, its tines vibrate (move to and fro) a certain number of times per second (Figure 10-1). The vibratory rate often is inscribed on the fork. For example, a fork bearing the number 512 will vibrate at the rate of 512 complete to-and-fro motions per second. Each complete to-and-fro movement is called a **cycle** of vibration. The word *cycle* implies a regular or periodic event, one that repeats itself in time. The number of cycles of vibration per unit of time is called the **frequency** of vibration and is expressed in units called **hertz (Hz)** when the number of cycles is counted for an interval of one second. Generally, as the frequency in hertz increases, the pitch of the sound, as perceived by the human ear, goes up. Thus, a tuning fork that vibrates at 1024 Hz will be perceived as having a higher pitch than one that vibrates at 512 Hz. In brief, the frequency of a sound refers to its rate of vibration, with higher frequencies being heard as having a higher pitch.

Depending on how hard the tuning fork is struck, the tines of the fork undergo different degrees of movement as they vibrate. As the fork is struck more forcefully, the tines have a larger movement, or **displacement.** As the displacement of the fork tines increases, a louder sound is heard. The amplitude (magnitude) of displacement relates roughly to the loudness of the sound. Actually, what a person hears is not directly the displacement of the tines but rather the effect of fork vibration on the air molecules between the fork and the person's ear. Because air is elastic, a displaced air particle

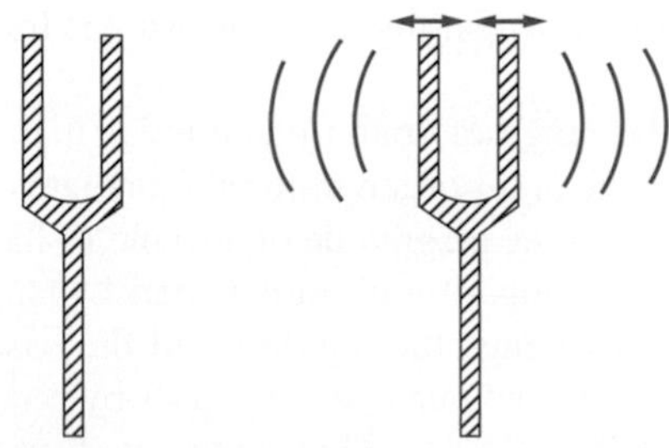

FIGURE 10-1
A tuning fork and its vibration. When the fork is struck, its tines undergo a to-and-fro vibration.

tends to return to its original position. As a tuning fork vibrates, the air particles also undergo a to-and-fro motion, causing the energy of the fork to be carried from particle to particle. In acoustic terms, the vibratory energy of the fork is propagated, or carried, by the air molecules. As the air molecules vibrate in response to the tuning fork, the air pressure at a person's eardrum varies in relation to the fork's frequency. The variations in pressure occur as molecules of air move to and fro, in a kind of chain reaction, with the vibrating fork.

The magnitude of a sound can be expressed in several different ways. Of primary importance are amplitude, intensity, and sound pressure. **Amplitude,** as just mentioned in relation to the vibrating tuning fork, is the displacement of particles subjected to vibration. Amplitude is difficult and inconvenient to measure for general purposes because the motions of particles are minute. **Intensity** is a measure of the energy that passes in unit time through unit area taken perpendicularly at any point to the direction of propagation at that point. Intensities of sound typically are measured in microwatts (energy) per square centimeter (area). The intensity of a sound wave is proportional both to the square of its amplitude and to the square of its frequency. This fact should be understandable on intuitive grounds if you recognize that (1) more energy is required for vibrations of greater displacement (amplitude), and (2) more energy is needed as frequency of vibration increases, because more to-and-fro motion occurs per unit of time. We judge the loudness of sounds more in accord with their intensity than their amplitude. Therefore, intensity is preferable to amplitude when discussing our reactions to sound. Because microphones respond to sound pressure changes rather than to intensity changes, sound pressure measurements have considerable practical value. **Sound pressure** is acoustic pressure in terms of force per unit of area. Although sound pressure now is specified by a unit called the pascal, an earlier and now outdated unit is easier to understand in terms of the measurement procedure. The earlier unit was the dyne per square centimeter (dyne/cm^2). The dyne is a measure of force, and the square centimeter is a measure of area. Tire inflation is specified by a similar unit: Air pressure in automobile tires is given in pounds (force) per square inch (area). In brief, we may summarize as follows: Amplitude is magnitude of particle displacement; intensity is energy flow per unit area; pressure is force per unit area.

Because the range of sound magnitudes that we hear is very large, on the order of ten million to one, it is more convenient to express the magnitude of a sound (either intensity or pressure) on a logarithmic rather than linear scale. For acoustic measurements, the logarithm to the base 10 is favored. This means that our scale increases by powers of ten: 1, 10, 100, 1000, and so on. Thus, the range from one to ten million can be covered in seven scale units rather than the ten million needed for a linear scale. The logarithmic scale is important for another basic reason. Judgments of the loudness of sounds are made more in relation to logarithmic units of intensity or pressure than to linear units of these variables.

The logarithmic unit used to measure sound intensity or pressure is the **decibel.** In fact, decibel is derived from the more fundamental unit, the **bel.** A decibel is one tenth of a bel (the morpheme *deci-* means "one tenth"). But a decibel is more than a simple logarithmic unit. In fact, *it is a logarithm of a ratio,* the ratio of two sound intensities or of two sound pressures. In the case of intensity, the number of decibels (dB) is given by the formula:

$$\text{No. of dB} = 10 \log_{10} \frac{\text{Intensity of one sound}}{\text{Intensity of a reference sound}}$$

That is, the intensity of one sound is expressed relative to the intensity of a standard or reference sound (usually 10^{-16} watts, where 10^{-16} means a decimal point followed by 15 zeros and a one). By analogy, we might express the weight of lumps of coal by comparing them to a reference lump. One lump might be twice as heavy as the reference lump, but another might be one hundred times as heavy. (In case you did not see it, the 10 immediately to the right of the equals sign is there because we are measuring *decibels* rather than *bels.*)

Because pressure is related to the square of intensity, the formula for decibels of sound pressure is different from that for intensity by a factor of two:

$$\text{No. of dB} = 20 \log_{10} \frac{\text{Pressure of one sound}}{\text{Pressure of a reference sound}}$$

The reference most commonly used for sound pressure is 0.0002 micropascal (or 0.0002 dyne/cm^2), which is the sound pressure of the faintest sound we can hear.

The tone generated by the tuning fork is of special importance in acoustics, because the description of other kinds of sounds is based on this elemental sound pattern. Essentially, more complex sounds are described as combinations of the elemental pure tones. The pure tones sometimes are called **sinusoids,** in recognition of a feature illustrated in Figure 10-2. This drawing shows a pencil attached to one tine of a fork. (In fact, this demonstration is more theoretical than practical, because the pencil would interfere with fork vibration.) Imagine that the tuning fork is drawn along from right to left so that the vibrating pencil leaves a trace on the paper. This trace takes the form of the trigonometric sine function, and that is why the pure tone is called a sinusoid. The trace shown in the figure is called a **waveform,** a graph of displacement against time. Figure 10-3 shows how the waveform of a sinusoid changes as frequency (rate of vibration) and amplitude (magnitude of vibration) are altered.

An important concept related to the waveform of a sound is that of **wavelength,** which is the linear distance between one point on a wave and the same point on the next wave. A simple analogy is one of waves on an ocean. The wavelength of the water waves is the distance between, for example, the crest of one wave and the crest of the following wave. This distance also could be measured between the troughs of two successive waves (see Figure 10-4). So long as the waves repeat at regular intervals, the wavelength can be measured as the distance between any two corresponding points of successive waves. The wavelength (symbol λ) is equal to the speed of sound *(c)* divided by the frequency of the sound *(f)*: $\lambda = c/f$. At sea level and a temperature of about 70° Fahrenheit, the speed of sound is about 1130 feet/second. Thus, the wavelength of a 100-Hz sinusoid would be equal to 1130 feet/second divided by 100 Hz, or 11.3 feet. A sinusoid of 100 Hz repeats itself over a physical distance of 11.3 feet. In this way, we can think of sound waves as being distributed spatially.

Actually, the wave motion for water waves and sound waves is not of the same type. A water wave is a **transverse wave,** or a wave in which particle motion is at right angles to the direction in which the wave travels. By way of illustration, a duck sitting on a lake bobs up and down with the wave motion, that is, it moves at a right angle to the direction of the moving wave. A sound wave is a **longitudinal wave,** or a wave in which particle motion is a back-and-forth oscillation along the line of the wave. The sound wave is a kind of chain reaction in which one particle strikes its neighbor, which in turn strikes its neighbor, and so on. However, the general idea of wavelength applies to both types of wave motion.

Figure 10-5 illustrates a very important graph called a **spectral plot** or a **spectrum.** The vertical axis represents amplitude and the horizontal axis represents frequency. A pure tone or sinusoid is represented as a single line on this graph. The frequency of the tone is given by the value on the (horizontal) *x*-axis, and the amplitude is given by the (vertical) *y*-axis value (or the height of the line). More sinusoids can be added to make **complex tones,** so that more lines appear in the spectrum. When several tuning forks sound together, the spectral plot of the complex result is shown in Figure 10-6. This spectrum is similar to that of the tone produced by the vibrating larynx before this tone is modified by the vocal tract. The laryngeal tone of voiced speech has energy at several frequencies that are **harmonically** related. That is, the frequencies are integer multiples of the lowest, or fundamental, frequency. If a speaker has a fundamental frequency of 125 Hz, then his or her laryngeal tone also will have energy at 250 Hz, 375 Hz, 500 Hz, etc. (125 Hz × 2, 125 Hz × 3, 125 Hz × 4, . . .).

We emphasize that the waveform (time pattern) and spectrum (frequency pattern) are alternative displays for the analysis of a given sound. It is possible by certain mathe-

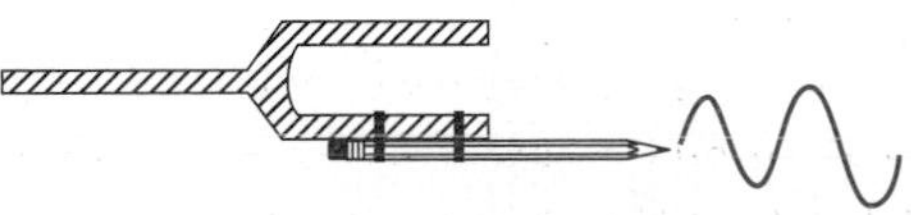

FIGURE 10-2
An imaginary demonstration in which a pencil attached to a vibrating tuning fork traces a sinusoidal pattern as the fork is drawn across a writing surface.

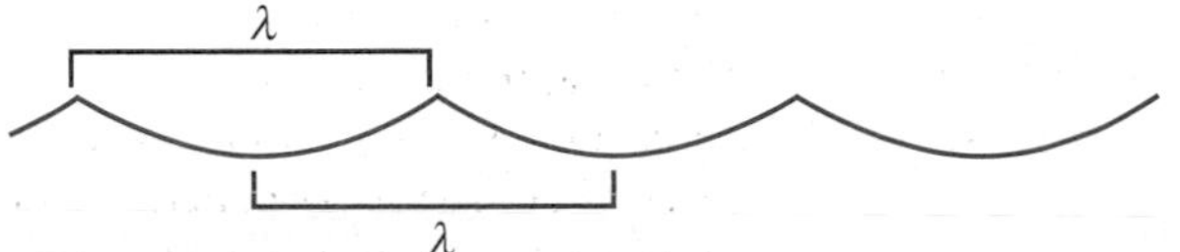

FIGURE 10-4
Concept of wavelength (λ) illustrated by analogy to water waves. The analogy is not exact, because water waves are transverse waves, whereas sound waves are longitudinal waves.

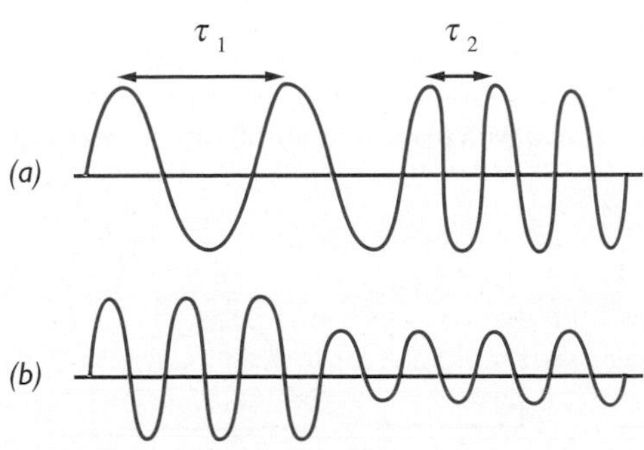

FIGURE 10-3
Changes in waveform as frequency *(a)* and amplitude *(b)* of sinusoidal vibration are changed. The tone in *(a)* would be perceived to increase in pitch, and the tone in *(b)* would be perceived to decrease in loudness. The symbols τ_1 and τ_2 designate the fundamental period of vibration ($\tau = l/f_0$).

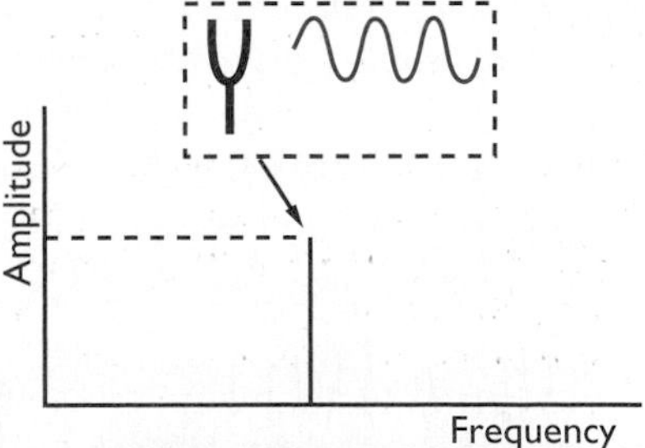

FIGURE 10-5
Spectrum, or amplitude-by-frequency plot of sound energy. The spectrum of a pure tone or sinusoid is a straight line, indicating that the acoustic energy is located at one frequency. The height of the line represents peak amplitude (intensity or sound pressure could be used instead of amplitude). The dashed line projects the height or magnitude of the line onto the amplitude axis. The insert shows a tuning fork and a sinusoidal waveform.

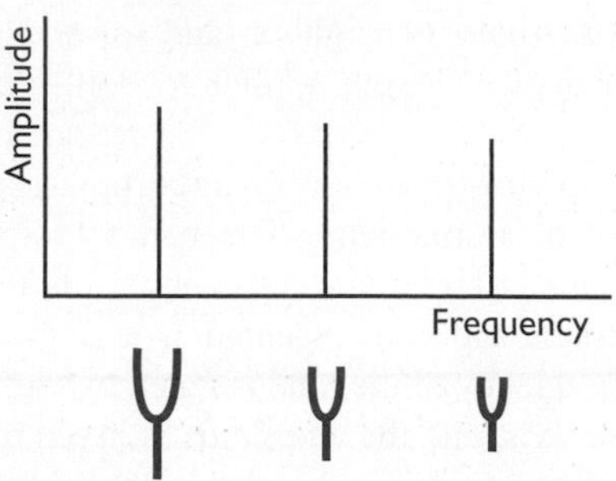

FIGURE 10-6
Spectrum for three tuning forks sounding simultaneously. Each fork is associated with one line of the spectrum. The resulting sound is a complex tone.

matics to calculate the spectrum if the waveform is known and to calculate the waveform if the spectrum is known. But for present purposes, it is sufficient to know that waveform and spectrum are complementary in the sense that time and frequency are related (frequency is the reciprocal of time). Periodic sounds have waveforms that repeat themselves at some regular intervals and spectra that contain separate and distinct lines of acoustic energy. Nonperiodic sounds have random structure in both their waveforms and their spectra. Examples of a waveform and spectra for nonperiodic sounds are shown in Figure 10-7.

Resonance

One other basic concept is that of **resonance.** *Resonance is a frequency-selective reinforcement of sound energy.* In other words, energy at only certain frequencies is strengthened. The frequency at which resonance occurs depends on the physical characteristics of the resonating object. A sketch of a very simple resonator is given in Figure 10-8. A tuning fork is placed near the mouth of a tube containing a plunger. The plunger allows the effective length of the tube to be adjusted so that it resonates at different frequencies. When the plunger is adjusted at just the right position, the tone from the tuning fork will increase in loudness. The nature of this process goes beyond the scope of this chapter, but a general explanation is that when the tube is of a certain length, an air molecule at its mouth is subjected to two vibratory forces at the same instant, one force directly from the tuning fork (a direct sound wave) and another force that bounces back from the closed end of the tube (a reflected sound wave). The combination of these two forces causes the air molecule to be displaced more greatly than it would be from one force alone.

A basic principle of resonance is that a body oscillates (vibrates) with greater amplitude for applied frequencies that are near its own natural frequency. In the case of air-filled tubes, the natural frequency is determined by the length and shape of the tube. Air-filled tubes are of special interest because the human vocal tract behaves acoustically as an air-filled tube. To illustrate this principle, we will consider a special case in vowel production, in which the tongue is so positioned that the cross-sectional area of the vocal tract is uniform along its length. That is, a cross section taken at any one place is equal to one taken anywhere else. We can make matters even simpler by straightening the vocal tract (by

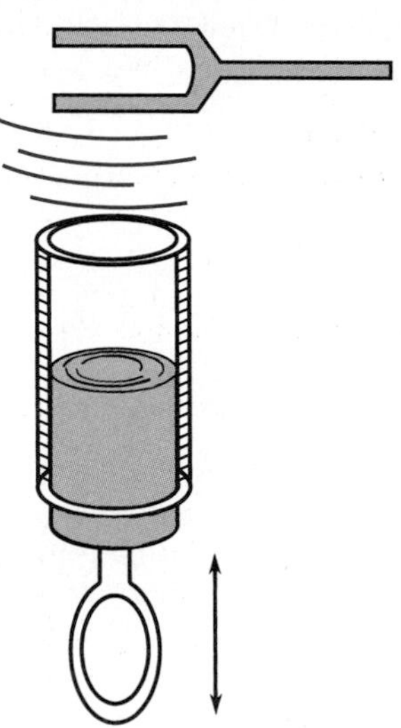

FIGURE 10-8
Demonstration of resonance, using the tuning fork as an energy source and a tube with plunger as an adjustable resonator.

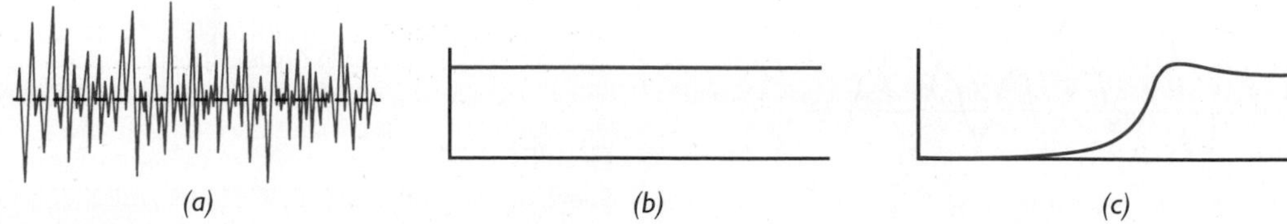

FIGURE 10-7
Examples of waveform and spectra for nonperiodic sounds. The waveform shown in *(a)* is nonperiodic because it does not repeat itself at regular intervals. The spectra shown in *(b)* and *(c)* represent two different kinds of noise—"white" noise in *(b)* and "colored" (frequency-shaped) noise in *(c)*. Because energy is continuously distributed over the frequency axis for these noise sounds, it is sufficient to draw the spectral envelope. Note that these continuous spectra are quite different from the line spectra shown in Figures 10-5 and 10-6.

imagination!) so that we have a straight tube rather than a curved one (the acoustic principles remain essentially the same despite this change in geometry).

The vowel of which we speak is the mid-central /ə/, or schwa. Vowel /ɛ/ also is fairly close to this configuration, particularly if the tongue position is somewhat retracted from its normal front carriage. The important feature is that the cross-sectional area of the vocal tract is essentially constant along its length. If this property is satisfied, this vowel is acoustically equivalent to a straight tube or pipe of uniform diameter. The vocal tract for vowel production is effectively closed at one end (the laryngeal end), because the vibrating vocal folds (the source of sound energy) act as a tube closure. Therefore, we also require that our pipe model be closed at one end and open at the lips.

A uniform pipe closed at one end and open at the other has resonance frequencies determined by the formula:

$$f_n = (2n - 1)c \div (4 \times le)$$

where f_n is a particular resonance frequency

n is an integer (1, 2, 3, . . .)

c is the speed of sound (let's take it to be 34,000 centimeters/second)

le is the length of the vocal tract (about 17 centimeters for an adult male)

The first resonance frequency of this pipe is calculated as follows:

$$f_1 = (2 - 1)\ 34{,}000\ \text{cm/s} \div (4 \times 17\ \text{cm})$$

$$= 34{,}000\ \text{cm/s} \div 68\ \text{cm}$$

$$= 500\ \frac{\text{cm/s}}{\text{cm}}$$ (the centimeter units cancel to leave seconds in the divisor)

$$= 500\ \text{Hz}$$ (we convert from reciprocal time to the equivalent frequency unit)

Continuing these calculations for the integers 2, 3, and 4, we learn that the first four resonances of this tube have the frequencies of 500, 1500, 2500, and 3500 Hz. Acoustic measurements on vowel /ə/ produced by adult male speakers yield values that agree with this result. Hence, this one special vowel can be modeled by a pipe of uniform diameter. Like the pipe, the human vocal tract has multiple resonances.

What happens if the tongue is not exactly in the center of the vocal tract, so that the cross-sectional area changes over the length of the tract? The major consequence is that the resonance frequencies no longer occur at regular intervals (note that for the central vowel /ə/, the resonance frequencies for an adult male occur with a spacing of 1000 Hz). For other vowels, the resonances are not uniformly spaced. For example, for vowel /i/, the first resonance has a low frequency (less than 500 Hz), and the second resonance has a high frequency (above 1500 Hz). For vowel /ɑ/, the first resonance has a high frequency (above 500 Hz), but the second resonance has a low frequency (below 1500 Hz). Thus, each vowel can be described by its particular pattern of resonance frequencies.

The formula given above sometimes is called the odd quarter-wavelength relationship. The term *odd* derives from the fact that the expression $(2n - 1)$ yields only odd numbers. The term *quarter wavelength* refers to the fact that the resonance frequency of the pipe is determined by the divisor $(4 \times le)$. What this expression means is that such a pipe will vibrate with maximum amplitude a sinusoid whose wavelength is four times as long as the pipe. The number four comes into consideration because when the pipe is just one-fourth as long as the wavelength of the tone, an air molecule sitting at the mouth of the pipe is subjected simultaneously to two forces that cause particle vibration in the same direction, one force from the direct sound wave and the other force from a reflected sound wave. The coincidence of direct and reflected sound waves occurs only when the pipe is of just the right length in relation to the tone. Under this same condition, a fixed pattern of vibration, called a **standing wave,** develops in the pipe. In this pattern, particles located at some points in the pipe do not vibrate at all, whereas particles at other points are subjected to a strong vibration. Standing waves occur only under the condition of resonance. A pipe that resonates to a tone of 500 Hz may not resonate to one of 710 Hz, because a standing wave occurs only when the wavelength of the tone has a certain relation to the length of the pipe.

Because physical objects have certain natural frequencies, or frequencies at which they tend to resonate, we will hear the effects of resonance only if sound energy of the appropriate frequency is applied. You might have heard a piano vibrate in response to another sound, such as a singer's voice. The resonance (or sympathetic vibration) occurred because the piano had a natural frequency equal to some component of the external sound.

VOWEL ACOUSTICS

Vowel production is a matter of shaping the vocal tract so that its resonance frequencies reinforce selected harmonic components of the laryngeal tone. The human vocal tract has several effective resonance frequencies, and their combined effect on the laryngeal tone yields a vowel sound. As the vocal tract is changed in shape and length, its resonance frequencies change and the vowel quality therefore changes. In brief, vowels are made by adjusting the resonator (vocal tract) to shape the laryngeal tone in certain ways.

In our classes, we have used the following demonstration of sound production. As shown in Figure 10-9, a cow larynx, secured from a local meatpacking plant, is attached to a shop vacuum cleaner that can be reversed to serve as a blower. We use the vacuum cleaner to blow air through the larynx and use our fingers to close and tense the cow's vocal folds. When the proper closing and tensing force is applied, the vocal folds vibrate. The resulting sound is not particularly interesting, being little more than a flat buzz. However, if a wastebasket is placed over the vibrating cow larynx, the sound is transformed to something that much more closely resembles a cow's bellow. The wastebasket acts like the cow's vocal tract to produce resonances. The same experiment might be done with an electrolarynx (an electrically driven artificial larynx) in place of the cow larynx.

The cow larynx–wastebasket demonstration summarizes the basic acoustic properties of vowel production. In human speech, the sound energy produced by the vibrating vocal folds is shaped by the resonances of the vocal tract. Human vowel sounds have several resonances, ranging from low frequency to high frequency. When the vocal tract is reshaped by a change in articular positions, the pattern of resonances changes. Thus, a particular combination of articulator positions is associated with a vocal tract shape, which is in turn associated with a particular pattern of resonances. The resonances of the vocal tract are called **formants.**

Formants are visible on an acoustic display of speech as pronounced bands of energy. A commonly used acoustic display in speech is the **spectrogram,** which is illustrated in Figures 10-10 and 10-11. This display is a three-dimensional pattern representing time from left to right on the horizontal dimension, frequency (closely related to our perception of pitch) from bottom to top on the vertical dimension, and intensity (related to amplitude and to our perception of loudness) as variations in the degree of blackness (sometimes called the gray scale).

Conventionally, spectrograms are of two types, **wide band** and **narrow band,** and the difference between them is important to the most effective analysis of speech sounds. These terms apply to the size of the analyzing filters. Basically, a **filter** is a kind of acoustic "window" through which we view a sound. More precisely, a filter is a frequency-selective system for sound transmission. Sounds of certain frequencies are passed by the filter, while sounds of other frequencies are not. Filters are basic to many techniques of spectral analysis, and the spectrograph is a good example. What the spectrograph does is to show by means of a black

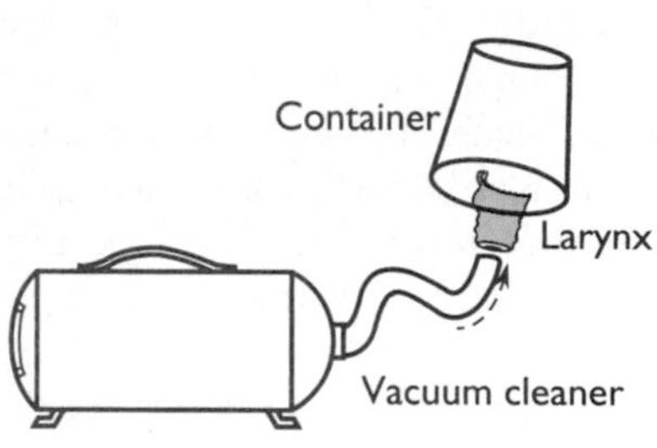

FIGURE 10-9
Laboratory demonstration of source–resonator concept of vowel production, using a vacuum cleaner, cow larynx, and wastebasket container.

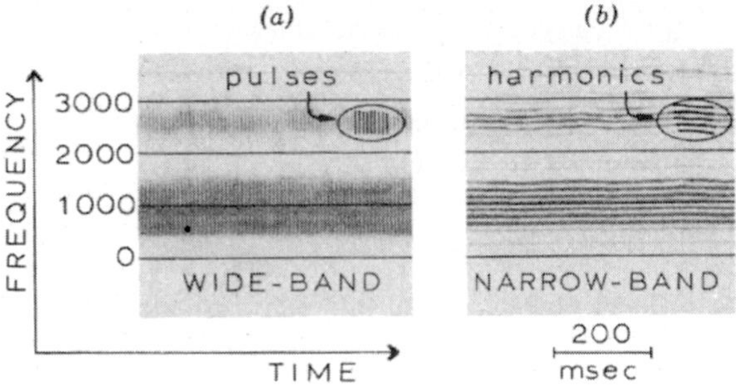

FIGURE 10-10
Wide-band *(a)* and narrow-band *(b)* spectrograms of vowel /ɑ/. Frequency in Hz is scaled on the vertical axis.

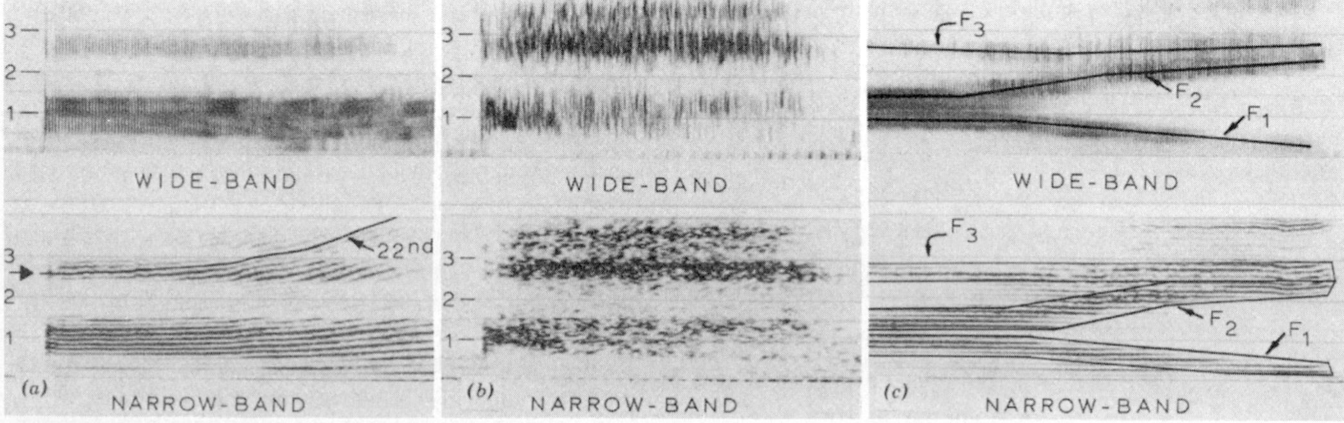

FIGURE 10-11
Part *(a)* shows wide-band and narrow-band spectrograms of vowel /ɑ/ produced with a rising f_0 (increasing vocal pitch). Part *(b)* shows a whispered /ɑ/, and part *(c)* shows a deliberately slow production of diphthong /ɑ͡ɪ/ (note formant-frequency changes: F_1 decreases, and F_2 increases). Frequency is scaled in kilohertz (kHz).

trace on a piece of paper the amount of energy that is detected in a certain frequency region, or band. When the analyzing filter is narrow (usually meaning 45 Hz in width), the spectrogram gives us a fine resolution in frequency, because we are using many narrow bands to study the sound. When the analyzing filter is wide (usually meaning 300 Hz in width), the spectrogram gives us a much coarser frequency analysis. We might put it this way: A narrow-band filter can distinguish two sounds that are only about 45 Hz apart in frequency, but a wide-band filter will "see" these two sounds as one.

Whether we use a wide-band or narrow-band filter depends on our objective in acoustic analysis (see Figure 10-10). If our interest is in harmonics, which are uniformly spaced at intervals equal to the fundamental frequency, then we usually want to use a narrow filter, because the harmonics are sometimes closely spaced in frequency and are individually narrow in frequency range. But if we are interested primarily in formants, then we usually will choose a wide filter, because the formants are so broad as to extend over two or more harmonics. Furthermore, the choice of narrow versus wide filter depends on whether we want fine resolution in frequency or time. As mentioned earlier, frequency and time are inversely related. This inverse relation is not just a mathematical fancy, for it has strong implications for the physical analysis of sound. When we narrow our "frequency window" to get a fine look at frequency, we necessarily enlarge our "time window" so that detail about events in time is somewhat lost. Conversely, when we narrow the "time window" to look at very brief events in time, we necessarily enlarge our "frequency window" so that detail about frequency is somewhat lost. For the most detailed analysis of time, a wide filter is needed. For the most detailed analysis of frequency, a narrow filter is needed.

A good illustration of this principle concerns how vocal fold vibration is represented in wide-band and narrow-band spectrograms. In the wide-band pattern, resolution is better in time than in frequency. As a result, vocal fold vibration usually appears as vertical striations, each one of which represents a glottal pulse (Figure 10-10). Because the pulses appear as long streaks along the frequency axis, their characterization by frequency is crude. In the narrow-band pattern, resolution is better in frequency than in time. Therefore, vocal fold vibration appears as a harmonic pattern in which the individual harmonics appear one on top of the other along the frequency axis (Figure 10-10). However, this resolution in frequency is gained by a loss of detail in time, as the individual glottal pulses are no longer evident in the spectrogram. Thus, we have a trade-off: When we want fine frequency detail, we must sacrifice time detail; and when we want fine time detail, we must sacrifice frequency detail. We cannot have both in the same analysis.

A general principle is to use the wide-band spectrograms to detect formants and to study acoustic changes that occur over very short intervals (like voice onset times). The narrow-band spectrogram is better for frequency-oriented analyses, such as harmonic patterns associated with the voicing source or noise patterns that remain spectrally stable over long periods of time.

Wide-band and narrow-band spectrograms of three speech utterances are shown in Figure 10-11. Part *(a)* of this figure represents a sustained vowel /ɑ/ produced with a rising vowel pitch by an adult male. Notice the closely spaced vertical lines in the wide-band spectrogram. Each of these lines represents a pulse of air from the vibrating vocal folds. Counting the number of air pulses in a one-second interval gives the rate, or frequency, of vocal fold vibration. As discussed in Chapter 3, the average frequency of vocal fold vibration is about 120 Hz for men, 250 for women, and 400 to 500 Hz for newborns. The narrow-band spectrogram displays the laryngeal energy as a harmonic pattern. Each of the closely spaced, horizontally oriented lines is a harmonic of the source spectrum. Because this vowel was produced with a rising f_0, all of the harmonics increase in frequency toward the end of the utterance. Thus, the harmonic pattern is a visual representation of a rising inflection. The 22nd harmonic is highlighted in ink to emphasize the f_0 change in this pattern.

The pulses of air escaping from the vibrating vocal folds provide the sound energy for voiced sounds, like vowel /ɑ/. The oral and nasal cavities are resonators that reinforce or strengthen some sound waves at the expense of energy of other sound waves. For the human vocal tract, several of these resonances usually are visible in a spectrogram. These vocal tract resonances are the formants referred to earlier and are denoted as the first, second, third, and so on, formants moving up the frequency scale. On the spectrogram, each formant appears as a dark band oriented horizontally on the page. Each vowel has a particular pattern of formants, called its **formant structure,** and in most cases just the lowest two formants—the first and second—are needed to identify the vowel. For the vowel in Figure 10-11*(a),* the first formant (F_1) has a center (or middle) frequency of about 750 Hz, and the second formant (F_2) has a center frequency of about 1200 Hz. It is important to understand that formants are a feature of the resonating cavities lying above the vocal folds. As these cavities are reshaped by changes in the positions of the tongue, jaw, and lips, the formant structure also changes. *Hence, formant structure is determined by the length and shape of the vocal tract.* On the other hand, the frequency of vocal fold vibration (fundamental frequency) is determined by the length and tension of the vocal folds. Notice that as the vocal frequency in Figure 10-11*(a)* is raised dramatically, the formant structure is unchanged, but the vertical lines representing vibration of the folds become closer together.

The spectrograms in part *(b)* of Figure 10-11 show a whispered vowel /ɑ/. Because the vocal folds are not vibrating, vertical striations and harmonics are not visible. The acoustic energy that activates the formants is derived from turbulence or friction noise that is developed at the larynx. Notice that the formants are apparent as bands of energy in which certain noise components are reinforced. These spectrograms confirm that formants are a property of the vocal tract and do not require voicing (vocal fold vibration) for their excitation. Any type of acoustic energy in the appropriate frequency bands will excite the formants.

Part *(c)* of Figure 10-11 shows spectrograms of the diphthong /aɪ/ as in the word *eye*. Because a diphthong is a vowel–vowel complex, its production is marked by a change in vocal tract shape and therefore a change in formant structure. Notice that the formants assume a bending pattern in which F_1 gets lower in frequency and F_2 gets higher in frequency. The change in shape of the resonating cavities is reflected as a change in formant structure. Notice that the vocal frequency changes only slightly during the change in formant structure: The vertical lines retain a similar spacing through most of the sound. The formants in the wide-band spectrogram are highlighted by the lines drawn through the center of each formant (such center lines are taken as the estimate of formant frequency). The formants in the narrow-band spectrogram are highlighted by the lines that enclose the reinforced harmonics.

The narrow-band spectrogram of an evenly intoned vowel /ɑ/ in Figure 10-12 shows us a picture of the reinforcement that formants give to certain harmonics. This spectrogram was made with an analyzing filter narrow enough to resolve the individual harmonics of the speaking voice. These harmonics are the horizontal bands numbered 1 to 9 in the illustration. Note that the ninth harmonic slightly exceeds 1 kHz[1] in frequency, meaning that the fundamental frequency is somewhat higher than 100 Hz (that is, 1000 Hz divided by 9). The first formant, F_1, is apparent as an emphasis or reinforcement of the sixth and seventh harmonics (note the darkening of these harmonics relative to the others). In fact, the center frequency for this vowel was estimated to be 750 Hz. The spectrogram shows that the formant reinforces the acoustic energy that lies in its frequency region. The effects of F_2 are only weakly evident, because the higher frequencies were deemphasized in making this spectrogram.

The first and second formants, F_1 and F_2, have frequencies for different vowels that reflect in a general way the differences in tongue articulation. The relationships are depicted in Figure 10-13, in which different vowels are plotted on a graph that has two labels on each axis. One set of labels applies to tongue position (high–low and front–back), and the other set applies to F_1 and F_2 frequency values. The graph shows that vowels with a high tongue position have a low F_1 frequency, whereas vowels with a low tongue position have a high F_1 frequency. *In other words, F_1 frequency is related primarily to the articulatory feature of tongue height.* The graph also shows that vowels with a back tongue position have a low F_2 frequency, whereas vowels with a front tongue position have a high F_2 frequency. *Thus, F_2 generally is related to the feature of tongue advancement (position of the tongue body on a back–front dimension).* Table 10-1 gives the first three formant frequencies for several vowels and diphthongs (averages for adult male speakers).

The formant frequency values given in Figure 10-13 and Table 10-1 are averages for an adult male. Values for adult females are about 20 percent higher, and values for young children are higher yet. These differences with sex and age occur because the formant frequencies vary with differences in the length of the vocal tract. The longer the vocal tract, the lower the formant frequencies. Consequently, the same vowel (a vowel with the same phonemic identity) is acousti-

[1] k = *kilo* as in *kilometer; kilo* means "1000," so 1 kHz = 1000 Hz, 2 kHz = 2000 Hz, and so on.

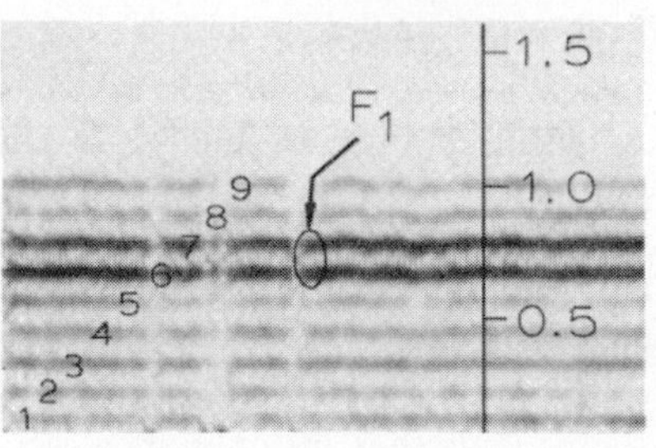

FIGURE 10-12
Narrow-band spectrogram showing the laryngeal harmonics (numbered 1 to 9) and the reinforcement of the sixth and seventh harmonics by the first formant, F_1. Frequency in kilohertz (kHz) is scaled on the vertical axis.

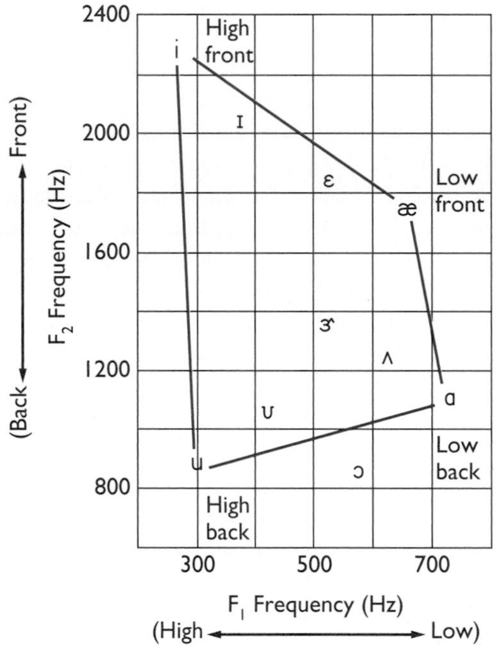

FIGURE 10-13
F_1–F_2 plot of selected vowels. The double labeling of the axes indicates that the horizontal axis (F_1 frequency) carries an articulatory interpretation of tongue position along the high–low dimension and that the vertical axis (F_2 frequency) carries an articulatory interpretation of tongue position along the back–front dimension.

TABLE 10-1
The First Three Formant Frequencies for Selected English Vowels and Diphthongs Produced by an Adult Male

Vowel Symbol	F_1	F_2	F_3
/i/	275	2250	3000
/ɪ/	400	2000	2550
/ɛ/	525	1850	2500
/æ/	650	1750	2400
/ɑ/	750	1150	2450
/ɔ/	575	850	2400
/ʊ/	450	1050	2250
/u/	300	875	2250
/ʌ/	650	1200	2400
/ɝ/	500	1350	1700
Diphthong Symbol	**F_1**	**F_2**	**F_3**
/a͡ɪ/	750–500	1250–1950	2500–2800
/ɔ͡ɪ/	550–500	830–1900	2525–2500
/a͡ʊ/	750–575	1325–900	2700–2250
/e͡ɪ/	550–400	1900–2100	2650–2700
/o͡ʊ/	575–450	900–800	2400–2350

Note: For diphthongs, formant values are given for onglide and offglide.

cally quite different when uttered by men, women, and children. Examples of vowel formant frequencies for different age and sex groups are shown in Figure 10-14.

Formant frequencies also can be used to compare and contrast the vowels in different languages. The F_1–F_2 plot is a convenient way of showing the similarity or dissimilarity between two vowels. A particular application of this approach is to study how well the vowels of one language are learned by the native speaker of another language. When the vowels in a first language (L1) and the vowels in a second language (L2) are plotted together in a F_1–F_2 plot, it is easy to judge the degree of their acoustic similarity. Research has shown that when an L1 and L2 vowel are acoustically similar but not identical, it is difficult for people to learn the "new" L2 vowel, apparently because they hear this vowel as equivalent to the similar vowel in L1 (Flege, 1987). The "new" L2 vowel is absorbed into the L1 system and treated to be identical to an "old" L1 vowel, even though the "new" vowel is acoustically distinct from the "old" vowel. The language learner's auditory perception of the L2 vowel overlooks the acoustic differences between the two vowels and considers them to be identical. In contrast, when a vowel in L2 has no counterpart in L1, it is usually fairly easy to learn the new L2 vowel.

An example of L2 vowel learning is the case of a native speaker of American English learning French (Flege, 1987). Both languages have a vowel symbolized as [u] (as in the

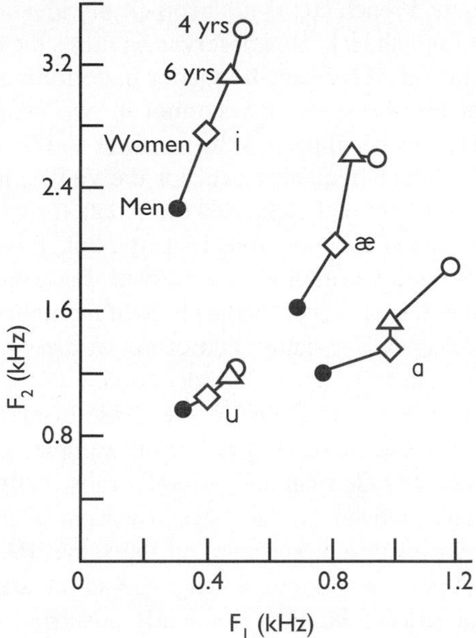

FIGURE 10-14
F_1 and F_2 frequencies for the vowels /i u ɑ æ/, showing mean values for men, women, six-year-old children, and four-year-old children.

English word *two* and the French word *tous*), but the two vowels are not acoustically identical. The vowel [u] as produced by a native speaker of French has a lower F_2 frequency than the supposedly "same" vowel produced by a native speaker of English. When native speakers of American English try to learn the French vowel, they tend to produce it with a relatively high F_2 frequency appropriate for the English [u]. Consequently, it does not sound like a French [u]. But now consider the French vowel /y/ (as in the French word *une*), which is unlike any vowel in American English. The French /y/ would be located approximately at the midpoint between vowel [i] and vowel [u] in the F_1–F_2 plot of Figure 10-13. It is not acoustically similar to any vowel in American English. The French vowel /y/ is learned relatively easily by native speakers of American English, presumably because of its acoustic distinctiveness.

These principles also apply to a native speaker of American English who tries to learn Spanish (or vice versa). Although Spanish has five vowels (/i e o a u/) that might appear to be the same as five nominal IPA vowels in American English, none of the Spanish vowels is a perfect match to a vowel from American English (Dalbor, 1980; Quiles, 1981; Flege, 1989). Flege (1989) observed that the tongue body has a higher position for Spanish /i/ than for English /i/ and that the tongue body is lower and farther back for Spanish /u/ than for English /u/.

This issue brings up an interesting point. It may seem reasonable that if a pair of languages have a vowel that is represented with the same IPA symbol, then the vowels in the two languages should be acoustically identical. But as we just discussed, the French [u] is not acoustically identical to the American English [u]. This observation raises the question: Is there a universal formant-frequency pattern for any given vowel that has the same IPA symbol in two or more languages? The answer appears to be *no*. Kent and Read (2002) compiled formant-frequency data for the vowels in several different languages and compared these data for vowels that were represented by the same IPA symbol. Rather large acoustic differences often were observed. For example, the F_2 frequency for [i] vowels had a range of more than 700 Hz across languages. The nature and origin of these cross-language differences are not well understood, but it is possible that languages have a distinctive **base-of-articulation** (Honikman, 1964; Bradlow, 1995). For example, back vowels in French and German are generally more extreme (and therefore have a lower F_2) than back vowels in English, even when the vowels are represented by the same IPA symbol. The base-of-articulation of a language is an articulatory setting that reflects the most frequently occurring segments and segment combinations in that language. The base-of-articulation concept may help to explain some of the differences in learning a new language.

CONSONANT ACOUSTICS

The acoustics of consonant articulation are complex. Because consonants are of several kinds, some vowel-like, some noise-like, some voiced, some voiceless, some long in duration, and some very brief in duration, a fairly large set of acoustic descriptors is required to discuss the details of consonant acoustics. However, the basic acoustic properties can be discussed broadly with respect to (1) the source of energy (voicing, frication noise, burst noise); (2) the manner or degree of vocal tract constriction (for example, complete closure for stops and affricates, narrow constriction for fricatives, nasal radiation for nasal consonants, or vowel-like oral radiation for liquids and glides); and (3) the place of vocal tract constriction (place of articulation as described in Chapter 5).

Source of Energy

If the vocal folds are vibrating while a sound is produced, the sound is called voiced. A voiced sound has as its acoustic property the quasiperiodic (meaning almost equally spaced in time) pulses of energy created as puffs of air escape through the vibrating vocal folds. Therefore, voiced consonants, like voiced vowels, are associated with vertical striations or voicing pulses on a spectrogram. Notice that, in the wide-band spectrogram of the simple sentence *The sunlight strikes raindrops in the air* in Figure 10-15, voicing pulses continue without interruption from the first vowel /ʌ/ in *sunlight* through the diphthong /a͡ɪ/ in the same word. Because the /n/ and the /l/ are voiced consonants, they show evidence of voicing pulses. However, for voiceless sounds like /t/, /s/, /k/, and /p/, the voicing pulses cease.

The voiceless sounds derive their energy from either frication (continued noise) or burst (brief transient noise). The /s/ sound, which recurs frequently in the spectrogram of Figure 10-15, is an example of a sound with a frication energy source. As air is forced through the narrow groove formed by the tongue tip and the alveolar ridge, noise is generated. A clear example of burst or transient noise can be seen for the /t/ in *strikes*. This burst noise immediately follows the brief stop gap (silent period) that in turn immediately follows the frication segment for the /s/. The stop gap, which is located just above the /t/ in the phonetic transcription, is a silent interval that results from complete closure of the vocal tract. As the lingua-alveolar closure for the /t/ is released, the air pressure that was contained behind the tongue closure escapes in an explosive burst. The brevity of the noise for the /t/ release contrasts with the much longer frication noise for the /s/.

For voiced fricatives, there are two energy sources: The voicing pulses associated with vocal fold vibration and the frication generated at the site of vocal tract constriction. The appearance of these sounds on a spectrogram is that of noise modulated by voicing (in other words, noise that is regulated in time by the puffs of air from the larynx). Examples of voiced fricatives are shown in Figure 10-16.

The voicing contrast (voiced versus voiceless) for stops in word-initial position frequently is described in terms of voice onset time (VOT), which is the temporal interval between the release of the stop closure and the onset of voicing. On a spectrogram, the release of the closure is signified by a brief burst of noise, and the onset of voicing is marked by the appearance of vertical striations in the voice bar (fundamental frequency) and formants. Thus, VOT is measured as the time separation between the release burst and the first appearance of vertical striations. Examples are shown in Figure 10-17 for the words *tame–dame* and *came–game*. Note that the voiceless stop always has a longer VOT than the voiced stop. Essentially, the difference in VOT between the voiced and voiceless categories means that the voiceless stop has a longer aperiodic (nonvoiced) interval. For voiced stops, voicing begins shortly after release, simultaneously with release, or slightly before release. For voiceless stops, voicing begins an appreciable time after release. The VOT for voiced stops is less than 20 ms, whereas the VOT for voiceless stops usually ranges between 30 and 80 ms, depending on a number of phonetic factors, including speaking rate, stress, and place of articulation.

Manner or Degree of Vocal Tract Constriction

This aspect of consonant production is represented by a number of different spectrographic features, some of which are illustrated in Figure 10-15. Note the spectrographic appearance of the following sounds, arranged roughly *in order of increasing openness of the vocal tract.*

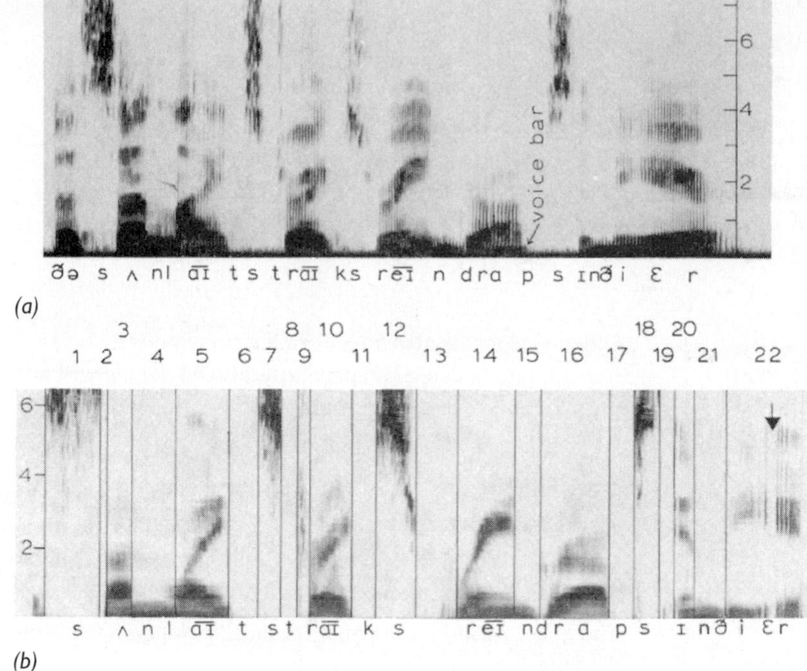

FIGURE 10-15

Spectrogram *(a)* is a man's recitation of the sentence *The sunlight strikes raindrops in the air.* Frequency in kHz is scaled on the vertical axis. The phonetic transcription at the bottom of the spectrogram can be used as a guide to segmentation. Spectrogram *(b)* is a woman's recitation of the sentence. The numbers at the top identify the following vertical slices or segments: 1—frication noise for [s]; 2—brief silent period; 3—vowel [ʌ]; 4—[n] + [l] sequence; 5—diphthong [ɑ͡ɪ]; 6—stop gap for [t]; 7—frication noise for [s]; 8—stop gap for [t]; 9—release burst and voiceless interval for [t]; 10—[r] + [ɑ͡ɪ] sequence; 11—stop gap for [k]; 12—combined noise segment: release burst for [k] and frication for [s]; 13—pause segment showing onset of voicing for following [r]; 14—[r] + [e͡ɪ] sequence; 15—nasal murmur for [n]; 16—[d] + [r] + [ɑ] sequence; 17—stop gap for [p]; 18—frication for [s]; 19—pause or silent interval; 20—vowel [ɪ]; 21—nasal murmur for [n] and weak fricative segment for [ð]; and 22—[i] + [ɛr] sequence (arrow points to glottal stop).

Stops: /t/ and /k/ in *strikes;* /d/ and /p/ in *raindrops.*

Fricatives: the two /s/ sounds in *strikes;* /ð/ in *the.*

Nasals: /n/ in *sunlight, raindrops,* and *in.*

Liquids: /l/ in *sunlight* and /r/ in *strikes* and *raindrops.*

The essential articulatory feature of a stop is articulatory closure, and the corresponding spectrographic feature is a **stop gap,** which is an interval of silence or greatly attenuated (decreased) sound energy. The /t/ in *strikes* has a silent stop gap, but the stop gap for /d/ in *raindrops* contains the low-frequency energy of voicing (the so-called **voice bar** at the extreme low-frequency region of the spectrogram) and, because of the influence of the abutting nasal /n/, a certain amount of nasally radiated energy. The release of a stop usually is associated with a burst of energy, as just discussed. This burst can be seen in the spectrogram of Figure 10-17.

The essential acoustic feature of a fricative is an interval of frication noise, which is conspicuous for the /s/ sounds in Figure 10-15. The intensity of this noise varies with place of production, as will be discussed in more detail in the following section. However, the great difference in intensity between /s/ and /ð/ can be seen from Figure 10-15 in the comparison of the /s/ in *raindrops* with the /ð/ in *the.* The frication noise for the latter is so weak as to be barely visible.

The nasal consonants /m n ŋ/ are the only phonemes uniquely identified with nasal radiation of the sound energy. Other phonemes are orally radiated. The nasal transmission of acoustic energy has major consequences on the overall intensity of the sound. As can be seen in Figure 10-15, nasal consonants tend to be weaker than surrounding vowels. For example, the /n/ in *sunlight* is markedly less intense (less overall blackness in the spectrogram) than the preceding vowel /ʌ/. Thus, even though the nasal tract is open as a route for radiation of the sound energy, this tract is not as efficient a path as the oral tract. Nasal consonants are weaker than vowel sounds and typically have a region of pronounced low-frequency energy (500 Hz or below).

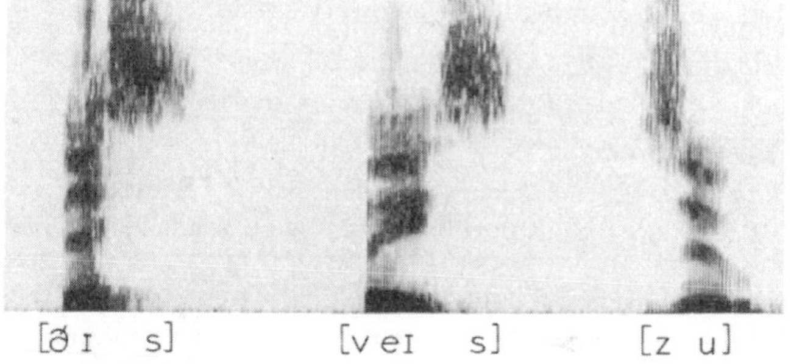

FIGURE 10-16

Spectrograms of words containing the voiced fricatives [ð], [v], and [z]. The noise energy for [ð] and [v] is so weak that it barely appears on the spectrogram.

The lateral /l/ and rhotacized /r/ (sometimes called liquids) are somewhat vowel-like in that they are sounds having a well-defined formant structure. They differ from vowels in that they have less overall energy and a lower frequency F_1. In Figure 10-15, the /l/ in *sunlight* and the /r/ in *strikes* and *raindrops* have bands of energy superimposed on the vertical striations of voicing. The liquids are less intense than surrounding vowels, but they are more intense than most other consonants.

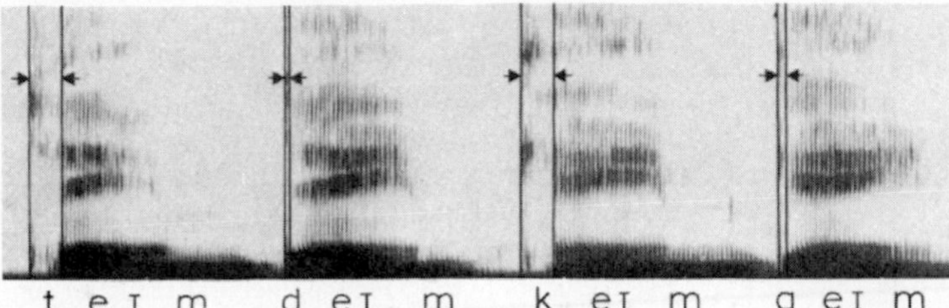

FIGURE 10-17
Spectrograms showing voice onset time (interval marked by arrows) for the initial stop consonants in the words *tame, dame, came,* and *game*.

These acoustic features demonstrate that as the vocal tract constriction for a consonant becomes less severe (more open), the consonant looks more like a vowel. In the extreme case of complete closure for a stop, there is little or no radiated acoustic energy during the stop gap. The fricatives have a continuous sound energy, but this energy does not have the well-defined formant structure of the vowels. Liquids and glides are more like vowels and have a distinctive formant pattern.

Place of Constriction

This property has many different acoustic correlates, but two of the most important are **formant transition** and **burst and frication spectra** (noise shaping). Formant transitions are bends or changes in formant structure. Whenever the articulators change position, the formant patterns also change, and transitions simply reflect articulatory movements, such as those between consonants and vowels. Formant transitions for the three CV syllables, /bɑ/, /dɑ/, and /gɑ/ are shown in Figure 10-18. These syllables were produced by a talking computer but are much like human speech and are easy to use for purposes of illustration. The only difference among these syllables lies in the transition for the second and third formants. The first formant, the one lowest in frequency, has the same shape for all three syllables. When we listen to these syllables, it is only the small difference in the transitions for the second and third formants, occurring over an interval of 50 ms, that allows us to distinguish /b/, /d/, and /g/. The pattern of the second and third formants in CV and VC transitions carries information about the place of articulation.

For a given consonant, the formant transition varies with vowel context, as illustrated in Figure 10-19. Notice that for these stylized /d/ + vowel syllables, the direction of the second formant can be either increasing or decreasing in frequency. One way of explaining these various patterns for a given stop is to hypothesize that all second-formant transitions begin at the same characteristic value (the small circle in the illustration) and then move to the second-formant frequency typical for the vowel. The characteristic value for the consonant is called the **second-formant locus,** or $\mathbf{F_2}$ **locus.** As a general principle, the F_2 locus increases in frequency as place of articulation moves back in the mouth.

Other consonants also have formant transitions associated with them; but, because of space limitations, details will not be given here. Some general points of importance are:

- Formant transitions are rapid changes in formant pattern, especially between consonants and vowels.
- These transitions carry information about place (and to some extent manner) of articulation and therefore play a significant role in the intelligibility of speech.
- The exact form of a formant transition depends on both the vowel and consonant involved.

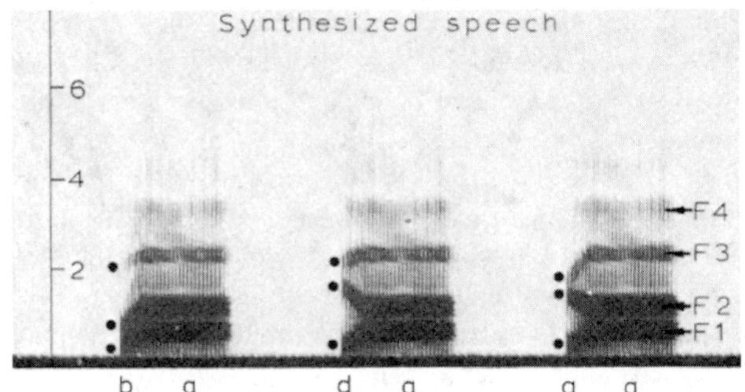

FIGURE 10-18
Spectrograms of the syllables [bɑ], [dɑ], and [gɑ] produced by a talking computer, or speech synthesizer. The small dots show the approximate starting frequencies of the first three formants. Frequency is scaled in kHz.

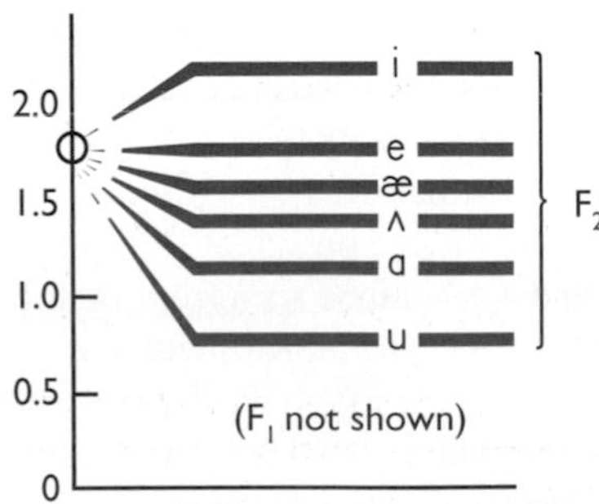

FIGURE 10-19
Composite of the F_2 patterns for [d] + vowel syllables, shown as a stylized spectrogram. Notice that the F_2 transition assumes different shapes depending on the vowel that follows the [d]. Frequency is scaled in kHz.

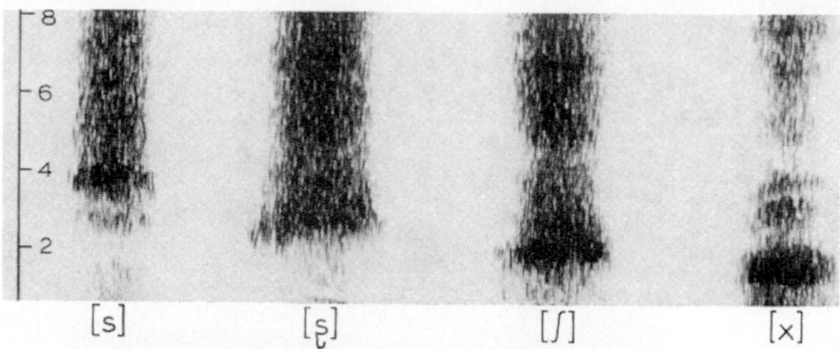

FIGURE 10-20
Spectrograms for the four fricatives [s], [ʂ], [ʃ], and [x]. Frequency in kHz is scaled on the vertical axis.

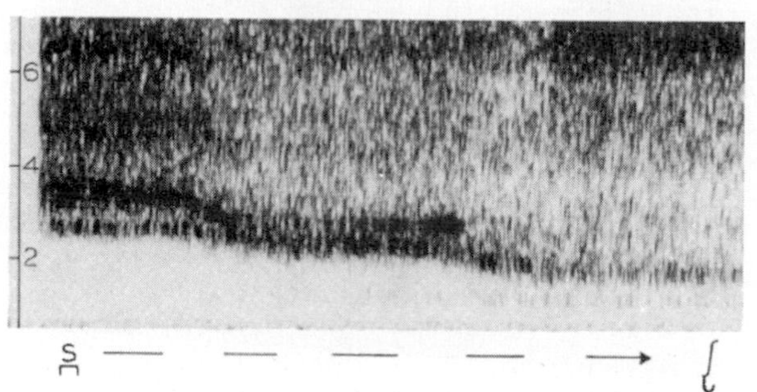

FIGURE 10-21
Spectrogram of the changing frication noise produced as a speaker gradually moves the point of articulation from front to back, beginning with a dentalized [s] and ending with a rhotacized [ʃ]. Frequency is scaled in kHz.

The noise of fricative and stop bursts also has characteristics that vary with place of articulation. Both the overall intensity of noise and the intensity-by-frequency (spectral) shaping of the noise depend on where the noise is generated. The most frontal fricatives /f v θ ð/ and the glottal fricative /h/ are the weakest. The stronger fricatives /s z ʃ ʒ/ are sometimes called sibilants. The spectral shaping for some lingual fricatives is illustrated in Figure 10-20, which shows spectrograms for a normal lingua-alveolar [s], a rhotacized [ʂ] (made with the tongue tip turned up), the lingua-palatal [ʃ], and the lingua-velar [x] (which is not a fricative phoneme in English but occurs in some other languages, such as German). This sequence of fricatives, for which the point of constriction moves progressively backward from /s/ to /x/, illustrates how the noise characteristics of fricatives are influenced by place. Notice in particular that, for this sequence of sounds, the low-frequency limit of the noise is progressively lower, moving from left to right. In part, this difference reflects the length of the resonating cavity in front of the point of constriction. The longer this cavity, the lower in frequency the resonances can be. For /s/, the front cavity is short, so the resonances are relatively high in frequency. For /ʃ/, the front cavity is longer, so the resonances are lower in frequency.

Another illustration of the change in noise spectrum as place of articulation is varied is given by the spectrogram in Figure 10-21. This spectrogram shows the acoustic result as a speaker gradually moves the point of constriction backward in the vocal tract, beginning with a dentalized [s̪] and ending with a rhotacized [ʃ].

Figure 10-22 summarizes the articulatory and acoustic properties of the places of articulation for English fricatives

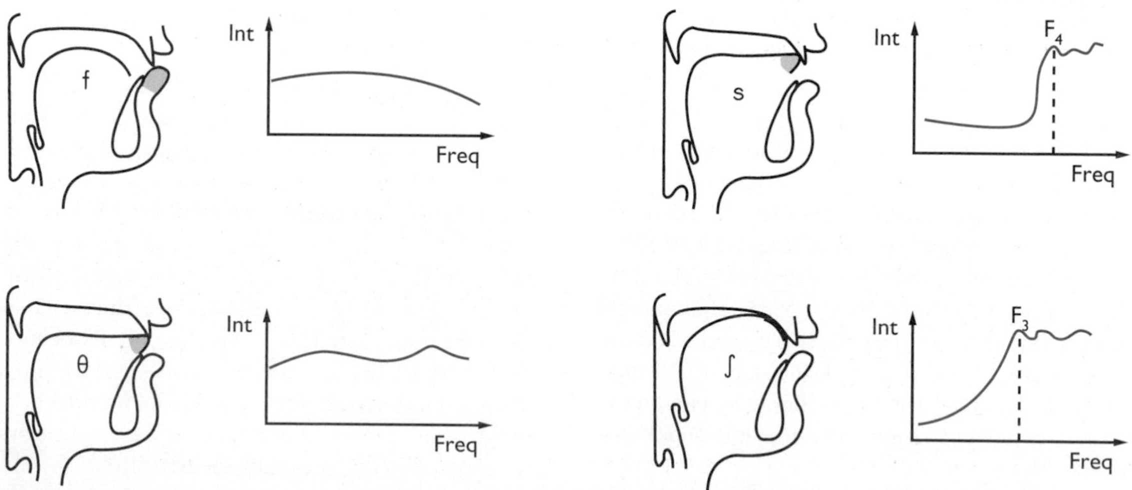

FIGURE 10-22
Articulatory configuration and acoustic spectrum for each of the fricatives [f], [θ], [s], and [ʃ].

(excluding /h/, which is acoustically similar to /f/). The drawings show the vocal tract configuration for each fricative and the general shape of the noise spectrum. The labiodental /f/ is of low intensity and has a "flat" spectrum (that is, with few peaks and valleys). Because the cavity in front of the labiodental constriction is very short, the resonances associated with this cavity are very high in frequency and of little importance to the auditory quality of the sound. Thus, /f/ is weak and flat.

Linguadental /θ/ is similar to /f/ but has a somewhat more important spectral shaping (note the peak at the high-frequency end of the spectrum). Because the anterior cavity, or the cavity in front of the constriction, is longer than that for the /f/, the associated resonances are lower in frequency. Still, like /f/, /θ/ is essentially a weak and flat fricative.

Lingua-alveolar /s/ has a longer front cavity than either /f/ or /θ/, and this factor accounts in part for the prominent spectral shaping of /s/. Most of the energy for /s/ is in the higher frequencies (above 4 kHz for an adult male). As a rule of thumb, the major concentration of acoustic energy for /s/ lies above the frequency value of the fourth formant (F_4) of an adjacent vowel. Both /s/ and lingua-palatal /ʃ/ are sibilants, a term that recognizes their intense noise energy. The /s/ is an intense, high-frequency fricative.

Lingua-palatal /ʃ/ has a longer front cavity than /s/ and has a greater amount of energy in the mid-frequency region. Generally, the major concentration of noise energy lies just above the frequency of the third formant (F_3) for an adjacent vowel (approximately 3 kHz for an adult male). Given these spectral properties, and the fact that /ʃ/ is a sibilant (high-energy fricative), the /ʃ/ may be described as an intense, mid-frequency sound.

SPEECH DISORDERS: SOME EXAMPLES OF ACOUSTIC ANALYSIS

Acoustic analyses of disordered speech help to illustrate further some of the concepts introduced in this chapter. The wide-band spectrogram in Figure 10-23 illustrates a breathy voice quality in a young hearing-impaired girl. In fact, her voice was so breathy as to have almost no tone of voicing. Note that the spectrogram, unlike those in Figures 10-11 and 10-15, does not have the vertical striations that represent vocal fold vibrations. Instead, the source energy is noise, which has a random, rather than periodic, fine structure in frequency and time. A narrow-band spectrogram would show an almost total loss of laryngeal harmonic pattern. However, it should be clear that formants are still readily visible in the wide-band spectrogram. Formants can be excited by either the periodic energy of voicing or the aperiodic energy of noise.

The spectrogram in Figure 10-24 illustrates the excitation of formants first by voicing energy and then, in the final portion, by noise energy without voicing. This spectrogram

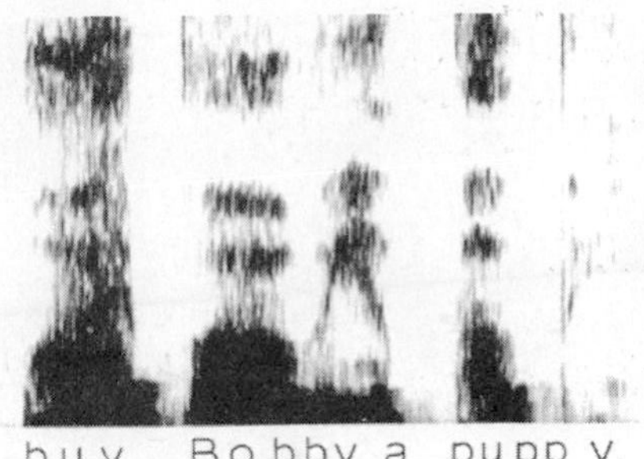

FIGURE 10-23
Spectrogram of the sentence *Buy Bobby a puppy,* as spoken by a young hearing-impaired girl. Her breathy voice quality appears as noise energy in the spectrogram. Note the absence of the finely spaced vertical striations that are visible in Figures 10-10, 10-11, and 10-15.

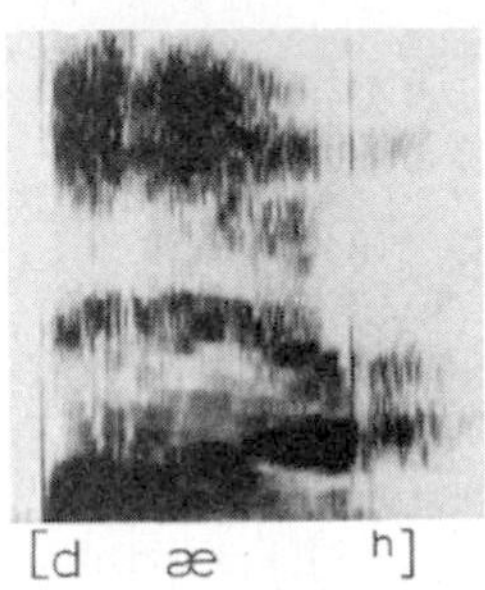

FIGURE 10-24
Spectrogram of the word *dad,* as spoken by a five-year-old boy with severely delayed speech and language. An aspirated interval replaces the final stop [d]. This utterance can be transcribed either [dæ æ̤] or [dæʰ].

shows the attempted production of the word *dad* /dæd/ by a five-year-old boy who consistently omitted word- or syllable-final consonants. However, spectrograms showed that he usually produced a breathy final segment in place of the consonant. Figure 10-24 is an example and shows the replacement of normal voicing by voiceless noise at the end of the utterance.

Voicing errors for the stop /p/ are illustrated in Figure 10-25 for a four-year-old boy. The spectrograms show two recitations of the words *took a spoon* /tʊk ə spun/. In both recitations, the /s/ of *spoon* was omitted. The /p/ that follows the (deleted) /s/ is produced as two different allophones. In spectrogram *(a),* the allophone is the aspirated [pʰ], which normally occurs in all released positions except those following /s/. The allophone shown in spectrogram *(b)* is the unaspirated [p⁼], which normally occurs following /s/. Perhaps because this boy consistently omitted /s/, his phonological system was unstable in the selection of the appropriate allophone. But whatever the reason for the inconsistency, this spectrogram clearly illustrates the acoustic differences between aspirated and unaspirated stops.

Spectrograms of glottal stops [ʔ] are shown in Figure 10-26. Part *(a)* of this figure is a spectrogram of the word

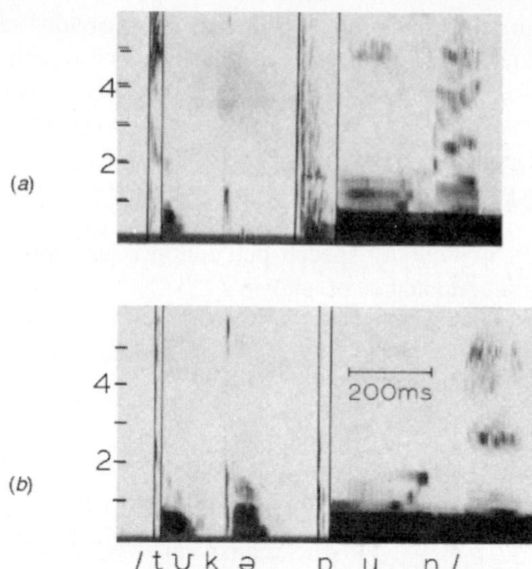

FIGURE 10-25
Spectrograms for two productions of the phrase *took a spoon* by a four-year-old boy. The /s/ in *spoon* is omitted in both productions, and the following /p/ appears as an aspirated stop in *(a)* but as an unaspirated stop in *(b)*. Frequency is scaled in kHz.

cake produced with an initial glottal stop. The spectrogram in part *(b)* shows a production of the word *hot* initiated with a glottal stop. The arrows in both spectrograms point to the instant of release of the laryngeal stricture; shortly after this release, vocal fold vibration begins. Superimposed on part *(b)* of Figure 10-26 is the f_0 curve for the utterance, showing that the f_0 begins at a relatively low value, then increases rapidly, and finally falls rapidly.

Errors in the articulation of vowels, liquids, and voiced glides frequently are evident as abnormalities in formant pattern. An example is shown in Figure 10-27, which shows spectrograms of an examiner's /ɝ/ and an imitation by a child with an /ɝ/ error. As the formant labels indicate, the examiner's /ɝ/ is characterized by a near convergence of F_2 and F_3. In fact, proximity of these two formants is distinctive of the English vowel /ɝ/. In contrast, F_2 and F_3 in the

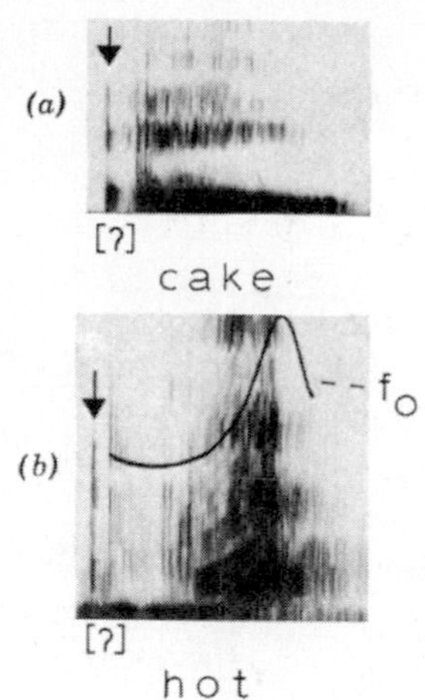

FIGURE 10-26
Spectrograms of glottal stops occurring in the words *cake (a)* and *hot (b)*. The speakers were children with cleft palates.

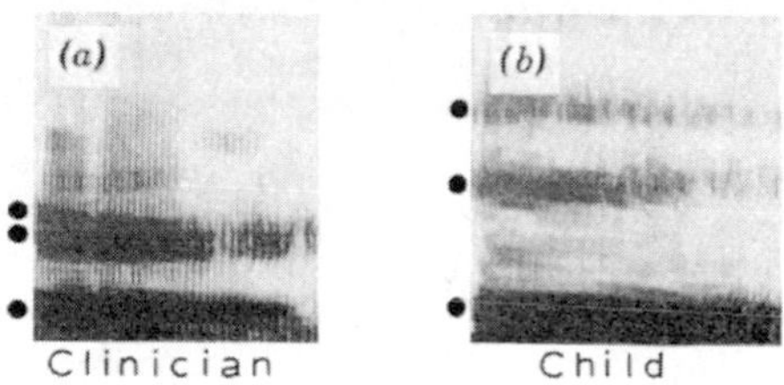

FIGURE 10-27
Spectrograms of correct /ɝ/ production by a clinician *(a)* and an imitation by a child with an /ɝ/ error *(b)*. The black dots show the starting frequencies of the first three formants. Note wide separation of F_2 and F_3 in the child's error production.

child's production are widely separated. Convergence of F_2 and F_3 also is characteristic of consonantal /r/, as can be seen in the word *strikes* and *raindrops* in Figure 10-15.

The importance of velopharyngeal closure is illustrated in Figure 10-28, which shows spectrograms for the sentence *I took a spoon and a dish* produced by a man with normal

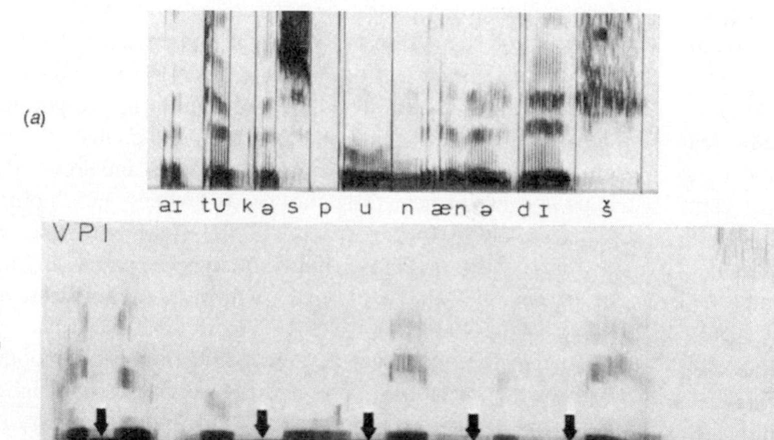

FIGURE 10-28
Spectrogram of the sentence *I took a spoon and a dish* as produced by an adult with normal speech *(a)* and by a child with severe velopharyngeal incompetence *(b)*. The arrows point to intervals of nasal resonance during oral closures.

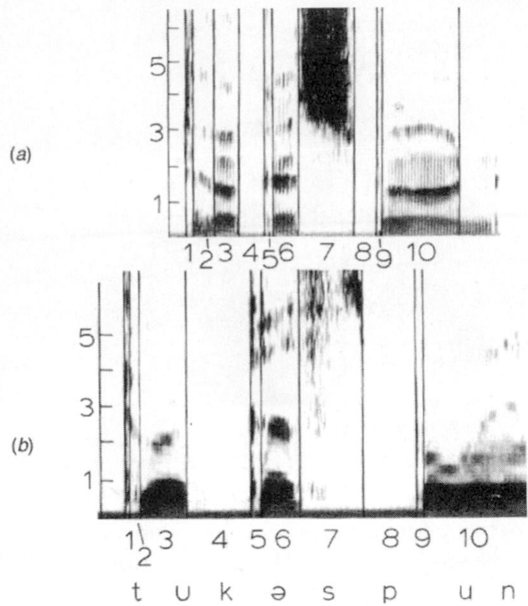

FIGURE 10-29
Spectrograms of the phrase *took a spoon* produced by an adult *(a)* and four-year-old boy *(b)*. Frequency is scaled in kHz. The numbered segments are: 1—release burst for [t]; 2—aspiration for [t]; 3—vocalic nucleus of the word *took*; 4—stop gap for [k]; 5—release burst and aspiration for [k]; 6—schwa vowel; 7—[s] frication; 8—[p] stop gap; 9—voice onset time for [p]; and 10—vocalic nucleus for [u] in *spoon*.

speech *(a)* and by a young boy *(b)* with severe velopharyngeal incompetence (that is, inadequate closure of the velopharynx). The boy's speech was highly nasal and unintelligible. In contrast to the normal pattern, with its well-defined vowel formants and conspicuous segments of frication noise, the pattern for the boy with velopharyngeal incompetence contains mostly low-frequency energy attributable to nasal resonance. Furthermore, the spectrogram for the boy shows that voicing was not interrupted as it should have been for voiceless segments. This abnormal continuation of voicing can be seen in the intervals marked by arrows. Obviously, this boy's spectrogram shows a serious degradation of the acoustic features needed for intelligible speech.

Spectrograms contain a very large amount of acoustic information that can be used for clinical purposes. However, the effective use of spectrograms as a clinical tool requires considerable practice in their interpretation. Acoustic features for individual speech sounds vary across speakers, especially as a function of age and sex of speakers. A comparison of the speech of an adult male and a four-year-old boy is shown in Figure 10-29. Notice that the child tends to make all segment durations longer than does the adult and that the child's acoustic energy for a given phonetic feature generally lies at a higher frequency than it does for the adult. For example, notice that the /s/ in *spoon* (segment number 7) is of longer duration and has higher frequency noise energy in the child's production. Despite the differences in segment durations and sound spectra, it is possible to segment the child's spectrogram in a fashion that accords fairly well with the segmentation of the spectrogram of the adult.

SPEECH PERCEPTION: AN INTEGRATIVE PROCESS

One way of viewing speech perception is as a process involving several stages of analysis:

Semantic-syntactic analysis
(meaning and grammar)
↓↑
Morphological analysis
(words)
↓↑
Phonetic analysis
(linguistically relevant sound contrasts)
↓↑
Auditory analysis
(general sound pattern)

The different levels of analysis are not independent in operation, but rather they interact as perceptual decisions are made. The interaction can be described by saying that speech perception is both a top-down and bottom-up process. A **top-down process** proceeds in the downward direction, moving from higher levels of analysis, such as word recognition, to lower levels of analysis, such as recognition of phonetic segments. A **bottom-up process** goes the other way, from lower to higher levels. Both processes seem to be involved when we listen to speech, because we make some decisions at lower (auditory and phonetic) levels but other decisions almost simultaneously at higher (morphologic and semantic-syntactic) levels.

This combined analysis is perhaps best illustrated by what happens when someone tries to speak to you in a very noisy room. Because the room interferes with the person's message, you might hear only a part of the total acoustic speech signal. From this residual portion, you extract some basic acoustic patterns and, in turn, some of the phonetic segments. Given this partial reconstruction of the phonetic sequence, you then attempt to guess or hypothesize about the higher-level organization of the message—the individual words or their structural relationship. In doing so, you rely on several sources of information: the social context, the linguistic context, the words in your language, and so on. Perhaps you might hear only the words "when" and "going," separated by a period of noise interference, but these two words, together with your linguistic hypotheses, are enough to decide that the actual message was "When are you going?"

Therefore, to say that the perception of speech is both a top-down and bottom-up process is to say that some higher-level and lower-level decisions are made at essentially the same time and in an interactive way. A listener probably makes enough lower-level auditory-phonetic decisions to provide basic data, or "food for thought," to be used by the higher-level stages of analysis. This process offers both efficiency and noise-resistance. If speech perception depended on a complete set of auditory-phonetic decisions before a linguistic interpretation were attempted, just one misarticulated phoneme or one brief noise interference might hamper the entire process. However, if higher-level linguistic decisions are formed as partial lower-level analyses are accomplished, the listener is freed from complete reliance on an error-free and undisturbed acoustic speech signal. The extent to which minor errors or interferences in the acoustic signal are ignored is demonstrated by experiments in which a speech sound on a recording of a spoken sentence is replaced (by editing of the recording) with an extraneous sound, such as a cough. The listener often is totally unaware of the alteration because his or her linguistic interpretation of the message overrides slight discrepancies at the acoustic level.

The combined top-down and bottom-up operations in speech perception sometimes can make it easy to overlook errors in the articulation of long phonetic strings. The speech-language clinician should be aware of this possibility and should never forget that there are auditory as well as visual illusions. Another example is that a listener often has a changing perception of a constant speech stimulus (say, a syllable or word) when the stimulus is presented repeatedly at brief intervals. This phenomenon is known as **verbal** (or **phonetic**) **transformation.** A similar change in auditory perception, called **phonetic adaptation,** occurs for individual phonemes or phonetic features in one stimulus following presentation of another stimulus. For example, a given sound may be perceived either as voiced or voiceless, depending on the immediately preceding auditory experience with stimuli of similar characteristics. That is, the auditory system can be *biased* by exposure to sound patterns.

It has been proposed that speech perception has a dual nature, in which some sounds are perceived categorically and others continuously. **Categorical perception** has been demonstrated most successfully for stop consonants and other sounds with rapid spectral changes, while **continuous perception** has been demonstrated primarily for vowels. Categorical perception for the stops /b d g/ is illustrated in Figure 10-30. The actual acoustic patterns of CV (stop + vowel) stimuli are shown at the left in the form of stylized formant patterns (F_1 and F_2). As discussed earlier, the formant transitions or bends often are sufficient cues for stop perception, and the differences in direction of F_2 transition for a given vowel context signal different places of production (/b/ versus /d/ versus /g/). The symbols at the right side of the figure show the majority **identification** responses of subjects for the acoustic patterns shown. The identifications are simply the phonemic labels (/b/, /d/, or /g/) that listeners assign to the patterns. Depending upon the particular form of the F_2 transition, listeners tend to hear one of the three stops. Shown at the middle of the figure are discrimination responses for pairs of the stimuli. **Discrimination** is a test of whether a listener can reliably distinguish a particular pair of the acoustic patterns. In the figure, patterns that cannot be discriminated (those that sound the same) are connected by a brace. Notice that all pairs within a phoneme category sound alike and that sharp or reliable discrimination of stimulus pairs occurs only at phoneme category boundaries (the dotted lines). Hence, discrimination performance is predicted by identification performance (or vice versa), such that *discrimination is poor for pairs within a category but good for pairs that cross a category boundary.*

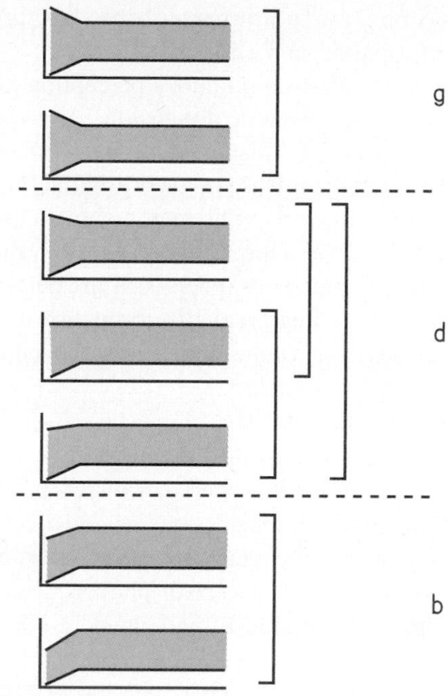

FIGURE 10-30
Representation of categorical perception. Stylized formant patterns (F_1 and F_2) are shown at the left for CV syllables. The brackets join stimuli that cannot be discriminated (they sound alike). The phonemic symbols at the right are the identification responses listeners attach to the stimuli. Note that any two stimuli heard as the same sound (/b/, /d/, or /g/) are not discriminated.

Continuous perception is illustrated for vowel sounds in Figure 10-31. A number of different vowels are shown by the points along a line in the F_1–F_2 plane. These sounds differ from one another only in the frequencies of the first two formants, F_1 and F_2. When individual vowels are presented to listeners for identification (phonemic labeling), categories are assigned as shown in the illustration. However, unlike the results for stop consonants, pairwise tests of discrimination for the vowels do not show a sharpening of discrimination at category boundaries. Listeners often can discriminate vowel sounds from within the same phoneme category as well as they can discriminate vowel sounds that cross a phoneme boundary. For example, any pair of vowels enclosed within the same ellipse might be discriminated as easily as an adjacent pair that fall in neighboring ellipses. Thus, in continuous perception, discrimination performance does not predict identification performance, or vice versa.

Tests of categorical versus continuous perception can be applied to many acoustic–phonetic dimensions. Voice onset time (VOT) is an example. As discussed earlier, VOT is the time difference between the release of a word-initial stop and the onset of voicing. Although VOT may assume a continuum of values, the phonetic interpretation of these values is binary, or two-valued: voiced or voiceless. If the perception of the voicing contrast is categorical, discrimination of VOT values should be best for values that cross the phonetic (voiced versus voiceless) boundary.

Another important characteristic of speech perception is that the perceptual significance of a given acoustic feature often depends on the phonetic context in which it occurs. That is, the feature is more conspicuous in some contexts than others. This characteristic means that articulatory errors are very likely to be noticed in certain phonetic contexts, whereas they might not be readily perceived in others. A good deal of research on speech perception points to the idea that many perceptual decisions for individual phonetic segments are made within at least a syllable-sized context. In fact, some theorists propose that the syllable is the basic unit within which speech perception decisions are made. The evidence for this idea is complex and comes from several sources. One particular line of support is that when formant transition segments are presented in isolation, they are not identified as speech sounds; but when the transition segments are combined with vowel segments, they are readily heard as stops. It seems that the formant transitions can be interpreted in a syllable context but not in isolation.

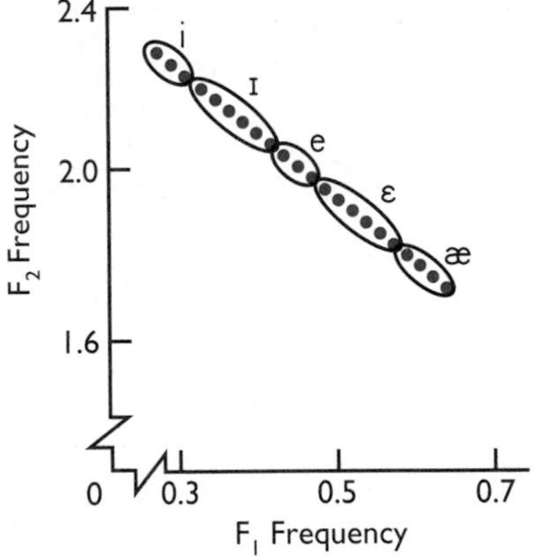

FIGURE 10-31
Representation of continuous perception. The small filled circles represent vowel sounds plotted according to the F_1 and F_2 frequencies. The ellipses enclose stimuli that are identified as the same vowel, /i/, /ɪ/, /e/, /ɛ/, or /æ/. In continuous perception, a stimulus pair within an ellipse (assigned to the same phoneme category) can be discriminated about as well as a pair of stimuli that lie in adjacent phoneme categories. Thus, identification (phoneme category) does not predict discrimination, or conversely.

Let us consider a clinically relevant example. Suppose that a clinician is listening to a child's /r/ production in C-/r/ clusters, such as those in the words *drain, train,* and *crane*. As discussed in Chapter 6, a liquidlike /r/ is partially devoiced when it follows a voiceless stop like /t/ or /k/. The acoustic illustration of this devoicing is shown in Figure 10-32, which presents wide-band spectrograms for each word. Of particular importance to the perception of /r/ are the formant transitions for F_2 and F_3. The voiced F_3 transition in Figure 10-32 has been highlighted in ink to show that the duration of the F_3 transition activated by voicing is quite different across the three words. The longer activation of F_3 by voicing in the word *drain,* as opposed to the two-stage noise + voicing activation in the words *train* and *crane,* could have implications for the ease and accuracy with which an articulatory error can be identified. Figure 10-32 shows that all /r/'s are not acoustically equal and that the information available to the listener's ear varies with phonetic context.

Figure 10-33 summarizes some of the durational and spectral features that are important to speech perception. Time is represented along the horizontal axis and frequency is represented logarithmically along the vertical axis. The frequency patterns apply to the speech of an adult male; higher frequency values should be assumed for women and children. The block labeled f_0 shows the range of fundamental frequency that might occur during emotional speech (the duration shown is simply one that is appropriate for stressed vowels in sentence context). The blocks labeled F_1 and F_2 show the frequency ranges associated with these two vowel formants, as well as the articulatory correlates of tongue height (F_1) and tongue advancement (F_2). The durations for F_1 and F_2 represent an average duration for a stressed vowel

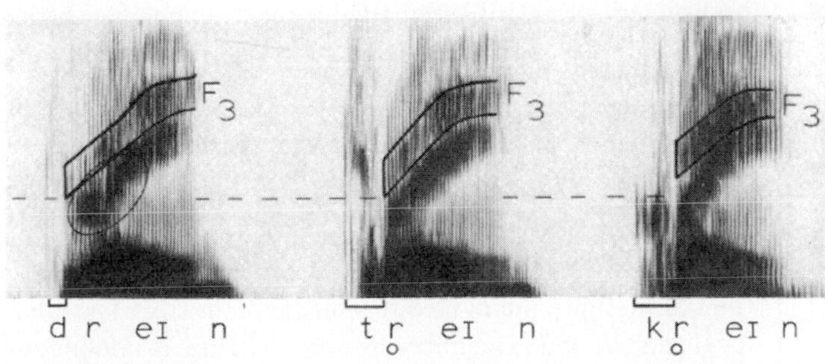

FIGURE 10-32
Spectrograms of the words *drain, train,* and *crane* showing how the extent of F_3 transition varies with voice onset time (bracketed interval at base of patterns). F_3 is bounded by inked lines, and the first part of the F_2 transition is highlighted for the word *drain*.

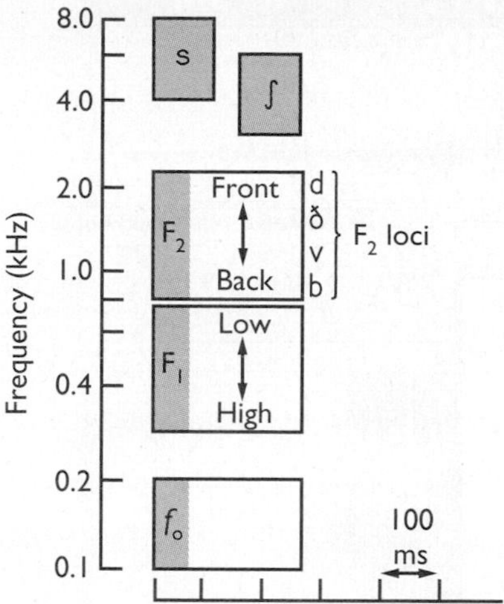

FIGURE 10-33
Graphic summary of spectral and temporal properties of some major sound classes. Vowels are represented by the blocks labeled f_0, F_1, and F_2. A duration of 250 ms is about average for stressed vowels in sentence context. The frequency ranges for F_1 and F_2 are appropriate for an adult male and correspond to the articulatory dimensions shown. The shaded part of the f_0, F_1, and F_2 blocks is the compression limit for vowels, that is, the minimum vowel duration. The approximate F_2 loci for four consonants with different places of articulation are shown on the side of the F_2 block. Finally, the blocks labeled [s] and [ʃ] indicate the primary acoustic energy concentration and average duration for these fricatives.

in sentence context. The shaded portion of the blocks for f_0, F_1, and F_2 represents what has been called the "compression limit" for a vowel, the shortest duration that a reduced vowel (typically schwa) can assume. F_2 loci for consonants are indicated along the right side of the F_2 block: Note that the F_2 locus frequency increases as place of articulation moves back in the mouth. Finally, the blocks labeled with the fricative symbols [s] and [ʃ] represent the primary concentration of noise energy of these sounds. The fricatives are shown with a duration of 100 ms, which is fairly typical of their occurrence in conversational speech.

Acoustic information for the perception of consonants is reviewed in the following section and organized by the major acoustic features of silence, voicing, noise, and transitions.

SUMMARY OF THE ACOUSTIC PROPERTIES OF VOWELS AND CONSONANTS

Acoustic analysis of speech entails a number of issues and a number of measurement possibilities. Pickett (1980) and Kent and Read (2002) are sources of extended information. The objectives of this chapter are rather modest: (1) to outline the central issues in acoustic analysis and (2) to point to some acoustic principles that have direct clinical relevance. This section of the chapter speaks to the latter objective.

The day likely will come when speech-language clinicians routinely use microcomputer-based systems to display and analyze the acoustic signal of speech. The essential hardware and software components are readily available (Read, Buder, and Kent, 1990, 1992) and affordable for many applications. The same personal computer that the clinician uses for analyzing language samples, phonologic patterns, and phonetic records can also be used to run programs for acoustic analysis. In fact, modern personal computers can run fairly powerful programs for acoustic analysis that only a few years ago required large laboratory computers. Figure 10-34 is an analysis display from one system, Computer Speech Lab (CSL) from Kay Elemetrics Corporation, that runs on personal computers. The screen display includes the signal waveform at the top, spectrogram at the bottom, and spectral analysis and formant values overlaid in boxes on the screen. Some other systems display the results of acoustic analysis in videographics suitable for children—colorful cartoon games, for example. These developments hold promise for a variety of clinical applications, including quantitative measurement of speech change and computer-based therapy in which the client interacts with a computer program. Some acoustic analysis systems and vendor addresses are listed at the end of this chapter.

Only a minority of clinicians use these systems in contemporary practice. A knowledge of some basic correlates between phonetic description and the acoustic features of speech is a first step in anticipating the future of machine-aided assessment and management in speech-language pathology and audiology. In addition, an understanding of these correlates can have immediate application to more traditional clinical practices. The following discussion summarizes some major acoustic phonetic principles and highlights clinical implications. This information by no means is a broad coverage of this topic, but it should suffice as an introduction.

Articulatory–Acoustic Relations for Vowels

Figure 10-35 is a summary of the basic relations between the articulation and acoustic patterns for vowels. Formant pattern is usually taken as the best overall description of the vowel's acoustic structure. Vowels in voiced speech have most of the energy in the so-called main formants (F_1, F_2, and F_3). F_1 is typically the most intense formant and therefore correlates highly with loudness estimates. Because vowels have predominantly low-frequency energy, their perception tends to be less affected than consonant perception by high-frequency hearing losses. Vowel /i/ has a particularly high F_2 frequency, which makes it difficult to hear for some persons with severe hearing losses. Vowels are the most intense components of speech and therefore define the overall energy pattern of most utterances. Figure 10-36 summarizes the basic articulatory–acoustic relations for diph-

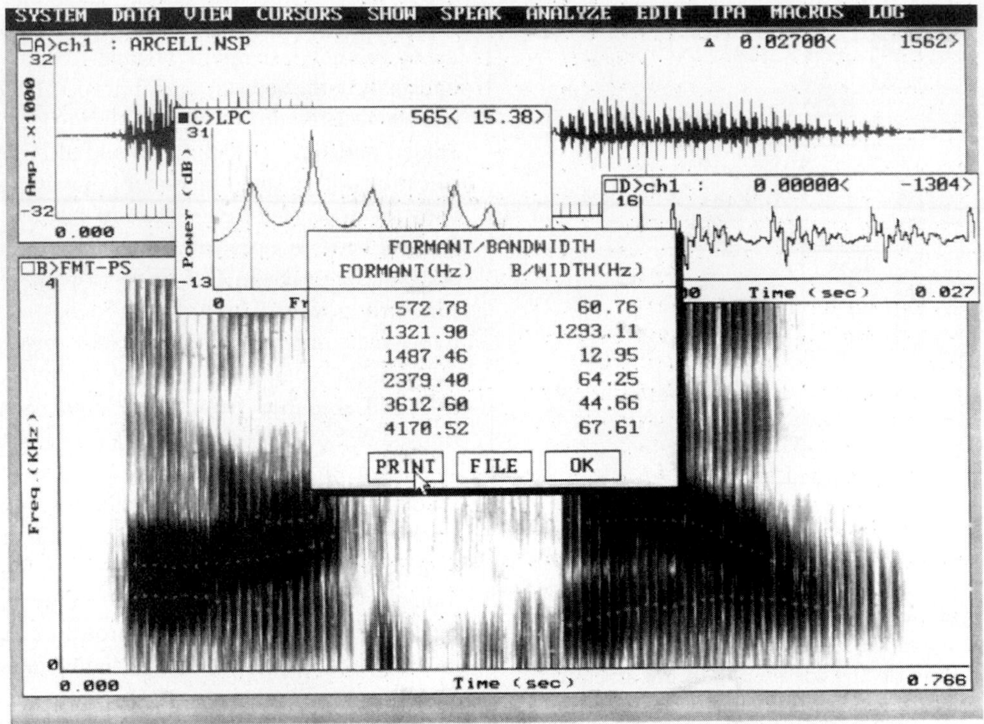

FIGURE 10-34
Display of speech analysis from Kay Elemetric Corporation's Computer Speech Lab (CSL). This display includes a spectrogram, waveform, spectrum, and measurements of formant frequencies and bandwidths. Reprinted with the permission of Kay Elemetric Corporation.

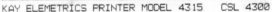

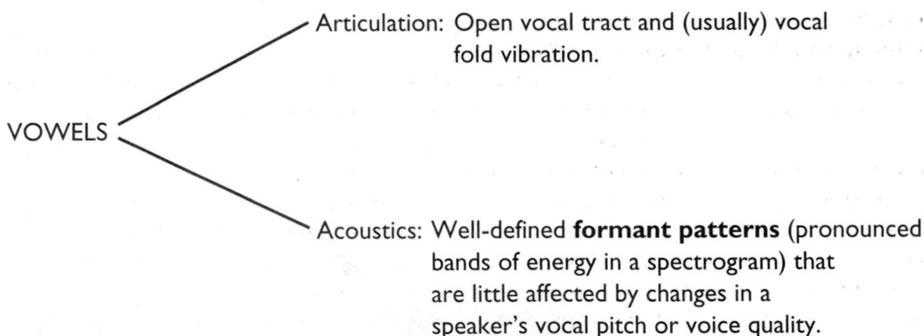

FIGURE 10-35
Basic articulatory–acoustic relations for vowels.

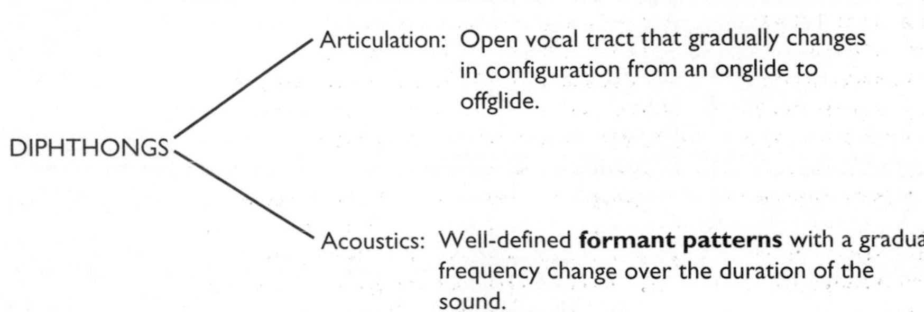

DIPHTHONGS
Articulation: Open vocal tract that gradually changes in configuration from an onglide to offglide.
Acoustics: Well-defined **formant patterns** with a gradual frequency change over the duration of the sound.

FIGURE 10-36
Basic articulatory–acoustic relations for diphthongs.

TABLE 10-2
Matrix of Acoustic Features for the Four Corner Vowels: High-Front, High-Back, Low-Front, and Low-Back

	Front	Back
High	Low F_1 frequency High F_2 frequency Large F_2–F_1 difference Small F_3–F_2 difference Short duration Weak intensity High f_0	Low F_1 frequency Low F_2 frequency Small F_2–F_1 difference Large F_3–F_2 difference Short duration Weak intensity High f_0
Low	High F_1 frequency High F_2 frequency Large F_2–F_1 difference Small F_3–F_2 difference Long duration Strong intensity Low f_0	High F_1 frequency Low F_2 frequency Small F_2–F_1 difference Large F_3–F_2 difference Long duration Strong intensity Low f_0

thongs, which differ from vowels in having a formant pattern that changes over time.

Some basic articulatory–acoustic correlates for the corner vowels are summarized in Table 10-2. This matrix can be helpful in selecting a vowel with particular acoustic features. For instance, if it is desired to use a vowel with a long inherent duration and strong intensity, then the low vowels /æ/ and /ɑ/ are good candidates.

Articulatory–Acoustic Relations for Consonants

The consonants are reviewed here by the major classes of obstruents and sonorants. A summary of acoustic information is provided in Table 10-3.

Obstruents. Recall that obstruents include the stops, fricatives, and affricates. The basic articulatory–acoustic relations for these sounds are shown in Figure 10-37 (stops), Figure 10-38 (fricatives), and Figure 10-39 (affricates). The acoustic description highlights the major acoustic cues for each type of obstruent.

Table 10-4 on page 328 is a summary of the aerodynamic and acoustic properties of obstruent consonants. Aerodynamic variables considered are airflow and air pressure. The acoustic correlates are described for both prevocalic and postvocalic positions.

The individual obstruent types are further discussed as follows.

Stops (/b/, /d/, /g/, /p/, /t/, /k/)

1. **Silence.** A silent interval or stop gap occurs before the release of the stop. This interval is truly silent for voiceless stops, as no energy is radiated from the oral cavity during the obstruction for the stop. However, voiced stops often have a small amount of low-frequency energy attributable to voicing. This energy appears as a low-frequency voice bar on a spectrogram. The duration of the stop gap generally falls in the range of 50 to 100 ms, depending on speaking rate, stress, voicing, and phonetic context.
2. **Voicing.** Vocal fold vibrations occur during most or all of the obstructed interval for voiced stops in medial position. Vocal fold vibrations may not be evident during the closure phase of initial or final stops. Voiced and voiceless stops in initial position are distinguished by voice onset time, or the time that intervenes between the release of the constriction and the beginning of voicing. Voiced stops have short voice onset times, meaning that voicing begins just before, simultaneously with, or just after consonantal release. Voiceless stops have long voice onset times, meaning that voicing begins relatively longer after consonantal release. Frequently, voiced and voiceless stops in final position are distinguished largely by the duration of a preceding vowel. Vowels that precede voiced stops are lengthened relative to vowels that precede voiceless stops. These are not the only cues that signal stop voicing, but they are among the most frequently cited in the literature. One other cue for voicing—aspiration noise for voiceless stops—is discussed in the following paragraph.
3. **Noise.** A burst of noise usually accompanies a stop release, with the duration of the burst varying from about 10 to 30 ms, depending on speaking rate, stress, voicing, and perhaps phonetic context. The noise burst is more prominent for voiceless than for voiced stops, because the former usually have a greater intraoral air pressure and, therefore, a stronger pulse of air upon release. In addition, voiceless stops are often produced with an aspiration noise that immediately follows the burst noise. The two segments of burst noise and aspiration noise usually occur for all voiceless stops except those that follow /s/ or those that are not released. Aspiration noise may be an important cue for voiceless stops. The noise burst for stops has a spectral shape determined by place of articulation. Even a brief noise burst may be sufficient for listeners to categorize place of articulation for stops. A general rule is that bilabials have a spectrum that is flat or gently falling, alveolars have a rising spectrum, and velars have a mid-frequency dominance.
4. **Transitions.** As the vocal tract shape is changed from that for a vowel to one for a consonant (or vice versa), the acoustic resonances also change, so that formant shifts are evident for VC (or CV) articulatory transitions. The duration of the transitions are on the order of about 40 to 60 ms for stops. This interval reflects the major phase of

TABLE 10-3
Primary Acoustic Cues for Various Consonants Produced in Syllable-Initial, Prevocalic Position[a]

	Bilabial	Labiodental	Linguadental	Lingua-alveolar	Lingua-palatal	Lingua-velar	Glottal
Stops	[b] [p] F_1 increases. F_2 increases. Burst has flat or falling spectrum.			[d] [t] F_1 increases. F_2 decreases except for high-front vowels. Burst has rising spectrum.		[g] [k] F_1 increases. F_2 increases or decreases. Wedge-shaped F_2–F_3. Burst has mid-frequency spectrum.	[ʔ] Little formant change.
Nasals	[m] F_1 increases. F_2 increases. Nasal murmur			[n] F_1 increases. F_2 decreases except for high-front vowels. Nasal murmur.		[ŋ] F_1 increases. F_2 increases or decreases. Nasal murmur.	
Fricatives		[v] [f] F_1 increases. F_2 increases except for some back vowels. Noise segment has weak and flat spectrum.	[ð] [θ] F_1 increases. F_2 increases except for some back vowels. Noise segment has weak and flat spectrum.	[z] [s] F_1 increases. F_2 decreases except for high-front vowels. Noise segment has intense, high-frequency (above 4 kHz) spectrum.	[ʒ] [ʃ] F_1 increases. F_2 increases or decreases. Noise segment has intense, high-frequency (above 3 kHz) spectrum.		[h] Little formant change. Noise segment has weak and flat spectrum.
Glides	[w] F_1 increases. F_2 increases.				[j] F_1 increases. F_2 decreases.		

[a]Formant transitions are described as increasing or decreasing in frequency during the consonant-to-vowel transition.

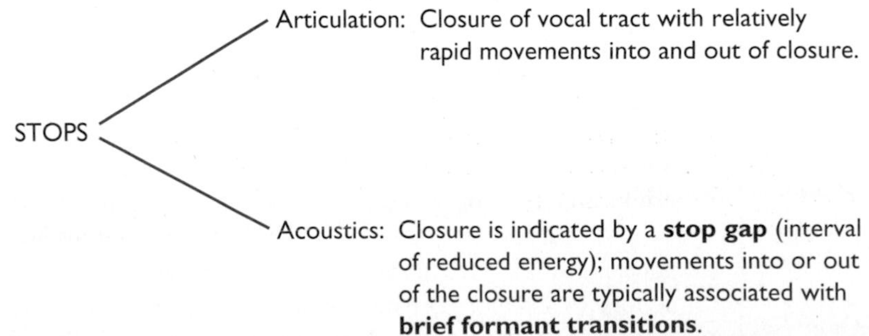

STOPS
Articulation: Closure of vocal tract with relatively rapid movements into and out of closure.
Acoustics: Closure is indicated by a **stop gap** (interval of reduced energy); movements into or out of the closure are typically associated with **brief formant transitions**.

FIGURE 10-37
Basic articulatory–acoustic relations for stops.

articulatory movement. The first-formant frequency during the vocal obstruction for a stop is nearly zero, so that VC transitions for F_1 are always falling and CV transitions are always rising in frequency. In other words, a very low F_1 frequency is an acoustic indicator of vocal tract closure. The direction of the second-formant frequency change is slightly more complicated, but the general pattern is shown in Table 10-3. To a first approximation, each place of articulation for stops can be associated with a particular F_2 locus, which specifies the frequency value at which the F_2 transition begins for CV syllables and ends with VC syllables (see Figure 10-33 and Table

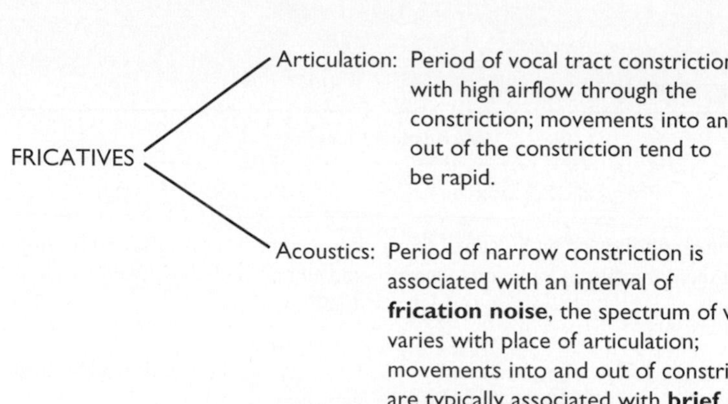

FRICATIVES
Articulation: Period of vocal tract constriction with high airflow through the constriction; movements into and out of the constriction tend to be rapid.
Acoustics: Period of narrow constriction is associated with an interval of **frication noise**, the spectrum of which varies with place of articulation; movements into and out of constriction are typically associated with **brief formant transitions**.

FIGURE 10-38
Basic articulatory–acoustic relations for fricatives.

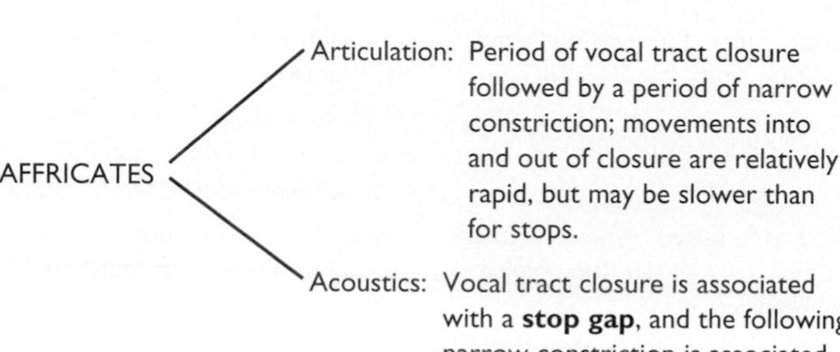

FIGURE 10-39
Basic articulatory–acoustic relations for affricates.

10-3). VC transitions tend to have longer durations than CV transitions.

Fricatives (/f/, /v/, /θ/, /ð/, /z/, /s/, /ʒ/, /ʃ/, /h/)

1. **Silence.** Usually none.
2. **Voicing.** Voiced fricatives are characterized by both periodic (or nearly so) vocal fold pulses and turbulence noise. The noise is essentially modulated by the vocal fold vibrations. That is, voiced fricatives have two energy sources—vocal fold vibration at the larynx and noise generated in the vocal tract.
3. **Noise.** Noise energy is the hallmark of the fricative. The noise duration is typically between 50 and 100 ms but can be longer in strongly stressed syllables or very slow speaking rates. Fricatives differ from one another in the intensity of the noise and its spectral shape. The fricatives /s/, /z/, /ʃ/, and /ʒ/ have much more energy than the others. These are sometimes called stridents or sibilants. The palatals /ʃ/ and /ʒ/ have lower-frequency energy than the alveolars /s/ and /z/. Figures 10-40 and 10-41 show the difference between /ʃ/ and /s/. Both the spectrum at the upper left and the spectrogram at the bottom of the illustrations show that the noise energy for /ʃ/ reaches down to about 2 kHz. The /s/ has energy that reaches to a lower limit of about 3.5 kHz. This spectral difference explains why /s/ seems to have a higher pitch than /ʃ/. The acoustic analyses in Figures 10-40 and 10-41 are for an adult male. Adult females and children would have higher frequency values for the two fricatives, but the relative differences between /s/ and /ʃ/ would be similar to those for the adult male speaker. The fricatives /f/, /v/, /θ/, /ð/, and /h/ are weak in overall energy and are therefore sometimes hard to identify from their noise segment alone. In some contexts, formant transitions may be more important than noise spectrum in the identification of these sounds. This can be an important point in clinical assessment.
4. **Transitions.** The formant transitions are similar to those for stops with corresponding places of articulation. See Table 10-3 for a summary. As previously noted, the perceptual significance of the noise segment versus the formant transitions depends to a large extent on the energy of the noise. If the noise is weak, the listener may rely more on the transitional information to identify the fricative.

Affricates (/tʃ/ **and** /dʒ/)

1. **Silence.** Affricates have a silent interval that is similar to the stop gap of stops.
2. **Voicing.** The vocal folds vibrate for the production of /dʒ/, but not for /tʃ/. Therefore, the noise segment is

TABLE 10-4
Summary of Aerodynamic and Acoustic Properties for Obstruents

Category	Aerodynamic Properties	Acoustic Properties	
		Prevocalic Position	Postvocalic Position
Voiceless stops	High intraoral air pressure and no oral flow during closure phase, followed by an oral pulse of high airflow upon release.	Stop gap followed by burst and then formant transition; long voice onset time.	Formant transition followed by stop gap and possible burst; short vowel duration.
Voiced stops	Moderate intraoral air pressure and no oral flow during closure phase, followed by an oral pulse of high airflow upon release.	Stop gap followed by burst and then formant transition; short voice onset time.	Formant transition followed by stop gap and possible burst; long vowel duration.
Voiceless fricatives	High intraoral air pressure and high oral airflow.	Noise segment followed by formant transition; voice bar absent.	Formant transition followed by noise segment; short vowel duration.
Voiced fricatives	Moderate intraoral air pressure and high oral airflow.	Noise segment followed by formant transition; voice bar present.	Formant transition followed by noise segment; long vowel duration.
Voiceless affricate	High intraoral air pressure maintained during two phases: (1) no airflow during closure and (2) high oral airflow upon release and frication.	Stop gap followed by noise segment and then formant transition; voice bar absent.	Formant transition followed by stop gap and then noise segment; short vowel duration.
Voiced affricate	Moderate intraoral air pressure maintained during two phases: (1) no airflow during closure and (2) high oral airflow upon release and frication.	Stop gap followed by noise segment and then formant transition; voice bar present.	Formant transition followed by stop gap and then noise segment; long vowel duration.

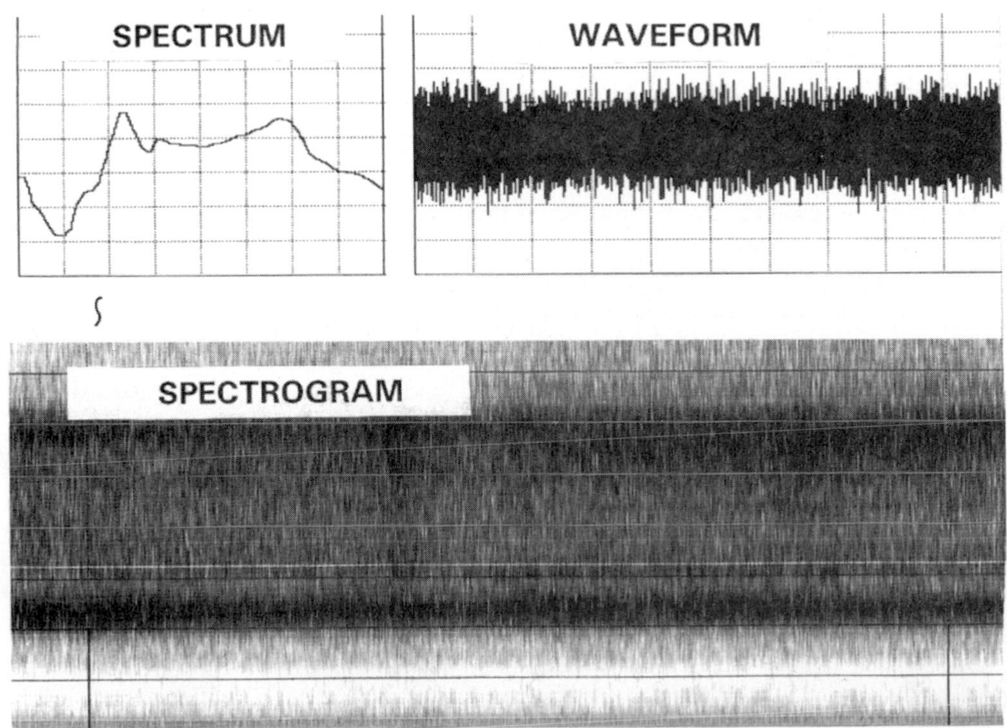

FIGURE 10-40
Spectrum, waveform, and spectrogram for the fricative /ʃ/. The spectrum at the top left is averaged over an interval represented by the vertical lines on the spectrogram.

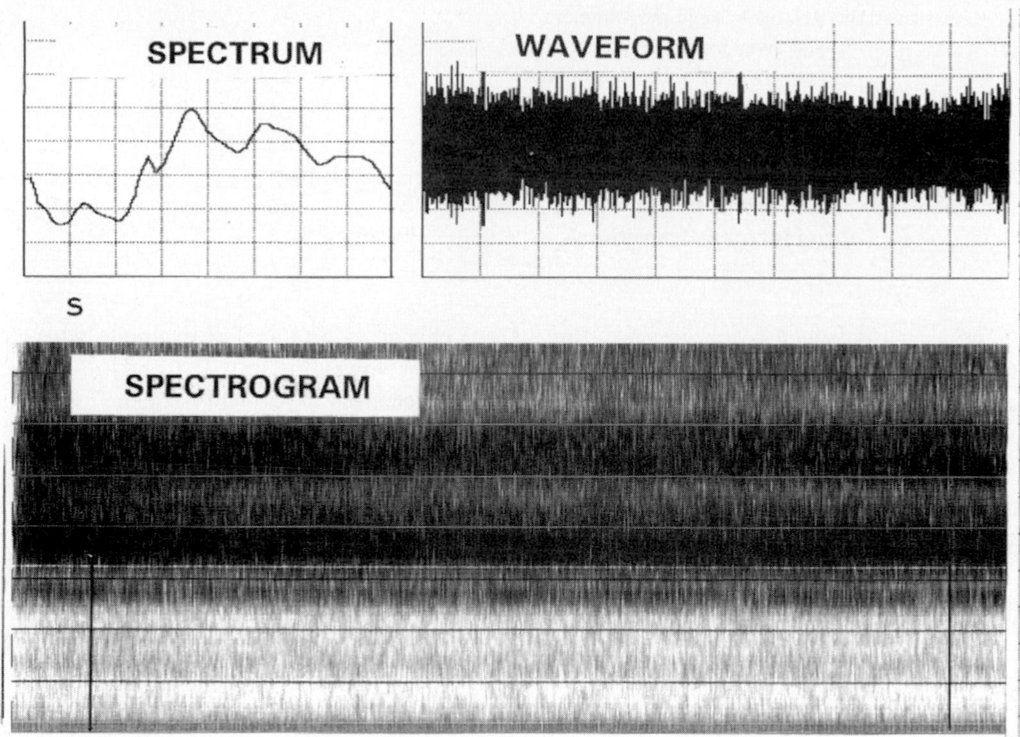

FIGURE 10-41
Spectrum, waveform, and spectrogram for the fricative /s/. The spectrogram at the top left is averaged over an interval represented by the vertical lines on the spectrogram.

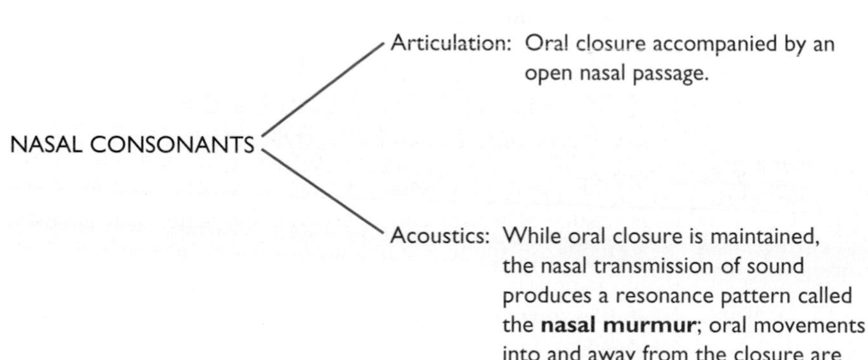

NASAL CONSONANTS
Articulation: Oral closure accompanied by an open nasal passage.
Acoustics: While oral closure is maintained, the nasal transmission of sound produces a resonance pattern called the **nasal murmur**; oral movements into and away from the closure are usually associated with **brief formant transitions**.

FIGURE 10-42
Basic articulatory–acoustic relations for nasals.

GLIDES

Articulation: Gradual movements away from a characteristic configuration.

Acoustics: **Moderate-duration formant transitions** away from a characteristic **formant pattern**.

FIGURE 10-43
Basic articulatory–acoustic relations for glides.

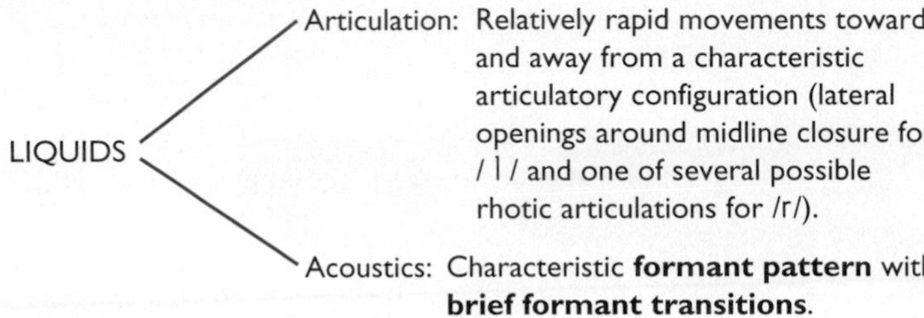

LIQUIDS
Articulation: Relatively rapid movements toward and away from a characteristic articulatory configuration (lateral openings around midline closure for /l/ and one of several possible rhotic articulations for /r/).
Acoustics: Characteristic formant pattern with brief formant transitions.

FIGURE 10-44
Basic articulatory–acoustic relations for liquids.

voiced for the former but is voiceless for the latter. But, like stops, affricates in final position may have as the primary voicing cue the relative duration of a preceding vowel—a longer vowel duration before the voiced affricate.

3. **Noise.** See description of fricatives /ʃ/ and /ʒ/. The spectral properties are similar.
4. **Transitions.** See discussion of stops and fricatives, especially /ʃ/ and /ʒ/.

Sonorants

Nasals (/m/, /n/, **and** /ŋ/). See Figure 10-42 for a summary of articulatory and acoustic characteristics.

1. **Silence.** No silent gap occurs. But the nasals have less energy than surrounding vowels and therefore may be associated with a dip in overall energy compared to vowel sounds.
2. **Voicing.** Nasals are completely voiced except for whispered speech.
3. **Noise.** None, except in unusual circumstances.
4. **Transitions.** The nasals are similar to stops in their articulatory dynamics and therefore have similar transitions. See Table 10-3 for details on formant patterns.

Glides or Semivowels (/w/, /ʍ/, /j/). See Figure 10-43 and Table 10-3 for a summary of articulatory–acoustic correlates.

1. **Silence.** None. Glides are typically weaker than neighboring vowels.
2. **Voicing.** Voicing continues throughout the glide articulation, except for whispered speech or the voiceless /ʍ/ (which may be disappearing from American English).
3. **Noise.** Rarely produced except for /ʍ/.
4. **Transitions.** As the vocal tract changes shape from glide to vowel (or vice versa), the acoustic resonances also change. Consequently, the formant frequencies undergo a gradual shift. These formant transitions for glides are longer in duration than those for stops, with continuous formant movements occurring for 100 ms or so. Glides can be distinguished from stops on the basis of transition durations, even when the extent of formant frequency change is similar. For example, when followed by the same vowel, the stop /b/ and the glide /w/ have similar changes in formant frequency values, but the change takes longer for the glide.

Liquids (/r/ **and** /l/). See Figure 10-44 for a summary of articulatory–acoustic correlates.

1. **Silence.** None, but liquids have lower energy than adjacent vowels.
2. **Voicing.** Except in whispered speech, /r/ and /l/ are voiced.
3. **Noise.** None, except in unusual circumstances.
4. **Transitions.** The liquids are generally similar to stops in their articulatory dynamics and therefore have relatively short durations of formant transitions. One major difference between /r/ and /l/ is that /r/ is associated with a very low third-formant frequency (the lowest of any sound in American English). Therefore, the F_3 transition is a reliable cue for identifying the /r/ sound.

ACOUSTIC CORRELATES OF SUPRASEGMENTAL PROPERTIES

To this point, the discussion pertains almost entirely to the acoustics of vowel and consonant segments. But acoustic methods are applicable to a host of issues in speech, including suprasegmental properties. We consider here acoustic studies relevant to loudness, vocal effort, and boundary effects.

Loudness and Vocal Effort

Loudness may seem to be a relatively straightforward aspect of speech, but an important complication should be noted. Current literature distinguishes loudness from vocal effort. Traunmuller and Eriksson (2000) defined vocal effort as "the quantity that ordinary speakers vary when they adapt their speech to the demands of increased or decreased communication distance" (p. 3438). In other words, vocal effort is the adjustment that we make when the distance between us and our listener(s) increases or decreases. Although vocal effort may be used for other purposes, it is the matter of distance between speaker and listener *(interlocutor distance)* that is of special concern. Now it may appear strange that we should speak of vocal effort rather than loudness when we try to account for adjustments in speech when there are changes in the distance between a speaker and listener. After all, intuition tells us that when people get farther away from us, we need to speak louder to be heard. This issue deserves some explanation.

Loudness is defined as the perception of the magnitude or strength of a sound and is usually scaled from soft to loud. To a first approximation, loudness is directly related to the physical measures of sound pressure level or intensity of a sound. So what happens when speakers adjust the loudness of their speech to be heard over varying distances from a listener? A very simple hypothesis is that speakers would follow the inverse square law, meaning that speakers would increase or decrease their vocal intensity by 6 dB for every doubling or halving of distance from the listener. If Listener A doubles his distance from Speaker B, then Speaker B should increase her vocal intensity by 6 dB. Interestingly, perceptual studies have shown that sound pressure level (or intensity) does not play a major role in judgments of vocal effort (Traunmuller and Eriksson, 2000). Although sound pressure level changes somewhat as speakers adjust their vocal effort, the relationship is variant, and the changes are often much smaller than would be predicted from the inverse square law. So what does change as the distance between speaker and listener increases? The most consistent changes that occur are those associated with increased vocal effort, specifically, increases in voice fundamental frequency (Rostolland, 1982; Traunmuller and Eriksson, 2000), increases in formant frequencies, especially for F_1 (Rostolland, 1982; Schulman, 1989; Junqua, 1993; Huber, Stathopoulos, Curione, Ash, and Johnson, 1999; Lienard and Di Benedetto, 1999; Traunmuller and Eriksson, 2000), increases in vowel duration (Fonagy and Fonagy, 1966; Bonnot and Chevrie-Muller, 1991), and changes in spectral emphasis or the tilt of the spectrum (Traunmuller and Eriksson, 2000). Vocal effort is a complex phenomenon that is not synonymous with loudness and is not directly related to physical measures of sound pressure level or intensity. The distinction between loudness and vocal effort is important when we try to understand what speakers actually do to make themselves understood to listeners who are positioned at various distances.

Boundary Cues

Boundary cues (or edge effects) are asymmetries in phonetic form that occur between internal positions and the edges of prosodic domains. In other words, a segment takes on different characteristics depending on whether it has an internal position as opposed to an edge or boundary position. The general pattern is that acoustic cues are enhanced for segments at the edges of prosodic domains. The enhancements take the form of lengthening of segments or pauses (Klatt, 1975, 1976; Beckman and Edwards, 1990; Wightman, Shattuck-Hufnagel, Ostendorf, and Price, 1992; de Pijper and Sanderman, 1994), strengthening (Fourgeron and Keating, 1997), changing the overlap between adjacent segments (Byrd, 1996; Byrd and Saltzman, 1998), and increasing the likelihood of glottalization of word-initial vowels (Dilley, Shattuck-Hufnagel, and Ostendorf, 1996). These effects distinguish a segment as occurring at a prosodic boundary and can help a listener to identify the boundary in question. De Pijper and Sanderman (1994) referred to the collective effects of these various cues as perceptual boundary strength. They showed that untrained listeners could reliably judge prosodic boundaries using these cues even when the lexical contents of the utterances were made unrecognizable.

A LOOK TOWARD THE FUTURE

The human ear is a marvelous sensory organ that has been the fundamental instrument in the history of phonetics research. Phoneticians have learned a great deal about speech by careful attention to the ear's auditory patterns. Similarly, auditory evaluation has contributed a great deal of information about speech disorders. But techniques for the physiologic and acoustic study of speech have expanded the potential of phonetic research and phonetic application, including the study of speech and language disorders. It is likely that many of the readers of this book will learn about phonetics and apply phonetic knowledge using acoustic analysis of some kind. Until fairly recently, acoustic analysis was found only in specialized laboratories. Today, the general user with a personal computer can perform some types of acoustic analysis with relatively low-cost software.

The essential step in using a personal computer to analyze speech is to digitize the speech waveform. Digitizing is a process of taking a continuously varying signal (the original speech waveform as recorded by a microphone) and converting it to a series of discrete samples. For a discussion of this process, see Kent and Read (2002). The digital signal processing that lies at the heart of modern systems for speech analysis offers a number of advantages, including the following:

- Visualization of speech patterns that are often too brief for confident perceptual analysis by the ear alone.
- Storage of speech samples as a digital file, which can be retrieved as desired.
- Editing of the digitized waveforms to extract an interval of special interest (such as isolating one fricative segment from a phonetic sequence).
- Measurement of speech features, including durations, fundamental frequency, formant frequencies, and various spectral features.
- Visual display of a client's speech pattern compared with a target pattern (for example, showing the /s/ sound produced by a child with an articulation disorder together with another /s/ sound that was correctly produced).

Extended discussion of these applications is outside the scope of this text. The interested reader is referred to Kent and Read (2002) for a general discussion of possibilities for acoustic analysis. We close this chapter with a list of speech analysis systems available for use with personal computers, either IBM-PC compatible or Apple Macintosh compatible. A vendor address is listed with each system.

Systems for IBM-PC computers

CSL (Computer Speech Lab) and Multi-Speech
Kay Elemetrics Corporation
12 Maple Avenue
Pine Brook, NJ 07058
Email: info@kayelemetrics.com

CSpeech and TF32
Professor Paul Milenkovic
Email: cspeech@chorus.net

CSRE (Computerized Speech Research Environment)
AVAAZ Innovations, Inc.
P.O. Box 8040
1225 Wonderland Rd. N.
London, Ontario
Canada N6G 2B0
Email: info@avaaz.com
http://www.icis.on.ca/hompages/avaaz

SpeechStation2
Sensimetrics Corporation
48 Grove Street, Suite 305
Somerville, MA 02144
Email: sensimetrics@sens.com

SpeechViewerIII
IBM Corporation
1133 Westchester Avenue
White Plains, NY 10604
IBM Special Needs Systems
1-800-426-4832 (voice) or 1-800-426-4833 (TTY)
Also visit Riverdeep Web site:
http://www.learningneeds.com

The following two systems use the Macintosh platform

Signalyze
Professor Eric Keller
University of Lausanne
Informatique-Lettres
1015 Lausanne
Switzerland
Email: 76357.1213@compuserve.com

SoundScope
GW Instruments, Inc.
35 Medford Street
Somerville, MA 02143-4237
Email: sales@gwinst.com

GLOSSARY

Amplitude the magnitude of a motion or displacement.

Base of articulation articulatory setting specific to an individual language that represents the most frequently occurring segments and segment combinations in that language.

Bel the basic unit of the logarithmic scale used to express sound magnitude (intensity or sound pressure); the bel is the logarithm of a ratio of sound intensities or sound pressures.

Bottom-up processor a system that operates by proceeding from lower levels to higher levels in a structure or model.

Burst and frication spectra the intensity-by-frequency characteristics of the noise that is generated during a stop burst or a fricative segment.

Categorical perception a perceptual phenomenon in which several similar, but not identical, stimuli are judged to belong to the same category; usually the stimuli within a category cannot be discriminated (as opposed to **continuous perception**).

Complex tones periodic sounds composed of two or more sinusoids.

Continuous perception a perceptual phenomenon in which similar or closely related stimuli can be discriminated (as opposed to **categorical perception**).

Continuous spectrum a spectrum in which the components are continuously distributed over a frequency region.

Cycle the basic periodic unit of a repetitive event; for example, the cycle of tuning fork vibration is one complete to-and-fro movement.

Decibel one tenth of a bel, the basic unit of the logarithmic scale used to express sound magnitude (intensity or sound pressure).

Discrimination the task of distinguishing between or among stimuli.

Displacement the movement in space of a particle or object. When the displacement of an acoustically vibrating particle is plotted against time, the result is called the waveform of a sound.

F_2 locus see Second-formant locus.

Filter a frequency-selective transmission system; some frequency components are passed with little or no loss of energy, whereas other frequency components are passed less well or not at all.

Formant a natural frequency or resonance of the vocal tract, often estimated by a peak in the acoustic spectrum. A particular formant is abbreviated F_n, where n is the formant number.

Formant structure the pattern of formants associated with a speech sound. Vowel sounds can be characterized by the frequencies of the first three formants, F_1, F_2, and F_3.

Formant transition a formant frequency change associated with phonetic transition.

Frequency rate of vibration, usually expressed as the number of cycles occurring in one second (see hertz).

Harmonic any component of a complex tone that is an integral multiple of the fundamental frequency of that tone.

Hertz (Hz) the unit of frequency, defined as one cycle of vibration per second.

Identification the task of assigning a different response to each stimulus in a set of stimuli.

Intensity the rate at which acoustic energy flows through a unit of area perpendicular to the direction of sound propagation.

Longitudinal wave a wave in which particle motion is a back-and-forth oscillation along the line of the wave; sound waves are longitudinal waves.

Narrow band a filter bandwidth that is relatively small in its frequency range. Conventionally, 45 Hz is narrow band for spectrograms of speech.

Phonetic adaptation a change in the perception of one stimulus caused by a recent presentation of another stimulus.

Pure tone a sound having a sinusoidal waveform and a single line as its spectrum; such tones are generated by tuning forks, for example.

Resonance a natural mode of vibration; generally, a resonance is any phenomenon in which a body (including an air-filled tube) is set into vigorous vibration by an energy source that has a period corresponding to one of the natural periods of the body.

Second-formant locus a characteristic frequency value of the second formant associated with a consonant sound or a place of articulation.

Sinusoid an acoustic waveform described by the trigonometric sine function; a pure tone has a sinusoidal waveform.

Sound pressure the physical magnitude of a sound expressed as the force per unit area, such as dynes per square centimeter or pascals.

Spectral plot or spectrum a graph of the magnitudes (amplitude, intensity, or sound pressure) of the frequency components of a sound.

Spectrogram a three-dimensional acoustic analysis, displaying frequency, amplitude, and time.

Standing wave the wave that results from the superposition of two oppositely directed wave trains of a similar nature; this wave does not have a progressive character but a stationary one.

Stop gap the acoustic interval associated with the closure period of a stop consonant; it appears on a spectrogram as an interval of silence (although a low-frequency voice bar might be evident for a voiced stop).

Top-down processor a system that operates by proceeding from higher levels to lower levels in a structure or model.

Transverse wave a wave in which particle motion is at right angles to the direction in which the wave travels; water waves are transverse waves.

Verbal transformation (or phonetic transformation) change in the perception of a stimulus that is repeatedly presented; e.g., a word that is heard over and over again may be heard as a different word even though the acoustic pattern is unchanging.

Voice bar a band of energy located on the extreme low-frequency portion of a spectrogram and associated with voicing.

Waveform a graph of amplitude as a function of time.

Wavelength the distance from one point on a periodic waveform to the corresponding point in the next cycle of the waveform.

Wide band a filter bandwidth that is relatively large in its frequency range. Conventionally, 300 Hz is a wide band for spectrograms of speech.

EXERCISES

1. Assume that a recording is obtained of a neutral (schwa) vowel produced by Sasquatch (or Bigfoot), the large humanlike creature reportedly seen in the Northwest and some other parts of the United States. If the first formant of the neutral vowel is determined to be 300 Hz, what is the estimate of the creature's vocal tract length? (Use the quarter-wavelength relationship discussed under the heading "Resonance.")

2. What is the fundamental period (the time required for one complete cycle of vibration) for each of the following frequencies?

   (a) 500 Hz

   (b) 1000 Hz

   (c) 5 kHz

3. Recalling that a logarithmic scale is an exponential scale, state which of the following is *not* a logarithmic scale or progression.

   (a) 0, 2, 4, 8, 16, 32

   (b) 0, 10, 100, 1000, 10000

   (c) 0, 2, 4, 6, 8, 10, 12

   (d) 0, 3, 9, 27, 81, 243

4. If the average second-formant (F_2) frequency for a particular vowel is 2000 Hz for adult male speakers, what is the expected average value for adult female speakers?

5. The voice onset time for word-initial stops varies with several factors. Generally, voice onset time is longer for velars than for alveolars and longer for alveolars than for bilabials. Also, as discussed in the text, voice onset time

is longer for voiceless stops than for voiced stops and longer for stops followed by liquids than for singleton stops. Using this information, arrange the following words in the expected order of increasing voice onset time, from the smallest to largest value of voice onset time.

par goat boat car glue

6. Circle the sounds in the following transcriptions that are associated with a nonperiodic waveform as part or all of their production.

   (a) [ɑ͡ɪ sɔ tɛn tre͡ɪnz]

   (b) [θɪn pipl̩]

   (c) [pɑlɪʃ me͡ɪks ɪt ʃɑ͡ɪn]

7. Assuming formant frequency values appropriate for an adult male speaker, draw the wide-band spectrograms (that is, formant structure) for the following sounds: /i/, /æ/, /u/, /ɔ͡ɪ/, /ɝ/, /ʌ/. Check your results against the frequency values given in Table 10-1.

8. Carefully study the spectrograms in Figure 10-15 and verify for each consonant represented the major acoustic features of silence, voicing, noise, and transitions discussed in the chapter.

Appendixes

Appendix A

Phonetics Symbols and Terms

At several places in the text, we have alerted the reader to the diversity of symbols and terms used to describe and classify speech sounds. The tables in this appendix should be useful for cross-referencing symbols, terms, and concepts found in a variety of sources read by students of phonetics. Table A-1 is the most recent update of the standard International Phonetic Alphabet (IPA), and A-8 includes IPA extensions for transcription of atypical speech.

CONTENTS

TABLE A-1

The International Phonetic Alphabet (revised to 1993, updated 1996). Copyright © 1996 The International Phonetic Association.

CONSONANTS (PULMONIC)

	Bilabial	Labiodental	Dental	Alveolar	Postalveolar	Retroflex	Palatal	Velar	Uvular	Pharyngeal	Glottal
Plosive	p b			t d		ʈ ɖ	c ɟ	k ɡ	q ɢ		ʔ
Nasal	m	ɱ		n		ɳ	ɲ	ŋ	ɴ		
Trill	ʙ			r					ʀ		
Tap or Flap				ɾ		ɽ					
Fricative	ɸ β	f v	θ ð	s z	ʃ ʒ	ʂ ʐ	ç ʝ	x ɣ	χ ʁ	ħ ʕ	h ɦ
Lateral fricative				ɬ ɮ							
Approximant		ʋ		ɹ		ɻ	j	ɰ			
Lateral approximant				l		ɭ	ʎ	ʟ			

Where symbols appear in pairs, the one to the right represents a voiced consonant. Shaded areas denote articulations judged impossible.

CONSONANTS (NON-PULMONIC)

Clicks		Voiced implosives		Ejectives	
ʘ	Bilabial	ɓ	Bilabial	ʼ	Examples:
ǀ	Dental	ɗ	Dental/alveolar	pʼ	Bilabial
ǃ	(Post)alveolar	ʄ	Palatal	tʼ	Dental/alveolar
ǂ	Palatoalveolar	ɠ	Velar	kʼ	Velar
ǁ	Alveolar lateral	ʛ	Uvular	sʼ	Alveolar fricative

VOWELS

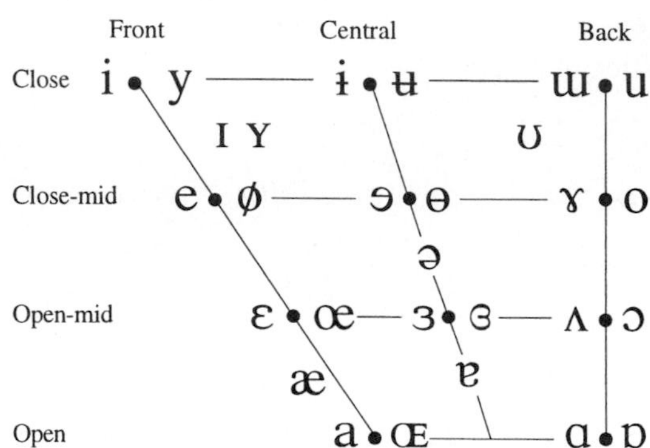

Where symbols appear in pairs, the one to the right represents a rounded vowel.

OTHER SYMBOLS

ʍ	Voiceless labial-velar fricative	ɕ ʑ	Alveolo-palatal fricatives
w	Voiced labial-velar approximant	ɺ	Alveolar lateral flap
ɥ	Voiced labial-palatal approximant	ɧ	Simultaneous ʃ and x
ʜ	Voiceless epiglottal fricative		
ʢ	Voiced epiglottal fricative		
ʡ	Epiglottal plosive		

Affricates and double articulations can be represented by two symbols joined by a tie bar if necessary. k͡p t͜s

SUPRASEGMENTALS

ˈ	Primary stress
ˌ	Secondary stress ˌfoʊnəˈtɪʃən
ː	Long eː
ˑ	Half-long eˑ
̆	Extra-short ĕ
|	Minor (foot) group
‖	Major (intonation) group
.	Syllable break ɹi.ækt
‿	Linking (absence of a break)

DIACRITICS Diacritics may be placed above a symbol with a descender, e.g. ŋ̊

̥ Voiceless	n̥ d̥	̤ Breathy voiced	b̤ a̤	̪ Dental	t̪ d̪
̬ Voiced	s̬ t̬	̰ Creaky voiced	b̰ a̰	̺ Apical	t̺ d̺
ʰ Aspirated	tʰ dʰ	̼ Linguolabial	t̼ d̼	̻ Laminal	t̻ d̻
̹ More rounded	ɔ̹	ʷ Labialized	tʷ dʷ	̃ Nasalized	ẽ
̜ Less rounded	ɔ̜	ʲ Palatalized	tʲ dʲ	ⁿ Nasal release	dⁿ
̟ Advanced	u̟	ˠ Velarized	tˠ dˠ	ˡ Lateral release	dˡ
̠ Retracted	e̠	ˤ Pharyngealized	tˤ dˤ	̚ No audible release	d̚
̈ Centralized	ë	̴ Velarized or pharyngealized	ɫ		
̽ Mid-centralized	e̽	̝ Raised	e̝ (ɹ̝ = voiced alveolar fricative)		
̩ Syllabic	n̩	̞ Lowered	e̞ (β̞ = voiced bilabial approximant)		
̯ Non-syllabic	e̯	̘ Advanced Tongue Root	e̘		
˞ Rhoticity	ɚ a˞	̙ Retracted Tongue Root	e̙		

TONES AND WORD ACCENTS

LEVEL			CONTOUR		
e̋ or	˥	Extra high	ě or	˩˥	Rising
é	˦	High	ê	˥˩	Falling
ē	˧	Mid	e᷄	˦˥	High rising
è	˨	Low	e᷅	˩˨	Low rising
ȅ	˩	Extra low	e᷈	˧˦˧	Rising-falling
↓		Downstep	↗		Global rise
↑		Upstep	↘		Global fall

TABLE A-2
Vowel and Diphthong Symbols in Several Transcription Systems[a]

Key Word	IPA (1979)	Symbol Name[b]	Shriberg and Kent[c] (this text)	Ladefoged (1975)	Prator and Robinett (1973)	Jones[d] (1966)
beat	i		i	i	iy	iː
bit	ɪ = ɩ		ɪ	ɩ	ɪ	i
bait	e		e, e͡ɪ	eɩ	ey	ei
bet	ɛ	"epsilon"	ɛ	ɛ	ɛ	ɛ
bat	æ	"ash"	æ	æ	æ	a
father	a		ɑ	ɑ	a	ɑː
bother	ɑ	"script A"	ɑ	ɒ	a	ɔ
bought	ɔ	"open O"	ɔ	ɔ	ɔ	ɔ, ɔː
boat	o	"closed O"	o, o͡ʊ	oɷ	ow	o, ou
put	ʊ = ɷ		ʊ	ɷ	ʊ	u
boot	u		u	u	uw	uː
but	ʌ	"caret" or "wedge"	ʌ	ʌ	ə	ʌ
above	ə	"schwa"	ə	ə	ə	ə
bite	ɑɩ		ɑ͡ɪ	aɩ	ay	ɑi
bout	ɑɷ		ɑ͡ʊ	aɷ	aw	ɑu
boy	ɔɩ		ɔ͡ɪ	ɔɩ	ɔy	ɔi
bird	ɝ	"reversed hooked epsilon"	ɝ	ər	ər	əː
better	ɚ	"schwar" or "hooked schwa"	ɚ	ər	ər	ə

[a]The format of this table was modified from Bronstein (1960, Appendix B) and from Ladefoged (1975, Table 4.1).

[b]Symbol names are only suggestive; alternative labels may be added by the reader. "Reversed hooked epsilon" refers to the Shriberg and Kent symbol in "bird." IPA alphabet does not differentiate stressed from unstressed [ɚ].

[c]Alternative symbols within a box represent allophonic variants by which phoneticians have symbolized tense vowels and diphthongs to indicate their increased duration and glide characteristics in certain environments (stressed syllables and open syllables [CV]).

[d]These symbols were taken from Jones's *The Pronunciation of English* (1966) and may differ somewhat from those used in his other works. They represent a Southern British form of English.

TABLE A-2
Vowel and Diphthong Symbols in Several Transcription Systems (continued)

Webster's New International							
3rd Ed. (1961)	2nd Ed. (1956)	Phonics Term[e]	Thomas (1958)	Kenyon and Knott (1953)[f]	Trager and Smith[g]	Hubbell (1950)[h]	Pike (1947)
ē	ē	"long e"	i, ɪ i	i	iy	i ĭ	i
i	ĭ	"short i"	ɪ	ɪ	i	i	ɩ
ā	ā	"long a"	e, e ɪ	e	ey	e ĭ	e
e	ē	"short e"	ɛ	ɛ	e	e	ɛ
a	ŏ	"short a"	æ	æ	æ	æ	æ
ä	ô		ɑ, a	ɑ	a	ɑə̆	a
ä	ō	"short o"	ɒ	ɑ	a	ɑ	ɑ
ȯ	ô		ɔ	ɔ	ɔ, ɔh, ɔw	ɔə̆	ɔ
ō	ō	"long o"	o, o ʊ	o	o, ow	ou	o
u̇	o͝o		ʊ	ʊ	u	u	ʊ
ü	o͞o	"long u"	u, ʊ u	u	uw	uŭ	u
ə	ŭ	"short u"	ʌ	ʌ	ə	ʌ	ʌ
ə	ȧ		ə	ə	ə	ə	ə
ī	ī	"long i"	a ɪ	aɪ	ay	a ĭ	a[i]
au̇	ou		ɑ ʊ	aʊ	aw	aŭ	a[u]
ȯi	oi		ɔ, ɪ	ɔɪ	oy	ɔĭ	o[i]
ər	ûr		ɜ, ɝ	ɝ	əhr	ɜ ə̆	r̩
ər	ẽ r		ə, ɚ	ɚ	ər	ə, r	r̩

[e]Phonics terms are presented as familiar referents from traditional reading instruction that relate to the common dictionary symbols in the two columns. *Phonics* refers to standard orthography only and must be kept distinct from *phonetics*.

[f]Kenyon and Knott base their system on a Midwestern dialect of American English.

[g]Trager and Smith base their system on an Eastern dialect of American English.

[h]Hubbell bases his system on a dialect of English spoken in New York City. The semicircular diacritic conveys a nonsyllabic value to the vowel below; it may also be used to indicate the weaker element of a diphthong (IPA convention).

TABLE A-3
Consonant Symbols in Several Transcription Systems

Consonant Symbol IPA (1979)	Example	Symbol Name[a]	Kenyon and Knott (1953)	Trager and Smith (1951)	Bloch and Trager (1942)	Pike (1947)	Webster[c] (1956)
θ	thing	"theta"	θ	θ	θ	θ	th "voiceless th"
ð	this	"ethe" [ɛð]	ð	ð	ð	đ "bar-d"	t̶h̶ "voiced th"
ʃ	she	"esh" [ɛʃ]	ʃ	š "s-wedge"	š	š	sh
ʒ	beige	"ezh" [ɛʒ]	ʒ	ž "z-wedge"	ž	ž	zh
ʧ[b]	church		ʧ	č "c-wedge"	tš	č	ch "cha"
ʤ[b]	judge		ʤ	ǰ "j-wedge"	dž	ǰ	j "ja"
ʍ	which	"voiceless w"	hw	hw	hw	hw	hw
j	you	"palatal glide"	j	y	j	y	y
ɹ[d]	red	"consonant R"	r	r	r	r	r
ŋ	sing	"eng"	ŋ	ŋ	ŋ	ŋ	ng

[a]The names in this column apply to the first column of symbols (IPA, 1979). Names for alternative symbols appear in the box with that symbol where it first appears.

[b]Variations among the affricate symbols are due to the attempt by some systems to denote the phonemic status of these two sounds as a single phoneme of English.

[c]Common dictionary symbols for most of these consonant phonemes are letter combinations known as "digraphs" (two graphemes).

[d][r] may be substituted for any retroflex sound, including the approximant [ɹ], so long as no ambiguity with the trill [r] results (*The Principles of the IPA*, 1978, p. 13).

TABLE A-4
Articulator Terms[a]

Articulator	Combining Term: Prefixal	Combining Term: Suffixal
Lips:	labio-	-labial
Tongue:	lingua-	-lingual
	glosso-	-glossal
Tip		
(apex)	apico-	-apical
Front	fronto-	-frontal
(lamina or blade)	lamino-	-laminal
Center	centro-	-central
Back		
(dorsum)	dorso-	-dorsal
Pharynx:	pharyngo-	-pharyngeal
Larynx:	laryngo-	-laryngeal
(glottis)		-glottal

[a]See Table A-5 for use of combining form with place of articulation. This table (Table A-4) was adapted from information presented in Mackay (1978, p. 116).

TABLE A-5
Point of Articulation Terms in Six Phonetic Systems

Place of Articulation	Shriberg and Kent (this text)	Catford (1977)	Peterson and Shoup (1966)	Gleason (1961)	Hockett[a] (1958)	Bloch and Trager (1942)
Lips	Bilabial	Exolabial Endolabial	Bilabial	Bilabial	Bilabial Apico-labial	Protruded Bilabial
Teeth	Labiodental Interdental Linguadental	Labiodental Dental	Unilabial Linguadental	Labiodental Dental	Labiodental Apico-interdental Apico-dental	Labiodental Dental
Alveolum (alveolar ridge)	Alveolar	Alveolar Post-alveolar	Alveolar Palatal-1	Alveolar Retroflex	Apico-alveolar Lamino-alveolar	Alveolar Cacuminal
Palate (vault)	Palatal	Pre-palatal Palatal	Palatal-2 Palatal-3 Palatal-4 Palatal-5 Palato-velar	Alveopalatal Palatal	Apico-domal Lamino-domal	Pre-palatal Medio-palatal Post-palatal
Velum (soft palate)	Velar	Velar Post-velar	Velar-1 Velar-2 Uvular	Velar Uvular	Front dorso-velar Back dorso-velar Dorso-velar	Pre-velar Medio-velar Post-velar
Laryngo-pharynx	Glottal	Pharyngeal Laryngeal	Pharyngeal Glottal	Glottal	Glottal	Pharyngeal Glottal Laryngeal

[a]Hockett typically describes both the part of tongue involved as well as the point of articulation.

TABLE A-6
Manner of Articulation Terms and Classification of Sounds in Twelve Phonetic Systems

1. Shriberg and Kent (this text):

Oral Closures			Oral Continuants						
Nasals	Stops	Affricates	Fricatives			Liquids		Glides	Vowels
			Nonsibilants	Sibilants		Lateral	Rhotic		
				Grooves (Blades)					
m n ŋ	p b t d k g ɾ ʔ	tʃ ʤ	f v θ ð h	s z	ʃ ʒ	l	r	w j	

2. Calvert (1980):

Stops (Aspirates)	Fricatives (Spirates)	Affricates (Stop fricatives)	Resonants				
			Orals				Nasals
			Semivowels			Vowels	
			Glides	Lateral	Retroflex		
p b t d k g	f v θ ð s z ʃ ʒ	tʃ ʤ	w j	l	r		m n ŋ

3. International Phonetics Association (1989):[a]

Plosives	Nasals	Lateral	Flap	Fricatives	Alveolar Approximant	Palatal and Velar Approximants	Vowels
p b t d k g ʔ	m n ŋ	l	ɾ	f v θ ð s z ʃ ʒ h	ɹ	j ɰ	

[a]For complete place manner chart based on the International Phonetic Alphabet (revised to 1996), see Table A-1 on p. 338.

4. Fromkin and Rodman (1978):[b]

Consonantals						Nonconsonantals	
Nonvocalics					Vocalics	Nonvocalics	Vocalics
Sonorants	Nonsonorants				Sonorants		
Continuants	Noncontinuants	Continuants					
Nasals	Nonnasals						
		Stridents		Nonstridents	Liquids	Glides	Vowels
m n ŋ	p b t d k g	tʃ ʤ	s z ʃ ʒ	f v θ ð h	l r	w j	

[b]Adaptation of a distinctive feature system. See Appendix C.

TABLE A-6
Manner of Articulation Terms and Classification of Sounds in Twelve Phonetic Systems (continued)

5. Tiffany and Carrell (1977)

Nonsyllabics						Syllabics		
Obstruent Consonants				Sonorant Consonants			Vowels	
Stops	Fricatives			Nasals and Lateral	Glides	Syllabic Consonants	Diphthongs	Vowels
	Nonsibilants	Sibilants						
		Concentrated	Distributed					
p b t d k g tʃ dʒ ʔ	f v θ ð h	s z	ʃ ʒ	m n ŋ l	j r w hw	m̩ n̩ l̩		

6. Ladefoged (1975, 1993):[c]

(Son.)	Obstruents			Sonorants					
Stops		Continuants							
(Nasals)	Orals	Fricatives		Approximants			Syllabics		Nasals
		Nonsibilants	Sibilants	Centrals		Lateral	Nasals	Approximants	
				Glides					
(m n ŋ)	p b t d k g	f v θ ð	s z ʃ ʒ	w j	ɹ	l	m̩ n̩ ŋ̩	ɹ̩ l̩	m n ŋ

[c]Ladefoged considers nasals to be classifiable in the stop category because they entail complete obstruction of the oral cavity.

7. Malmberg (1963):

Consonants											Vowels
Momentary		Continuous									
Stopped Passage of Air		Constricted Passage of Air								Free Passage of Air	
Stops	Nasals	Liquids			Frictional Continuants					Frictionless Continuants	Vowels
		Lateral	Trills		Flat	Round					
			Rolled	Flapped		Sibilants	Sibilants				
p b t d k g ʔ	m n ŋ	l	r ʀ	ɾ	f v θ ð	s z	ʃ ʒ	ɹ	h	ɹ w j	

TABLE A-6
Manner of Articulation Terms and Classification of Sounds in Twelve Phonetic Systems (continued)

8. Hockett (1958):

Contoids					Contoid-Vocoids	Vocoids			
Obstruents					Sonorants				Pure Vocoids (vowels)
Stops	Spirants				Nasal Continuants	Liquids		Glides	
	Slit	Rill	Surface			Lateral	Retroflex		
p b t d k g	f v θ ð	s z	ʃ ʒ	h	m n ŋ	l	r	w j	

9. Pike (1943):

Contoids (nonvocoids)							Vocoids	
Nonresonants (rarely syllabic)					Resonants (frequently syllabic) (syllabic)			
Stops			Frictionals		Nonfrictionals			
Number of Articulator Closures			Orals	Nasals	Nasal Resonants	Oral Resonants		
						Lateral	Central	
1	2	3					Glides	Vowels
p	p b t d k g	pʰ tʰ kʰ	f v θ ð s z ʃ ʒ h	"snorts"	m n ŋ	l	w j r	

10. Bloomfield ([1933] 1984):[d]

Noisy Sounds					Musical Sounds					
Stops	Trills	Spirants			Nasals		Lateral	Inverted	Semivowels	Vowels
Plosives	Tongue Flip	Nonsibilants	Sibilants							
			Hisses	Hushes						
						m n	l	r	w j	
p b t d k g	ɾ	h f v θ ð	s z	ʃ ʒ	ŋ	Consonatoids		Vocaloids	Nonsyllabics	
						Semiconsonants			Semivowels	Vowels
Mutes (always nonsyllabic)						Sonants (sometimes syllabic)				(syllabic)
Consonants										Vowels

[d]For phonetic terms, read down; for phonemic terms, read up.

TABLE A-6
Manner of Articulation Terms and Classification of Sounds in Twelve Phonetic Systems (continued)

11. Jesperson (1913):

Increasing Degree of Sonorancy ⟶								
Voiceless (surd)		Voiced (sonant)						
Stops	Fricatives	Stops	Fricatives	Nasals and Lateral	Trills and Flap	Vowels		
						Closed	Semiclosed	Open
p t k	f θ s ʃ h	b d g	v ð z ʒ	m n ŋ l	r̬ ʀ ɾ			

12. Sweet (1877):

Consonants						Vowels			
Open		Divided	Shut		Nasals	Nonround		Round	
Voiceless	Voiced		Voiceless	Voiced		Wide	Narrow	Wide	Narrow
f ʍ ʃ s θ h	v w ʒ z ð r j	l	p t k	b d g	m n ŋ				

TABLE A-7
Viseme Classes of the Phonemes of American English[a]

Class 1 (bilabials): /p/ /b/ /m/
Class 2 (labiodentals): /f/ /v/
Class 3 (linguadentals): /θ/ /ð/
Class 4 (rounded sonorants): /w/ /r/
Class 5 (palatals): /tʃ/ /ʤ/ /ʃ/ /ʒ/
Class 6 (alveolars): /t/ /d/ /s/ /z/
Class 7 (velars and alveolar sonorants): /k/ /g/ /n/ /l/
Class 8 (glottal): /h/

[a]Sounds in a viseme class share visual features. Sounds from different viseme classes can be distinguished from visual cues, such as jaw opening or lip configuration.

TABLE A-8
extIPA Symbols for Disordered Speech (revised to 2002)

CONSONANTS (other than on the IPA Chart)

	bilabial	labiodental	dentolabial	labioalv.	linguolabial	interdental	bidental	alveolar	velar	velophar.
Plosive		p̪ b̪	p͆ b͆	p̳ b̳	t̼ d̼	t̪͆ d̪͆				
Nasal			m͆	m̳	n̼	n̪͆				
Trill					r̼	r̪͆				
Fricative median			f͆ v͆	f̳ v̳	θ̼ ð̼	θ̪͆ ð̪͆	h̪͆ ɦ̪͆			ʩ
Fricative lateral+median								ʪ ʫ		
Fricative nareal	m͋							n͋	ŋ͋	
Percussive	ʬ						ʭ			
Approximant lateral					l̼	l̪͆				

Where symbols appear in pairs, the one to the right represents a voiced consonant. Shaded areas denote articulations judged impossible.

DIACRITICS

͍	labial spreading	s͍	͈	strong articulation	f͈	͊	denasal	m͊
͆	dentolabial	v͆	͉	weak articulation	v͉	͋	nasal escape	v͋
̪͆	interdental/bidental	n̪͆	\	reiterated articulation	p\p\p	͌	velopharyngeal friction	s͌
̳	alveolar	t̳	͎	whistled articulation	s͎	↓	ingressive airflow	p↓
̼	linguolabial	d̼	→	sliding articulation	θ͢s	↑	egressive airflow	!↑

CONNECTED SPEECH

(.)	short pause
(..)	medium pause
(...)	long pause
f	loud speech [{$_{f}$ lɑʊd $_{f}$}]
ff	louder speech [{$_{ff}$ lɑʊdɚ $_{ff}$}]
p	quiet speech [{$_{p}$ kwaɪət $_{p}$}]
pp	quieter speech [{$_{pp}$ kwaɪətɚ $_{pp}$}]
allegro	fast speech [{$_{allegro}$ fɑst $_{allegro}$}]
lento	slow speech [{$_{lento}$ sloʊ $_{lento}$}]
crescendo, ralentando, etc. may also be used	

VOICING

ˬ	pre-voicing	ˬz
ˬ	post-voicing	zˬ
(̥)	partial devoicing	(z̥)
(̥	initial partial devoicing	(z̥
̥)	final partial devoicing	z̥)
(̬)	partial voicing	(s̬)
(̬	initial partial voicing	(s̬
̬)	final partial voicing	s̬)
=	unaspirated	p⁼
h	pre-aspiration	ʰp

OTHERS

(◯), (C̲)	indeterminate sound, consonant	(( ))	extraneous noise ((2 sylls))
(V̲), (P̲l̲.v̲l̲s̲)	indeterminate vowel, voiceless plosive, etc.	¡	sublaminal lower alveolar percussive click
(N̲), (v̲)	indeterminate nasal, probably [v], etc.	!¡	alveolar and sublaminal clicks (cluck-click)
( )	silent articulation (ʃ), (m)	*	sound with no available symbol

REFERENCES FOR PHONETIC SYMBOL SYSTEMS

All of the phonetic symbol systems described in this appendix have been widely used in some area of linguistics or communicative disorders. The following references provide additional information on phonetic symbolization, including several systems developed for special needs. The Internet resources for more information on the International Phonetic Association additional learning materials and IPA fonts were courteously provided by Thomas Powell.

Ball, M. J. 1988. The transcription of phonation types. *Clinical Linguistics and Phonetics, 2:* 253–56.

Bernhardt, B., and Ball, M. J. 1993. Characteristics of atypical speech currently not included in the Extension to the IPA. *Journal of the International Phonetic Association 23:* 35–38.

Bronsted, K., Grunwell, P., Henningsson, G., Jansonius, K., Karling, J., Meijer, M., Ording, U., Sell, D., Vermeij-Zieverink, E., and Wyatt, R. 1994. A phonetic framework for the cross-linguistic analysis of cleft palate speech. *Clinical Linguistics and Phonetics 8:* 109–25.

Grunwell, P., and Russell, J. 1987. Vocalisations before and after cleft palate surgery: A pilot study. *British Journal of Disorders of Communication 22:* 1–17.

International Phonetic Association. 1999. *Handbook of the International Phonetic Association: A guide to the use of the International Phonetic Alphabet.* Cambridge, UK: Cambridge University Press.

Laver, J. 1980. *The phonetic description of voice quality.* Cambridge, UK: Cambridge University Press.

Miller, S. 2000. *Targeting pronunciation: The intonation, sounds and rhythm of American English.* Boston: Houghton Mifflin.

PRDS Working Party. 1980. The phonetic representation of disordered speech. *British Journal of Disorders of Communication 15:* 217–23.

PRDS Working Party. 1983. *The phonetic representation of disordered speech: Final report.* London: The King's Fund.

Pullum, G. K., and Ladusaw, W. A. 1996. *Phonetic symbol guide.* 2nd ed. Chicago: The University of Chicago Press.

Trost, J. E. 1981. Articulatory additions to the classical description of the speech of persons with cleft palate. *Cleft Palate Journal 18:* 193–203.

Woodard, M. 1991. The use of diacritics for visual articulatory behaviours. *British Journal of Disorders of Communication 26:* 125–28.

INTERNET RESOURCES

Home Page of The International Phonetic Association

http://www2.arts.gla.ac.uk/IPA/ipa.html

IPA Learning Materials

http://www2.arts.gla.ac.uk/IPA/cassettes.html
http://www.sil.org/computing/catalog/ipahelp.html
http://hctv.humnet.ucla.edu/departments/linguistics/VowelsandConsonants/

IPA Fonts

http://www2.arts.gla.ac.uk/IPA/ipafonts.html
http://www.sil.org/computing/fonts/encore-ipa.html
http://www.chass.utoronto.ca/~rogers/fonts.html

Appendix B

Distributional, Structural, and Proportional Occurrence Data for American English Sounds, Syllables, and Words

The 15 tables in this appendix provide comprehensive statistical information on English speech sounds. These data have been compiled and arranged as a handy reference source for the clinician. It is important to note that the statistical studies cited have used many different approaches; original sources should be consulted for full details of sampling, counting procedures, and other important methodological information.

CONTENTS

TABLE B-1
Some Distributional Characteristics of American English Phonemes[a, b]

Phoneme	Characteristics
/ʒ, ŋ/	These never occur in word-initial position; all other consonants do.
/h, j, w/	These never occur in word-final position; all other consonants do.
/r/	In word-final singleton position, /r/ is generally preceded only by a tense vowel, such as *near, nor.*
/ʃ, ŋ/	In word-final singleton position, /ʃ/ and /ŋ/ are generally preceded only by a lax vowel, such as *mesh, mash; ring, rung.*
/ɪ, ɛ, æ, ʊ, ʌ/	These lax vowels never occur in open syllable words; they can only occur before consonants or consonant clusters.
/i, e, ɑ, ɔ, u/ /o͡ʊ, ɑ͡ɪ, ɑ͡ʊ, ɔ͡ɪ/	All tense vowels and all diphthongs can occur in open syllables, such as *see, saw, sew.*

[a]For a complete description of the distributional characteristics of English speech sounds, see Gimson (1970). This work is based on British pronunciation; there is nothing comparable in breadth and depth for American pronunciation, but Kenyon (1964) provides background for certain dialects (Traugott and Pratt, 1980).

[b]Exceptions to distributional characteristics in English words are indicated in the text (e.g., some proper nouns).

TABLE B-2
Distributional Characteristics of Initial and Final Consonant Clusters[a]

Word-Initial Clusters[b]		Word-Final Clusters[c]		
CC-	CCC-	-CC	-CCC	
p+l, r, j	s+p+l, r, j	p+ t, θ, s	p+ t, θ	+s
t+ r, j, w	s+t+ r, j	t+ θ, s	t+ θ	+s
k+l, r, j, w	s+k+l, r, j, w	k+ t, s	k+ t	+s
b+l, r, j		b+ d, z	m+p, f	+s
d+ r, j, w		d+ z	n+ t, θ	+s
g+l, r, j, w		g+ d, z	ŋ+ k	+s
m+ j		tʃ+ t	l+p, t, k, f, θ	+s
n+ j		dʒ+ d	f+ t, θ	+s
l+ j		m+p, d, f, θ, z	s+p, t, k	+s
f+l, r, j		n+ t, tʃ, dʒ, θ, s, z		
v+ j		ŋ+ k, d, z	p+s	+t
θ+ r, j, w		l+p, t, k, b, d, tʃ, dʒ, m, n, f, v, θ, s, z	t+s	+t
s+l, j, w, p, t, k, m, n		f+ t, θ, s	k+s	+t
ʃ+ r		v+ d, z	d+s	+t
h+ j		θ+ t, s	m+ p	+t
		ð+ d, z	n+s, tʃ	+t
		s+p, t, k	ŋ+ k	+t
		z+ d	l+s, p, k, tʃ	+t
		ʃ+ t	s+ p, k	+t
		ʒ+ d		
			n+ d	+z
			l+b, d, m, n, v	+z
			n+dʒ, z	+d
			l+dʒ, m, v	+d
			k+ s	+θ
			n+t	+θ
			ŋ+ k	+θ
			l+ f	+θ

[a]Initial and final consonant clusters do not precede or follow all vowels in English. For representative information on British English, see Gimson (1970), from which the data in Table B-2 were taken.

[b]Glides and liquids are the only consonants permitted in the third position of word-initial CCC clusters.

[c]Final CCCC patterns are formed using /t/, /d/, /s/, or /z/ as a final element to represent the grammatical morpheme for past tense or plural *(glimpsed)*.

TABLE B-3
Structural Characteristics of Monosyllabic Words[a]

Syllable Type	Example	Broad Phonetic Spelling
V	a	[ə] or [ʌ]
CV	the	[ð ə] or [ð i]
CCV	tree	[t r i]
CCCV	screw	[s k r u]
VC	is	[ɪ z]
VCC	its	[ɪ t s]
VCCC	asks	[æ s k s]
CVC	cup	[k ʌ p]
CCVC	plane	[p l e͡ɪ n]
CCCVC	strain	[s t r e͡ɪ n]
CVCC	sits	[s ɪ t s]
CVCCC	sixth	[s ɪ k s θ]
CVCCCC	sixths	[s ɪ k s θ s]
CCVCC	stacks	[s t æ k s]
CCCVCC	stripped	[s t r ɪ p t]
CCVCCC	spanked	[s p æ ŋ k t]
CCVCCCC	glimpsed	[g l ɪ m p s t]
CCCVCCC	sprints	[s p r ɪ n t s]
CCCVCCCC	strengths	[s t r ɛ ŋ k θ s]

[a]See Moser (1969) for a thorough compendium of monosyllabic words in English. For information on the numerous structural types of polysyllabic words, see Roberts (1965).

TABLE B-4
Proportional Occurrence of Phonetic Classes in Adults' Speech[a]

Phonetic Class	Proportion of All Phonemes
Vowels/Consonants	
Vowels and diphthongs	38.10
Retroflex vowels	2.21
Consonants	58.50
Syllabic consonants	1.19
Vowels Classified	
by Place:	
Front	14.28
Centralized	13.51
Back	7.26
Back to front: [a͡ɪ] [ɔ͡ɪ]	3.05
by Height:	
High	13.87
Mid	13.70
Low	6.84
Low to high: [a͡ɪ] [a͡ʊ] [ɔ͡ɪ]	3.69
Consonants Classified	
by Voicing:	
Voiceless	20.63
Voiced	37.87
by Manner:	
Stops	18.82
Fricatives	16.47
Affricates	1.05
Nasals	10.80
Liquids and Glides	11.36
by Place:	
Labial and labiodental[b]	12.78
Dental and alveolar[c]	35.64
Palatal[d]	2.79
Velar and glottal	7.29

[a]These data are adapted from Mines et al. (1978).

[b]Includes /w/ and /ʍ/.

[c]Includes /r/ and /θ/ and /g/.

[d]Includes /j/.

TABLE B-5
Proportional Occurrence of Phonetic Classes in Children's Speech[a]

Phonetic Class	Proportion of All Phonemes		
	1st Grade	3rd Grade	5th Grade
Vowels/Consonants			
Vowels and diphthongs[b]	40.07	39.94	40.00
Consonants	59.93	60.06	60.00
Vowels Classified			
by Place:			
Front	16.11	16.27	16.14
Central	14.31	14.34	14.73
Back[c]	5.20	5.40	5.60
Back to front: [a͡ɪ] [ɔ͡ɪ]	3.78	3.25	2.88
by Height:			
Closed (high and mid)	16.54	17.14	17.52
Open (low)	18.98	18.80	18.90
Low to high: [a͡ɪ] [a͡ʊ] [ɔ͡ɪ]	4.54	4.00	3.60
Consonants Classified			
by Voicing:			
Voiceless	20.45	21.02	20.65
Voiced	39.48	39.04	39.35
by Manner:			
Stops and Affricates	19.57	19.89	19.44
Fricatives	15.00	15.05	15.77
Nasals	13.29	12.58	11.64
Liquids and Glides	12.08	12.54	13.15
by Place:			
Labial and labiodental[d]	16.58	15.78	15.53
Dental and alveolar[e]	31.49	32.01	32.02
Palatal[f]	11.29	12.52	16.57
Velar and glottal	9.89	9.88	9.27

[a]These data are adapted from Carterette and Jones (1974).

[b]For separate diphthong data, see "Vowels Classified by Height: Low to High."

[c]Includes the diphthong [a͡ʊ].

[d]Includes /θ/ and /ð/ and /w/.

[e]Includes /r/.

[f]Palatal glide [y or j] not reported in Carterette and Jones's data summary.

TABLE B-6
Proportional Occurrence of Vowels and Diphthongs Overall and in Initial, Medial, and Final Position of Words in Adults' Speech[a]

Rank Order	Vowel Phoneme	Percent of All Vowels and Diphthongs	Percent within Phoneme			
			Initial	Medial	Final	Single
1	ə	18.10	18.80	34.71	25.28	21.18
2	ɪ	12.76	31.13	67.25	1.16	0.05
3	i	9.15	2.56	36.44	60.01	0.01
4	ɛ	7.95	0.21	76.79	2.31	0.02
5	ɑ͡ɪ	7.36	7.82	40.17	12.30	39.71
6	æ	5.59	30.65	67.72	1.50	0.01
7	o	4.58	10.64	41.08	43.27	5.01
8	e	3.90	3.85	64.36	30.07	1.72
9	ʌ	3.63	14.54	82.11	0.05	2.83
10	ɑ	3.54	22.17	74.93	1.75	1.15
11	u	2.81	0	50.77	49.06	0.02
12	ɔ	1.90	35.26	62.48	2.26	0
13	ʊ	1.88	1.40	68.91	29.06	0.06
14	ɑ͡ʊ	1.60	17.91	65.82	16.12	0.02
15	ɔ͡ɪ	0.20	4.65	58.14	37.21	0
Alternates:						
Front		1.57	44.92	47.65	6.98	0.05
Central[b]		6.48	12.98	74.49	10.59	2.03
Back		1.70	16.27	68.72	14.87	0.01
Retroflex vowels[c]		5.49	0.01	41.13	50.91	7.48

[a]These figures combine vowel, vowel alternate, and retroflex vowel data as originally reported by Mines et al. (1978).

[b]Central alternates include both front and back vowels, which alternate with central vowels.

[c]Retroflex vowels include ɚ, ɝ, and alternates ɚ ~ ɝ, ɚ ~ ur, ɚ ~ ər.

TABLE B-7
Proportional Occurrence of Consonants Overall and in Initial, Medial, and Final Position of Words in Adults' Speech[a]

Rank Order	Consonant Phoneme	Percent of All Consonants	Percent within Phoneme		
			Initial	Medial	Final
1	n	11.49	12.42	40.97	46.48
2	t	9.88	20.68	30.04	49.18
3	s	7.88	37.09	29.35	30.75
4	r	6.61	14.64	63.26	22.06
5	l	6.21	23.72	51.92	24.31
6	d	5.70	25.18	24.55	49.99
7	ð	5.37	90.23	8.46	1.26
8	k	5.30	34.38	41.76	23.77
9	m	5.11	37.87	28.02	33.91
10	w[b]	4.81	88.29	11.40	0.01
11	z	4.70	0.06	10.72	86.41
12	b	3.24	65.25	32.78	1.83
13	p	3.07	47.77	35.96	16.00
14	v	2.97	10.53	39.41	50.00
15	f	2.65	63.15	23.49	12.87
16	h	2.23	92.18	7.82	0
17	g	2.02	68.16	23.84	7.84
18	j	1.87	78.84	20.81	0
19	ŋ	1.85	0.01	30.76	69.15
20	θ	1.19	57.44	20.52	21.35
21	ʤ	0.95	49.22	31.54	19.24
22	ʃ	0.95	32.76	58.23	8.32
23	ʧ	0.85	15.71	24.39	44.19
24	ʒ	0.15	10.11	84.27	5.62
	Allophonic Alternates				
1	ɾ	1.76	7.02	56.13	36.86
2	ʔ	0.85	15.78	20.62	61.85
3	t ~ ʔ	0.21	0	52.94	47.06
4	t ~ ɾ	0.13	17.95	46.15	35.90

[a]The data presented here are adapted from Mines et al. (1978).

[b]Both /w/ and /hw/ are combined here.

TABLE B-8
Proportional Occurrence of Vowels and Diphthongs in First Grade, Third Grade, and Fifth Grade Children's Speech[a]

		Proportion of All Vowels and Diphthongs		
Rank Order	Vowel or Diphthong	1st Grade	3rd Grade	5th Grade
1	ə	31.87	32.03	32.70
2	ɪ	11.13	11.46	11.40
3	i	9.51	9.94	10.34
4	ɑ͡ɪ	9.27	7.93	6.98[b]
5	æ	8.09	7.68	7.60
6	ɛ	7.34	7.60	6.82
7	o͡ʊ	5.09	5.49	5.63
8	e	4.15	4.05	4.20
9	ɑ	3.83	3.88	4.11
10	ɔ	3.59	3.48	3.60
11	u	3.03	3.12	3.33
12	ɑ͡ʊ	1.92	1.89	1.78
13	ʊ	1.04	1.25	1.29
14	ɔ͡ɪ	0.15	0.20	0.23

[a]The data presented here are adapted from Carterette and Jones (1974).

[b]/ɑ͡ɪ/ is out of rank order by one place here. Otherwise, the rank orderings remain constant across the three grades sampled.

TABLE B-9
Proportional Occurrence of Consonant Phonemes in First Grade, Third Grade, and Fifth Grade Children's Speech[a]

	Percent of All Consonants					
	1st Grade		3rd Grade		5th Grade	
Rank	Consonant	Percent	Consonant	Percent	Consonant	Percent
1	n	13.63	n	13.46	n	12.59
2	r	8.20	r	8.73	r	9.01
3	t	7.91	t	7.77	t	7.69
4	m	7.49	s	7.48	s	7.31
5	s	6.94	d	6.53	d	6.81
6	d	6.31	m	6.30	m	5.43
7	w	5.57	w	5.22	l	5.33
8	l	4.96	l	5.05	w	5.05
9	k	4.96	ʔ	4.92	k	4.82
10	z	4.58	k	4.76	z	4.62
11	ʔ[b]	4.49	ð	4.58	ð	4.52
12	ð	4.42	z	4.28	ʔ	3.65
13	h	3.37	b	3.13	h	3.04
14	b	3.18	h	3.07	b	2.94
15	g	2.90	g	2.52	g	2.56
16	f	2.21	p	2.34	j	2.53
17	p	2.12	f	2.18	p	2.49
18	v	1.64	j	1.88	f	2.30
19	j	1.41	v	1.58	v	2.12
20	ŋ	1.05	ŋ	1.19	ŋ	1.38
21	θ	1.03	θ	0.96	ʃ	1.33
22	ʃ	0.84	ʃ	0.94	θ	1.04
23	ʤ	0.53	tʃ	0.57	tʃ	0.74
24	tʃ	0.51	ʤ	0.57	ʤ	0.69
25	ʒ	0	ʒ	0	ʒ	0

[a]These data are adapted from Carterette and Jones (1974).

[b]/ʔ/ is included as a "phoneme" of English in the original data.

TABLE B-10
Proportional Occurrence of Consonants in Initial, Medial, and Final Position of Words in First Grade, Second Grade, and Third Grade Children's Speech[a]

Rank Order	Consonant Phoneme	Percent of Consonants	Percent Initial	Percent Medial	Percent Final
1	n	13.14	7	62	31
2	t	11.74	22	22	55
3	d	10.25	15	12	73
4	r	7.83	14	46	40
5	s	6.50	50	20	30
6	ð	6.40	93	7	0
7	l	5.55	23	41	36
8	w[b]	5.33	94	6	0
9	m	4.63	35	26	39
10	k	4.25	41	29	30
11	z	3.70	0	6	94
12	h	3.33	99	1	0
13	b	2.97	76	23	1
14	p	2.73	52	23	25
15	g	2.38	77	13	10
16	v	1.91	4	36	60
17	f	1.83	64	17	19
18	ŋ	1.61	0	22	78
19	θ	0.93	45	22	33
20	ʃ	0.84	76	17	7
21	j	0.77	98	2	0
22	ʤ	0.69	78	12	10
23	ʧ	0.55	31	24	45
24	ʒ	0.01	0	100	0

[a]These data are adapted from data originally reported by Mader (1954).

[b]The percent reported for /w/ also includes the frequency of /ʍ/, as reported in the original data.

TABLE B-11
Proportional Occurrence of the 25 Most Frequent Word-Initial and Word-Final Consonant Clusters in Adults' Speech in Three Studies

	Word-Initial Clusters							Word-Final Clusters					
	Dewey[a] (1923)		French[b] et al. (1930)		Roberts (1965)			Dewey (1923)		French et al. (1930)		Roberts (1965)	
Rank	Cluster	%	Cluster	%	Cluster	%	Rank	Cluster	%	Cluster	%	Cluster	%
1	hw-	1.63	pr-	1.06	hw-	1.64	1	-nd	4.67	-nt	4.40	-nt	1.87
2	pr-	1.31	hw-	0.91	pr-	1.06	2	-nt	1.61	-nd	2.56	-st	1.68
3	tr-	1.06	st-	0.87	fr-	0.69	3	-st	1.50	-st	1.18	-nd	1.06
4	fr-	0.76	tr-	0.69	st-	0.80	4	-rd	0.66	-ts	1.11	-rz	0.80
5	st-	0.76	fr-	0.62	pl-	0.76	5	-ns	0.65	-ŋk	0.76	-nts	0.72
6	pl-	0.57	pl-	0.36	tr-	0.56	6	-nz	0.61	-ld	0.75	-rd	0.60
7	gr-	0.41	kw-	0.28	gr-	0.34	7	-ks	0.53	-rz	0.57	-ld	0.43
8	kw-	0.35	bl-	0.23	kl-	0.28	8	-kt	0.52	-ks	0.47	-rn	0.42
9	sp-	0.35	sp-	0.19	kw-	0.27	9	-ld	0.45	-kt	0.42	-kt	0.41
10	str-	0.32	kl-	0.18	gl-	0.24	10	-rt	0.42	-rd	0.37	-ŋk	0.39
11	nj-	0.27	others	1.01	sk-	0.23	11	-ts	0.39	others	3.73	-nz	0.37
12	kl-	0.26			θr-	0.22	12	-rn	0.32			-zd	0.29
13	dr-	0.24			br-	0.21	13	-nts	0.20			-rt	0.28
14	θr-	0.23			kr-	0.21	14	-rs	0.19			-ks	0.28
15	kr-	0.22			sp-	0.20	15	-lf	0.18			-ts	0.25
16	dj-	0.20			fj-	0.20	16	-rst	0.18			-vd	0.25
17	br-	0.18			dr-	0.15	17	-ŋk	0.17			-rk	0.20
18	bl-	0.14			str-	0.11	18	-zd	0.16			-lz	0.18
19	tw-	0.13			bl-	0.11	19	-rk	0.16			-mz	0.17
20	fj-	0.12			sm-	0.06	20	-ŋz	0.15			-rs	0.14
21	tj-	0.12			sl-	0.06	21	-rm	0.14			-rst	0.14
22	sj-	0.09			fl-	0.05	22	-ndz	0.13			-pt	0.13
23	fl-	0.09			sw-	0.05	23	-mz	0.13			-kst	0.12
24	kj-	0.08			tw-	0.04	24	-lz	0.12			-rm	0.11
25	mj-	0.07			bj-	0.04	25	-gz	0.11			-dz	0.11

[a]Dewey (1923) data are reported for prevocalic and postvocalic positions rather than word-initial and word-final positions.

[b]French, Carter, and Koenig (1930) data are reported for the top ten clusters only. The remainder are grouped under "others."

TABLE B-12
Syllable Types and Most Frequent Syllables in Adults' Speech

Syllable Types[a]			Most Frequent Syllables[b]		
Rank Order	Syllable Type	Proportional Occurrence	Syllable	Morpheme	Proportional Occurrence
1	CVC	33.5	ðə	the	7.3
2	CV	21.8	ʌv	of	4.0
3	VC	20.3	ɪn	in	3.3
4	V	9.7	ænd	and	3.3
5	CVCC	7.8	ɪ	-y	3.2
6	VCC	2.8	ə	a	3.2
7	CCVC	2.8	tu	to	3.2
8	CCV	0.8	ɪŋ	-ing	2.4
9	CCVCC	0.5	ɚ	-er	2.1
			rɪ	-ry	1.6
			ɪt	-it	1.4
			ðæt	that	1.3
			ɪz	is	1.3
			a͡ɪ	I	1.3
			lɪ	-ly	1.2
			fɔr	for	1.1
			others		<1.0

[a]French et al. (1930). C = Consonant; V = Vowel.

[b]Dewey (1923).

TABLE B-13
Word Types and Most Frequent Words in Adults' Speech

Word Types[a]				Ten Most Frequent Words in Four Studies			
Rank Order	Type	Proportional Occurrence	Number of Words of This Type	I[b]	II[c]	III[d]	IV[e]
1	VC	14.51	29				
2	CVC	9.52	307	the	I	I	I
3	CV	8.12	14	of	you	the	and
4	CVS	7.55	85	and	the	a	to
5	SVC	5.48	104	to	a	it	the
6	VS	5.07	10	a	on	to	a
7	CVSC	3.83	394	in	to	you	of
8	SVS	3.59	24	that	that	of	in
9	SV	2.94	6	it	it	and	we
10	CVCC	2.36	298	is	is	in	for
11	V	2.32	1	I	and	he	it
12	SVSC	1.40	103				
13	VSS	1.38	4				
14	CVCVC	1.12	266				
15	VSC	1.05	28				
16	CVCVS	1.04	86				
		71.28	1759				

Proportional Occurrence of One-, Two-, and Three-Syllable Words		
Syllables per Word	Proportional Occurrence	Number of Words
one	76.92	2747
two	17.05	3969
three	4.55	2247
	98.52	8963

[a]Roberts (1965). C = Consonant; V = Vowel; S = Semivowel.
[b]Dewey (1923).
[c]French et al. (1930).
[d]Denes and Pinson (1963).
[e]Roberts (1965).

TABLE B-14
Most Frequent Phonemic Words in Children's and Adults' Speech[a]

Rank	1st Grade	3rd Grade	5th Grade	Adult
1	ʔ ə m	ʔ ə m	ə m	j ɛ ɑ
2	ə m	ə m	j ə n o͡ʊ	j ə n o͡ʊ
3	ə	æ n	n o͡ʊ	w ɛ l
4	n o͡ʊ	j ə n o͡ʊ	j ɛ ɑ	n o͡ʊ
5	æ n	ʔ ə	æ n	o͡ʊ
6	æ n d	w ɛ l	w ɛ l	ə ʰ
7	w ɛ l	n o͡ʊ	o͡ʊ	æ n
8	ɑ͡ɪ	ʔ æ n	ə	ə
9	o͡ʊ	o͡ʊ	j ɛ ə	ɑ͡ɪ
10	ʔ ə	s o͡ʊ	æ n d	s o͡ʊ
11	æ n ð ɛ n	ə	ə ʰ	ə n
12	j ɛ ə	j ɛ ə	ʔ ə m	j ɛ ə
13	s ə m t ɑ͡ɪ m z	ɑ͡ɪ	h ɪ	ə h ə
14	ð ə n	j ɛ ɑ	s o͡ʊ	ɑ͡ɪ m i n
15	ə n	ʔ æ n d	ə n	ɑ͡ɪ n o͡ʊ
Types	4569	4815	5796	3447
Tokens	5528	5963	7187	4146

[a]Carterette and Jones (1974) define *phonemic words* in terms of a prosodical feature: a pause in the flow of sound. A phonemic word is a sound group or pattern that occurs between pauses (p. 26).

TABLE B-15
Summary of Findings on the Proportional Occurrence of Speech Sounds in Children's and Adults' Speech

Factor	Finding
Phoneme and phonetic class	(1) Four consonant sounds /n, t, s, r/ account for 25 percent of all phoneme occurrences (Dewey, 1923); ten phonemes /ə, n, t, ɪ, s, r, i, l, d, ɛ/ account for nearly half (47 percent) of all phoneme occurrences (Mines et al., 1978).
	(2) Approximately two-thirds of consonant occurrences are voiced (Mines et al., 1978).
	(3) The majority of consonant and vowel occurrences are articulated at the front of the mouth. Labial and labiodental sounds (21.6) and dental and alveolar sounds (60.9) account for over 80 percent of consonant occurrences. Front and central vowels account for nearly 75 percent of vowel occurrences (Mines et al., 1978).
	(4) The majority of vowels (over 71 percent) are articulated in the high (36.4 percent), high-mid (2.9 percent), or mid (32 percent) sections of the oral cavity (Mines et al., 1978).
	(5) Of all occurrences of syllabic consonants in adult conversational speech (1.2 percent), /n̩/ is most frequent, followed by /l̩/ and then /m̩/.
Position in word	(6) Four sounds /s, ð, w, h/ comprise more than 46 percent of the initial consonant occurrences in words said by young grade-school children; five sounds /n, d, t, r, z/ comprise more than 69 percent of the final consonant occurrences in words said by young grade-school children (Mader, 1954).
	(7) Five sounds /ð, h, w, dfʍ, j/ occur in the initial position in over 90 percent of their occurrences in children's conversational speech; /z/ occurs in the final position in over 90 percent of its occurrences in children's conversational speech (Mader, 1954).
Structural forms	(8) Clusters are formed by phonemes whose distinctive features are neither very similar nor very different (Saporta, 1955). The most frequent clusters are sound pairs with the same alveolar place of articulation, but different manners of articulation (Denes and Pinson, 1963).
	(9) Simple syllable shapes—vowel syllables and those released and/or arrested by a simple consonant—comprise 87 percent of the syllables used in conversational speech (Faircloth and Faircloth, 1973).
	(10) The 16 most commonly occurring syllables and 10 words in adult speech (see Tables B-12 and B-13) make up more than 25 percent of our verbal behavior (Dewey, 1923).
Demographics	(11) Overall frequency of occurrence or positional frequency of occurrence of consonant sounds is not associated with grade in school or sex of children.
	(12) Frequency of occurrence of phonemes is only slightly related to age, sex, level of education, or early place of residence of adult speakers; moreover, ". . . frequency of occurrence of phonemes in English is primarily a function of the structure of the English language itself, and its relation to form (either spoken or written) or to style is very slight" (Mines et al., 1978, p. 223).

Appendix C

Distinctive Features

Distinctive features are an alternative system to the one described in this book. But this is not to say that distinctive features are incompatible with, or in opposition to, the phonetic system we have developed in this text. In fact, many of the general principles we have discussed could be described using distinctive features. First, we will examine what a distinctive feature is, and then we will show how distinctive features relate to the phonetic system of this book.

To illustrate the concept of distinctive features, we will start with a nonphonetic example. Imagine that we have a group of people of both sexes and different ages and our task is to group them into men, women, boys, and girls. To form the groups, we could ask people to stand in a single line and then separate them on the basis of two questions: Is the sex of this person male or female? Is this person an adult (for example, using a cutoff age of 18 years) or a child? We can cast these questions into the form of a coding tree as follows.

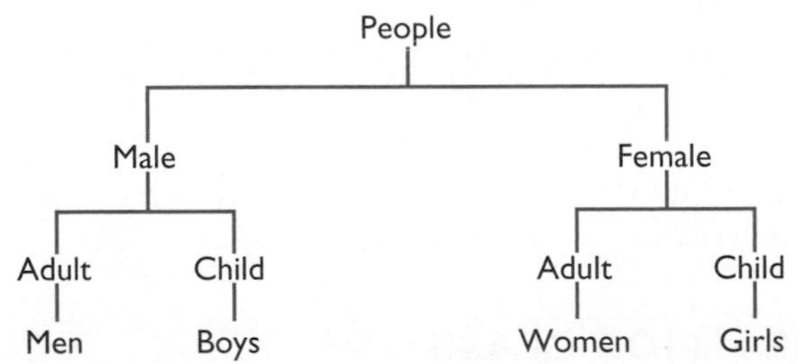

The first decision line, or branch, of this tree divides the people into two groups—male and female. The second branch divides each sex group into two age groups—adults and children. The final line gives us the desired final grouping into the classes of men (MALE + ADULT), boys (MALE + CHILD), women (FEMALE + ADULT), and girls (FEMALE + CHILD).

Because MALE versus FEMALE, and ADULT versus CHILD, are dichotomous, or divided into mutually exclusive groups, we could cast the coding tree into the form shown in the following figure. That is, each person is either male (+MALE) or female (–MALE) and either adult (+ADULT) or child (–ADULT). The terms we use to form each "plus" and "minus" group are arbitrary. The division into gender groups could just as well be made by changing the first

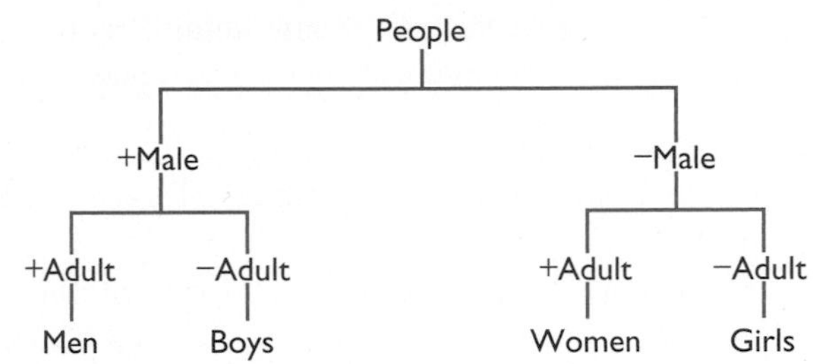

branch to –FEMALE versus +FEMALE. The essential point is that we form our groups by making binary (two-way) decisions at each branch of the coding tree. If we make correct binary decisions at each branch, we end up with the desired classes of men, boys, women, and girls. The branch names MALE (+MALE or –MALE) and ADULT (+ADULT or –ADULT) can be regarded as distinctive features for the classification of the people.

Distinctive features used in linguistic phonetics also are usually binary, although one could develop a system involving decisions that are three-way, four-way, and so on. Binary features often are preferred because of convenience in coding and a belief that the pertinent classes of sounds really can be formed of dichotomous groups. Binary features are best suited and most easily applied to attributes having opposing traits. For example, it is fairly easy to conceive of sounds as being either nasal (+NASAL) or nonnasal (–NASAL). Consonants described as +NASAL would be /m n ŋ /; other consonants would be –NASAL. Other attributes of sounds, such as place of articulation, might not be as inherently binary.

Ideally, distinctive features should fulfill three functions:

1. They should be capable of describing the systematic phonetics (a phonetic function).
2. They should serve to differentiate lexical items (a phonemic function).
3. They should define natural classes of sounds, that is, segments that as a group undergo similar phonological processes.

In addition, distinctive features are particularly advantageous for a linguistic purpose if a given set of features can be applied to all languages of the world. Although this criterion is not of primary importance to clinical phonetics, the speech-language clinician does have a similar concern, namely, that the features be widely applicable to patterns of developing and disordered speech. Whether or not distinctive features described in the literature are satisfactory for this purpose is perhaps controversial, but the authors would argue for the negative. Nonetheless, distinctive features have a general relevance to the study of phonetics and phonology and also offer significant advantages for some kinds of phonetic analysis. Therefore, speech-language clinicians should be familiar with them.

What is a distinctive feature? Some definitions or descriptions found in the literature are quoted as follows.

(*a*) *"A distinctive feature is any property that separates a subset of elements from a group"* (Blache, 1978, p. 56).

(*b*) *"Distinctive features are those indispensable attributes of a phoneme that are required to differentiate one phoneme from another in a language"* (Singh and Singh, 1976, p. 177).

(*c*) *"Distinctive features are really distinctive categories or classes within a linguistic system but just like in accepted analysis it is required that they are consistent with the phonetic facts and these phonetic facts on various levels [articulatory, acoustic, perceptual, or linguistic] have lent their names to the features"* (Fant, 1973, p. 152).

(*d*) *"It should be appreciated that distinctive features in the sense utilized by Jakobson, Fant and Halle (1952) primarily constitute a system for subdividing phonemes and other components of the message ensemble. A distinctive feature has certain correlates on each stage of the speech communication chain and these correlates are described in terms of various parameters and cues. . . . A distinctive feature is thus a unit of the message ensemble rather than a property of the signal ensemble. The term 'distinction' or 'minimal category' would have been more appropriate and might have led to less confusion concerning their nature and use"* (Fant, 1973, p. 162).

(*e*) *"A theory of distinctive features constructs category systems for phonemes; the categories are intended to cover all languages. Each feature category is derived by joint consideration of three levels of linguistic analysis: the perceptual level, the acoustic level, and the articulatory level. Thus the purpose of distinctive feature theory is to provide a single consistent framework for specifying the phonology, i.e., the communicative sound structure, of any language."* (Picket, 1980, p. 103).

(*f*) *"In recent years, phonological theory has moved to a system of distinctive feature classification based upon articulatory contrasts among phonetic segments. Here the aim has been to identify a system which differentiates every sound segment from every other segment by a phonetic or distinctive feature. Relative to phonological theory, it is intended that this system be universal to the languages of the world. It is most important to note that distinctive features systems are not intended as refinements in the descriptions of articulation already available from research in acoustic and physiological phonetics. Instead they are intended as the most economical description of phonemic (rather than phonetic) contrasts, and as such, may differ in some cases from the details of the phonetician's description of articulation"* (Williams, 1972, pp. 34–35).

From this sampling of remarks, it should be clear that distinctive features are pertinent to phonemic and not phonetic contrasts and that the names assigned to individual features do not always come from the same level of analysis or observation (articulatory, acoustic, perceptual, or linguistic). Partly because of the abstract nature of distinctive features and partly because of the inadequacy of definitions of their articulatory correlates, some of the early writings, especially those of Chomsky and Halle, have been criticized (for example, see Ladefoged, 1971, and Pak, 1971). Furthermore, some clinical applications of distinctive feature theory have been seriously questioned (Walsh, 1974; Parker, 1976). We point out these problems because we believe that the speech-language clinician should be aware that distinctive feature theory should be applied cautiously to the actual phonetic behavior of their clients.

The distinctive features described in this appendix are largely those proposed by Chomsky and Halle (1968) in their book *The Sound Patterns of English*. Departures from the Chomsky and Halle system are taken from Fant (1973) and Hyman (1975).

THE MAJOR CLASS FEATURES (TABLE C-1)

The major class features of syllabic, consonantal, and sonorant define the five major sound classes of vowels, syllabic nasals and liquids, nonsyllabic nasals and liquids, obstruents, and glides or semivowels. (Hyman also used nasal as a class feature to distinguish the liquids and nasals.) Definitions of the major class features are as follows.

Syllabic–Nonsyllabic

Syllabic characterizes the role that a segment plays in the structure of a syllable. A +syllabic sound serves as a nucleus or peak of a syllable; a –syllabic (nonsyllabic) sound does not. Vowels are +syllabic, whereas most, but not all, consonants are –syllabic. Some consonants, the liquids and nasals, can serve as syllable nuclei in words like *battle* /b æ t l̩/ and *button* /b ʌ t n̩/.

TABLE C-1
Distinctive Features for Major Sound Classes

Feature	Oral Cavity Obstruents	Nasals and Liquids	Syllabic Nasals and Liquids	Glides	Vowels
Syllabic	–	–	+	–	+
Sonorant	–	+	+	+	+
Consonantal	+	+	+	–	–

Sonorant–Nonsonorant

This feature refers to the resonant quality of most sounds produced with a relatively open vocal tract. Vowels, nasals, liquids, and semivowels (glides) are +sonorant. The obstruents are –sonorant.

Consonantal–Nonconsonantal

Consonantal sounds have a narrowed constriction in the oral cavity—either total occlusion or a narrowing sufficient to create frication. Stops, fricatives, affricates, nasals, and liquids are +consonantal. Vowels and semivowels are –consonantal.

The three major class features can be used in a coding tree to define the major sound classes as follows. Note that each branch of the tree is associated with one of the three features and that the left and right directions at each branch are labeled with the + and – feature values.

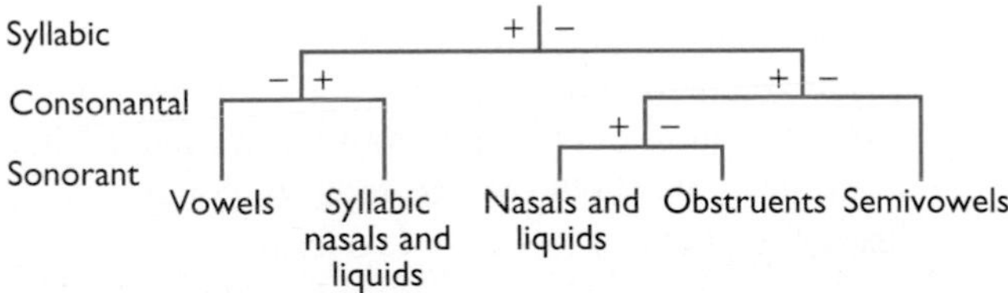

The same information can be represented in table form as shown in Table C-1. The table shows which values (+ or –) of each feature are associated with a given sound class. For example, vowels can be identified in bracket convention as

$$\begin{bmatrix} +\text{ syllabic} \\ +\text{ sonorant} \\ -\text{ consonantal} \end{bmatrix}$$

The enclosure of all three features within brackets indicates that they are taken together to define the sound or sounds in question.

MANNER OF ARTICULATION FEATURES (TABLE C-2)

Additional classes of sounds are determined by features having generally to do with manner of articulation. The following features fall into this group.

Nasal–Nonnasal

Nasal sounds are produced with an open velopharynx so that air can escape through the nose. Nonnasal sounds are produced with a closed velopharynx so that air pushed out from the lungs can escape only through the mouth. The only nasal consonants in English are /m n ŋ /.

Continuant–Noncontinuant

For continuant sounds, the primary constriction in the vocal tract does not completely block the flow of air. But for noncontinuants, or stops, the flow of air is completely blocked for some period of time. The stops /p t k b d g / and affricates / tʃ ʤ / are the noncontinuants in English.

Instantaneous Release–Delayed Release

With an instantaneous or abrupt release of the primary closure in the vocal tract, little or no turbulence is generated as the constriction widens. But with a delayed release, significant turbulence is generated upon release, causing an acoustic similarity to a fricative produced at the same point. The stops /b d g p t k / are produced with instantaneous release; the affricates /ʤ tʃ / are produced with delayed release.

Strident–Nonstrident

Strident sounds are produced with a greater intensity of noise than nonstridents. The noise intensity is determined by characteristics of the constriction, including roughness of the articulatory surface, rate of airflow over it, and angle of incidence between the articulatory surfaces. The strident sounds are /s z ʃ ʒ tʃ ʤ /.

Lateral–Nonlateral

This feature is restricted to coronal consonantal sounds. Lateral sounds are produced by lowering the midsection of the tongue at both sides or at only one side, so that air flows around the midline closure. Nonlateral sounds do not have such a side passage. The only lateral in English is /l/.

TABLE C-2
Distinctive Features of Selected Consonants[a]

	m	b	p	h	d	t	ŋ	g	k	z	s	ʃ
Nasal	+	–	–	+	–	–	+	–	–	–	–	–
Low				–	–	–	–	–	–	–	–	–
High				–	–	–	+	+	+	–	–	+
Back				–	–	–	+	+	+	–	–	–
Anterior	+	+	+	+	+	+	–	–	–	+	+	–
Coronal	–	–	–	+	+	+	–	–	–	+	+	+
Continuant	–	–	–	–	–	–	–	–	–	+	+	+
Strident										+	+	+
Delayed Release		–	–		–	–		–	–			
Voiced	+	+	–	+	+	–	+	+	–	+	–	–

[a]An empty cell means that the feature is either not relevant to the sound classification or is redundant with other features for that sound. For example, the features "Low," "High," and "Back" are unspecified for /m/, because tongue position of /m/ varies with context. The feature "Strident" is unspecified for /ʍ/, because nasals cannot be strident.

CAVITY (PLACE OF ARTICULATION) FEATURES (TABLE C-2)

The following features describe cavity configuration, or place or articulation. Some of them are defined relative to a neutral position of the tongue, which is essentially the position for [ɛ] in *bed*.

Coronal–Noncoronal

Coronal sounds are produced with the blade of the tongue raised from its neutral position; noncoronal sounds are produced with the blade of the tongue in the neutral position. For example, /t d n l θ/ are coronals; /p f k g / are noncoronal.

Anterior–Nonanterior

Anterior sounds are produced with an obstruction that is located in the front of the palato-alveolar region of the mouth; nonanterior sounds are produced without such an obstruction. The palato-alveolar region is that where the ordinary English /ʃ/ (or /š/) is produced. For example, /b f θ s / are anterior; /ʃ k g / are nonanterior.

High–Nonhigh

High sounds are produced by raising the body of the tongue above the level that it occupies in the neutral position; nonhigh sounds are produced without such a raising of the tongue body. For example, /i u k g / are high; /ɛ æ ɑ / are nonhigh.

Low–Nonlow

Low sounds are produced by lowering the body of the tongue below the level that it occupies in the neutral position; nonlow sounds are produced without such a lowering of the body of the tongue. For example, /æ ɑ / are low; /ɛ ɪ k u / are nonlow.

Back–Nonback

Back sounds are produced by retracting the body of the tongue from a neutral position; nonback sounds are produced without such a retraction of the tongue body from the neutral position. For example, /u ɑ o ʊ k / are back; /i ɛ æ / are nonback.

Rounded–Nonrounded

Rounded sounds are produced with a narrowing of the lip orifice; nonrounded sounds are produced without such a narrowing. For example, /u o w ɝ / are rounded; /i ɛ æ / are nonrounded.

Distributed–Nondistributed

Distributed sounds are produced with a constriction that extends for a considerable distance along the direction of the airflow; nondistributed sounds are produced with a constriction that extends only for a short distance in this direction. In English, this feature is useful to differentiate /s z / from /θ ð/.

SOURCE FEATURES

Only one source feature is considered here. Other features described by Chomsky and Halle either have been contradicted by acoustic and physiological data or simply have too many difficulties to be useful for the phonetic description of English sounds. A better treatment of source features is needed.

Voiced–Nonvoiced

Voiced sounds are associated with vibration of the vocal folds and, therefore, with a low-frequency periodic component of the acoustic signal. Nonvoiced sounds are not produced with vibration of the vocal folds.

RELATIONSHIPS BETWEEN DISTINCTIVE FEATURES AND TERMS USED IN THIS BOOK

Some relationships between distinctive features and phonetic descriptions used in this book are shown in the following list of phonetic terms and their associated distinctive features. For example, the phonetic term *bilabial* used in this book is associated with sounds that have the distinctive features +anterior, –coronal, and +distributed.

Place of Articulation

Bilabial: [+anterior, –coronal, +distributed]

Labiodental: [+anterior, –coronal, –distributed]

Linguadental: [+anterior, +coronal, α distributed[1]]

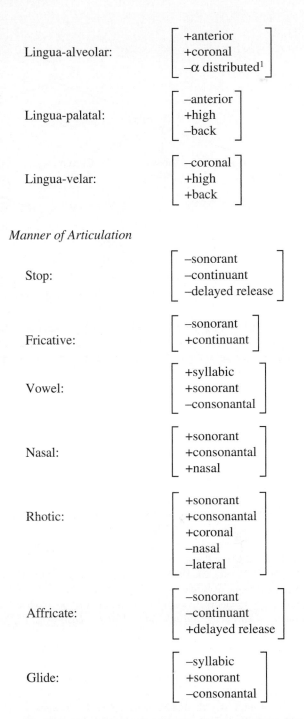

Lingua-alveolar: [+anterior, +coronal, –α distributed[1]]

Lingua-palatal: [–anterior, +high, –back]

Lingua-velar: [–coronal, +high, +back]

Manner of Articulation

Stop: [–sonorant, –continuant, –delayed release]

Fricative: [–sonorant, +continuant]

Vowel: [+syllabic, +sonorant, –consonantal]

Nasal: [+sonorant, +consonantal, +nasal]

Rhotic: [+sonorant, +consonantal, +coronal, –nasal, –lateral]

Affricate: [–sonorant, –continuant, +delayed release]

Glide: [–syllabic, +sonorant, –consonantal]

In the interest of conciseness, we have considered in this review the distinctive features described by Chomsky and Halle (1968). Other systems of distinctive features have been proposed, and revisions have been suggested for some of the features introduced by Chomsky and Halle. Moreover, unlike the linear arrangement of features as shown here, alternative feature systems organized in nonlinear or hierarchical patterns have also been proposed. Figure C-1 is an example of one such nonlinear arrangement of phonetic features. The use of various feature systems is discussed by several contributors in the book edited by Ball and Kent (1997).

[1]The symbol α is a "dummy variable" used to show that the Chomsky-Halle features can distinguish dental and alveolar consonants only if they differ with respect to the feature distributed. For example, if interdentals are –α distributed, then alveolars must be +α distributed. (See Ladefoged, 1971.)

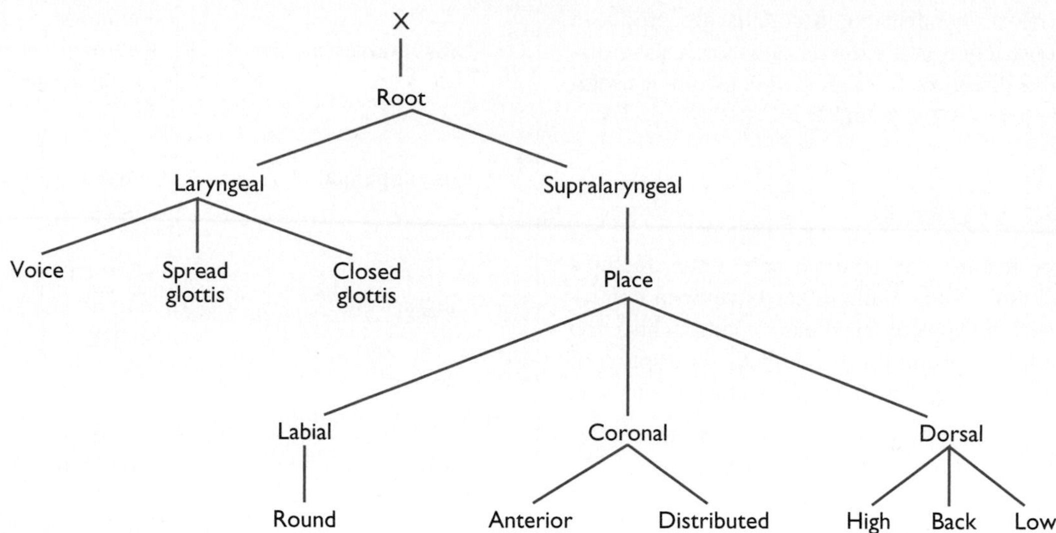

FIGURE C-1
One example of feature geometry, in which phonetic features are arranged in a hierarchy. The root subdivides into laryngeal and supralaryngeal levels, each of which is associated with additional features at lower levels. Feature geometry, unlike linear systems, readily allows some features to be subsumed under others, i.e., they are not independent. For more information, see: McCarthy, J. 1988. Feature geometry and dependency: A review. *Phonetica 45:* 84–108.

For additional reading on distinctive features, see the following widely cited sources.

RECOMMENDED READING AND REFERENCES

Ball, M. J., and Kent, R. D. (Eds.). 1997. *The new phonologies.* San Diego: Singular Publishing Group, Inc.

Blache, S. 1978. *The acquisition of distinctive features.* Baltimore, MD: University Park Press.

Chomsky, N., and Halle, M. 1968. *The sound patterns of English.* New York: Harper & Row.

Compton, A. 1970. Generative studies of children's phonological disorders. *Journal of Speech and Hearing Disorders 35:* 315–37.

Fant, G. 1973. *Speech sounds and features.* Cambridge, MA: MIT Press.

Hyman, L. 1975. *Phonology: Theory and analysis.* New York: Holt, Rinehart & Winston.

Jakobson, R., Fant, C. G. M., and Halle, M. 1952. *Preliminaries to speech analysis: The distinctive features and their correlates.* Acoustics Laboratory Technical Report 13, Massachusetts Institute of Technology, Cambridge, MA. Reprinted by MIT Press, Cambridge, 1967.

Jakobson, R., and Halle, M. 1956. *Fundamentals of language.* The Hague, Netherlands: Mouton.

Ladefoged, P. 1971. *Preliminaries to linguistic phonetics.* Chicago: University of Chicago Press.

Leonard, L. 1973. Some limitations in the clinical application of distinctive features. *Journal of Speech and Hearing Disorders 38:* 141–43.

Pak, T. 1971. Convertability between distinctive features and phonemes. *Linguistics: An International Review 66:* 97–114.

Parker, F. 1976. Distinctive features in speech pathology: Phonology or phonemics? *Journal of Speech and Hearing Disorders 41:* 23–39.

Picket, J. 1980. *The sounds of speech communication.* Baltimore, MD: University Park Press.

Singh, S. 1976. *Distinctive features: Theory and validation.* Baltimore, MD: University Park Press.

Singh, S., and Singh, K. 1976. *Phonetics: Principles and practices.* Baltimore, MD: University Park Press.

Trubetzkoy, N. S. 1969. *Principles of phonology.* Translated by C. Baltaxe. Berkeley: University of California Press.

Walsh, H. 1974. On certain practical inadequacies of distinctive feature systems. *Journal of Speech and Hearing Disorders 39:* 32–43.

Wheeler, M. 1972. Distinctive features and natural classes in phonological theory. *Journal of Linguistics 8:* 87–102.

Williams, F. 1972. *Language and Speech.* Englewood Cliffs, NJ: Prentice-Hall.

Appendix D

Procedures to Calculate Transcription Reliability and Research Findings

THE TERM *RELIABILITY*

The primary goal of this training series is to teach clinicians to produce reliable clinical data using two-way scoring, five-way scoring, and phonetic transcription. What are *reliable* data?

Reliable data, like reliable friends, can be depended on. Specifically, reliable data can be depended on to *agree with* some criterion measure, such as other data taken by the same person or data taken by a criterion judge. The degree of reliability or dependability, however, is entirely a matter of practicality. Just as a person's being a few minutes late may be tolerable in certain situations, a mere "ballpark" estimate of a particular phenomenon may be sufficient for making certain clinical decisions. In other situations, however, a person's dependability within a few seconds may make the difference between life and death. The point is that the degree of reliability or dependability—the amount of agreement we require between our data and criterion measurements—is entirely an individual matter. To illustrate this point, consider the following clinical situation.

Suppose we have a child learning to say /s/ by repeating a list of ten words containing an /s/ target. Every time the child says /s/ correctly, as judged by the clinician, the child gets a point toward some favorite play activity. In this clinical situation, how *reliable* does the clinician need to be in making two-way ("correct–incorrect") scoring decisions? 100 percent? 95 percent? 90 percent? 85 percent? How critical is it that the clinician reinforce all and only correct /s/'s in order for the child to acquire the correct /s/?

This question has never been studied. However, most learning theorists would agree that less than 70 percent reliability would not be fair to the child in this learning situation. At the upper end, however, 100 percent reliability may not be necessary either. Notice that if only ten items were being trained, 70 percent reliability would mean that to three of the ten responses the child makes, the clinician would say "correct" when the child was really "incorrect," or vice versa. Would a child acquire a correct /s/ under these feedback conditions? Again, it depends on the situation. The degree of reliability required of a person or of an instrument depends entirely on permissible tolerance under particular conditions. Measurements made by means of a micrometer are more precise than those made with the common ruler; however, each tool has its own error factor in terms of its quality of construction and in terms of the person doing the reading. Similarly, although five-way scoring may be more precise than two-way scoring, each system has its own error factors. The next section will show you some ways to assess your own error factor so that you can calculate your dependability, when using the three systems presented in this training series. The last section summarizes research findings on factors that influence the reliability of clinical transcription.

PROCEDURES TO CALCULATE TRANSCRIPTION RELIABILITY

Four Types of Reliability Checks

Table D-1 is a representation of the four types of reliability checks that should be familiar to clinicians.

Intrajudge agreement, how well a person agrees with himself or herself, can be assessed in two ways. As indicated in Table D-1, one way is to record a live session; scoring or transcription done later from the recording is compared to that which was done live. This way of assessing reliability is efficient for the working clinician because it requires the least amount of time. As described in Chapter 7, however, comparison of judgments made live with those made from recordings introduces uncontrolled factors. The second type of intrajudge assessment (Table D-1), recording-to-recording, compares responses made to the same recording scored on two separate occasions. This controls the stimulus conditions, as long as comparable playback conditions are maintained.

Interjudge agreement, agreement between two or more persons, can be assessed either live or from a recording, as described in Table D-1. In this series, your interjudge agreement is assessed each time you compare your scores of transcription to the key. Your agreement with the consensus key is a measure of how often you agree with the "experts." If you assume that our keys are valid (!), your relative compe-

TABLE D-1
Four Types of Reliability Assessment

Type of Reliability	Assessment Conditions	
	Live–Recording	Recording–Recording
Intrajudge	One clinician scores/transcribes both live and from a recording of the same session and compares the results.	One clinician scores/transcribes the same recording on two occasions and compares the results.
	Live	Recording
Interjudge	Two or more clinicians score/transcribe the same session live and compare their results.	Two or more clinicians score/transcribe a recording at same or different times and compare their results.

tence for each type of clinical task can be represented by a percentage figure. The next section describes several ways to calculate your percentage of agreement with each key.

How to Calculate Percentage of Agreement

Reliability of transcription is assessed as the **percentage of agreement** with an established source. As just discussed, this other source can be the same examiner, another examiner, or a group of examiners. Obtaining a percentage of agreement is not a difficult task. The formula is:

$$\textit{Percentage of agreement} = \frac{\textit{Number of units scored similarly}}{\textit{Total number of units scored}} \times 100$$

In this general formula, the "units" used are defined in terms of the variable of interest. For example, units could be all /s/ sounds, all fricatives, all /r/ sounds, or all dentalized /s/'s. Whichever unit is chosen, it is the comparison between each established criterion unit and each comparison judgment that is of interest.

How to Calculate Reliability in This Text

We now confront the issue of how much reliability we should expect when people score or transcribe disordered speech. We know that 100 percent agreement, whether intrajudge or interjudge, is not realistic to expect, nor is it generally necessary to achieve. In this section, we will provide some guidelines for how to compare your scoring and transcription of the recorded materials to the answer keys provided in this manual. Two concepts underlie the strategies we suggest.

The first concept is that of functional equivalence between different phonetic transcriptions. In this situation, two transcribers may perceive similar speech events but elect to use somewhat different phonetic symbols to capture this essentially similar perceptual event. If one transcriber symbolizes a sound as [i̞] (lowered /i/) and the other transcriber hears it as [ɪ̝] (raised /ɪ/), do they really disagree? For all but the most fine-grained analyses, the two transcriptions are functionally equivalent. Now consider a slightly different situation, the transcription [s] versus [t͓]. These transcriptions are nearly functionally equivalent, in that each symbolizes a frictionalized sound made in the area of the dental-alveolar ridge. Certainly, these two symbols are more nearly equivalent than, for example [s] versus [t]. These examples illustrate the point that transcriptions may "agree" to different degrees: (1) They may be *identical,* (2) they may be *functionally equivalent,* or (3) they may be *nearly functionally equivalent.*

The second and related concept concerns the arbitrary nature of reliability criteria, discussed earlier in terms of a person's dependability. In some measurement situations, we can justly afford to set a liberal (low) standard of agreement. In other situations, we must set a more strict (high) criterion for an acceptable level of agreement. Specifically, in some situations, transcriptions that are functionally equivalent or nearly functionally equivalent may be usefully considered to be in agreement. In other situations, only identical transcriptions should be scored as agreements. Consider three transcriptions of a child's response for the word *pan:*

Transcriber 1 [p æ̃ n]
Transcriber 2 [p æ]
Transcriber 3 [p æ̃]

Does Transcriber 2 agree with Transcriber 1 on the final segment? We would have to say by a strict criterion that they do not agree. Transcriber 1 has used a final /n/, whereas Transcriber 2 has not. Transcriber 3 also disagrees with Transcriber 1 in that /n/ is not present, but Transcriber 3 has symbolized the vowel as nasalized. By a strict criterion, each transcriber disagrees with the others on the final segment. But by a more liberal criterion, Transcriber 3, who has marked nasalization on the vowel, may be considered to be more in agreement with Transcriber 1 than Transcriber 2 is, because Transcriber 2 has marked neither the nasal segment nor the nasalization on the vowel. Because we know that hearing word-final /n/ can be difficult, we may elect to call the transcriptions of Transcriber 1 and Transcriber 3 **nearly functionally equivalent** on the basis of their vowel transcriptions.

You can use these two concepts—**functional equivalence** and setting a **strictness criterion**—in calculating your agreement with the answer keys. Each time your transcription differs from that given in the key, ask yourself whether your transcription is functionally equivalent or nearly functionally equivalent with that provided in the key. You may then want to calculate your percentage of agreement both in terms of a strict criterion (perhaps identical transcription with that given in the key or in the consensus column) and also by a more liberal criterion (functional or near functional equivalence). To parallel the previous example, the fact that you recognize the presence of a stop—although you may disagree with the key on the exact nature of the stop—should be more highly valued than missing the stop altogether. These matters should be discussed with your instructor.

To summarize, for any given speech event, there are several ways to transcribe its major characteristics. Particularly in clinical transcription, which uses many diacritic markings, alternate transcriptions of an event may be functionally equivalent. You can be "right on," "close," "in the ballpark," or "off by a mile." To get useful feedback on your learning, you should calculate your percentage of agreement with the experts using both strict and liberal criteria. In clinical situations, you will need to keep aware of how dependable you are in your phonetic skills. Just as you need to calibrate periodically an instrument such as an audiometer—to ensure validity and reliability of measurement—you also need to check regularly the reliability of your scoring and phonetic transcription.

RELIABILITY FINDINGS IN CLINICAL TRANSCRIPTION

Chapter 7 introduced several factors associated with the reliability of phonetic transcription in clinical settings. Because transcription is basic to the validity of assessment and management, the reliability of phonetic transcription has been the source of many studies. For your interest as a student of phonetics, we provide two summaries of this research.

The first research review, Table D-2, summarizes findings sampled from over a dozen studies crossing a variety of clinical settings. The right-most column of conclusions provides wide-ranging perspectives on the reliability of phonetic transcription. You may find it interesting to review some of these generalizations with your instructor, perhaps arranging to pursue your own research for an extra credit project. References for all papers cited in Table D-2, plus some core references in phonetic transcription, are included in the bibliography at the end of this appendix.

A second research review, Table D-3, is taken from a series of studies conducted in one research setting (Shriberg and Lof, 1991). These reliability findings were obtained from five two-person phonetic transcription teams. Each team learned to do phonetic transcription using the symbols and procedures described in *Clinical Phonetics*. They also learned procedures to reach a consensus between their individual judgments (Shriberg et al., 1984). As you look at the generalizations from these studies, you will see that not all teams were able to develop clinically reliable narrow phonetic transcription. Specifically, the interjudge agreements of some teams (i.e., their consensus agreements assessed on the same recorded speech samples at two different times) was less than 70 percent.

The challenge of increasing intrajudge and interjudge agreement has been the source of several studies and reviews in the years since the data summarized in Tables D-2 and D-3. Essentially, estimates of transcription agreement on consonants, vowels, and especially diacritics continue to be often unacceptably low, especially among researchers and speech-language pathologists with more limited training and with children who have significant speech involvements (e.g., Cucchiarini, 1996; Grunwell and Harding, 1996; Ingrisano, Klee, and Binger, 1996; Maassen, Offerninga, Vieregge, and Thoonen, 1996; Vieregge and Maassen, 1999; Gooch, Hardin-Jones, Chapman, Trost-Cardamone, and Sussman, 2001; Howard and Heselwood, 2002). Moran and Fitch (2001) have recently demonstrated that phonetics students' phoneme awareness, as assessed by a battery of measures, may be significantly associated with their scores on transcription quizzes. These authors speculate on the possibility of improving transcription skills by providing students with activities designed to increase their phoneme awareness. Such strategies, as well as the availability of new transcriptions systems and audio training programs, may help in teaching skills that may increase the reliability of clinical transcription (e.g., Ball, Code, Rahilly, and Hazlett, 1994; Ball, Rahilly, and Tench, 1996; Small, 1999; Ball, Esling, and Dickson, 2000; Hoffman and Buckingham, 2000; Louko and Edwards, 2001; Pollock and Berni, 2001; Powell, 2001; Snow, 2001; Stoel-Gammon, 2001). Moreover, it is likely that substantial improvement in transcription agreement may be achieved using procedures that provide online acoustics information (see Chapter 10) on segmental and suprasegmental aspects of speech production. Until such potentially effective systems become readily available, however, it is important to acknowledge the reliability challenges associated with broad and narrow phonetic transcription as an auditory-perceptual skill.

TABLE D-2
Sample Findings and Conclusions Categorized by 12 Sources of Variance in Phonetic Transcription Reliability

Source	Variable	Study	Mean Agreement Findings[a]	Conclusions
A. Subjects	1. Intelligibility	Philips and Bzoch (1969)	Interjudge variability with intelligibility: $r = 0{\cdot}19$	There is little association between interjudge agreement and intelligibility.
	2. Severity of involvement	Irwin (1970)	Interjudge: correct sounds = 88%; misarticulated sounds = 66%	Agreement is considerably higher when calculated on correct, compared to misarticulated, sounds.
	3. Type of error	Philips and Bzoch (1969)	Agreement on error type (five classifications): intrajudge = 50–91%; interjudge = 6–19%	Judges have low levels of agreement on each of five categories of error classifications.
		Norris, Harden, and Bell (1980)	—	Interjudge agreement on omissions was higher than on substitutions.
	4. Clinical significance	Shriberg, Kwiatkowski, and Hoffmann (1984)	Exact retest consensus reliability was 68%; with nonerror diacritics removed, exact agreement was 76%.	Consensus transcription agreement is higher when based only on sound changes that have clinical significance.
B. Analyses	5. Transcribers	Siegel (1962)	Interjudge: $r = 0{\cdot}92$	Transcribers can be trained to high agreement levels in making correct/incorrect judgments of sounds in isolated words, but differences on scores assigned by individual transcribers can be considerable.
		Burkowsky (1967, 1971)	Intrajudge = 64%; interjudge = 36%	"The field of speech pathology does not produce students with proven competence in listening to speech sound production" (p. 1).
		Irwin (1970)	Interjudge = 87%	"Undergraduate majors in speech pathology were relatively [reliable]" (p. 554).
		Diedrich and Bangert (1976, 1981)	—	Sounds may be judged as correct more often by judges who also are functioning as the child's clinician.
	6. Type of agreement	Schissel and Flournoy (1978)	—	Intrajudge agreement was higher than interjudge agreement for both experienced and inexperienced listeners.
	7. Type of system	Amorosa, von Benda, Wagner, and Keck (1985)	Interjudge: live = 56%; tape = 72%	Transcription procedures that do not allow for unlimited replays will result in over-diagnosis of phonologic disability because "all other information on phonetic detail has either been omitted or must be considered unreliable" (p. 286).
		Pye, Wilcox, and Siren (1988)	—	Broad transcriptions were used because "the frequency with which two or more individual transcribers chose to use the same diacritic marker for the same segment was quite small" (p. 21).
	8. Agreement criteria	—	—	—
C. Contexts	9. Sampling mode	Irwin and Krafchick (1965)	—	Identification of misarticulations was better in words than in phrases.
		Pye, Wilcox, and Siren (1988)	—	Interjudge agreement was higher for articulation test responses than for continuous speech.
	10. Structural, grammatical, and stress forms	McCauley and Skenes (1987)	Significantly more unstressed than stressed /r/'s scored as correct	(Among other interpretations), listeners may have a more lenient standard for correct /r/ in unstressed, compared to stressed, contexts.
	11. Word position	Philips and Bzoch (1969)	Interjudge: word-initial = 80%; word-medial = 78%; word-final = 67%	". . . sounds in final positions account for a greater portion of the disagreements" (p. 28).
	12. Target environment	Ruscello, Lass, Posch, and Jones (1980)	6–24% judgment shifts on correct, moderate errors, and severe errors on /r/ and /s/	". . . alterations in judgment . . . occur when individuals listen repeatedly to the same stimuli" (p. 5).
		Norris, Harden, and Bell (1980)	—	Syllabic function contributed little to interjudge agreement.

[a]Blank entries in this column reflect situations in which single agreement figures would not be representative.

TABLE D-3
Summary of Generalizations about Sources of Variance for Further Research[a]

Source	Variable	Sample Levels	Generalization
A. Subjects	1. Intelligibility	High, medium, low	Transcriber agreement on consonants and vowels has a low to moderately positive association with the subjects' severity of involvement, as indexed by percentage of consonants correct and intelligibility.
	2. Severity of involvement	Mild, moderate, severe	
	3. Type of error	Deletion, substitution, distortion	Neither the absolute nor relative percentages of each of the primary error types—deletions, substitutions, or distortions—are highly associated with transcription agreement.
	4. Clinical significance	Articulation error, acceptable allophone	Transcriber agreement is not associated with the clinical significance of diacritical description of speech.
B. Analyses	5. Transcribers	Background, training	No generalization
	6. Type of agreement	Intrajudge, interjudge, consensus	The two types of transcription agreement—interjudge and intrajudge—have essentially similar average percentages of agreement, ranging from the mid-60s to the mid-high-90s.
	7. Type of system	Broad, narrow (International Phonetic Alphabet, other)	The two systems of phonetic transcription—broad (93%) and narrow (74%)—differ in average transcription agreement by approximately 20 points.
	8. Agreement criteria	Exact, within-class, other	The three types of transcription agreement criteria for diacritics—exact (33%), within-class (40%), and any diacritic (48%)—differ in average transcription agreement (uncorrected for chance agreement) by a range of approximately 15 points.
C. Contexts	9. Sampling mode	Continuous speech, articulation test	Transcription agreement based on continuous speech samples is somewhat higher than agreement based on articulation test responses.
	10. Structural, grammatical, and stress forms	Canonical, grammatic, stress	No generalization
	11. Word position	Initial, medial, final	Of the three word positions, word-initial consonants are generally transcribed most reliably, with word-final consonants typically associated with the lowest reliability.
	12. Target environment	Stimulus context, phonetic context	No generalization

[a]Shriberg and Lof, 1991.

TABLE D-3 (Continued)

Source	Variable	Sample Levels	Generalization
D. Units	13. Class 14. Features	Consonants, vowels Manner, place, voicing, height	Average transcription agreement at the level of phonetic features and classes is within acceptable levels for broad transcription and generally below acceptable levels for narrow phonetic transcription.
	15. Sounds	24 consonants, 17 vowels/diphthongs	The reliability of broad transcription of vowels in a sample is essentially independent of their rank order of occurrence and percentage correct. For consonants, transcription agreement is independent of rank order of occurrence and lower, but within an acceptable range, for the 12 most frequently misarticulated sounds. Average transcription agreement percentages for each of the 41 sounds are within acceptable levels for broad transcription but generally below acceptable ranges for narrow phonetic transcription.
	16. Diacritics	35 symbols for narrow transcription	There are substantial differences in the average number of diacritics per word used by different consensus transcription teams within and between sampling modes and subject groups. There is fairly stable consistency in the average number of diacritics per word used by the same consensus transcription team doing narrow phonetic transcription on the same speech sample. The proportional occurrence of individual diacritic symbols in narrow phonetic transcription ranges from low to moderately high depending on consensus transcription teams, subject groups, and sampling modes. Transcription agreement on an individual diacritic is essentially independent of its proportional occurrence in a speech sample. The average interjudge and intrajudge percentage of agreement estimates for diacritic transcription are below acceptable reliability boundary levels, even at the least strict agreement criteria.

GLOSSARY

Functional equivalence essentially equivalent phonetic transcriptions of a target behavior that uses alternative symbolization.

Interjudge agreement the extent to which two or more clinicians make similar judgments about a target behavior.

Intrajudge agreement the extent to which a clinician makes similar judgments on different occasions about the same target behavior.

Near functional equivalence nearly equivalent phonetic transcriptions of a target behavior in terms of place and manner features.

Percentage of agreement the number of target units scored or transcribed similarly divided by the total number of units scored (multiplied by 100).

Strictness criteria an arbitrary basis for determining agreement between transcriptions. *Liberal criteria* might allow transcriptions that are nearly functionally equivalent to be counted as agreements; *strict criteria* might allow only identical transcriptions to be counted as agreements.

EXERCISES

1. To assess her intrajudge reliability, a clinician gives a child an articulation test on two separate occasions. She then compares her score sheets taken from the two sessions. Is this a good way for the clinician to assess her intrajudge reliability? Why or why not?

2. To assess his interjudge reliability, a clinician scores a child live, then brings a recording of the session to his clinical supervisor. The clinician then calculates a percentage of agreement between his scores and those of his supervisor for all /s/ words in the sample. Is this a correct way for the clinician to assess his interjudge reliability? Why or why not?

3. A clinician scores a recorded audio sample on two separate occasions and finds that she agrees with herself on 22 out of a possible 25 items. What is her percentage of intrajudge agreement?

4. A clinician scores a recording of a child on two separate occasions. He finds that he agrees with himself on 22 items and disagrees on 8 items. What is his percentage of intrajudge agreement?

5. On a 67-item test scored by two examiners, Examiner 2 disagrees with Examiner 1 on 11 items. What is the percentage of agreement between Examiner 1 and Examiner 2?

A BIBLIOGRAPHY ON TRANSCRIPTION RELIABILITY

Amorosa, H., von Benda, U., Wagner, E., and Keck, A. 1985. Transcribing phonetic detail in the speech of unintelligible children: A comparison of procedures. *British Journal of Disorders of Communication 20:* 281–87.

Bailey, C. J. N. 1978. Suggestions for improving the transcription of English phonetic segments. *Journal of Phonetics 6:*141–49.

Ball, M. J., Code, C., Rahilly, J., and Hazlett, D. 1994. Nonsegmental aspects of disordered speech: Developments in transcription. *Clinical Linguistics and Phonetics 8:* 67–83.

Ball, M. J., Esling, J., and Dickson, C. 2000. The transcription of voice quality. In R. D. Kent and M. J. Ball (Eds.), *Voice quality measurement* (pp. 49–58). San Diego, CA: Singular.

Ball, M. J., Rahilly, J., and Tench, P. 1996. *The phonetic transcription of disordered speech.* San Diego, CA: Singular.

Buckingham, H. W., and Yule, G. 1987. Phonemic false evaluation: Theoretical and clinical aspects. *Clinical Linguistics and Phonetics 1:* 113–25.

Burgi, E. J., and Matthews, J. 1960. Effects of listener sophistication upon global ratings of speech behavior. *Journal of Speech and Hearing Research 3:* 348–53.

Burkowsky, M. R. 1967. A study of the perception of adjacent fricative consonants. *Phonetica 17:* 38–45.

Burkowsky, M. R. 1971, November. A question of perceptual competence. Paper presented at the Annual Convention of the American Speech-Language-Hearing Association, Chicago.

Cole, R. A. 1973. Listening for mispronunciations: A measure of what we hear during speech. *Perception and Psychophysics 1:* 153–56.

Crystal, D. 1985. Things to remember when transcribing speech. *Child Language Teaching and Therapy 2:* 235–39.

Cucchiarini, C. 1996. Assessing transcription agreement: Methodological aspects. *Clinical Linguistics and Phonetics 10:* 131–55.

Diedrich, W. M., and Bangert, J. 1976. Training speech clinicians in recording and analysis of articulatory behavior. Washington, D.C.: U.S. Office of Education Grant No. OEG-0-70-1689 and OEG-0-71-1689.

Diedrich, W. M., and Bangert, J. 1981. *Articulation learning.* Houston: College Hill Press.

Edwards, J., Fourakis, M., Beckman, M. E., and Fox, R. A. 1999. Characterizing knowledge deficits in phonological disorders. *Journal of Speech, Language, and Hearing Research 42:* 169–86.

Faircloth, M. A., and Blasdell, R. C. 1979. Conversational speech behaviors. In N. J. Lass (Ed.), *Speech and language: Advances in basic research and practice* (Vol. 2, 283–320). New York: Academic Press.

Gooch, J. L., Hardin-Jones, M., Chapman, K. L., Trost-Cardamone, J. E., and Sussman, J. 2001. Reliability of listener transcriptions of compensatory articulations. *Cleft Palate-Craniofacial Journal 38:* 59–67.

Grunwell, P., and Harding, A. 1996. A note on describing types of nasality. *Clinical Linguistics and Phonetics 10:* 157–61.

Henderson, F. M. 1938. Accuracy in testing the articulation of speech sounds. *Journal of Educational Research 31:* 348–56.

Hoffman, P. R., and Buckingham, H. W. 2000. Development of a computer-aided phonetic transcription laboratory. *American Journal of Speech-Language Pathology 9:* 275–81.

Hoffman, P. R., and Schuckers, G. H. 1978. Audio-recording effects upon judgment reliability of children's /r/ misarticulation. *Perceptual and Motor Skills 47:* 451–56.

Howard, S. J., and Heselwood, B. 2002. The contribution of phonetics to the study of vowel development and disorders. In M. J. Ball and F. E. Gibbon (Eds.), *Vowel disorders* (pp. 37–82). Boston: Butterworth-Heinemann.

Ingrisano, D., Klee, T., and Binger, C. 1996. Linguistic context effects on transcription. In T. W. Powell (Ed.), *Pathologies of speech and language: Contributions of clinical phonetics and linguistics*. New Orleans: International Clinical Phonetics and Linguistics Association.

Irwin, R. B. 1970. Consistency of judgments of articulatory productions. *Journal of Speech and Hearing Research 13:* 548–55.

Irwin, R. B., and Krafchick, I. P. 1965. An audio-visual test for evaluating the ability to recognize phonetic errors. *Journal of Speech and Hearing Research 8:* 281–90.

Johnson, C., and Bush, C. N. 1971. A note on transcribing the speech of young children. *Papers and Reports on Child Language Development 3:* 95–100.

Kearns, K. P., and Simmons, N. N. 1988. Interobserver reliability and perceptual ratings: More than meets the ear. *Journal of Speech and Hearing Research 30:* 131–36.

Louko, L. J., and Edwards, M. L. 2001. Issues in collecting and transcribing speech samples. *Topics in Language Disorders 21:* 1–11.

Maassen, B., Offerninga, S., Vieregge, W., and Thoonen, G. 1996. Transcription of pathological speech in children by means of extIPA: Agreement and relevance. In T. Powell (Ed.), *Pathologies of speech and language: Contributions of clinical phonetics and linguistics* (pp. 37–43). New Orleans, LA: International Clinical Phonetics and Linguistics Association.

McCauley, R. J., and Skenes, L. L. 1987. Contrastive stress, phonetic context, and misarticulation of /r/ in young speakers. *Journal of Speech and Hearing Research 30:* 114–21.

Moran, M. J., and Fitch, J. L. 2001. Phonological awareness skills of university students: Implications for teaching phonetics. *Contemporary Issues in Communication Science and Disorders 28:* 85–90.

Norris, M., Harden, J. R., and Bell, D. M. 1980. Listener agreement on articulation errors of four- and five-year old children. *Journal of Speech and Hearing Disorders 45:* 378–89.

Oller, D. K., and Eilers, R. E. 1975. Phonetic expectation and transcription validity. *Phonetica 31:* 288–304.

Perrin, E. H. 1954. The rating of defective speech by trained and untrained observers. *Journal of Speech and Hearing Disorders 19:* 48–51.

Philips, B. J. W., and Bzoch, K. R. 1969. Reliability of judgments of articulation of cleft palate speakers. *Cleft Palate Journal 6:* 24–34.

Pollock, K. E., and Berni, M. C. 2001. Transcription of vowels. *Topics in Language Disorders 21:* 22–40.

Powell, T. W. 2001. Phonetic transcription of disordered speech. *Topics in Language Disorders 21:* 52–72.

Pye, C., Wilcox, K. A., and Siren, K. A. 1988. Refining transcriptions: The significance of transcriber 'errors.' *Journal of Child Language 15:* 17–37.

Riley, K., Hoffman, P. R., and Damico, S. K. 1986. The effects of conflicting cues on the perception of misarticulations. *Journal of Phonetics 13:* 481–87.

Ruscello, D. M., Lass, N. J., Posch, V., and Jones, C. L. 1980, November. The verbal transformation effect as studied in judgments of misarticulations. Paper presented at the Annual Convention of the American Speech-Language-Hearing Association, Detroit.

Schissel, R. J., and Flournoy, J. E. 1978. An investigation of the variability of judgments of experienced and inexperienced listeners in their use of a screening test of articulation. *Journal of Communication Disorders 11:* 459–68.

Schliesser, H. F., Stevens, C. A., and Bruce, C. E. 1973. Interobserver reliability of direct magnitude estimation of articulatory defectiveness. *Perceptual and Motor Skills 36:* 63–66.

Sharf, D. J. 1968. Distinctiveness of 'defective' fricative sounds. *Language and Speech 11*(Pt. 1): 38–45.

Shaw, S., and Coggins, T. E. 1991. Interobserver reliability using the phonetic level evaluation with severely and profoundly hearing-impaired children. *Journal of Speech and Hearing Research 34:* 989–99.

Shelton, R. L., Johnson, A., and Arndt, W. B. 1974. Variability in judgments of articulation when observers listen repeatedly to the same phone. *Perceptual and Motor Skills 39:* 327–32.

Sherman, D., and Morrison, S. 1955. Reliability of individual ratings of severity of defective articulation. *Journal of Speech and Hearing Disorders 20:* 352–58.

Shockey, L. R. 1973. Phonetic and phonological properties of connected speech. *Working Papers in Linguistics 17:* 1–143. (Doctoral dissertation, Ohio State University, 1974).

Shriberg, L. D. 1972. Articulation judgments: Some perceptual considerations. *Journal of Speech and Hearing Research 15:* 876–82.

Shriberg, L. D., Hinke, R., and Trost-Steffen, C. 1987. A procedure to select and train persons for narrow phonetic transcription by consensus. *Clinical Linguistics and Phonetics 1:* 171–90.

Shriberg, L. D., Kwiatkowski, J., and Hoffmann, K. 1984. A procedure for phonetic transcription by consensus. *Journal of Speech and Hearing Research 27:* 456–65.

Shriberg, L. D., and Lof, G. L. 1991. Reliability studies in broad and narrow phonetic transcription. *Clinical Linguistics and Phonetics 5:* 225–79.

Siegel, G. 1962. Experienced and inexperienced articulation examiners. *Journal of Speech and Hearing Disorders 27:* 28–35.

Siren, K. A., and Wilcox, K. A. 1990. The utility of phonetic versus orthographic transcription methods. *Child Language Teaching and Therapy 6:* 127–46.

Small, L. H. 1999. *Phonetics: A practical guide for students.* Boston: Allyn & Bacon.

Snow, D. 2001. Transcription of suprasegmentals. *Topics in Language Disorders 21:* 41–51.

Stephens, M. I., and Daniloff, R. 1977. A methodological study of factors affecting the judgment of misarticulated /s/. *Journal of Communication Disorders 10:* 207–20.

Stitt, C. L., and Huntington, D. A. 1963. Reliability of judgments of articulation proficiency. *Journal of Speech and Hearing Research 6:* 49–56.

Stockman, E. J., Woods, D. R., and Tishman, A. 1981. Listener agreement on phonetic segments in early infant vocalizations. *Journal of Psycholinguistic Research 19:* 593–617.

Stoel-Gammon, C. 2001. Transcribing the speech of young children. *Topics in Language Disorders 21:* 12–21.

Van Borsel, J. 1989. The reliability of phonetic transcriptions: A practical note. *Child Language Teaching and Therapy 5:* 327–33.

Van Demark, D. R. 1964. Misarticulations and listener judgments of the speech of individuals with cleft palates. *Cleft Palate Journal 1:* 232–45.

Vieregge, W. H., and Maassen, B. 1999. ExtIPA transcriptions of consonants and vowels spoken by dyspractic children: Agreement and validity. In B. Maassen and P. Groenen (Eds.), *Pathologies of speech and language: Advances in clinical phonetics and linguistics* (pp. 275–84). London: Whurr.

Weismer, G. 1984. Acoustic analysis strategies for the refinement of phonological analysis. In M. Elbert, D. Dinnsen, and G. Weismer (Eds.), *Phonological theory and the misarticulating child* (ASHA Monographs. No. 22, 30–52). Rockville, MD: American Speech-Language-Hearing Association.

Wertz, R. T., and Rosenbek, J. C. 1992. Where the ear fits: A perceptual evaluation of motor speech disorders. *Seminars in Speech and Language 13:* 39–54.

Witting, C. 1962. On the auditory phonetics of connected speech: Errors and attitudes in listening. *Word 18:* 221–48.

Appendix E

Procedures for Audio Recording and Speech Sampling

Consider your *purposes* for obtaining a speech sample.

- What type of phonological analysis do you intend to accomplish?
- What kind of speech sample is needed for the analysis?
- Will you be able to transcribe the speaker while you obtain the speech sample, or will you need to record the sample for later transcription?
- Does the speaker present any behavioral or linguistic difficulties that will affect the quality or representativeness of the sample?
- What stimulus materials will you need?
- What technical aspects of recording will you need to know about prior to and during the recording?

This barrage of questions was to get your attention! Consider all the information that follows—then be sure to *prepare* and *practice* everything needed to obtain speech samples that are appropriate and efficient for phonetic transcription. The next section provides some background on technical issues in audio recording, followed by a step-by-step list.

SOME TECHNICAL INFORMATION ON AUDIO RECORDING

It is helpful to think of a speech signal as having three potential forms: an *airborne acoustic signal* that is produced by the talker and that rapidly fades as its energy is lost, an *analog signal* that is stored on magnetic tape (such as that used in conventional cassette and open-reel analog tape recorders), or a *digital signal* that is stored on magnetic tape, a diskette, a compact disc (CD), or a Mini-Disc. When we analyze speech, we generally work from one of these three forms. Because the actual acoustic signal of speech (the airborne signal) vanishes as soon as it is produced, we need to store the signal if we are to listen to it again or to analyze it with acoustic techniques. The acoustic signal is an analog signal, meaning that its amplitude varies continuously with time. A microphone is used to convert this acoustic signal to an electrical signal that is then fed to a storage device. An analog magnetic recording, such as that done with ordinary (nondigital) cassette recorders, stores the signal as variations in a magnetic field. The magnetic tape recorder is a device that converts the electrical energy from a microphone to magnetic energy. As the tape passes by the record heads of the tape recorder, the metallic particles in the tape retain a magnetic field that represents a signal. When we want to play this signal, the reproduce heads convert the magnetic field to an electrical signal. The whole process depends critically on the movement of magnetic tape past the record and reproduce heads of a tape recorder.

Recordings of speech go back more than 100 years, beginning in 1877 with Thomas Edison, who recorded his voice on a cylinder phonograph with the intention of developing a dictation machine. The first flat disc recording was made by Emile Berliner in 1887, and the first magnetic recorder was invented in 1898 by Valdemar Poulsen, who used a steel wire as the recording medium. The technology of digital audiotape (DAT) was first used in recording studios in the late 1970s, and the CD became popular in the early 1980s. Because of the shift in recording technology to digital methods, it is important to understand some of the basics about digital signal processing (DSP).

A digital recording leaves the analog world and is stored as a series of numbers (hence, digits) in a digital computer or in a digital storage of some kind (e.g., DAT, CD, Mini-Disc). The process of digitization is discussed later in this appendix (but for extended discussion, see Baken and Orlikoff, 2000; Kent and Read, 2002). For present purposes, we note simply that a digital computer stores numbers; if we want to store a speech waveform in a computer, we must convert the analog waveform to a series of numbers that represents the waveform. The digital information can be stored on a magnetic tape (called a digital magnetic tape) or on a disk. When we want to hear this stored signal, we rely on a process that converts the stored digital information to an analog signal. Therefore, the use of digital technology for storing a speech signal requires two kinds of conversion: Analog to digital (A/D) conversion and digital to analog (D/A) conversion. The three different forms of the speech signal are essentially interchangeable in that a given airborne acoustic signal can be recreated from either an analog or digital recording.

The goal in high-fidelity recording is to make a stored version of the signal that is as faithful as possible to its original production. To accomplish this goal, it is necessary to use proper equipment and techniques to minimize noise and distortion. The discussion that follows is organized to consider (a) the physical environment in which a recording is made, (b) the recording microphone, (c) the recording device (either analog or digital), and (d) recording procedures and pitfalls.

Arranging the Recording Environment

General Considerations. A first step that is all too often neglected is to evaluate the physical setting in which a recording will be made. A few small efforts can greatly enhance the quality of recordings. The primary goal is to determine if there are any obstacles to successful recording and, if possible, to remedy those that are found. A common problem is *background noise* that may contaminate speech recordings. Unfortunately, many recordings are diminished in value because of excessive noise on the tape that could have been prevented by a few easy steps. Some sources of noise include heating and air conditioning systems, fluorescent lighting, paging systems and telephones, bathrooms, corridors, elevators, playgrounds or parks, heavily traveled roadways, and electronic equipment (including personal computers that may generate fan noise). One source of noise that is sometimes overlooked is the recorder itself, especially when an internal microphone is used. If a source of noise is discovered and cannot be eliminated, it may be necessary to choose a different location (such as another room or building) for the recording or to record at times when the noise is less likely to occur (such as early mornings or evenings). Sometimes, it helps simply to move the recording equipment to a different position in the room (for example, away from a fan in a ventilating unit). As discussed later, the choice of microphone also can be important in reducing noise in a recording situation.

Reverberations (Reflections). A second potential problem relating to room acoustics is *reverberation,* or sound reflected within the recording room (Bachety, 1998). Reverberation is most likely to occur in rooms that have hard parallel surfaces (a typical situation in most buildings), on which sound waves can bounce back and forth. The result is a condition known as *slap echo,* which is especially disruptive for high frequencies. Use of drapes or other wall treatments can reduce reverberation. Another reflection problem is called *near-field reflections.* This problem occurs when a recording microphone is located close to a hard surface, such as a wall. Therefore, it is often better to place a microphone near the center of a room rather than close to one of its walls.

Recording Equipment: Microphones

There are many types of microphones from which to choose. In addition to cost issues, your choice of a microphone for phonetic transcription purposes depends on the type of recording you intend to make. Pressure zone microphones (PZM) and omnidirectional microphones are similar in that they can sense sounds produced at various locations in a room. A typical application might be a small room in which a child is free to move about, when the goal is to record what the child says wherever he or she may be. Unidirectional microphones with cardioid or hypercardioid pickup are designed for recordings of near sound and are therefore ideal for applications in which a particular sound target is of interest, such as one talker in a group. Parabolic microphones not only can record at large distances but also can pick up particular sounds if desired.

The technical terms for the different recording situations described earlier are *ambient room recording,* referring to recordings done in a general room environment, and *close recording,* referring to a microphone placement in close proximity to the person being recorded. Both types of recording may be of interest in a particular site. For example, ambient room recording may be preferred when the goal is to record the vocalizations from several children who are playing together, but a close recording is needed when the objective is to record one child only and there is little interest in surrounding acoustic events. To achieve these two different goals, it would be best to use two different microphones.

One common choice of microphone in the clinic is a full-size microphone that is mounted on a wall or ceiling or positioned on a microphone stand on a table top. Although this kind of microphone serves well for many purposes, there are some potential problems, especially when young children are being recorded. A common problem with both placements is that children may turn their heads so that the mouth-to-microphone distance is highly variable. Consequently, the strength of the signal will wax and wane with head movements. Although this variation in signal strength is not damaging for all applications, it can present serious obstacles to analyses that require close attention to sound patterns. Another problem that may occur when a table-mounted microphone is used is that children may bump against the table or pound it with their hands. Obviously, such noises will interfere with speech recordings.

The problems just described can be avoided by using specialized microphones. A *lavaliere microphone,* which attaches to a talker's clothing, is well suited to applications in which one person is being recorded closely and there is relatively little movement. Lavaliere microphones do not always work well with young children who are highly active because body movements create motion noises that are readily picked up by the microphone. Another specialized microphone that works well in the clinic is a *miniature head-mounted condenser microphone.* Modern microphones of this type can ensure high-quality recordings even when the talker changes head or body position, because the microphone follows head movement. Winholtz and Titze (1997) described a microphone of this type that is well suited to general recording needs. These microphones and their head mounts are light and usually can be worn comfortably for long periods. Of course, not all children will be eager to wear a contraption of any kind on their heads, but the enterprising clinician can often make a game of it to encourage cooperation. Finally, many general-purpose tape recorders have their own built-in microphones that vary widely in quality. It is wise to determine the characteristics of these microphones to be certain that they are suitable for a particular application. Although they are easy to use, internal microphones (located within the recorder) may not provide a signal of the desired quality. A particular problem is that they readily pick up noise produced by the recorder itself. In general, it is better to avoid using an internal microphone.

Recording Equipment: Analog and Digital Devices

The microphone must be connected to some kind of recording equipment. Among the choices are: (1) analog tape recorders with either reel-to-reel tapes or cassette tapes, (2) a DAT recorder, (3) a CD writer, (4) a digital disk device, or (5) a direct recording to computer disk. There are variations in quality within most of these choices, especially among analog tape recorders. As discussed earlier, analog recorders preserve the analog (continuous) nature of the signal to be recorded. In contrast, a digital recorder (DAT, CD, digital disk) stores a signal that has been converted to digital form. You are probably familiar with audiocassette recorders and CDs through your personal use. CDs offer large storage capability and good durability, making them popular for musical recordings. CDs function by recording a stream of data as tiny pulses on a plastic-coated aluminum disc. A laser beam then reads the data for playback. This method greatly reduces the potential for physical wear, which is another reason for the current popularity of CDs for musical recordings. For professional speech recordings, such as clinical recordings, a DAT recorder has become an increasingly popular choice. Because DAT recorders have controls that resemble those on analog tape recorders, most users adapt quickly to digital recording technology. We discuss next several factors that are essential to making a successful recording.

Choosing a Tape Recorder. When purchasing a recorder or choosing among recorders that may be available in an equipment room, users should keep in mind some minimum specifications regarding performance of the recorder (Baken and Orlikoff, 2000). The *frequency response* or *frequency characteristic* is a graph of the response of the system as a function of frequency. This graph shows the relationship between input and output of the system for different frequencies. A flat response is desirable, meaning that the response should not vary more than 3 dB over the frequency range of 30 to 15,000 Hz. Poor-quality recorders may have a limited frequency range and/or a highly variable frequency response. *Signal-to-noise ratio* (S/N) is the ratio of energy between the signal to be recorded and the background noise. Generally, the S/N should be at least 55 dB, meaning that the signal is 55 dB greater than the noise. *Wow* and *flutter* are variations in the speed of tape transport and should be less than 0.15 percent (unweighted) or 0.10 percent (weighted). Wow is a low-frequency variation, and flutter is a higher-frequency variation. Finally, the *signal leakage* between channels (left and right) should be less than or equal to 40 dB. If your recorder meets these specifications, it should be suitable for professional recordings.

Digital Recording (Digital Signal Processing). When a digital recording is made, it is important to know some basic information about digitization. *Sampling rate* relates to the frequency range available for recording and storing a signal. DAT recorders are available with different sampling rates (the rate at which the signal is sampled for conversion from analog to digital signal). The higher the sampling rate, the wider the frequency range (bandwidth) of recording. As a rule of thumb, the frequency range that can be represented is about half the sampling rate. Most DAT recorders offer a sampling rate of 44.1 kHz, which affords a highest frequency of about 20 kHz (excellent for most speech applications). For recordings of moderately high quality, sampling rates should be higher than 8 kHz. Bettagere and Fucci (1999) reported that listener-rated quality was superior for digitized speech sampled at 16 kHz than for analog tape-recorded speech. When a sampling rate of 8 kHz was used for digitized speech, the quality was essentially equal to that of analog tape-recorded speech. With modern equipment, there is very little reason to use a sampling rate of less than 16 kHz unless the objective is to record very long samples of speech, such as conversation. Especially when recording the speech of young children, a sampling rate of less than 25 kHz will very likely exclude the higher-frequency energy in fricatives (Kent and Read, 2002).

The other consideration in A/D conversion is *quantization,* which is expressed in bits. Quantization is the representation of signal amplitude, which changes in time during speech. The idea is to quantize (break into small pieces or "quanta") the amplitude dimension so that changing values of amplitude can be represented as a series of numbers. Most modern DAT recorders offer 16- or 32-bit conversion. A 16-bit conversion permits 65,536 levels of amplitude to be represented in the digitized speech sample. This means that the amplitude variations that occur in a speech sample can be stored with up to 65,536 different numbers. Such a level of quantization ensures a high-quality signal free of the quantization noise that can occur with lower levels of conversion.

In short, the important thing to remember is that a 16-bit conversion should be used at minimum.

Magnetic Tapes. Recording tape consists of a thin (5 to 50 microns) plastic base that is coated with fine magnetic particles in a binder that allows these particles to change their orientation (and thereby store a signal). The base is commonly made of a synthetic material such as acetate, polyester (under the trademark name Mylar), polyvinylchloride (PVC), or certain polyesters (especially PET film, the current standard for magnetic tapes). A primary concern in tape manufacture is to make tapes that resist stretching. Although Mylar is much stronger than acetate, it tends to stretch when pulled. This stretching destroys information recorded on the tape. Acetate tape breaks before it stretches, so that it can be repaired by splicing, with good potential for preservation of the recorded signal. The more recent types, PVC and tensilized-type PET, have high tensile strength that resists stretching. Another difference is durability: Mylar, PVC, and PET tapes hold up quite well, but acetate tapes disintegrate after about 15 years (Cudahy, 1988; Strong and Plitnik, 1983).

Cassette tapes come in formats such as C-60 or C-120. The number after the "C" indicates the total playing time in minutes. A C-60 tape plays 30 minutes on each side. Open reel tapes are gauged in mils. A standard 7-inch reel of 1.5 mil tape plays for 30 minutes at a tape speed of 7.5 inches per second (ips). The same tape plays for twice as long at a tape speed of 3.75 ips and for half as long at a tape speed of 15 ips.

Choose a magnetic tape that is suited to individual applications. If low cost is the primary factor, quality of recording may be sacrificed. Inexpensive tapes are often thin and subject to deterioration with use. More expensive tapes generally have a better composition of metal particles that retain the magnetic field. Analog tape comes in different types, three of which are commonly used: Type I (normal bias, ferric oxide), Type II (high bias, chromium dioxide), and Type IV (high bias, metal). Cost and quality increase across this series. Type I tape is suitable for routine purposes. Type II offers a better frequency response and is preferred when signal energy above 12 kHz is important (as in music or fricatives in the speech of young children). Type IV also affords a good frequency response but is the most expensive.

The design and manufacture of tapes are constantly improving. Newer technologies for digital tapes involve the production of metal-evaporated (ME) tape, which may provide better durability than metal particulate (MF) tapes.

Recording Procedures and Pitfalls

The following suggestions pertain to obtaining a recording of high quality with potential for long-term storage.

Recording Level. Generally, tape recorders allow the user to control the amplitude of the signal to be recorded with a knob or slide that is labeled *recording level* or *input level.* Better-quality recorders have a VU (volume units) needle or LCD lights that indicate the recording level. The VU meter was specifically designed so that engineers working at telephone or radio terminals could monitor the transmission of speech or musical programs (Beranek, 1988). The standard VU meter is a colored scale that is graduated in either volume units or in percentages. Volume units should not be confused with decibels, which are used on other types of meters (such as sound-level meters). The red part of the VU meter's scale corresponds to positive VU values (0, +1, +2, +3) or to percentages greater than 100 percent and is generally avoided in making recordings. The remaining part of the scale (usually yellow or white) corresponds to negative VU values (–1, –2, –3) or percentages less than 100 percent. For most recordings with analog recorders, the VU meter should not peak higher than 0 VUs or 100 percent on the VU meter. When the signal strength is highly variable, occasional peaks into the "red" zone are acceptable, so long as the average reading is in the "yellow" zone. However, the "red" zone should be avoided entirely when recording with a DAT recorder to prevent distortion.

Automatic Level Control (ALC). Many recorders are equipped with this function, also called automatic gain control (AGC). In general, *do not use this function,* because it distorts the actual strength of recorded signals. For example, consider a situation in which recordings are being made of a child who only occasionally produces speech and often does so with explosive bursts of short duration. When the child is silent, the ALC automatically adjusts the input volume to a maximum level. But when the child produces a sudden exclamation, the ALC circuitry quickly reduces the input volume, which may cause a loss of signal. ALC does have some benefits (particularly when the objective is to record sounds in a noisy environment and there is no interest in actual sound levels), but these rarely apply to phonetic transcription. We recommend purchase of recorders with ALC only if this function can be turned on or off as needs dictate. Although ALC may be desirable in some circumstances, it is not a good idea to use it without careful consideration of its consequences for particular applications.

Noise Reduction Systems. Because tape recorders generate noise, there has been a long-term interest in finding ways to reduce noise inherent to the recording process. Of the various approaches that have been developed, the two most successful are *Dolby* and *DBX*. The discussion of these systems is necessarily quite technical, and they are described only briefly here.

Dolby is named after the engineer who invented this process. There are different types of Dolby, only two of which are discussed here. Dolby-A uses two signal paths, a linear amplifier and a differential network. The output of the differential network is added to the "straight-through" signal for recording the signal and subtracted for reproducing the signal. The differential network divides the frequency spectrum into four bands and applies its action only for the band(s) where it is needed. Dolby-B is a simpler process and is commonly used to reduce background noise in analog cassette recorders, which typically operate with a low tape speed and a narrow recording track. Dolby-B is similar to Dolby-A in that it uses a main signal path and a side chain. The effect of the side chain is to record low-level, high-frequency signals at a higher level, thereby improving the S/N. DBX is similar to Dolby-A in that it is a complementary system. DBX uses compression to improve the high-frequency S/N.

Distortion and Ghosting. As noted earlier, magnetic tape holds the signal of interest in a magnetic field. The primary goal in magnetic tape recording is to saturate the tape with the desired signal and to avoid underrecording and overrecording. The former produces more noise than signal, and though it may seem strange that one can have too much recording level, excessive levels can result in distortion of sound quality and *ghosting* (or print-through). Ghosting occurs when a strong magnetic field on a portion of the tape "ghosts over" (or "prints") onto the underlying or overlying portion of the tape on the spool. In effect, another part of the tape receives an additional and unintended magnetic field because it is wound over a very strong field. What does this sound like? Frequently, you will hear the ghosting as background sounds or as a kind of double recording ("echoes") in which recorded samples are heard twice. In conclusion, it is always wise to refer to the operating manual to determine the optimal adjustment of recording level.

Tape Stretch. Another problem with tapes is stretch, especially with Mylar tapes. A new tape is wound at high tension on its spool. The first time it is used, this tension is partially released. With rewinds and replays, a section of the tape can be stretched, potentially causing "dropouts" (a noticeable drop in signal strength) or a change in tone quality. Remember that the tape must pass by the heads of the tape recorder if we are to record or reproduce a signal. If the tape is stretched after a signal is recorded, the signal will be altered on playback. Although some degree of tape stretch is unavoidable with repeated use of a tape, there are some steps that can reduce it:

1. Before a tape is used to make a recording, it should be fully fast-forwarded and then rewound. The purpose is to set the tension at a lower level than that set by the manufacturer and also to set the tension in accord with the tape deck under use.
2. It is better to use tapes that are thicker. This may mean avoiding tapes with longer play times (90 minutes or more), because they are typically thinner. These problems are not as severe with DAT as with analog tapes, but all magnetic tapes are susceptible to some mechanical wear and tear.
3. Be gentle: Avoid abrupt, vigorous, and unnecessary rewinds and replays. Stretch is particularly severe on the leading portion of a tape, which is subject to large forces developed during rapid rewinds.

Note that a permanent acoustic archive would have to be based on other recording media that are not typically used in general-purpose speech recordings. However, for most purposes, one can get satisfactory long-term storage from recording on digital disks or CDs or directly on to the hard drive of the computer. The major drawback to the latter is that speech samples consume large amounts of computer memory, and few of us want to fill our computer memories with stored speech samples. Therefore, a reasonable means of long-term storage is to use diskettes or CDs. These offer still another advantage, as discussed next.

Although we might like to think that tape recordings last indefinitely, they do not. In general, recordings deteriorate with time, particularly so when stored in an environment with high temperature and humidity. Both analog and digital tapes are metal particle tapes that are subject to eventual deterioration (Speliotis and Peter, 1991). For most magnetic media, deterioration can be detected within 5 to 8 years after recordings are made (Leek, 1995). Although control of temperature and humidity will extend the accuracy of the recorded information, errors ultimately will contaminate the quality of the recorded data. For short-term applications, these degradations may not be of much concern, but anyone who hopes to build a library of magnetic tapes for long-term use should be aware that magnetic tapes are susceptible to deterioration.

Summary

Making a high-quality recording is more than just pushing a "record" button. It is worth taking some extra time to observe the basic principles discussed in this appendix. With proper attention to a few details, you can make a recording that is virtually free of noise and distortion.

SPEECH SAMPLING PROCEDURES

Step-by-Step Procedures

1. Based on all the considerations reviewed in the previous discussion, select the appropriate recorder.
2. Learn the basic features of the recorder.
   a. Where does the power cord plug into the recorder?
   b. Where does the remote microphone plug into the recorder?
   c. How do you set the recording speed?
   d. What knobs or buttons control loudness of recording and/or playback?

e. Does the recording mode require simultaneous depression of two buttons?
f. How does the pause control work?
g. How does the remote off/on switch on the microphone work?

3. As underscored previously, use the *manual* volume control, not the *automatic* volume control. Automatic volume controls will distort beginnings and endings of speech and include unwanted background noise.
4. To avoid recording any noise emanating from the machine during recording, carefully position the recorder on a different surface and as far as possible from the microphone.
5. Prior to recording, announce the speaker's name and the complete date on the tape. It is also useful to record this information at the end of the tape or disc when you have finished recording. Be sure to write this information clearly on the media container and on the label.
6. Use the identification recording as an opportunity to test your setup. Do you hear any other noise on the recording? Are all the buttons and dials working correctly? Recheck all settings!
7. When you are ready to record the speaker, place the microphone no more than six to eight inches from the speaker's lips. To avoid "popping" noises, angle the microphone to point at the speaker's nose, rather than mouth. Adjust the volume control so that the speaker's vowels cause the needle on the VU meter to peak just below the distortion area. The consonants should be sufficiently audible to discriminate subphonemic features, such as unaspirated and frictionalized stops. Volume levels between one-third and two-thirds of full scale usually yield the signal-to-noise ratios required for narrow or broad phonetic transcription. Be sure that your utterances can be heard easily upon playback, with the speaker's voice somewhat louder than yours.
8. If you must record in a noisy environment, minimize negative effects by reducing the mouth-to-microphone distance when the noise is constant. Have the speaker repeat any words that might have been obscured by a transient noise.

Evoking the Speech Sample

Procedures to evaluate or "test" speech usually include specific directions about how to obtain responses from the speaker. Standardized administration procedures are central to the validity of data obtained from articulation tests and word-repetition tasks. Free speech sampling should also be accomplished using standardized procedures with each speaker. The following recommendations will help you obtain rich conversational speech samples from young children with phonological disorders.

1. Be casual about the presence of the microphone so that periodic adjustments of the volume level or the placement of the microphone do not disturb the speaker. Most children can be trained to respect equipment (e.g., to not touch the microphone). Explain why you need cooperation. Adults are often more self-conscious about being taped than children, but children will accommodate to the tape recorder if you are matter of fact.
2. Use a variety of materials and introduce different topics as needed to keep the speaker talking and to obtain representative proportions of parts of speech, word shapes, and phonemes. Medial and final /ʤ/ do not regularly occur in spontaneous conversational speech, and, therefore, no special procedures are used to evoke them. (See Shriberg and Kwiatkowski, 1985, for procedures and findings using five types of continuous speech samples: free, story, routines, interview, and scripted.)
3. If you are obtaining a free speech sample from a speaker who is difficult to understand, plan to gloss (repeat what the speaker says using a natural conversational style) after each utterance. It is not necessary to gloss every word—just those that the speaker intended to say that will be difficult to understand from the recording. Be sure to allow the speaker opportunities to clarify utterances to increase intelligibility for later transcription.
4. Make notes on articulatory behaviors that may not be perceptible on the audio recording, such as lip rounding or unrounding, unreleased stops, fricative distortions, and any facial gestures that may accompany speech production.
5. Make summary notes on the speaker's general health, motivation, and physical state (e.g., whether congested or irritable during the recording); these factors could affect the validity of the speech sample.

Some Transcription Alternatives

One final aspect of sampling and recording to consider is the level of phonetic detail you intend to transcribe. For example, if you will be transcribing prosody, the speech sample needs to be representative of natural speech, rather than a narrative. Following are six other transcription choices discussed in this text (see Chapter 7) and in Ohde and Sharf (1992). You may not be able to make decisions on each of these and other transcription alternatives until you have some familiarity with the speaker's error pattern.

1. *Aspiration* [ʰ], [⁼]. Aspirated and unaspirated stops are predictable in English and therefore can be omitted when a speaker's use of stops is not in question.
2. *Stop release* [˺]. The release of postvocalic stops is optional (i.e., in free variation). Thus, it is not necessary to transcribe the release unless it is exaggerated or unless no release occurs where expected (e.g., *past* [pæstʰ]).
3. *Nasality* [˜]. Nasal assimilation is predictable in nasal

consonant contexts and may not need to be transcribed unless noticeably greater than normal.

4. *Duration* [ː], [˃]. Predictable vowel duration may be omitted, using duration symbols only when they may provide information on consonant deletion or devoicing.
5. *Devoicing* [̥]. Predictable devoicing of final obstruents or consonants preceded by voiceless consonants (e.g., /ɾ̥/ in *try*) may not need to be transcribed.
6. *Vowel neutralization.* The precise vowel used in unstressed syllables (e.g., [ə] or [ɛ] or [ɪ]) may not be important to capture for phonological analysis.

REFERENCES

Bachety, M. 1998, September. Bouncing reverb out of the lab. *Sound Communications 44:* 96–7, 126.

Baken, R. J., and Orlikoff, R. F. 2000. *Clinical measurement of speech and voice,* 2nd ed. San Diego: Singular.

Beranek, L. L. 1988. *Acoustical measurements.* Woodbury, NY: Acoustical Society of America.

Bettagere, R., and Fucci, D. 1999. Magnitude-estimation scaling of computerized (digitized) speech under different listening conditions. *Perceptual and Motor Skills 88:* 1363–78.

Cudahy, E. 1988. *Instrumentation in speech and hearing.* Baltimore: Williams & Wilkins.

Kent, R. D., and Read, C. 2002. *The acoustic analysis of speech.* Albany, NY: Singular/Thomson Learning.

Leek, M. R. 1995, November. Will a good disc last? *CD-ROM Professional 8:* 102–10.

Modaff, J. V., and Modaff, D. P. 2000. Technical notes on audio recording. *Research on Language and Social Instruction 33:* 101–18.

Ohde, R. N., and Sharf, D. J. 1992. *Phonetic analysis of normal and abnormal speech.* New York: Merrill/Macmillan Publishing Company.

Shriberg, L. D., and Kwiatkowski, J. 1985. Continuous speech sampling for phonological analyses of speech-delayed children. *Journal of Speech and Hearing Disorders 50:* 323–34.

Shriberg, L. D. 1993. Four new speech and prosody-voice measures for genetics research and other studies in developmental phonological disorders. *Journal of Speech and Hearing Research 36:* 105–40.

Speliotis, D. E., and Peter, K. J. 1991. Corrosion study of metal particle, metal film, and BA-ferrite tape. *IEEE Transactions on Magnetics 27:* 4724–26.

Strong, W. J., and Plitnik, G. 1983. *Music, Speech, High Fidelity,* 2nd ed. Soundprint (no city given).

Tomes, L. 2001, October. "Testing, testing, one, two, three": Making high fidelity recordings of speech. *Newsletter, Special Interest Division 5, Speech Science and Orofacial Disorders 11:* 1–13. Rockville, MD: American Speech-Language-Hearing Association.

Utz, P. 1989. *Recording great audio.* Radio Shack Corporation. An inexpensive, well-illustrated manual containing useful instructions on all facets of audio recording.

Winholtz, W. S., and Titze, I. R. 1997. Miniature head-mounted microphone for voice perturbation analysis. *Journal of Speech, Hearing, and Language Research 40:* 894–99.

Westbury, J. R., Hashi, M., and Lindstrom, M. J. 1999. Differences among speakers in lingual articulation of American English /ɾ/. *Speech Communication 26:* 203–26.

Appendix F

Dialect: Language Variations across Cultures[1]

Speech-language pathologists learn phonetics as a tool for recording the speech productions of clinical populations. Although we may think of clinical populations as limited to individuals with communication *disorders,* many individuals who demonstrate communication *differences* or *dialects* also seek the services of speech-language clinicians. The purpose of this appendix is to introduce students of clinical phonetics to the topic of dialect, which was briefly introduced in Chapter 2. The following sections will define dialect, highlight the relationship between dialect and culture, describe dialect types, introduce the myth of a standard dialect, and address strategies for applying clinical phonetics to dialect management.

DIALECT

Dialect refers to variations in speech and language patterns across groups of people. Known as *speech communities,* these groups are in constant internal communication. Essentially, speech communities constitute groups of speakers who share a set of norms and rules for the use of language (Romaine, 1982) as well as language characteristics and communication habits. Examples of speech communities include native speakers of a language who are from different geographic regions, speakers who represent different social groups within the same language, and speakers who have learned the language of a region as a nonnative form. In addition, speech communities such as families, school classes, peer groups, professional or occupational groups, as well as groups defined by gender, sexual orientation, or drug use also demonstrate their own varieties of a given language. Thus, all language speakers demonstrate dialect variations—even though we may perceive ourselves to be dialect-free (Esling, 1998).

Because dialects represent variations of a particular language, they are typically mutually intelligible yet distinctly different from each other. For example, native speakers of English within the United States, the United Kingdom, Canada, and Australia typically can communicate with one another, despite obvious differences in these varieties of English. Similarly, American English speakers who are native to New York, Atlanta, and Boston may notice differences in each other's speech but will still be able to communicate effectively. Dialect has an impact on all components of the language system, reflecting variations in phonology, morphosyntax, semantics, and pragmatics. These variations lead speakers with different dialects to demonstrate variations in pronunciation, grammatical forms, word choice and usage, and discourse and interaction style.

Variations in *phonology* are referred to as *accents* and are heard as differences in articulation and prosody. Articulation differences relate primarily to variations in vowel productions, but they include some consonant differences as well. For instance, people from the northern portion of the United States are likely to produce the word *greasy* as [g r i s ɪ], whereas speakers from the southern portion are likely to produce it as [g r i z ɪ]. In addition, prosodic variations reflect some of the most overt and pervasive aspects of accent. It has been shown, for example, that phonology in general plays a crucial role in ethnic identification, but intonation patterns alone may be sufficient to identify a speaker from an ethnic minority (Bailey and Thomas, 1998).

Variations in *morphosyntax* typically include changes in verb tenses, noun plurals, prepositions, pronouns, adjectives, adverbs, conjunctions, and word order. An example of morphosyntactic variation can be observed in the sentence "Are you coming over?" in which the pronoun *you* could be formed as "you," "youse," or "you all." Each of these pronunciations is an acceptable marking of the pronoun in different regions of the United States.

Variations in *semantics* refer to the different words used to label objects and events in the speaker's environment. For example, a carbonated soft drink that comes in a can is called *pop, soda,* or *tonic* in various parts of the United States. Similarly, *skillet* and *frying pan* are used in different geographic locations to refer to the same cooking utensil. The semantic domain poses some of the greatest dialect challenges for

[1]This appendix was written by Linda J. Carpenter, Ph.D. Dr. Carpenter is a Professor in the Department of Communication Disorders, University of Wisconsin–Eau Claire. She has had extensive experience with the challenging clinical and professional issues associated with regional, social, and foreign dialects. In this appendix Dr. Carpenter provides the broad sociocultural perspectives on dialects and specific procedures needed to transcribe the speech of persons who seek clinical assistance to modify an accent.

nonnative English speakers, particularly with respect to idiomatic and figurative expressions.

Variations in *pragmatics* refer to the numerous ways language is used in context to carry out communication functions. While all languages have rules governing functions such as greeting, requesting, persuading, and protesting, dialect groups vary in how they accomplish these and other communication functions. For example, speakers of African American Vernacular English (AAVE) engage in several unique discourse patterns, such as *call-response* and *signification.* Call-response refers to the "spontaneous verbal and nonverbal interaction between speaker and listener in which all of the speaker's statements *(calls)* are punctuated by expressions *(responses)* from the listener" (Smitherman, 1977, p. 104). As such, call-response serves an acknowledgement function in discourse. Signification is a speech act "in which a speaker humorously puts down, talks about, needles—that is, signifies on—the listener. Sometimes it is done to make a point; sometimes it's only for fun. This type of folk expression in the oral tradition has the status of a customary ritual that's accepted at face value. That is to say, nobody who's signified on is supposed to take it to heart" (Smitherman, 1977, pp. 118–19). Both call-response and signification allow discourse partners to relate to and interact with each other in culturally acceptable ways.

Dialect variations are also systematic and rule-governed. Sound substitutions, sound omissions, and differences in prosody that are characteristic of accents are all examples of variations in the rules governing the phonological code. Specifically, sound substitutions reflect differences in phonemic repertoire, sound omissions reflect phonotactic variations, and differences in prosodic variables, such as stress, reflect variations in suprasegmental rules. To illustrate an example of differences in phonemic repertoire, consider that although all speakers of American English are expected to articulate words such as *red, robin, crown,* and *trace* with the consonantal /r/, a speaker from eastern New England may drop the rhotic consonant in post-vocalic contexts and derhotacize the vocalic forms (/ɝ/, /ɚ/). In this case, a speaker might say [pa:k] for /pɑrk/, or [faðə] for /fɑðɚ/. The speaker may also demonstrate /r/ intrusion when words that end in vowels come before words that begin with vowels. Thus, the speaker might say, "This is a really good *idea*" but "The *idear* is good."

DIALECTOLOGY

General dialectology is the branch of linguistics concerned with the geographic and social distribution of language. Dialectologists describe the linguistic and social variables associated with language differences, typically focusing on linguistic phenomena as they are observed in the community. That is, dialectologists describe the language form (i.e., phonology, morphosyntax), content (i.e., semantics), and use (i.e., pragmatics) of languages in geographic and social contexts, without judging the quality of these differences.

Beginning in the 1920s, American dialectologists focused their efforts on mapping linguistic geography in the United States. Using interview methodology, dialect fieldworkers gathered data on lexicon or vocabulary, grammatical structures (primarily verb forms), and speech forms (articulation) across geographic regions. Locations of individual speakers were plotted on maps to indicate use and nonuse of the particular linguistic feature under study. By connecting these plot points, lines known as *isoglosses* were drawn to define dialect boundaries. After more than 40 years of research, these efforts resulted in linguistic atlases of New England, the Mid-Atlantic and South Atlantic states, the North Central States, the Upper Midwest, the Gulf Coast States, and the Pacific Coast.

The earliest and most comprehensive linguistic atlas data were collected in the New England states and along the eastern seaboard. Because of the depth and breadth of the raw data available for the eastern regions of the United States, later studies were designed to analyze the lexicon (Kurath, 1949), verb forms (Atwood, 1953), and speech forms (Kurath and McDavid, 1961) within these areas.

During the last century, dialectologists have compiled a substantial body of information on dialect regions in the United States and their historical origins. From this rich database, others have been intrigued by the links between dialect and culture.

DIALECT AND CULTURE

The language variations of dialect are closely tied to the concept of *culture,* or the learned behaviors of mankind. Cultural learning is accomplished through both enculturation and socialization. *Enculturation* is the process of acquiring the characteristics of a given culture, such as skill in the culture's language. *Socialization* is the process of learning to function as a member of a society by adopting culturally prescribed roles. The socialization process begins at birth, as a person learns the culture in which he or she is raised. Cultural learning is shared throughout the lifespan, usually with a group of people who have common living patterns that bind them together. Cultural learning is also dynamic, because it adapts to surrounding conditions and needs within the environment. Given these characteristics, manifestations of culture may include foods, clothing, housing, etiquette patterns, values, attitudes, belief systems, child-rearing practices, educational systems, nonverbal communication, and dialectal aspects of language and speech.

As a cultural artifact, language reflects the culture from which it arises; the language and speech variations of dialect are culturally learned and transmitted behaviors. In studying dialects, sociolinguists explore the relationships between language use and social patterns, and examine the underlying

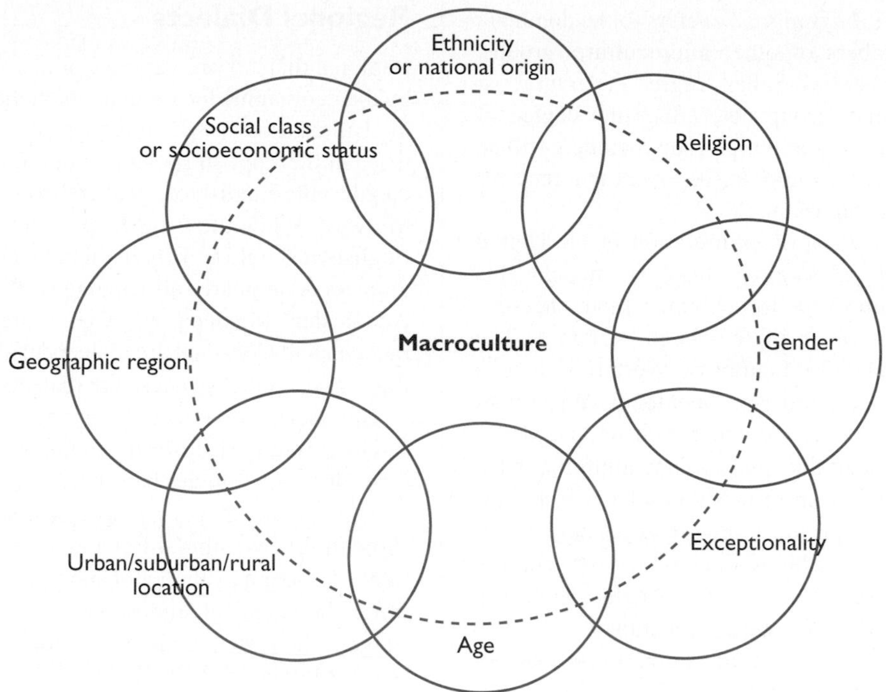

FIGURE F-1
Cultural identity of an individual (adapted from Carpenter, 1990).

sociocultural drives of linguistic use. Because of its focus on the social and cultural aspects of language, a sociolinguistic perspective emphasizes the concept of speech as an act of individual identity.

The cultural identity of an individual is determined by a macroculture and several microcultures (Carpenter, 1990). Figure F-1 represents this concept. *Macroculture* refers to the core, or universal culture, of a society. Originally, white Anglo-Saxon Protestant groups dominated the American macroculture. American values and political institutions are still strongly related to these values. However, the American macroculture is no longer limited to whites, Anglo-Saxons, or Protestants—it now includes a large and varied membership, many of whom are ethnic minorities. The American macroculture, while host to a growing multitude of ethnicities, still demonstrates several basic values, such as the belief that status should be based on occupation, education, and/or financial worth; the preference for achievement over inheritance; and the emphasis on a middle-class work ethic.

In addition to the macroculture, a society is composed of several microcultures, each characterized by unique values and behaviors. *Microcultures* may relate to age, exceptionality or disability, gender, religion, ethnicity or national origin, socioeconomic status, geographic region, and urban/suburban/rural locations. Although exceptionality or disability status has not been traditionally conceptualized as a microculture, it is included here because a historical view of the treatment of people with disabilities suggests parallels with the treatment of minorities. For example, children who were deaf and used sign language, as well as Native American children, were at one time removed from their families and placed in boarding schools in which they were prevented from using their native languages.

The various microcultures overlap with one another as well as with the macroculture; thus, the scheme in Figure F-1 is a bit misleading, because microcultures do not overlap with only adjacent groups. Nevertheless, this overlapping relationship models the following four points:

1. The behavior of any individual is a function of the macroculture in addition to any number of microcultures.
2. A behavior cannot be attributed to membership in a particular microculture alone.
3. There exists a potential for tension among overlapping microcultures, as well as between a microculture and the macroculture.
4. Sociocultural variables within the microculture, such as ethnicity and socioeconomic status, are often confounded.

The relationship between macroculture and microcultures develops through the process of assimilation, which generally refers to blending into the dominant culture. *Cultural assimilation* (also known as *acculturation*) refers to an individual's acquisition of the characteristics of another cultural group. This kind of assimilation can be reflected in language use, dress, hairstyle, and the like. Not everyone acculturates: One's degree of cultural assimilation is personally determined.

In contrast, *structural assimilation* refers to the dominant group accepting members of other microcultural groups. Whereas individuals determine their degree of cultural assimilation, the dominant group determines the degree of structural assimilation. Microculture group members will be assimilated into the macroculture to the extent that they are accepted by the dominant group.

Traditionally, the pattern of assimilation in the United States has suggested an Anglo-conformity model. This model encourages minorities to renounce their ancestral values and culture in favor of the Anglo versions. The Anglo-conformity model also focuses on Western European traditions and leads to a melting-pot metaphor: When constituents come together, they surrender their unique identities. Under the influence of this model, many minorities have strived for total acculturation in the hope of being assimilated into the dominant group, although most have never been fully accepted. Often, after giving up their own culture, minorities can't "go back." Thus, the Anglo-conformity model can lead minorities to cultural alienation.

A multicultural model serves as an alternative to total acculturation and structural assimilation. Such a model acknowledges and encourages the validity and visibility of various microcultures, including their languages and dialects, and reduces pressures for conformity created by structural assimilation forces. In contrast to the Anglo-conformity model, a multicultural model leads to a salad-bowl metaphor: All constituents come together, but they also retain their unique identities and complement one another.

Speech-language pathologists who provide dialect management services must be mindful of the links between language and culture and of the dangers of providing services under an Anglo-conformity model. Rather than eradicating all evidence of dialect and accent, instruction under a multicultural model aims to facilitate effective communication within the parameters of the dialect. When language is treated as an aspect of culture, dialect variations are accorded due respect as cultural artifacts.

TYPES OF DIALECT

Historically, dialectologists in the United States have pursued two primary lines of inquiry: analyzing regional differences and examining social variations. These are not mutually exclusive categories, because social variations cut across geographic regions. These categories do, however, represent differences in research emphasis and focus. Linguistic geographers emphasize dialect boundaries and focus on mapping variations, whereas sociolinguists emphasize speakers' social and cultural backgrounds and focus on linguistic use. In addition, investigators of nonnative language learning have explored language and speech variations in the English produced by nonnative speakers. These approaches to linguistic variation reflect three major dialect types: *regional, social,* and *foreign.*

Regional Dialects

Regional dialects are varieties of a single language, defined by the geographic location in which the variety is spoken. In the United States, we can recognize some unique characteristics in the English spoken by people from the South compared to the English of speakers from the Northeast and the Midwest. While the focus here is on variations in American English, it should be kept in mind that dialects defined by region occur in nearly all languages. For example, Castilian, Andalusian, Mexican, and Cuban are dialects of Spanish; Parisian and Canadian are dialects of French; and Mandarin, Cantonese, and Taiwanese are dialects of Chinese.

Boundaries drawn for regional variations of American English were derived from studies based on linguistic atlas data. Numerous studies have been conducted to examine lexical, grammatical, and phonological boundaries, and results show significant similarities across studies in the regions defined. Although a number of subregions have also been identified, the results of studies based on these linguistic atlases suggest three major dialect regions in the United States: North, Midland, and South. Figure F-2, drawn from Kurath's (1949) study of lexical variations in the East Coast, illustrates these major regions as well as their subregions. Figure F-3, drawn from Carver's (1987) nationwide study of lexical variation, illustrates expansion of the major regions across the country.

Causes of Regional Dialects. Although native speakers can easily recognize regional variations in their language, the reasons for these variations are less transparent. Wolfram and Schilling-Estes (1998) proposed two sets of factors—sociohistorical and linguistic—to explain the existence of regional variations.

Sociohistorical factors include settlement patterns, migration routes, geography, language contact, social stratification, group reference, and personal identity. Each of these factors is nonlinguistic but leads to substantial linguistic consequences. A brief, selected history of American English dialects will illustrate this point.

American English dialects are rooted in the regional speech and language variations of 17th century England. Colonists emigrated from northern and southern England and settled in various locations on the Atlantic Coast. Settlers from northern England established themselves in the Mid-Atlantic region, whereas settlers from southern England tended to cluster in New England and in the southern coastal states. The speech patterns that evolved in these regions of the United States are similar to the patterns of the English settlers—notably, the phonological variations in the rhotic phonemes described previously in this appendix and elsewhere in this text. In New England, the Connecticut River served as a natural geographic barrier to communication, and the differences in speech patterns east and west of that line are dramatic, with /r/-lessness prevalent in eastern New

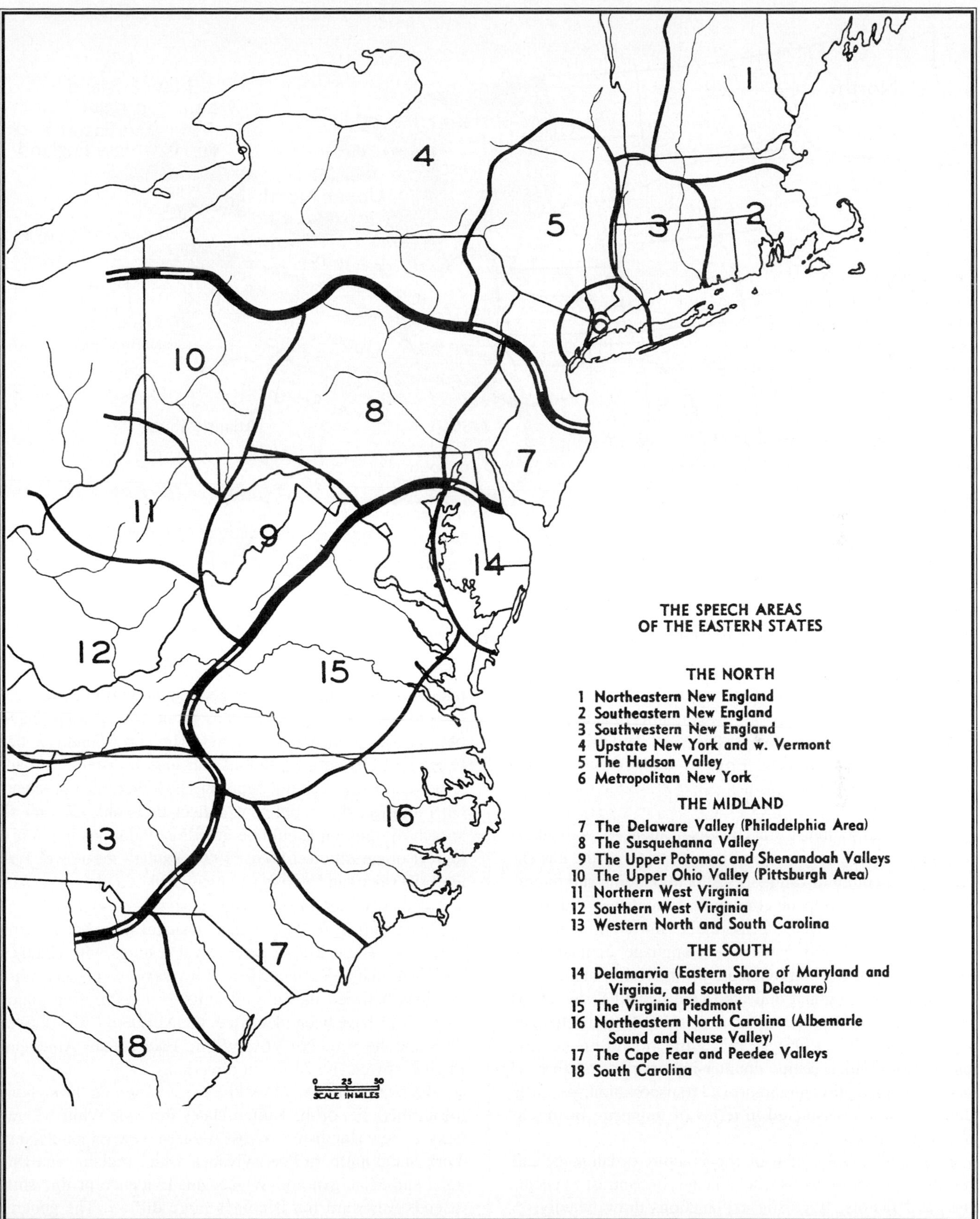
1
2
3
4
5
6
7
8
9
10
11
12
13
14
15
16
17
18
THE SPEECH AREAS
OF THE EASTERN STATES
THE NORTH
1 Northeastern New England
2 Southeastern New England
3 Southwestern New England
4 Upstate New York and w. Vermont
5 The Hudson Valley
6 Metropolitan New York
THE MIDLAND
7 The Delaware Valley (Philadelphia Area)
8 The Susquehanna Valley
9 The Upper Potomac and Shenandoah Valleys
10 The Upper Ohio Valley (Pittsburgh Area)
11 Northern West Virginia
12 Southern West Virginia
13 Western North and South Carolina
THE SOUTH
14 Delamarvia (Eastern Shore of Maryland and Virginia, and southern Delaware)
15 The Virginia Piedmont
16 Northeastern North Carolina (Albemarle Sound and Neuse Valley)
17 The Cape Fear and Peedee Valleys
18 South Carolina
0 25 50
SCALE IN MILES

FIGURE F-2
Lexically defined dialect regions of the eastern United States.

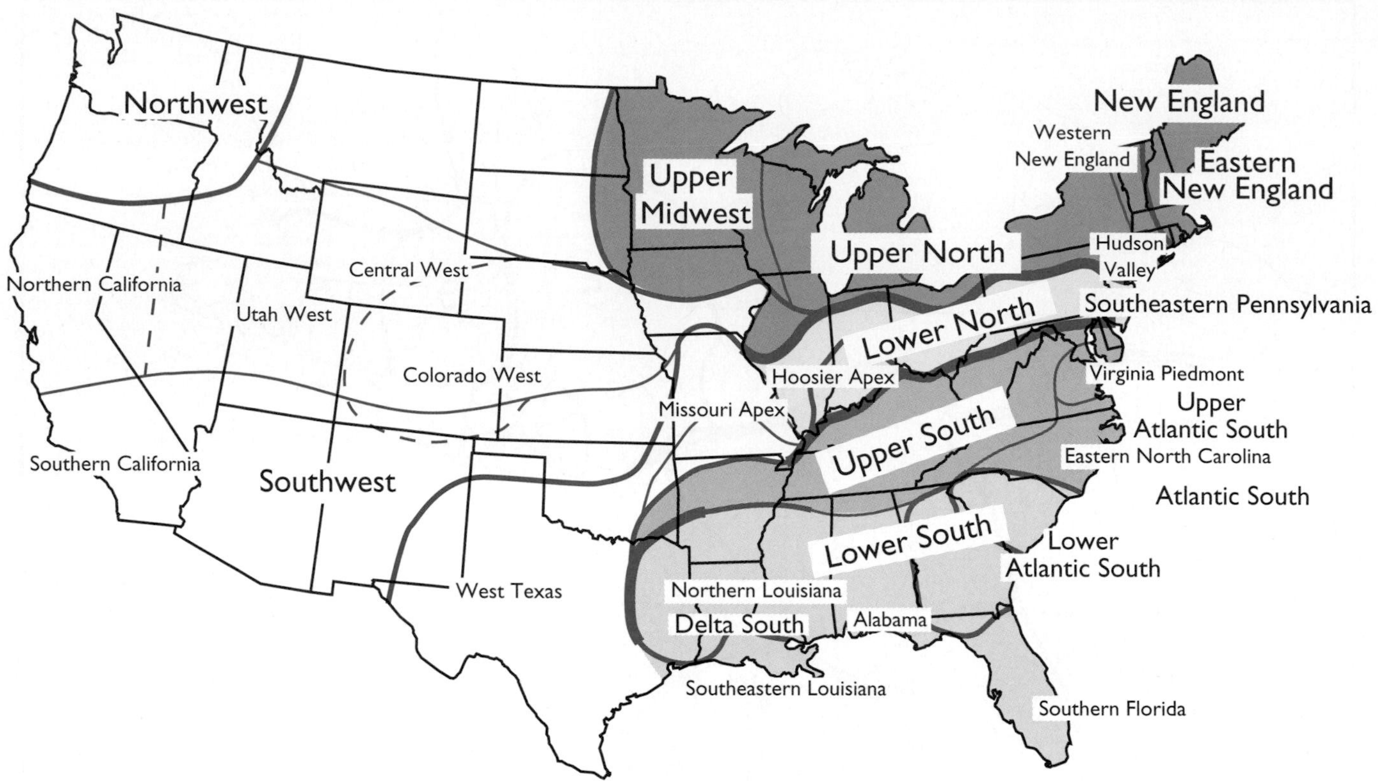

FIGURE F-3
Major lexically defined dialect regions of the continental United States.

England and /r/-fullness prevalent in western New England. Moreover, while the /r/-less quality persists in the eastern portion of this region, it is the westward migration of people from western New England—and their /r/-full speech—that contributed to the full /r/ productions in the Midwest.

Whereas all sociohistorical factors influenced regional dialects in the past, they are no longer barriers in the current age of mass communication. Settlement patterns and migration routes do not impede communication as they did in the past, because improved transportation and communication systems have altered patterns of language contact. The prevalence of mass communication might also suggest the possibility that regional dialects in the United States could become less differentiated. In fact, phonological changes (e.g., Labov, 1991, 1996) are in the direction of greater differentiation, which seems counter-intuitive in the face of mass communication and improved transportation, yet quite plausible when considered in terms of linguistic factors in language variation.

Linguistic factors focus on the structure of language and the rules governing its use and change. In contrast to sociohistorical factors, linguistic explanations draw heavily on phonological data and provide evidence for dialects as artifacts of linguistic change over time. Interest in the development of speech recognition systems drives investigations of phonological variation across geographic regions. Most efforts to determine dialect regions in the United States have been based on vocabulary studies. The correspondence between lexically defined regions and speech patterns that are important in speech recognition, however, is not clear. Operating on the belief that dialect divisions relevant to speech recognition should be based on variations in phonological organization, Labov (1991) studied the vowel systems of American English and identified two major types of sound changes: *chain shifts* and *mergers.*

Chain shifts reflect systematic changes in vowel systems over time. These shifts rotate vowel features with changes operating like a domino effect. They serve to preserve distinctions between meaningful units of speech. Two major chain shifts have been identified: the Northern Cities Vowel Shift and the Southern Vowel Shift. Each rotates American English vowels in a different direction.

The Northern Cities Vowel Shift is observed throughout the northern tier of the United States from the White Mountains of New Hampshire across western New England; New York State; northern Pennsylvania, Ohio, Indiana, and Illinois; and Michigan and Wisconsin. Evidence of this shift extends westward but becomes more diffuse. The general pattern of this chain shift, referenced to the vowel quadrilateral (see inside front cover), is illustrated in Figure F-4. The numbers on the diagram indicate the order of change, showing that the shift begins when the /æ/, as in *cad,* moves front and up to the position of /iə/, as in *idea.* The /ɑ/, as in *cod,* then shifts forward to sound like /æ/, and the /ɔ/, as in *cawed,* moves down to the former position of /ɑ/. The /ɛ/, as in *Keds,* moves back and down, sounding like the /ʌ/ in *cud,* and the /ʌ/ then moves back to the former position of /ɔ/. Finally, the /ɪ/, as in *kid,* moves back, parallel to the shift noted for /ɛ/.

The Southern Vowel Shift is observed in the Mid-Atlantic States and throughout the southern states, the southern mountain states, and the Upper and Lower South. It moves in a different direction than the Northern Cities Shift, and the general pattern, again referenced to the vowel quadrilateral, is shown in Figure F-5.

As the numbered arrows indicate, the Southern Shift begins when the diphthong /ɑ͡ɪ/ becomes a monophthong and the first element of the original diphthong moves slightly forward. The nucleus of the tense vowel /e͡ɪ/ then drops in a nonperipheral direction from the periphery of the system, and /i/ drops parallel to /e͡ɪ/ but occupying a higher final position. The three front lax vowels move, with /ɪ/ and /ɛ/ moving up to the positions formerly held by /i/ and /e͡ɪ/, and /æ/ moving parallel to the others. Then /u/ moves to the front, and the nucleus of /o͡ʊ/ moves to the center. Finally, /ɔr/ moves to a high-back position, and /ɑr/ moves up to take its place.

These Northern and Southern chain shifts have radically altered the positions of the vowels in relation to each other. The effect is that the phones (i.e., sounds actually produced) that represent a particular phoneme in one dialect represent a different phoneme in another dialect.

Mergers represent the consolidation of two phonemes into one. In contrast to chain shifts, mergers neutralize contrasts between vowel sounds and collapse meaning distinctions. Two primary mergers have been identified: ɔ/ɑ in all contexts and ɪ/ɛ before nasals. In the ɔ/ɑ merger, words such as *caught* /k ɔ t/ and *cot* /k ɑ t/, and *dawn* /d ɔ n/ and *Don* /d ɑ n/ become homophones. This collapse of the distinction between /ɔ/ and /ɑ/ is considered an *unconditioned merger* because it affects the sounds wherever they appear. The only unconditioned merger in the American English vowel system, the ɔ/ɑ merger is characteristic of speakers in the western half of the United States, eastern New England, western Pennsylvania, and northern Minnesota. Speakers in the most heavily populated areas in the Mid-Atlantic States, the North, and the north midland retain the distinction between these sounds. In contrast, *conditioned mergers* occur in a particular phonemic environment. One of the most widespread conditioned mergers involves the distinction between /ɪ/ and /ɛ/ before the nasals /m/ and /n/, which causes words such as *pin* and *pen* to become homophones. Traditionally, this merger has been characteristic of speakers in the southern region of the United States, but recent analyses suggest that this merger is spreading north and west from its southern base.

Because language is a dynamic system, there is an interactive and complementary relationship between the two explanations for the existence of regional dialects. In fact, the

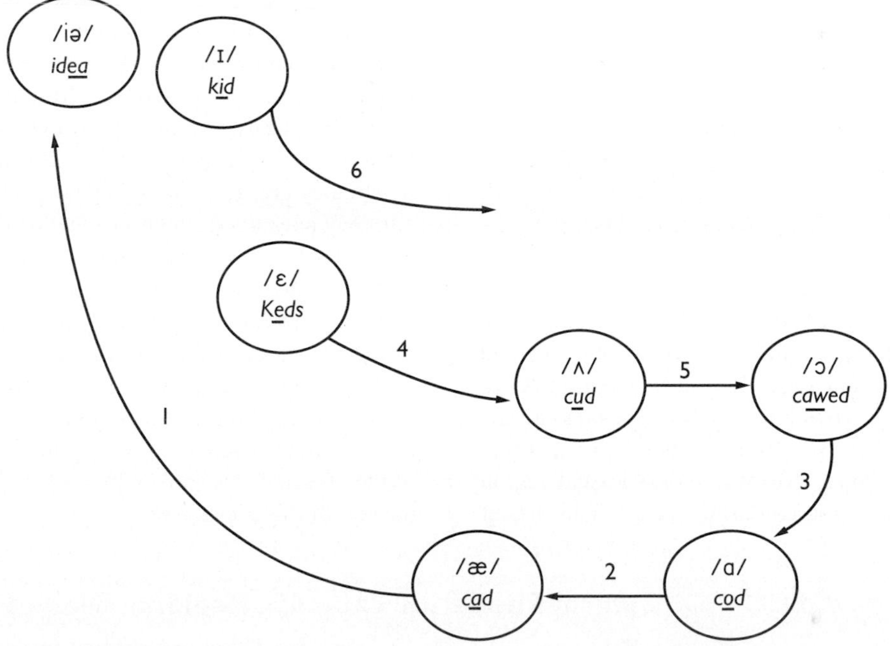

FIGURE F-4
The Northern Cities Vowel Shift (adapted from Labov, 1991, 1996). Figure from "The Three Dialects of English," by W. Labov, in *New Ways of Analyzing Sound Change: Quantitative Analyses of Linguistics Structure*, edited by P. Eckert, copyright 1991, Elsevier Science (USA), reproduced by permission of the publisher.

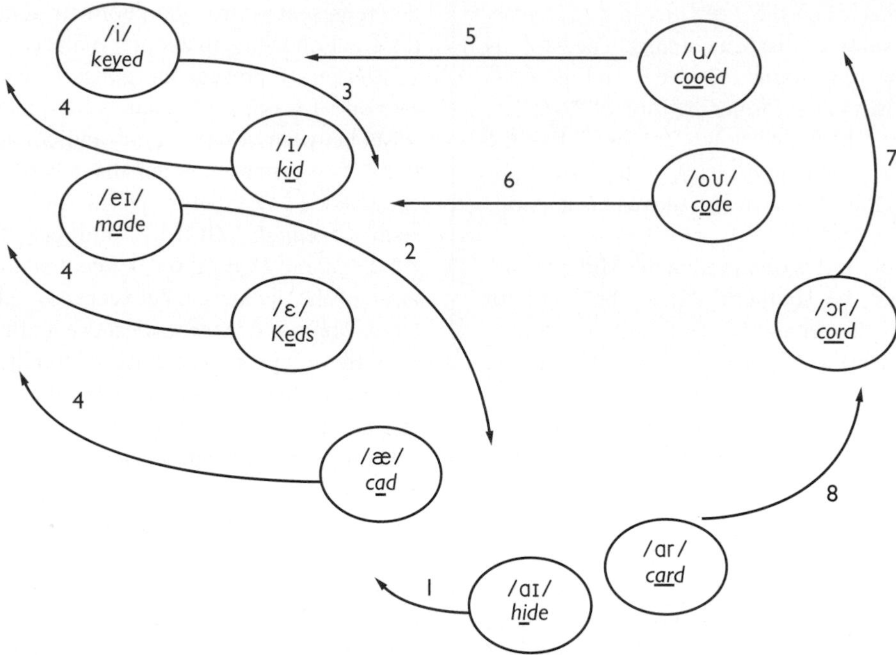

FIGURE F-5
The Southern Vowel Shift (adapted from Labov, 1991, 1996). Figure from "The Three Dialects of English," by W. Labov, in *New Ways of Analyzing Sound Change: Quantitative Analyses of Linguistics Structure*, edited by P. Eckert, copyright 1991, Elsevier Science (USA), reproduced by permission of the publisher.

combination of sociohistorical and linguistic factors explains the origins of American English, how the varieties of English spoken in the United States have changed in ways that contrast with British varieties, why speakers in different regions of the United States have unique accents, and why these differences persist and increase.

American English Regional Accents. Results of Labov's (1991, 1996) vowel studies define three accent regions for American English phonology: North, Midland, and South. Although the correspondence is close, the geographic regions defined by phonology and lexicon do not completely overlap. The North area for phonology corresponds roughly to the Upper North region described in the lexicon by Carver (1987), excluding eastern New England and Minnesota (see Figure F-3). This accent region is defined by variations in vowel productions related to the Northern Cities Shift. Labov's Midland phonology area corresponds roughly to Carver's Lower North lexical region but also extends to the West, excluding Texas. This accent region is defined in part by the occurrence of the ɔ/ɑ merger. The South area begins south of the Ohio River and corresponds to the Upper and Lower South lexical regions defined by Carver. Vowel variations related to the Southern Vowel Shift define this region.

In the accompanying audio examples, speakers originally from the North (New York), the Midland (Montana), and the South (Tennessee) represent some accent regions in the United States. Speakers begin with an introduction about where they are from, how long they have lived there, where else they have lived, and how long they have spoken their dialect. Keep in mind that these samples are provided as opportunities for listening to and transcribing dialect variations, and not as prototypes. Listen to these speakers for evidence of the vowel shifts and mergers characteristic of their geographic regions, and try to capture their productions using your skills in phonetic transcription. Additional suggestions for listening to each of the six audio samples, including a list of the 16 sentences spoken by each speaker, are provided at the end of this appendix.

PROCEED TO: Clinical Phonetics Tape 4B: Regional Dialects
Audio Example #1: A Northern Dialect
Audio Example #2: A Midland Dialect
Audio Example #3: A Southern Dialect

Social Dialects

Social dialects are the varieties of a language spoken by definable social groups, and the study of social variations examines the relationships between language and social class, race, sex, and occupation (Williams, 1977). The very notion of dialect defined in social terms implies a standard against which all varieties are judged. Such standards are not defined by linguists but are a product of social fact, because groups with higher status often impose their own behaviors, including language, as the standard for other groups. Generally speaking, upper classes in cultural centers often define and represent standard behavior.

Even though a standard variety exists for some languages (such as Received Pronunciation of British English and Parisian French), with respect to American English, the idea of a single standard is a myth (e.g., Esling, 1998; Preston, 1998). Interestingly, even in the absence of a universal standard for American English, there is widespread belief—held by speakers rather than linguists—that some regional varieties are more consistent with a standard than others and that some social varieties are so far from standard as to be socially stigmatized (Preston, 1999).

In the United States, every region has its own social stratification and its own distribution of mainstream and nonmainstream varieties, referred to as *prestigious* (or *mainstream*) versus *vernacular* (or *nonmainstream*). All socially differentiated dialects represent rule-governed systems and serve the same communication functions that are characteristic of any language. The major difference between prestigious and vernacular varieties is that speakers of all varieties hold many vernacular dialects in low esteem.

Although sociolinguists have explored an array of socially defined varieties, primary interest has focused on stigmatized vernacular dialects. A number of vernaculars have been studied, such as Appalachian English, Southern White Non-Standard English, Northern White Non-Standard English, and African American Vernacular English (AAVE). Of these varieties, AAVE has received the greatest attention both from linguists and from the general public.

African American Vernacular English. *African American Vernacular English* (*AAVE*) is currently the preferred term for an American English dialect that has also been referred to as *vernacular Black English, nonstandard English, Negro dialect, Black dialect,* and *Ebonics,* among other terms. This variety is spoken by approximately 80 percent of Americans of African descent, the majority of whom are members of lower socioeconomic groups that reside in urban areas. Wolfram (1994) refers to AAVE as "the paradigm case of vernacular dialect phonology" (p. 227), in part because focus on this variety launched modern social dialectology and caused educators, including speech-language pathologists, to confront the deficit/difference controversy surrounding language diversity.

Older notions of the origins and persistence of AAVE were heavily couched in racist views. Speech and language patterns of African Americans had been attributed to purported differences in anatomical, cognitive, and motivational factors. More modern, although still racist, explanations of differences between AAVE and standard English described the former as an incomplete or limited language or as an immature form of English. Under this view, speakers of AAVE were described as deficient in language and concept formation.

In contrast to these older views, AAVE is now widely recognized as a linguistic code distinct from standard English and capable of serving all the functions routinely carried out by language systems. Yet the relationship between AAVE and standard English still presents challenges in several areas. Almost 40 years ago, Stewart (1964) discussed this issue in an educational context and referred to the "quasi-foreign language relationship" between AAVE and standard English:

> *Although the structural correspondences between the language of the learner [AAVE] and the language being taught [Anglo American English] might, at some linguistic levels (such as their respective vocabularies), be so close that the learner could justifiably be considered as already having a native or near-native command of that aspect of the language being taught . . . there would still be enough differences between the two linguistic systems at other levels (such as their grammars) to warrant the use of at least some foreign-language teaching procedures* (p. 11).

This position was echoed in 1979 by a court order in Ann Arbor, Michigan (*Martin Luther King* v. *Ann Arbor*) and in 1997 by a school board proposal in Oakland, California (Board of Education). Both of these actions acknowledged the legitimacy of AAVE as a distinct dialect rather than as a substandard form—a position held by many sociolinguists for some time—and called for teaching standard English to speakers of the dialect in an effort to improve academic achievement of African American students. While the logic of this argument is intuitively sensible, and the linguistic data on which it is based are robust, heated reactions to both the Ann Arbor decision and the Oakland proposal suggest widespread misconceptions about and bias against AAVE. Such inclinations are not due to inherent structural weakness in the variations themselves but rather to the societal position of the dialect's speakers. Thus, the low social regard associated with AAVE persists, maintaining the dialect as a stigmatized vernacular.

Origins of AAVE. Sociolinguists propose two hypotheses about the origins of AAVE. The *Creolist hypothesis* traces the origins of AAVE to European maritime expansion and slave trade in West Africa. According to this perspective, AAVE is derived from African languages that evolved into Plantation Creole in the southern region of the United States. In contrast, the *Anglicist hypothesis* traces the origins of AAVE to Britain and the same varieties that led to the major dialects of Anglo American English.

The Creolist hypothesis represented the prevailing view in the 1970s and still enjoys popularity—due in part to sociohistorical forces such as social stratification, group reference, and personal identity, which appear to be more influential in maintaining social dialects today than they were in the past. However, evidence supporting the Anglicist hypothesis began to surface in the 1980s, driving sociolinguists to continue exploring the roots of AAVE. It may be that the Creolist position is correct, but forces of de-Creolization have eliminated differences that existed at one time. Furthermore, bi-directional language assimilation has resulted in the sharing of features from varieties spoken by African Americans and Caucasians, causing AAVE and standard English to be less different than they were in the past. It is also possible that the Anglicist position is the accurate historical explanation, but cultural identity and sociolinguistic segregation have led to and reinforced distinct varieties along ethnic lines.

It has been suggested that AAVE is eroding in the United States (Taylor, 1972), although AAVE is still different from other varieties of American English and continues to diverge from other vernaculars (Wolfram and Schilling-Estes, 1998). Structural features of modern AAVE cut across all linguistic components; contemporary AAVE demonstrates unique characteristics, yet remains intelligible to speakers of other American English dialects.

Characteristics of AAVE. Scholars have constructed a lengthy list of characteristics of AAVE. Most of these features have more recently been shown also to occur in other American English dialects defined either by region or social class. The differences appear to be more an issue of frequency of occurrence, with AAVE showing more prevalent usage of some features than is typically seen in Anglo American English varieties. The eight features presented in Table F-1 are considered unique to AAVE (Wolfram and Schilling-Estes, 1998).

Brief inspection of the entries in this list suggests that most of the unique features of AAVE are grammatical rather than phonological; only the first two features describe phonological production patterns. In addition, there are several features in which the language aspect involved is confounded. Features 3, 4, and 5, for instance, although defined in grammatical terms, may also be perceived as phonological variations.

With respect to phonological variations, AAVE and Standard English phonology use the same phonemes and similar syllable shapes. However, in AAVE vowels and diphthongs are more likely than consonants to be subjected to a combination of regional and social influences. Thus, vowel and diphthong patterns of AAVE are often similar to patterns noted in the speech of Caucasians living in the same locality. In terms of sentence intonation, AAVE speakers demonstrate a wider pitch range (extending to higher levels) than Anglo American English speakers. Furthermore, the falsetto register is used more often in AAVE, and more rising and level final contours are noted. It is important to emphasize, however, that both "standard" and "nonstandard" forms occur in the speech of most AAVE speakers. In addition, nonstandard features also occur in the speech of Standard English speakers, but less frequently. Pollock and Berni (2001) provide a comprehensive list of dialectal changes in AAVE (Table A-1) in their informative coverage of transcription procedures for vowels and diphthongs.

Audio Example #4 provides a sample of AAVE. Listen to this speaker, originally from Milwaukee, Wisconsin, for examples of consonant and vowel differences that are characteristic of AAVE. Try to transcribe her productions, using the guidelines discussed later and summarized at the end of this appendix.

TABLE F-1
Language Characteristics Unique to AAVE

Characteristic	Example
1. Devoicing of voiced stops in stressed syllables	[b ɪ t] for *bid;* [b æ k] for *bag*
2. Reduction of final consonant clusters when followed by a word or a suffix beginning with a vowel	[l ɪ̝ f ʌ p] for *lift up*
3. Absence of present tense, third person *-s*	*she walk* for *she walks*
4. Absence of plural *-s* in the general class of noun plurals	*four girl* for *four girls*
5. Absence of possessive *-s*	*man hat* for *man's hat*
6. Absence of copula and auxiliary in *is* forms	*He in the kitchen* for *He's in the kitchen*
7. Use of habitual *be*	*Sometimes my ears be itching*
8. Use of remote time stressed *been* to mark an action that took place or a state that began in the past and is still relevant	*I been known him a long time*

Source: Drawn from Wolfram and Schilling-Estes (1998). By permission of Blackwell Publishing.

PROCEED TO: Clinical Phonetics Tape 4B: Social Dialects
Audio Example #4: An AAVE Dialect

Foreign Dialects

Foreign language variations are noted in the productions of speakers for whom the local dominant language is a nonnative form. The term *nonnative language* rather than *second language* is preferred, because many speakers from outside the United States are proficient in numerous languages. In the United States, individuals from an array of non-English language backgrounds demonstrate foreign dialect variations in their production of English. For example, a young man seen in our university clinic for dialect management is from Laos. His native language is Hmong, but he also speaks Lao and Thai and can read and write in those two languages. Similarly, a woman from Haiti who sought accent management instruction speaks French and Haitian Creole as her native languages. As an adult, she has learned English as well as Spanish and speaks, reads, and writes in both of those languages.

Interest here focuses on the phonological variations that contribute to foreign accent. But keep in mind that foreign dialect speakers themselves may be more concerned about other aspects of language, particularly semantics (Egan, Serflek, and Carpenter, 2000), than about the speech aspects of accent.

Causes of Foreign Accent. The major "cause" of foreign accent variations is the speaker's native language. That is, the rules governing the native language compete with and intrude on the production of English. The author recalls, for example, a man from Nepal who sought services for dialect management at a university clinic. He was working on his doctoral degree and, as a teaching assistant, found that many of his students had difficulty understanding him. Among the variations in his English production was interchangeable use of /s/ and /ʃ/, so that his pronunciation of *sip* /sɪp/ was indistinguishable from that of *ship* /ʃɪp/. These two speech sounds, which are distinct phonemes in English, represented one phoneme class in his native language. Similarly, the French and Haitian Creole speaker mentioned previously tended to reduce American English diphthongs, for instance, /a͡ɪ/ was reduced to /ɑ/ or /ɑː/. This variation reflected the limited occurrence of diphthongs in her native language(s).

The Hmong speaker mentioned in the previous paragraph produced the words in Table F-2. Examination of these productions shows a tendency to delete final consonant singletons and to reduce final consonant clusters. Indeed, Hmong is an open-syllable language characterized by consonant-vowel (CV) syllable shapes. Moreover, the permitted syllable shapes are typically simple, without consonant clusters in either a syllable release or syllable arrest position. In contrast, as a closed-syllable language, English requires syllable-final consonants to be marked, requiring marking of all elements in consonant clusters, regardless of position. Thus, the pronunciation variations of the Hmong speaker can be directly traced to intrusion of his first language rules on his English productions. It is important to note that this phonological variation also intrudes on production of English morphological markers, as seen in the omission of the plural marker in *costumes.* This particular variation appears to be phonologically conditioned; however, it also has elements of morphosyntactic intrusion, because Hmong does not mark plurals on individual morphemes in the way such markings are accomplished in English. Rather, Hmong uses number indicators or classifiers (similar to the way plurality is marked, for example, in American Sign Language), which also contributes to differences in English production by Hmong speakers.

TABLE F-2
English Words Produced by a Native Speaker of Hmong

Target Word	Phonetic Target	Phonetic Production
boats	/bo͡ʊts/	[bo͡ʊs]
house	/ha͡ʊs/	[ha͡ʊ]
costumes	/kɑstumz/	[kɑstum]
tournament	/tɔrnəmɛnt/	[tɔrnəmɛn]
distance	/dɪstɪns/	[dɪstɪn]
taste	/te͡ɪst/	[te͡ɪs]
sports	/spɔrts/	[spɔrs]

Native language rules are considered the primary influence on accent variations in nonnative languages; however, Yavas (1998) proposes that the relative markedness of a sound also impacts a speaker's production of that sound in a nonnative language. Yavas uses the terms *marked* and *natural* to refer to unexpected versus expected phonological phenomena, respectively. For instance, the front, unrounded vowels /i/ and /e/ occur in most of the world's languages and are, therefore, considered natural. In contrast, a front-rounded vowel symbolized as /y/ occurs less frequently (it does not occur in English, for example) and is, therefore, considered marked. In the context of learning a nonnative language, Yavas proposes that speakers acquire acceptable production of natural, or unmarked, sounds more readily than marked sounds.

Another contributor to a nonnative speaker's variations in pronunciation relates to the conditions under which he or she learned the nonnative language. For example, most nonnative speakers whom we see in the clinic have learned English as a written form. If their instruction also included spoken English, most of their teachers were other nonnative speakers, many of whom spoke a variety of British English. As a result, our clients' productions tend to reflect their limited exposure to the sound of American English as spoken by native speakers. Moreover, a British English filter often confounds the phonological influence of the speaker's native language on American English.

Aspects of Foreign Accent. As is true of other types of accent, aspects of foreign accent can be described in terms of the phonemic repertoire and phonotactic, morphophonemic, and suprasegmental rules. The differences between the phonemic repertoires of a speaker's native language (L1) and the target language (L2) dictate which sounds will be produced in a nonnative accent. For example, though English and Spanish share several sounds (e.g., /p/, /b/, /t/, /d/, /s/, /f/), there are also sounds that are unique to each language: English includes /ʃ/ and /θ/, but Spanish does not; and Spanish includes the trilled /r/ and velar fricative /χ/, but English does not. As a result, native speakers of Spanish might be expected to have difficulty producing English words that contain /ʃ/ and /θ/; and, likewise, native speakers of English will likely have trouble producing a trilled /r/ and /χ/. Each speaker's productions will be most similar to sounds in the native language that are closest in phonetic features to the target sound.

Foreign accent is also reflected in allophonic variations within a language. For example, /d/ and /ð/ represent distinct phonemes in English, whereas Spanish treats these sounds as allophones of the phoneme /d/, with [d] occurring in word-initial position and after /n/, and [ð] occurring in intervocalic position. Thus, a native speaker of Spanish might apply this native language rule to English pronunciation and, at times, sound as if he or she was lisping.

Variations in how sounds function in syllables and how syllables are shaped also contribute to foreign accent. For example, whereas both English and Vietnamese allow the sound /ŋ/ (as in *si<u>ng</u>*) in their phonemic repertoires, /ŋ/ cannot function in a syllable-release position in English but can in Vietnamese. This difference is illustrated by the difficulty many Americans experience in pronouncing Vietnamese names such as Nguyen.

With respect to syllable shapes, although English and Spanish both include /s/ and /t/ in their phonemic repertoires, only English allows those sounds to combine in a CCV syllable shape. Therefore, the word *stew* may be produced as [s t u] by a native speaker of American English (depending on his or her regional dialect), but a native speaker of Spanish may produce it as [ɛ s t u], with a syllable break between /s/ and /t/. Similarly, all dialects of Chinese demonstrate highly constrained syllable structures: No dialect permits consonant clusters, and all dialects allow a restricted set of consonants in syllable-arrest position. Clearly, differences between the phonotactic rules of Chinese and English contribute to the difficulties that many Chinese speakers have with English pronunciation, and vice versa.

Consider, too, how English morphological markers are produced in Standard English, for example, the three regular plural morphemes listed in Table F-3. The morphophonemic rule that governs such productions might be stated as: The plural marker is realized as [s] following voiceless stops, [z] following all voiced consonants, and [ɪ z] or [ə z] following voiceless or voiced fricatives and affricates. Native speakers of German, a language characterized by final consonant devoicing, may produce /d ɔ g z/ as [d ɔ k s] and /w ɑ tʃ ɪ z/ as [w ɑ tʃ ɪ s]. These productions represent variations on an English morphophonemic production rule and, as such, are perceived as indicative of an accent.

Variations in prosodic elements such as lexical, sentential, and emphatic stress contribute heavily to all accents as well as to nonnative varieties. For instance, English uses pitch variations at the sentence level to distinguish statements from questions, whereas other languages vary pitch at the syllable level to contrast meaning. In *tone languages,* such as Chinese and Hmong, these pitch changes operate as phonemic segments. That is, just as the English words *bought* and *ball* have different meanings due to the differences in one phoneme, word meanings in tone languages vary as a function of the tone associated with each syllable. Thus, the meanings of two (or more) phonetically identical words depend on which of several tones are used in each syllable. This suprasegmental variation is often seen clinically in exaggerated pitch variability during English production. Yin (2001) found that native speakers of tone languages have wider frequency and intensity ranges than speakers of non-tone languages.

The accompanying audio samples provide examples of English as spoken by nonnative speakers. One is a native Spanish speaker who originally comes from Panama, and the other is a native Chinese speaker who originally comes from Taiwan. Tables F-4, F-5, F-6, and F-7 will help you identify the English phonological variations of these nonnative

TABLE F-3
The Three Regular English Plural Morphemes

Noun Morpheme	Singular	Plural
dog	/dɔg/	/dɔgz/
cat	/kæt/	/kæts/
watch	/wɑtʃ/	/wɑtʃɪz/

TABLE F-4
Sounds in Spanish

	Phoneme	Allophone(s)	Orthographic	
Vowels	i	i	i	*pipa*
	e	e	e	*mesa*
	u	u	u	*fútbol*
	o	o	o	*sopa*
	a	a	a	*llame*
Consonants				
Stops	p	p	p	*peso*
	b	b	b	*bailar*
		β		*llave*
	t	t	t	*toma*
	d	d	d	*dinero*
		ð		*nido*
	k	k	c, k	*vaca*
	g	g	g	*gato*
		ɣ		*lago*
Nasals	m	m	m	*mano*
	n	n	n	*nariz*
	ŋ	ŋ	ñ	*baño*
Consonants (continued)				
Fricatives	f	f	f	*foto*
		ɸ		*emfermo*
	x	x	j	*reloj*
		h		
	s	s	s	*sin*
Liquids	l	l	l	*limón*
	ɾ	ɾ	r	*martillo*
		l		
	r	r	r	*roto*
		ʀ		
Glides	w	w	u	*hueso*
		gw		
	j	j	y, ll	*llama*
		ʤ		
		ʒ		
Affricate	tʃ	tʃ	ch	*chavo*
		ʃ		

Source: After Iglesias and Anderson, 1993. From John H. Bernthal and Nicholas W. Bankson, *Articulation and Phonological Disorders*, 3rd ed. Copyright © 1993. Reprinted by permission by Allyn & Bacon. From *Cultural & Linguistic Diversity Resource Guide for Speech-Language Pathologists,* 1st edition. © 2000. Reprinted with permission of Delmar, a division of Thomson Learning. Fax 800 730-2215.

TABLE F-5
Phonological Characteristics of Spanish Dialects

Pattern	Example	English	Spanish Dialect
Stops			
/b/ → [v]	/boka/ → [voka]	mouth	M
/d/ → ø	/sed/ → [se]	thirsty	C, D
/d/ → ø	/dedo/ → [deo]	finger	M, C, PR, D
/k/ → ø	/doktoɾ/ → [dotoɾ]	doctor	M, D
/g/ → [ɣ]	/goma/ → [ɣoma]	tire	D
Nasals			
/n/ → [ŋ]	/amon/ → [amoŋ]	ham	C, PR, D
/n/ → ø	/amon/ → [amo]/[amõ]	ham	C, PR
Fricatives			
/f/ → ɸ	/kafe/ → [kaɸe]	coffee	PR, D
/s/ → ø	/dos/ → [do]	two	M, C, PR, D
/s/ → ^{h}	/dos/ → [do^h]	two	M, C, PR, D
/x/ → [h]	/xamon/ → [hamon]	ham	M, C, PR, D
Liquids			
/ɾ/ (flap) → ø	/koɾtaɾ/ → [kottaɾ]	to cut	C, PR, D
/ɾ/ (flap) → [l]	/koɾtaɾ/ → [koltaɾ]	to cut	PR, C, D
/ɾ/ (flap) → [i]	/koɾtaɾ/ → [koitaɾ]	to cut	PR, D
/r/ (trill) → [ʀ]/[x]	/pero/ → [peʀo/pexo]	dog	PR, D, (M; rare)
Glides			
/j/ → [ʤ]/[ʒ]	/jo/ → [ʤo/ʒo]	I	C, M, PR, D
/w/ → [gw]	/weso/ → [gweso]	bone	C, M, PR, D
Affricate			
/tʃ/ → [ʃ]	/mutʃo/ → [muʃo]	a lot	D

Key: M = Mexican; C = Cuban; PR = Puerto Rican; D = Dominican; ø = deleted; ^{h} = aspirated

Source: Adapted from Goldstein and Iglesias (in preparation). From *Cultural & Linguistic Diversity Resource Guide for Speech-Language Pathologists,* 1st edition. © 2000. Reprinted with permission of Delmar, a division of Thomson Learning. Fax 800 730-2215.

TABLE F-6
Phonological Characteristics of Mandarin and Cantonese Dialects of Chinese

	Mandarin	Cantonese
Initial Consonants		
Stops	/p, pʰ, t, tʰ, k, kʰ/	/p, pʰ, t, tʰ, k, kʰ/
Nasals	/m, n, ŋ/	/m, n, ŋ/
Fricatives	/f, s, s, z, ʃ, χ/	/f, s, h/
Affricates	/ts, tsʰ, tcʰ/	/ts, tsʰ/
Lateral	/l/	/l/
Glides	none	/j, w/
Final Consonants		
Stops	none	/pʰ, tʰ, kʰ/
Nasals	/n, ŋ/	/m, n, ŋ/
Glides	none	/j, w/
Tones	high-level, rising, falling-rising, falling	high-level, high-falling, high-rising, mid-level, low-falling, low-rising, low-level

Source: Adapted from Goldstein (2000). From *Cultural & Linguistic Diversity Resource Guide for Speech-Language Pathologists,* 1st edition. © 2000. Reprinted with permission of Delmar, a division of Thomson Learning. Fax 800 730-2215.

TABLE F-7
Phoneme Segments of the Xiamen Dialect of Chinese

Initial Consonants	p pʰ b m t tʰ n l ts tsʰ s k kʰ g ŋ h
Final Consonants	m n ŋ p t k ʔ
Vowels	i ɪ u a ɛ e o ɔ

Source: Adapted from Sung (1999).

speakers that are related to interference from their native languages. Tables F-4 and F-5 provide information on phonological characteristics of Spanish. Although several dialects of Spanish have been identified, the few phonological variations among them should not impede your recognition of those first-language features that influence English production. For future reference, Table F-6 provides information on the phonological characteristics of Mandarin and Cantonese dialects of Chinese—the most frequently spoken varieties of Chinese in the United States. Chinese dialects, unlike those of Spanish, are mutually unintelligible. Table F-7 provides information on the consonant and vowel phonemes of the Xiamen variety of the Min dialect, the native variety of Chinese most commonly spoken in Taiwan. The Xiamen dialect also includes eight tones, in contrast to the typical four tones in Mandarin and Cantonese. Table F-7 should be helpful in listening to Audio Example #6: A Speaker from Taiwan.

PROCEED TO: Clinical Phonetics Tape 4B: Foreign Dialects
Audio Example #5: A Speaker from Panama
Audio Example #6: A Speaker from Taiwan

PREVALENCE OF DIALECT VARIATIONS

Students are often interested in information about the types of persons who seek dialect management services from a speech-language pathologist (SLP) and how frequently an SLP might see such clients. Individuals who seek clinical services for dialect management are most often well-educated, cognitively intact, literate adults who refer themselves for service because of educational or professional demands for more effective English. Some are interested specifically in modifying an accent (such as an attorney who believes his southern accent has a negative impact on his effectiveness at trial), while others may request broad-based dialect management (such as an Ethiopian graduate student who wants assistance with professionally oriented English vocabulary, pronunciation, and syntax).

It is relatively easy to describe the type of person who seeks dialect management services but more difficult to specify how frequently SLPs might see such clients. People who seek dialect management services typically are not counted by government agencies, unlike children who are served in school settings, or children and adults who suffer specific medical conditions such as traumatic brain injury, stroke, or Alzheimer's disease. Therefore, the usual data sources are not likely to reflect the number of people who receive services for dialect variations.

Some U.S. census data may help estimate the number of adults *in need* of dialect management services. According to the 1990 Census (U.S. Bureau of the Census, 1990), the most recent date for which detailed information is available about foreign-born residents of the United States, 19.8 million people (7.9 percent of the population) were foreign-born. Of that number, approximately 80 percent spoke a language other than English at home, and more than half reported that they did not speak English "very well." Approximately 20 percent had earned at least a baccalaureate degree, and a similar proportion of those who were employed and over 16 years of age had worked in management or a professional specialty—an employment category that is likely to require superior spoken English skills.

A word of caution is important here. First, these figures reflect the number of adults in need of dialect management services, not the number who actually sought or received services. That number would likely be substantially smaller and even more difficult to estimate. However, factors such as geographic location within the United States and type of service setting will influence the frequency with which a clinician might see clients for dialect management. That is, clinicians in California, Texas, Florida, New York, New Jersey, and Connecticut are most likely to be called on to work with nonnative speakers of English: 10 percent or more of residents in those states are foreign-born. Clinicians in Washington, Michigan, Ohio, Pennsylvania, Maryland, Virginia, Massachusetts, and Rhode Island may also see clients who request dialect management services, because 3 to 9.9 percent of the populations in those states are foreign-born. Moreover, clinicians in private practice and student clinicians in university clinics are more likely to see clients for dialect management than are school-based clinicians or clinicians who work in medical settings.

A second caution concerns the types of dialect discussed in this appendix—regional, social, or foreign. This discussion has focused on foreign-born residents—individuals who might demonstrate foreign dialect variations—rather than native speakers of American English who might seek services to modify regional accents. The latter number is virtually impossible to estimate but is likely to be even smaller than the number of nonnative speakers who seek dialect management services.

DIALECT AND CLINICAL PHONETICS

Persons who seek clinical services should be evaluated across an array of communication domains, but the focus here in the appraisal of accent will be limited to speech issues. Clinical phonetics with such speakers involves the three separate but related activities of sampling, transcription, and analysis and interpretation.

Sampling

Regardless of the clinical area of interest, the goal of any speech sampling procedure is to obtain a systematic and representative sample of a speaker's productions. *Systematic* means that all targets of interest are included in the sample. In the context of sampling a dialect, a speaker must have opportunities to produce all consonant, vowel, and diphthong sounds allowed in American English, as well as the range of syllable shapes and prosodic patterns characteristic of the language. *Representative* means that the sample is reflective of the speaker's usual, rather than his or her best, productions.

Clinical sampling requires some trade-offs, because the most systematic sample may be the least representative. To obtain the required information, more than one sample may be needed with opportunities for spontaneous as well as spontaneous-evoked productions. *Spontaneous productions* are those generated by the speaker using conversational or narrative speaking tasks. Although most representative, spontaneous productions are not necessarily systematic, because the occurrence of desired targets is uncontrolled. In contrast, *spontaneous-evoked productions* result from having the speaker read or name predetermined stimulus materials.

With clients who demonstrate accents, spontaneous-evoked speech samples most frequently rely on having the speaker orally read printed materials. These may be in the form of a sentence articulation test, which contains sound-loaded sentences that target a particular English phoneme or phonemes. Because dialects vary more frequently in vowel than in consonant production, it is important to ensure that the stimulus materials include an adequate vowel sample. Although printed materials are the most appropriate for evoking speech samples from adult dialect clients, they are influenced by the person's oral reading fluency and his or her ability to read English. To control for difficulties in oral reading, an alternative procedure can be used. The speaker can be asked to orally read a single printed word and then use it in a spontaneously generated sentence. This procedure evokes a sample that is both systematic and representative of the speaker's production patterns, and it is used in some commercially available clinical assessment materials (e.g., Compton, 1983; Sikorski, 1997).

These sampling procedures will yield systematic and representative samples collected under focused, discrete, and controlled conditions. It is commonly recommended that clinicians also collect a completely spontaneous sample to compare productions under more systematic versus more representative conditions.

Transcription

Dialect samples should be transcribed narrowly, using diacritic markings to indicate the systematic variations that contribute to a speaker's accent. Such notation requires refined listening skills and well-developed abilities in phonetic transcription—the very hard-won skills you are acquiring in your phonetics class! It may not be clinically reasonable or feasible to narrowly transcribe each utterance in a continuous speech sample. In practice, clinicians are more likely to transcribe narrowly at the word or phrase level to highlight the variations that characterize a speaker's dialect.

It is also important that transcription reflect what the speaker actually said, unbiased by the transcriber's own dialect. Consider the example in the following paragraph, which invariably occurs in the author's phonetics classes.

In the Upper Midwest of the United States, particularly in west central Wisconsin, it is typical for speakers to shift pronunciation of the phoneme /æ/ to /e͡ɪ/ before the voiced velar stop /g/ and the voiced nasal /ŋ/. This variation suggests evidence of the Northern Cities Vowel Shift that is characteristic of the region, and it leads to pronunciation of words like *bag, wagon,* and *thank* as [b e͡ɪ g] rather than /b æ g/, [w e͡ɪ g ə n] rather than /w æ g ə n/, and [θ e͡ɪ ŋ k] rather than /θ æ ŋ k/. These variations are recognizable in daily communication, but they do not disrupt comprehension of meaning. However, in phonetics classes that include words like *thank* [θ æ ŋ k] on transcription quizzes, students from Wisconsin typically reauditorize the word to accord with their own dialect. As you probably have experienced in your own class, such situations make for "lively" exchanges about quiz grades! Clinically, this illustrates the need for speech-language pathologists to be thoroughly familiar with the implications of their own dialect for assessment and treatment.

Analysis and Interpretation

As reviewed in detail in the preceding appendix (Appendix E), we will assume that all samples for dialect analysis have been recorded using high-quality equipment and under good recording conditions. Similarly, they should be played back for transcription and analysis on good-quality equipment. Otherwise, the signal may not be sufficiently clear to hear the variations that define a speaker's accent. Note that it is risky to rely solely on a recorded sample for a first pass at transcription: If the equipment fails, the clinician will be left without any information. Therefore, if possible, it is prudent to complete at least some of the transcription of the sample live, using the recording for additional detail. Some additional guidelines for transcription are listed at the end of this appendix.

The transcribed sample can be analyzed in several ways. An initial analysis may focus on the variations produced, with the intent of identifying the ways in which the speaker's production differs from a desired standard. The resulting list of variant features can then be subjected to *contrastive* analysis, which evaluates the speaker's actual productions of English from the perspective of the characteristics of his or her native dialect or language. Contrastive analysis allows a clinician to determine the extent to which a speaker's variant productions can be explained or understood by the phonological rules governing the native dialect or language. Identifying competing rules facilitates an understanding of cross-dialect influence. This type of analysis is particularly important when evaluating young speakers of social dialects; without knowing the rules that govern their native varieties, clinicians are more likely to misidentify such speakers as having a language disorder.

As with the speech of a client with phonological disorder, the speech of a person with an accent should be assessed for intelligibility. This type of judgment estimates how much of a speech sample a listener understands and is typically assessed by having the listener transcribe orthographically what was said. With many dialect speakers, however, speech may be intelligible but noticeably accented. Researchers have addressed this issue by proposing the concept of *comprehensibility*—the extent to which a listener believes he or she will have difficulty understanding a speaker (Derwing and Munro, 1997; Munro and Derwing, 1999). Practically, comprehensibility translates to an estimate of distraction, and this estimate helps identify the extent to which an accent disrupts communication.

A Case Example

The following case example illustrates the application of phonetic transcription to clinical practice. The oral communication goals of this young man are typical of clients who seek the services of speech-language pathologists for dialect management.

A., a graduate student majoring in environmental and public health, referred himself to a university speech and hearing clinic, wishing to focus on the "weaker points" of his spoken English, specifically his pronunciation skills. At the time of his initial contact with the clinic, A. was 29 years old. Originally from Ethiopia, A. had been in the United States for 10 years, and he planned to remain in the United States after completing his graduate education. A.'s native language is Oromo, and he also speaks Amharic, Adre, and Arabic. He was taught to read and write English by Ethiopian teachers beginning in the sixth grade. A. has also taken English composition classes to enhance his language skills. He had not received formal instruction in spoken English.

A representative sample of A.'s spontaneous English production was collected. He gave a brief speech about tuberculosis, which had originally been a presentation for a university class in public health. While not a systematic sample, as previously defined, it did reflect his most usual speech patterns. The sample was first transcribed verbatim orthographically, with A.'s mazes or repetitions and revisions noted in brackets. Depicted below, this transcript gives a sense of A.'s oral English facility and fluency.

Today's presentation of us is on the topic of tuberculosis [and un] as you all know, tuberculosis is one of the classical diseases, which has been haunting humanity. [Un] it has been known as a disease for thousands of years. [And un] there is evidence in some Egyptian mummies that it was known to ancient pharaohs. Even though [the mortality of] the mortality rate is declining in Europe and North America, [in] in twentieth century America is still vulnerable to tuberculosis because America is the only industrialized countries which has broad border with underdeveloped countries.

In around 1850, TB was the chief cause of death in the United States and England, claiming about 25 percent of all deaths. Until 1909, tuberculosis was the number one cause of death in America. Unlike other infectious diseases, tuberculosis is an insidious and debilitating disease that afflict more people with death after a lingering sickness.

The clinician's impression was that morphological and syntactic variations were more disruptive to A.'s communication in English than were phonological variations. In that regard, intonational contours and stress patterns at the sentence level did not vary noticeably from patterns expected in American English. Consequently, no efforts were made to complete a narrow transcription of the entire sample. Rather, the clinician listened again to A.'s sample, noting those variations that distracted attention from the message. While the entire sample was not transcribed phonetically, clinical phonetics notation was used to indicate phones actually produced by A. as well as his stress variations. These transcriptions are provided in Table F-8. Several patterns of phonological variation are clear from this sample:

- Voicing shifts, including devoicing of final consonants on *is, of,* and *years* and assimilatory changes on *cases,* are likely due to interference from A.'s native language but may also be related to pronunciation of words as they are spelled rather than as they are spoken.
- Vowel shifts and stress variations, as seen in A.'s production of *Egyptian, vulnerable,* and *cause,* are likely due to his attempt to pronounce English words based on their orthographic spellings.
- Morphophonemic pronunciation rule variations, as seen in A.'s production of *deaths,* are likely due to his unfamiliarity with English pronunciation rules.

Instruction with A. took a broad-based dialect management approach. Work focused not only on these English phonological issues, but also addressed morphosyntactic concerns

TABLE F-8
Selected Productions of a Nonnative English Speaker

Target Word	Phonetic Target	A.'s Production
haunting	/hɔntɪŋ/	[hɑʊntʃɪŋ]
tuberculosis	/təb[2]ɝkjəl[1]osɪs/	[t[2]ɝbəkl[1]osɪs]
is	/ɪz/	[ɪs]
years	/jɪrz/	[jɪrs]
deaths	/dɛθs/	[dɛθɪs]
cause	/kɔz/	[k͡ɑʊz]
vulnerable	/v[1]ʌlnɚbl̩/	[v[2]ʌlnɚ[1]e͡ɪbəl]
Egyptian	/[2]idʒ[1]ɪpʃɪn/	[[2]idʒ[1]ɪpʃiən]
cases	/ke͡ɪsɪz/	[kezəz]
of	/ʌv/	[ʌf]

related to verb tenses and number agreements as well as semantic elements of word meaning and usage.

SUMMARY AND CONCLUSIONS

Language and speech variations associated with dialect add richness, depth, and color to the linguistic landscape. The challenge for speech-language pathologists and others who are interested in language learning and use is to know the variations characteristic of their own dialects as well as those of other dialects, and to apply that knowledge in a culturally sensitive manner.

Professional role definition also dictates that clinicians distinguish between communication disorders and communication differences. An individual from a linguistically and culturally diverse population can demonstrate both; differentiating between the two relies on knowing which aspects of linguistic variation reflect disorder and which reflect ethnic or cultural diversity. Moreover, awareness of underlying personal and social sources of variation also contributes to making appropriate decisions. The primary means to distinguish disorder from difference is to complete a phonetic transcription of a language sample and analyze the speech patterns in the context of the client's linguistic and cultural background. Developing an understanding of the potential impact of differences in speech-language patterns on effective communication is the task of speech-language pathologists in an increasingly diverse society.

SOURCES FOR FURTHER STUDY

Bauer, L., and Trudgill, P. (Eds.). 1998. *Language myths.* London: Penguin. This slim volume, written in nontechnical terms, is a collection of essays that address numerous myths about language and dialect.

Mufwene, S. S., Rickford, J. R., Bailey, G., and Baugh, J. 1998. *African-American English: Structure, history, and use.* London: Routledge. This comprehensive text presents well-documented information about African American Vernacular English (AAVE).

Preston, D. R. (Ed.). 1999. *Handbook of perceptual dialectology.* Amsterdam: John Benjamins. This collection presents the most recent ideas and data on relationships between language use and the social regard of people for one another.

Wolfram, W., and Schilling-Estes, N. 1998. *American English.* Malden, MA: Blackwell Scientific Publications. This book is a comprehensive treatment of language variations, particularly varieties of American English.

REFERENCES

Atwood, E. B. 1953. *A survey of verb forms in the Eastern United States.* Ann Arbor: University of Michigan Press.

Bailey, G., and Thomas, E. 1998. Some aspects of African-American vernacular English phonology. In S. S. Mufwene, J. R. Rickford, G. Bailey, and J. Baugh, (Eds.). *African-American English: Structure, history, and use* (pp. 85–109). London: Routledge.

Board of Education of the Oakland Unified School District. 1997, January. *Resolution of the Board of Education adopting the report and recommendations of the African-American task force.* Retrieved May 26, 2001, from the World Wide Web: http://www.linguistlist.org/topics/ebonics/ebonics-res2.html.

Carpenter, L. J. 1990. *Multicultural education and the undergraduate curriculum: A faculty workshop* [Workshop summary]. Eau Claire: Department of Communication Disorders, University of Wisconsin–Eau Claire.

Carver, C. M. 1987. *American regional dialects: A word geography.* Ann Arbor: University of Michigan Press.

Compton, A. J. 1983. *Compton phonological assessment of foreign accent.* San Francisco: Carousel House.

Derwing, T. M., and Munro, M. J. 1997. Accent, intelligibility and comprehensibility: Evidence from four L1s. *Studies in Second Language Learning 19:* 1–16.

Egan, L., Serflek, E., and Carpenter, L. J. 2000, November. *Learning English as a nonnative language: Learners' perspective.* Poster presented at the annual convention of the American Speech-Language-Hearing Association, Washington, DC.

Esling, J. H. 1998. Everyone has an accent except me. In L. Bauer and P. Trudgill (Eds.), *Language myths* (pp. 169–75). London: Penguin.

Fairbanks, G. 1960. *Voice and articulation drill book.* New York: Harper & Row.

Goldstein, B. 2000. *Resource guide on cultural and linguistic diversity.* San Diego: Singular.

Goldstein and Iglesias (in preparation). *Contextual probes of articulation competence—Spanish.*

Iglesias, A., and Anderson, N. 1993. Dialectal variations. In J. Bernthal and N. Bankson (Eds.), *Articulation and phonological disorders* (3rd ed., pp. 147–61). Englewood Cliffs, NJ: Prentice-Hall.

Kurath, H. 1949. *A word geography of the eastern United States.* Ann Arbor: University of Michigan Press.

Kurath, H., and McDavid, R. 1961. *The pronunciation of English in the Atlantic states.* Ann Arbor: University of Michigan Press.

Labov, W. 1991. The three dialects of English. In P. Eckert (Ed.), *New ways of analyzing sound change* (pp. 1–44). San Diego: Academic Press.

Labov, W. 1996, October. The organization of dialect diversity in North America. Paper presented at the Fourth International Conference on Spoken Language Processing, Philadelphia, PA. Retrieved November 6, 2000, from the World Wide Web: http://babel.ling.upenn.edu/phono_atlas/ICSLP4/BW/ICSLP4BW.html.

Martin Luther King Junior Elementary School Children, et al. v. *Ann Arbor School District Board,* 473 F. Supp. 1371 (E.D. Mich. 1979).

Munro, M. J., and Derwing, T. M. 1999. Foreign accent, comprehensibility, and intelligibility in the speech of second language learners. *Language Learning 49* (supp. 1): 285–310.

Pollock, K. E., Bailey, G., Berni, M. C., Fletcher, D. G., Hinton, L. N., Johnson, I. A., and Weaver, R. O. 1998. *Phonological characteristics of African-American vernacular English: An updated resource list.* Poster presentation at the annual convention of the American Speech-Language-Hearing Association, San

Antonio, TX. (Also available at http://www.ausp.memphis.edu/phonology.)

Pollock, K. E., and Berni, M. C. 2001. Transcription of vowels. *Topics in Language Disorders 21:* 22–40.

Preston, D. R. 1998. They speak really bad English down South and in New York City. In L. Bauer and P. Trudgill (Eds.), *Language myths* (pp. 139–49). London: Penguin.

Preston, D. R. (Ed.). 1999. *Handbook of perceptual dialectology* (vol. 1). Amsterdam: John Benjamins.

Romaine, S. (Ed.). 1982. *Sociolinguistic variation in speech communities.* London: Arnold.

Sikorski, L. D. 1997. *Proficiency in oral English communication,* 2nd ed. Santa Ana, CA: LDS Associates.

Smitherman, G. 1977. *Talkin' and testifyin': The language of Black America.* Boston: Houghton Mifflin.

Stewart, W. A. 1964. Urban Negro speech: Sociolinguistic factors affecting English teaching. In R. W. Shuy (Ed.), *Social dialects and language learning* (pp. 10–18). Champaign, IL: National Council of Teachers of English.

Sung, D. W. H. 1999. *The Chinese language.* Retrieved 12/12/01 from the World Wide Web: http://www.sungwh.freeserve.co.uk/chinese/ch-intro.htm.

Taylor, O. L. 1972. An introduction to the historical development of Black English: Some implications for American education. *Language, Speech, and Hearing Services in Schools 3:* 5–15.

U.S. Bureau of the Census. 1993, September. *We the American foreign-born.* Retrieved August 18, 2001, from the World Wide Web: http://www.census.gov/apsd/wepeople/we-7.pdf.

Williams, R. 1977. Challenge of social dialects. In I. K. Jeter (Ed.), *Social dialects: Differences versus disorders* (pp. 2–10). Rockville, MD: ASHA.

Wolfram, W. 1994. The phonology of a sociocultural variety: The case of African American vernacular English. In J. E. Bernthal and N. W. Bankson (Eds.), *Child phonology: Characteristics, assessment, and intervention with special populations* (pp. 227–44). New York: Thieme.

Wolfram, W., and Schilling-Estes, N. 1998. *American English: Dialects and variation.* Malden, MA: Blackwell Scientific Publications.

Yavas, M. 1998. *Phonology: Development and disorders.* San Diego: Singular.

Yin, S. J. 2001. *Voice range profiles of speakers of native Taiwanese-Mandarin and American-English.* Unpublished master's thesis, University of Wisconsin–Eau Claire.

SUGGESTIONS FOR LISTENING TO THE AUDIO EXAMPLES

The six audio examples that accompany this appendix are intended to demonstrate the varieties of accents that may require your skills in broad or narrow phonetic transcription. They provide you with an opportunity to hear and transcribe accented speech, perhaps as part of a class assignment, on your own, or with other members of the class. For instructors and students interested in transcriptions of these samples we have placed transcripts for both the conversation and the 16 sentences on the *Clinical Phonetics* Web site. As noted on our Web site, there are always valid alternative ways to represent what you hear.

The following four-step transcription guidelines might be useful:

1. Listen to each sample once or twice before attempting transcription. Try to determine what features are attracting your attention. As discussed in the text, which features are associated with possible reductions in intelligibility or comprehensibility?
2. Look at your main characters and diacritics charts (located on the inside front and back covers) and find the combination of symbols that may be used to capture the features that differ. Notice, in particular, how the diacritics are divided into the following eight symbol groups to modify differences you might perceive in: Stress, Nasality, Lip position and gestures, Offglides or stop release, Timing, Juncture, Tongue position and gestures, and/or Sound Source. That's a lot of possibilities! Going back to #1 above, what features really stand out as different?
3. As noted in the body of this appendix and elsewhere in the text, you'll probably find yourself looking for the right symbols to modify perceived differences for vowels and diphthongs—especially the tongue symbols that indicate changes of place, as well as stress symbols to indicate differences in primary, secondary, and tertiary stress. You will need diacritic symbols for consonants too, especially voicing changes within cognates (recall the difficulty with reliable transcription of such changes). In contrast, the frequent deletion and substitution of consonants, as described for some of the audio examples, should be much easier to transcribe reliably!
4. Transcribe some words, phrases, or whole utterances that are representative of the speakers' segmental and suprasegmental differences. It is typically not useful to transcribe an entire conversation sample or responses to all speech tasks. Rather, the goal is to provide representative transcription of those speech differences that may be candidates for accent reduction.

LIST OF AUDIO EXAMPLES ON CLINICAL PHONETICS TAPE 4B: AUDIO EXAMPLES

Regional Dialects: Audio Example #1: A Northern Dialect

Regional Dialects: Audio Example #2: A Midland Dialect

Regional Dialects: Audio Example #3: A Southern Dialect

Social Dialects: Audio Example #4: An AAVE Dialect

Foreign Dialects: Audio Example #5: A Speaker from Panama

Foreign Dialects: Audio Example #6: A Speaker from Taiwan

SENTENCES FOR PHONETIC INVENTORY (ADAPTED FROM FAIRBANKS, 1960)

/i/ 1. Some people reason that seeing is believing.

/ɪ/ 2. Bill saw a big fish swimming in the ripples.

/e͡ɪ/ 3. Late at night the agent made his way to the place where the sailors stayed.

/ɛ/ 4. Special regulations were necessary to help the selling of eggs.

/æ/ 5. Sally banged the black sedan into a taxicab.

/ʌ/ 6. I am unable to understand my Uncle Gus.

/ɑ/ 7. John started across the yard toward the barn.

/ɔ/ 8. Is Shaw the author of "Walking on the Lawn"?

/o͡ʊ/ 9. Don't go home alone in the snow.

/ʊ/ 10. Captain Hook pushed through the bushes to the brook.

/u/ 11. As a rule we go canoeing in the forenoon.

/ju/ 12. Hugh refused to join the musicians' union.

/ɑ͡ʊ/ 13. Fowler wants to plow all the ground around his house.

/ɑ͡ɪ/ 14. The tile workers were fighting for higher prices and more time off.

/ɔɪ/ 15. The boys enjoyed the work that Roy avoided.

/ɝ/ 16. First the girls turned on the furnace, then they burned the dirty curtains.

Appendix G
Infant Vocalizations

Why consider the phonetic transcription of infant vocalizations? A primary reason is that clinicians increasingly find they are involved in providing services to the birth-to-three population. Another reason is that research has shown that (1) babbling and other early vocal behaviors are continuous with (and can predict) later language accomplishments, and (2) characteristics of infant vocalizations can help to identify children who are at risk for communication disorders. Some studies of infant development consider babbling as a form of early language development (Vestergaard et al., 1999). It is increasingly recognized that babbling and other infant vocalizations are not strictly prelinguistic; even in the first year of life, children are making strides in language development.

WHAT IS THE ROLE OF THE IPA?

An immediate and important question is whether infant vocalizations can be satisfactorily transcribed with the symbols of the IPA. If they can, then there is no need for a special discussion geared to the sounds of infants. But a substantial opinion has formed on the opposite view—infant vocalizations are not adequately represented by the symbols of the IPA. One major reason is that infants do not produce only sounds that correspond to those of adult speech. Even when some similarity does occur, it is not certain that the infant sound is phonetically equivalent to the adult sound it resembles. There are several explanations for this. First, infants have a very different configuration of the speech production system (see Appendix H). The newborn infant has a vocal tract that is more like that of a chimpanzee than of an adult human. Second, there is no guarantee that infants produce sounds that have the status of phonemes or even phonetic segments. Presumably, phonemes and phones are established as units only when a phonetic and phonological system has been established. Third, it is not clear how an utterance or vocal unit of some kind should be defined in infant vocalizations such as multisyllabic babble. Utterances generally cannot be defined in terms of words, phrases, or sentences. What, then, is an utterance? We consider this issue next.

UNITS OF OBSERVATION: UTTERANCES AND SYLLABLES

One possibility is to consider the breath group (defined in Chapter 3) as a natural way of putting vocalizations together in an utterance. A logical reason for using breath groups is that all speakers, however old they may be, must interrupt vocalizations for the purpose of respiration. Or, to put it differently, speech is inherently a respiratory activity. Therefore, the respiratory cycle is an unavoidable structure in the organization of speech and speechlike sound patterns. In the task of breath-group marking, the listener tries to identify audible inspirations or pauses that are long enough to contain inspirations. Inspirations, whether audible or inferred, then mark the boundaries between different utterances. With this criterion, some utterances will include a single sound while others may include a string of syllables. Although the task of judging breath groups is not always easy, it appears to have satisfactory reliability (Nathani and Oller, 2001) and may often be the only practical way of identifying an utterance unit.

Typically, once utterances have been delineated, the next step is to determine their syllable composition. Like the breath group, the syllable is a unit that is nearly universal in vocal behaviors. An utterance can be described in terms of the total number of syllables and the number of different syllable shapes it contains. The syllable is an appealing unit of analysis because it is the minimal rhythmic unit of speech (Kent, Mitchell, and Sancier, 1991; Nathani and Oller, 2001) and because it is a unit within which smaller segments (vowel-like and consonant-like elements) can be detected. The syllable, then, is the means to a description of rhythmic patterns and complex organizations that extend across a multisyllabic series even as it permits an examination of intrasyllabic structure.

A TAXONOMY OF INFANT VOCALIZATIONS

It is fair to say that modern opinion is very guarded on the application of the IPA as a singular tool to represent vocal behaviors in infants. Although phonetic transcription with the IPA may have some value (as considered later in this appendix), there is concern that the transcriptions lack validity and reliability. For this reason, different systems have been developed for the representation of infant sounds. Even very young infants are capable of a variety of sounds that can be cataloged in different ways, depending on the purpose of the analysis and the assumptions made by the person doing the analysis. But many investigators have distinguished categories such as vegetative sounds, fixed vocal signals, grunts, and speechlike sounds (also called *protophones* by Oller, 2000). These types of vocalizations can occur with high frequency, and they are useful for an initial categorization of sounds. Each of these categories is defined here as a general introduction to the phonetic analysis of infant vocalizations.

1. *Vegetative sounds* include burps, coughs, and other sounds associated with basic biological processes. However, some sounds are ambiguous in this regard; see the following discussion of grunts, which may be construed as vegetative or communicative, depending on the circumstances of their production.
2. *Fixed vocal signals* include reflexive crying, laughing, and shrieking. These may be associated with particular affective states (e.g., distress, glee, surprise), and they may combine with speechlike vocalizations. Sounds of this kind are often discarded from analyses of vocalizations, but the distinction is not always easy. Particularly troublesome are fussy and whiny vocalizations, which are sometimes regarded as important prelinguistic vocal behaviors (Stark, 1989). It may be wise to classify fussy and whiny vocalizations separately from crying and laughter. Some infants frequently use a fussy or whiny vocal quality in a variety of situations and vocalization types, some of which may appear to have communicative value.
3. *Grunts* are interesting sounds that can be difficult to categorize. Some grunts, such as those accompanying movement or effort, might be placed in the vegetative category. However, grunts can occur with high frequency in some infants, and they may accompany acts of focal attention and may even be used communicatively (Kent and Bauer, 1985; Boliek, Hixon, Watson, and Morgan, 1996; McCune et al., 1996). Some infants will grunt as they point to a desired object, such as a toy or food item. From an acoustic perspective, grunts are produced with periodic vocal fold vibration and a stable vocal tract, and therefore can resemble prototypical human vowel sounds (Owren, Seyfarth, and Cheney, 1997). It is not clear how grunts differ from quasi-resonant nuclei defined later in this section, but it seems appropriate to designate a category for grunts.
4. *Speechlike vocalizations* are sounds that resemble adult speech in some manner, such as syllable structure, prosodic or rhythmic pattern, or phonetic variation. Sometimes these vocalizations are subcategorized. One system is based on protophones (Oller, 2000; Nathani and Oller, 2001). Because protophones are classified "differently on the basis of their resemblance to the characteristics of mature, canonical syllables" (Nathani and Oller, 2001, p. 324), the discussion of these sound categories begins with canonical syllables and then proceeds to the remaining categories. The canonical syllable is a standard against which other vocalization types are compared.
   a. *Canonical syllables* are defined as "mature, adultlike syllables that contain a vowel-like nucleus and consonant-like margin, have rapid formant transitions between the margin and the nucleus, and are produced with normal phonation" (Nathani and Oller, 2001, p. 325). This definition is a combination of perceptual and acoustic terms that is intended to describe a syllable like that occurring in adult speech. Such syllables are produced with a smooth phonation and with relatively rapid movements between consonantal and vocalic elements.
   b. *Marginal syllables* are similar to canonical syllables except that they have slow formant transitions. It is not clear that listeners can really detect slow formant transitions except as they might distinguish glides from stops (e.g., [w] from [b]). A formant transition is an acoustic concept and can be measured satisfactorily only in an acoustic analysis such as a spectrogram (and even then, infant vocalizations can be challenging in acoustic analysis; Kent and Read, 2002). It is probably sufficient to say that the marginal syllable lacks the rapid consonant-to-vowel and vowel-to-consonant articulation that typifies canonical syllables. As a consequence, they do not sound as mature or as accomplished as does the canonical syllable.
   c. *Fully resonant nuclei* possess only vowel-like elements that resemble mature, adult vowels. Typically, these sounds will have at least moderate duration and will have a resonant sound quality similar to vowels produced by adults.
   d. *Quasi-resonant nuclei* are similar to fully resonant nuclei except that the vowel-like elements are produced with a vocal tract that is at rest and therefore do not sound like adult vowels. Presumably, the "rest" position of the vocal tract is a neutral position that is maintained during rest breathing. Possibly, these elements are also nasalized, which alters the resonant quality and may distinguish them from fully resonant nuclei.

The use of these broad categories does not preclude more refined analyses. Even if the IPA is not entirely suitable, there are other transcription systems that offer information on sound patterns. Some possibilities are the following:

- *Vowel articulation* can be described in terms such as high-front, mid-front, low-front, central, high-back, mid-back, and low-back, whether or not phonetic symbols are used to identify individual vowel-like sounds.
- *Consonant articulation* can be described in terms of place of articulation (bilabial, labiodental, interdental, alveolar, palatal, dorsal, uvular, pharyngeal, glottal) and/or manner (stop, fricative, trill, affricate, nasal, lateral, rhotic, glide). The number of different consonants in babble appears to be a useful predictor of later language development (McCune and Vihman, 2001).

STAGE DESCRIPTIONS OF VOCAL DEVELOPMENT

Several different stage models have been proposed for vocal development in infants (Kent and Miolo, 1994). Two of the more influential models are shown in Tables G-1 and G-2. Table G-1 is based largely on vocalization types described earlier in this appendix. Note, for example, that quasi-resonant nuclei are typical of an early phonation stage (birth to 1 month) and that fully resonant nuclei are characteristic of the expansion stage (4 to 6 months). Stage models are useful in that they provide a general description of typical vocalization patterns for certain periods of development. However, it should be kept in mind that large individual differences occur and that stage models should be used with due caution. Some of the stages may be more reliably observed than others. Several studies show that the emergence of canonical babbling (also called repetitive, reduplicated, or multisyllabic babbling) is one of the most reliable milestones in vocal development (Oller, 1978, 2000; Roug, Landberg, and Lundberg, 1978; Koopmans-van Beinum and Van der Stelt, 1986).

PHONETIC ACCOMPLISHMENTS DURING THE FIRST TWO YEARS

Phonetic inventories are simply counts of the different sounds in a child's utterances. Inventories supply information on the types of sounds produced, as well as on the frequencies of occurrence of different types. Developmental indices that can be derived from inventories include inventory size (the total number of elements that occur), type–token ratio (the differences in the frequency of usage of different phonetic elements), and various phonetic ratios (e.g., the ratio of vowels to consonants, the ratio of canonical syllables to total number of syllables; the ratio of voiced to voiceless consonants). Despite the simplicity of phonetic inventories and the hazards of using IPA symbols to represent the sounds in infancy, the results from different studies show a general agreement that can be used to chart the development of speech sounds. The following summary is based on information in Oller (1978, 1995), Mowrer (1980), Locke (1983), Kent and Bauer (1985), Stoel-Gammon (1985), Dyson (1988), Kent and Miolo (1994), Robb and Bliele (1994), and Vihman (1996). Although the results should be used with due caution, they provide an overall perspective on phonetic accomplishments during the first two years of life. This account begins with the period of three to six months. Although phonetic data have been reported for the first three months of life, there are questions about the reliability of transcription and the suitability of IPA phonetic transcription for the vocal tract in early infancy.

Three to Six Months

At about this age, a major change occurs in vocal behavior. Oller (1978) identified the age of four months as the onset of an "expansion stage" that is characterized by an increase in the number and diversity of sounds. As explained in Appendix H, this is a time of major anatomic remodeling of the

TABLE G-1
Stages of Infant Speech Production[a]

Name of Stage	Typical Age	Characteristic Vocalization Types	Metaphonological Characteristics of Mature Language
Phonation	0–1 month	QRN (quasi-resonant nucleus)	Normal phonation in nonreflexive vocalizations
GOO	2–3 months	GOO (QRN plus velar or uvular consonant-like element)	Vocalizations with closure: alternation between opening and closure of the vocal tract
Expansion	4–6 months	FRN (fully resonant nuclei)	Use of resonance capacity for contrasts of resonance types
		RSP (raspberry)	Front as opposed to back (GOO) closures
		SQ (squeal)	Further manipulation of vocalizations during closure
		GRL (growl)	Pitch contrasts
		YEL (yell)	Amplitude contrasts
		IES (ingressive-egressive sequence)	Further control of vocal breath stream
		MB (marginal babble)	Alternation of *full* opening and closure of the vocal tract
Canonical	7–10 months	BB (canonical babbling)	Syllabic timing constraints on relationship of openings and closures (vocalic transitions)
Variegated	11–12 months	VAR (variegated babbling)	Contrasts of consonantal and vocalic types
		GIB (gibberish)	Contrasts of stress

[a]Adapted from Oller, D. K. (1980). The emergence of speech sounds in infancy. In *Child phonology,* eds. G. Yeni-Komashian, J. Kavanaugh, and C. Ferguson. Vol. 1, *Production,* 93–110. New York: Academic Press.

TABLE G-2
Levels of Prespeech Development, Description of Vocalizations, and Age of Anticipated Onset for Typically Developing Infants in an English-Speaking Environment[a]

Level	Onset	Vocalization
1. Reflexive	0–2 mos.	Cry; discomfort sounds; vegetative sounds; quasi- and fully resonant nuclei
2. Control of phonation	2–4 mos.	Nasalized sounds; segments with closants (e.g., trills, friction, raspberries); vocants/fully resonant nucleus; vocants (vowel-like productions); chuckles; sustained laughter
3. Expansion	4–6 mos.	Series of vocants; vowel glides; isolated closants; ingressive sounds; squeals
4. Control of articulation	5–8 mos.	Series of closants; series of closants plus vocants; series of squeals; marginal babbling
5. Babbling	6–12 mos.	Reduplicated babbling (more than two CV syllables in a series); nonreduplicated babbling (babbling with different C's and V's); single CV productions; whispered production of segments
6. Disyllables and vowels	12–18 mos.	Rounded vowels; point vowels; pairs of CV's produced separately; disyllables (CVCV)
7. Prewords and expressive jargon	15 mos.	CVC syllables; diphthongs; jargon; babbling with complex syllables (CCV, CVC, VCV)

[a]Adapted with permission from Stark, R. E. 1993. Early language intervention: When, why, how? *Infants and Young Children 1:* 44–53, with permission of Aspen Publishers, Inc., © 1989.

vocal tract, and the anatomic changes may contribute to an expanded phonetic capability. The vowel sounds that occur most frequently during this period are [ɛ ɪ ʌ] (Mowrer, 1980). The consonants that occur most frequently in the early part of this interval are the glottals [h ʔ] and the velars [g k] (Mowrer, 1980).

Six to Twelve Months

During this period, the vowel-to-consonant (V/C) ratio diminishes compared to its value in the first half-year of life, meaning that the number of consonants, compared to vowels, increases. For example, the V/C drops from 4.5 in the birth-to-two-month period to about 2.0 in the eight-to-twelve-month period (Mowrer, 1980). A relatively small number of sounds accounts for the great majority of phones transcribed in babbling (Kent and Miolo, 1994), and at least in the early part of this period, there is a pronounced similarity in the sounds produced by infants who are raised in different language environments (Locke, 1983, 1993). In other words, phonetic differences among languages are not reflected in the phonetic patterns of babbling, perhaps indicating that universal factors, such as biology, account for sound selections in babbling. The vowels that are most likely to occur in babbling during the second half-year of life are central, mid-front, and low-front. The consonants that are most likely to occur are voiced stops (primarily bilabial and apical), nasals (typically bilabial and apical), fricative [h], and glide [w]. One of the major differences between consonants produced in the first half-year and those produced in the second half-year is that glottals and velars predominate in the former, whereas alveolars and labials predominate in the latter (Mowrer, 1980; Smith and Oller, 1981).

12 to 18 Months

Inventory size does not appear to increase markedly from about 8 months to 18 months (Robb and Bliele, 1994). The average inventory of consonants is about six, selected especially from the set [b d g t m n h w l]. About two to three times as many consonants are used in syllable-initial position (five to ten in Robb and Bliele, 1994) than in syllable-final position (two to four in Robb and Bliele, 1994). Consonants in syllable-initial position tend to be voiced stops, the nasals [m] or [n], and the fricative [h]. Consonants likely to appear in syllable-final position are [t m h s].

18 to 25 Months

Inventory size increases at about 18 to 22 months. A typical two-year-old has an inventory of about 10 to 20 consonant phones. Consonants that are likely to be added during this period are from the set [p t k f s z ʃ ʤ j]. The inventory of syllable-initial consonants grows more rapidly than that for syllable-final consonants. Consonants in syllable-final position are more likely to be voiceless, whereas consonants in syllable-initial position are more likely to be voiced.

REFERENCES

Boliek, C. A., Hixon, T. J., Watson, P. J., and Morgan, W. J. 1996. Vocalization and breathing during the first year of life. *Journal of Voice 10:* 1–22.

Dyson, A. T. 1988. Phonetic inventories of 2- and 3-year-old children. *Journal of Speech and Hearing Disorders 53:* 89–93.

Kent, R. D., and Bauer, H. R. 1985. Vocalizations of one-year-olds. *Journal of Child Language 12*: 491–526.

Kent, R. D., and Miolo, G. 1994. Phonetic abilities in the first year of life. In P. Fletcher and B. MacWhinney (Eds.), *Handbook of child language* (pp. 303–34). Oxford, England: Basil Blackwell.

Kent, R. D., Mitchell, P. R., and Sancier, M. 1991. Evidence and role of rhythmic organization in early vocal development in human infants. In J. Fagard and P. Wolff (Eds.), *The development of timing control and temporal organization in coordinated action.* Amsterdam: Elsevier.

Kent, R. D., and Read, W. C. 2002. *The acoustic analysis of speech.* Albany, NY: Singular/Thomson Learning.

Koopmans-van Beinum, F. J., and Van der Stelt, J. M. 1986. Early stages in the development of speech movements. In B. Lindblom and R. Zetterstrom (Eds.), *Precursors of early speech* (pp. 37–50). Basingstoke, England: Macmillan Press.

Locke, J. L. 1983. *Phonological acquisition and change.* New York: Academic Press.

Locke, J. L. 1993. *The child's path to spoken language.* Cambridge, MA: Harvard University Press.

McCune, L., and Vihman, M. M. 2001. Early phonetic and lexical development: A productivity approach. *Journal of Speech, Language, and Hearing Research 44:* 670–84.

McCune, L., Vihman, M. M., Roug-Hellichius, L., Delery, C. B., and Gogate, L. 1996. Grunt communication in human infants (Homo sapiens). *Journal of Comparative Psychology 110:* 27–36.

Mowrer, D. E. 1980. Phonological development during the first year of life. In N. J. Lass (Ed.), *Speech and language: Advances in basic research and practice* (Vol. 4, pp. 99–137). New York: Academic Press.

Nathani, S., and Oller, D. K. 2001. Beyond ba-ba and gu-gu: Challenges and strategies in coding infant vocalizations. *Behavior Research Methods, Instruments, and Computers 33:* 321–30.

Oller, D. K. 1978. The emergence of the sounds of speech in infancy. *Allied Health and Behavioral Sciences 1:* 523–49.

Oller, D. K. 1995. Development of vocalizations in infancy. In H. Winitiz (Ed.), *Human communication and its disorders. A review* (Vol. IV, pp. 1–30). Timonium, MD: York Press.

Oller, D. K. 2000. *The emergence of the speech capacity.* Mahwah, NJ: Lawrence Erlbaum Associates.

Owren, M. J., Seyfarth, R. M., and Cheney, D. L. 1997. The acoustic features of vowel-like grunt calls in chacma baboons (*Papio cyncephalus ursinus*): Implications for production processes and functions. *Journal of the Acoustical Society of America 101:* 2951–63.

Robb, M. P., and Bleile, K. M. 1994. Consonant inventories of young children from 8 to 25 months. *Clinical Linguistics and Phonetics 8:* 295–320.

Roug, L., Landberg, I., and Lundberg, L.-J. 1989. Phonetic development in early infancy: A study of four Swedish children during the first eighteen months of life. *Journal of Child Language 16:* 19–40.

Smith, B. L., and Oller, D. K. 1981. A comparative study of premeaningful vocalizations produced by normally developing and Down syndrome infants. *Journal of Speech and Hearing Disorders 46:* 46–51.

Stark, R. E. 1989. Temporal patterning of cry and non-cry sounds in the first eight months of life. *First Language 9:* 107–36.

Stoel-Gammon, C. 1985. Phonetic inventories, 15–25 months: A longitudinal study. *Journal of Speech and Hearing Research 28:* 505–12.

Vestergaard, M., Obel, C., Henriksen, T. B., Sorensen, H. T., Skajaa, E., and Ostergaard, J. 1999. Duration of breastfeeding and developmental milestones during the latter half of infancy. *Acta Paediatrica 88:* 1327–32.

Vihman, M. M. 1996. *Phonological development: The origins of language in the child.* Cambridge, MA: Basil Blackwell.

Appendix H

Anatomic Bases of Developmental Phonetics

Why should a book on clinical phonetics be concerned with how the speech production system develops? The primary reason is that children's phonetic abilities relate in part to developmental issues, including the growth and maturation of the speech production system. The importance of this topic was mentioned in Appendix G, which cautioned about the uncritical use of the IPA in transcribing infant vocalizations. It is clear that infants have very different vocal tracts compared to adults, and these differences place limitations on the use of phonetic systems tailored to adult speech. Developmental phonetics refers to the acquisition of phonetic ability in children. This ability is acquired over a considerable span of childhood. In fact, changes in some aspects of speech production are evident even until young adulthood. Although it is usually assumed that a child has mastered all phonemes of the language by about eight years of age, speech production is refined at least until the age of puberty. This refinement includes increased precision and reliability of speech patterns. In addition, the child must adjust for continuous changes in the physical structures of speech production. These changes include increased size of individual structures, alterations in the shape of structures, changes in the relationship between different structures, and development of various tissues that comprise the speech production system. A primary point is that the child is not simply a small version of the adult.

The intent behind the information that follows is to provide a general background for the normal or typical development of speech production. Because speech depends on the growth and maturation of a biological system, it is important to understand how the developmental biology of speech relates to major advances in speech production. The information presented in Chapters 3, 4, and 5 is based largely on the adult system of speech production. Although this information carries over substantially to the speech production system of children, there are some developmental differences that should be taken into account when considering the phonetic capabilities of children. The following outlines highlight major developmental changes in the biological system of speech. These are keyed to overall patterns of phonetic development, to provide a perspective on how a child's phonetic accomplishments relate to maturation of the speech production system. The information that follows also is important in considering how craniofacial anomalies may affect the development of speech.

Note: The information presented here reflects a statistical average and should not be used to chart the growth and development of an individual child. Nonetheless, it is helpful to understand how the complex system of speech production reaches its mature form. For more detailed information, see papers cited in the references.

DEVELOPMENTAL BACKGROUND FOR SPEECH PRODUCTION IN CHILDREN

Major Developmental Milestones in the Respiratory System

The respiratory system is the source of energy for most speech sounds. The sounds of the English language are almost entirely produced on exhaled air, which is used to (1) set the vocal folds into vibration so that periodic energy is produced, and (2) create air pressures for stops, fricatives, and affricates so that aperiodic energy is generated. The respiratory system changes remarkably from infancy to adulthood; some of the major changes are summarized in the following. A major point to be noted is that respiratory capacity and coordination are developed during childhood.

- **Newborn.** The diaphragm of the newborn has bellowslike displacement, unlike the pistonlike effect in adults. Therefore, the newborn has a very different mechanical system for respiration. There is a gradual shift toward the mechanical pattern of adulthood.

  Rest breathing rate is 30 to 80 breaths/minute (compared to the 15 to 20 breaths/minute that is typical for adults).
- **Two months.** Development of the alveoli begins; until this time, the baby has virtually no small air sacs within the lungs. These sacs are important for effective gas exchange in respiration.
- **Three years.** Respiratory function is not closely geared to linguistic requirements until about this age, meaning that the child does not coordinate respiratory actions with the linguistic structure of an utterance until about 3 years of age.

  On average, a three-year-old child can prolong a vowel sound for no more than 10 seconds, compared to 20 or 30 seconds for adults. This difference is related partly to respiratory capacity and partly to differences in the efficiency of phonation.

Rest breathing rate is 20 to 30 breaths/minute.

Note: Functional maturation is especially evident during the period of three to seven years.

- **Four years.** The expiratory work in speech breathing is greater than for adults. To produce the same sound intensity, children's respiratory systems have to work harder, for example, by generating higher levels of subglottal air pressure to produce a comparably intense sound.
- **Seven years.** Lung architecture is essentially remodeled to adult pattern.

  By this age, there is an essential convergence on adult-like patterns of respiratory function.

  Children continue to use greater subglottal air pressures than adults for speaking, but the expiratory work in speech breathing is much reduced compared to four-year-olds.
- **Eight years.** The number of alveoli reaches the adult value of about 300,000.
- **Ten years.** There is refinement of respiratory patterns; functional maturation is achieved.

  Rest breathing rate is 17 to 22 breaths/minute.
- **Twelve to eighteen years.** Increase in lung capacity, especially in boys. Fifteen years is sometimes taken as the age of growth completion.

Major Developmental Milestones in the Laryngeal System

The larynx serves as a valve and as a source of vibration. The valving function is especially notable when we close the folds tightly for purposes such as lifting a heavy object or when we set the folds into vibration to produce the laryngeal tone. Because newborns typically cry within seconds of birth, we might think that the larynx has little to do between birth and adulthood, aside from becoming larger. In fact, the larynx changes in many ways that have only recently been described. Some developmental changes in the vocal tract and larynx are illustrated in Figures H-1 (newborn), H-2 (child of about four years of age), and H-3 (adult).

- **Newborn.** Laryngeal position is high in the neck, so that the laryngopharynx is relatively short. Vocal folds are 5 to 7 mm long (compare Figures H-1 and H-3.)

  Entire lamina propria is uniform (i.e., there is no lamination corresponding to adult histology). The lamina propria is the layered structure of the adult vocal folds, which is central to contemporary theories of vocal fold vibration. About one-half of the infant glottal length is cartilaginous, compared to about one-third in adults (compare Figures H-1 and H-3).

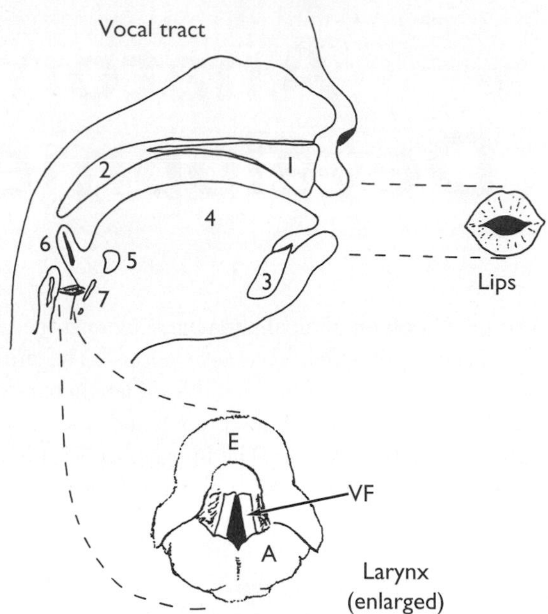

FIGURE H-1
Vocal tract (lateral view), lips (frontal view), and larynx (superior view) of a newborn. The numbers identify structures as follows: 1—hard palate; 2—soft palate (velum); 3—jaw (mandible); 4—tongue; 5—hyoid bone; 6—epiglottis; and 7—larynx (cartilages and vocal folds). The enlarged view of the larynx shows: E—epiglottis; VF—vocal folds; and A—arytenoid cartilage, to which the vocal folds attach. From *Journal of Medical Speech–Language Pathology.* © 1995. Reprinted with permission of Delmar, a division of Thomson Learning. Fax 800 730-2215.

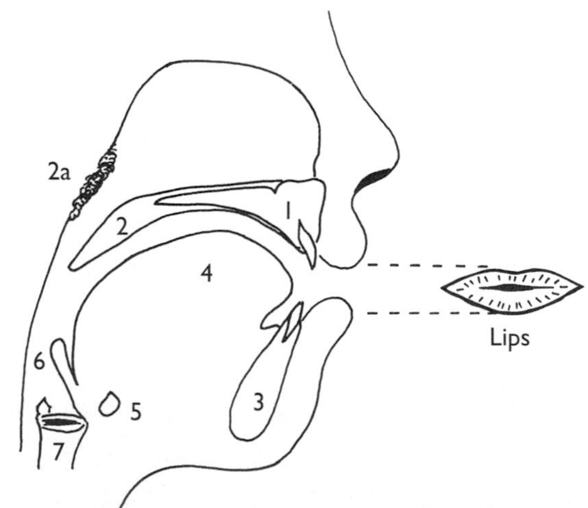

FIGURE H-2
Vocal tract (lateral view) and lips (frontal view) of a four-year-old child. The numbers identify structures as follows: 1—hard palate; 2—soft palate (velum); 2a—nasopharyngeal tonsil (adenoid); 3—jaw (mandible); 4—tongue; 5—hyoid bone; 6—epiglottis; and 7—larynx (cartilages and vocal folds). From *Journal of Medical Speech–Language Pathology.* © 1995. Reprinted with permission of Delmar, a division of Thomson Learning. Fax 800 730-2215.

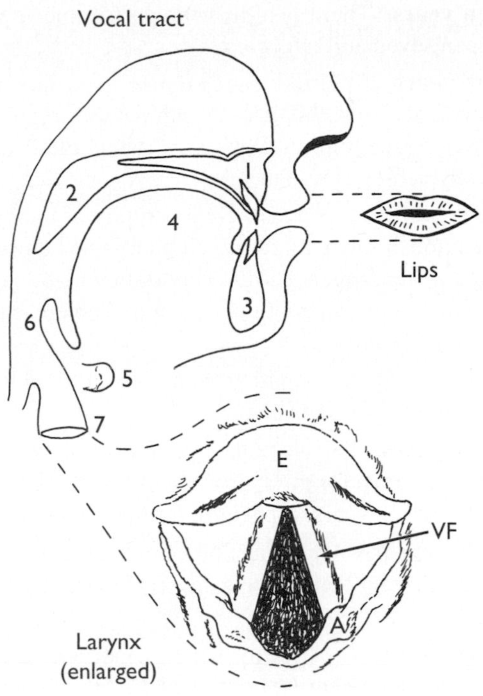

FIGURE H-3
Vocal tract (lateral view), lips (frontal view), and larynx (superior view) of an adult male. The numbers identify structures as follows: 1—hard palate; 2—soft palate (velum); 3—jaw (mandible); 4—tongue; 5—hyoid bone; 6—epiglottis; and 7—larynx (cartilages and vocal folds). The enlarged view of the larynx shows: E—epiglottis; VF—vocal folds; and A—arytenoid cartilage, to which the vocal folds attach. From *Journal of Medical Speech–Language Pathology.* © 1995. Reprinted with permission of Delmar, a division of Thomson Learning. Fax 800 730-2215.

- **Four years.** Vocal ligament appears between one and four years. This is a major development in the lamination of the vocal folds.
- **Six years.** Vocal fold length is about 8 mm in both sexes. The two layers of the vocal ligament become differentiated between six and fifteen years.
- **Eight years.** Sex differences begin to emerge in laryngeal tissues.
- **Twelve years.** Differentiation of lamina propria is now nearly complete, so that the layers of the vocal folds have an adultlike appearance.

  Adolescent voice change begins in males between 12.5 and 14.5 years.

  Length of vocal folds is 12 to 17 mm in pubescent girls and about 15 to 25 mm in pubescent boys.
- **Sixteen years.** Adult morphology of vocal folds is achieved.
- **Adult.** Vocal length is about 21 mm in women and about 29 mm in men.

Major Developmental Milestones in the Upper Airway (Vocal Tract) Subsystem of Speech Production

The upper airway is a complex system that has complex patterns of growth and development. It is not far from the truth to say that we are born with a vocal tract that resembles that of the nonhuman primates, such as the chimpanzee. The vocal tract is remodeled during the first few months and years of life so that it takes on the distinctive form of the human vocal tract. But even after the essential form is attained, the structures of this system continue to grow and develop. The following summary outlines the major changes that occur between birth and adulthood.

- **Birth.** The newborn has a vocal tract anatomy that resembles that of a nonhuman primate.

  With the descent of the larynx between one and four months, there is a disengagement of the soft palate and epiglottis (Figure H-1).

  The oral structures are adapted to sucking. The tongue can move pistonlike within the mouth, and the circular lips can seal effectively against a nipple. These features are apparent in Figure H-1.

- **Four months.** At about this age, the larynx has descended in the neck, and the infant's vocal tract more closely resembles that of the human adult. This corresponds to what some have called the "expansion stage" in phonetic development. Anatomic changes may contribute to this stage of increased phonetic ability.

- **Six months.** Primary dentition first emerges at about six months and continues until about twenty-four months. Usually, the mandibular central incisors are the first to erupt; these are closely followed by the maxillary central incisors.

  The dental arcade establishes boundaries and points of contact for lingual articulation. The lingua-dental and labio-dental sounds require frontal incisors for their production.

  Canonical babbling typically begins at about seven to nine months. The consonant sounds that are most likely to occur are voiced bilabial and apical stops, bilabial and apical nasals, the fricative [h], and the glide [w]. Vowels tend to be selected from the central, mid-front, and low-front regions of the vowel quadrilateral.

- **One year.** One year is the approximate age of first words, which usually have the same sounds and syllable shapes used in earlier babbling. By the age of eighteen months, most children have an inventory of about six consonants selected from the set [b d g t m n h w l]. First primary molars achieve occlusal contact at about sixteen months; this occlusal event marks the appearance of a stable jaw closing pattern, so that the jaw returns to about the same closing position. This may help to stabilize the articulatory patterns for speech.

The lateral incisors and first molars erupt at about this time. The lateral incisors erupt between seven and twenty months and the first molars between ten and sixteen months.

- **Two years.** The lips grow rapidly between one and two years.

  The second molars erupt between twenty and twenty-four months.

  By the age of two years, most children have an inventory of 10 to 20 consonant phones. Sounds that are typically added during the second year are selected from the set [p t k f s z ʃ ʤ j].
- **Three years.** The laryngopharynx is now well developed.
- **Four years.** Hypertrophy (enlargement) of nasopharyngeal tonsil (adenoid) commonly occurs at about this time (labeled 2a in Figure H-2). This can cause a constriction in the velopharyngeal port and a change in oral-nasal resonance. Some children may sound denasalized.

  The vocal tract essentially assumes adultlike geometry (Figure H-2).

  The vowel system is usually mastered except for rhotics; this accomplishment may result in part from the stability of tongue–jaw coordination and refined control of tongue body.
- **Six years.** The skull attains nearly adult size; the facial skeleton is still immature in size and shape. *Note:* The difference in growth rate between the skull and the facial bones means that most of the speech structures have substantial increases in size even after the skull has nearly stopped growing.

  Emergence of permanent (secondary) dentition occurs at about the age of six. The shedding of primary dentition may result in temporary changes in articulation, especially for lingua-dental and lingua-alveolar fricatives.
- **Seven years.** There is a growth spurt in the lower face between seven and ten years.
- **Eight years.** Adultlike precision of jaw movement is achieved at about this age. A comparable regulation of lips and tongue follows. Phonetic mastery of all sounds is typically achieved by this age.
- **Nine years.** At this age, there is atrophy of the nasopharyngeal tonsil; the pattern of velopharyngeal closure may change in consequence. Some children who do not adapt to this anatomic change may have a problem balancing oral/nasal resonance.
- **Ten years.** There is rapid growth in tongue and lips from about nine to thirteen years.
- **Twelve years.** Twelve is the age of essential maturation of the vocal tract for girls; growth continues for boys until about eighteen years, especially for lips, jaw, and tongue.
- **Fourteen years.** By the age of fourteen, there is eruption of all permanent dentition except wisdom teeth (third molars).
- **Sixteen years.** By sixteen, adult proportions are essentially developed; there is continued growth of some structures in boys.

SELECTED BIBLIOGRAPHY

Kent, R. D. 1999. Motor control: Neurophysiology and functional development. In A. J. Caruso and E. A. Strand (Eds.), *Clinical management of motor speech disorders in children.* New York: Thieme Medical and Scientific Publishers.

Kent, R. D., and Vorperian, H. K. 1995. Anatomic development of the craniofacial-oral-laryngeal systems: A review. *Journal of Medical Speech-Language Pathology 3:* 145–90.

Vorperian, H. K., Kent, R. D., Gentry, L. R., and Yandell, B. 1999. Magnetic resonance imaging procedures to study the concurrent anatomic development of vocal tract structures: Preliminary results. *International Journal of Pediatric Otorhinolaryngology 49:* 197–206.

Answers to Exercises

Chapter 1: Overview of Clinical Phonetics

Linguistic Complexity	System Complexity	Response Complexity
1. word	two-way scoring	single sound
2. continuous speech	two-way scoring	multiple sounds
3. sentences	five-way scoring	single sound
4. continuous speech	phonetic transcription	multiple sounds
5. word	five-way scoring	multiple sounds

Chapter 2: Linguistic Phonetics

1.

	Number of Morphemes	Morphemic Analysis
(a)	3	light + en +ed
(b)	1	table
(c)	3	morph + em(e) + ic
(d)	3	re + cruit + ment
(e)	3	dis + mis + (s)ed
(f)	3	tele + vis(e) + ion
(g)	1	finger
(h)	3	sing + er + s
(i)	3	re + veal + ing
(j)	4	im + pos(e) + it + ion

2. Some possibilities are:

expose	oppose	repose	dispose
exposition	appose	pose	purpose
impose	compose	suppose	propose
imposition	depose	Can you think of any others?	

3.

	Number of Phonemes	Phonetic Transcription
(a)	4	/d ɔ t ɚ /
(b)	5	/l æ f t ɚ /
(c)	3	/f o͡ʊ n /
(d)	5	/k ʌ b ɚ d /
(e)	7	/s ɛ l o f e͡ɪ n /
(f)	3	/n i d /
(g)	6	/ʃ ɪ k ɔ g o /
(h)	5	/f ɪ ŋ g ɚ /
(i)	4	/s ɪ ŋ ɚ /
(j)	4	/s ɪ k s /

4. Real Words:
   - (b) grith (security, protection, or peace)
   - (d) scute (a bony plate)
   - (e) trave (a cross beam)
   - (g) skeg (naut., after part of keel)
   - (k) spile (a plug or spigot)
   - (l) knar (a knot in wood)

   Note that the made-up words contain the following sequences: *fs, sr, kt, dl, shl, gv.* Can you think of any English words that start with these sound sequences?

Chapter 3: The Three Systems of Speech Production

1. See Figure 3-7 and Figure 3-13.
2. See text.
3. (a) p—lips
   (b) g—dorsum of tongue; s—tip of tongue
   (c) f—lower lip; m—lips
   (d) l—tip of tongue; k—dorsum of tongue
   (e) th—tip of tongue; ng—dorsum of tongue
   (f) ch—blade of tongue; s—tip of tongue
   (g) c—tip of tongue; ph—lower lip
   (h) b—lips; th—tip of tongue
4. Although the tongue is (v)ery i(m)(p)ortant in speech articulation, there are several re(p)orts of (p)ersons who produce intelligible speech e(v)en a(f)ter (m)ost of the tongue has (b)een surgically remo(v)ed (often because of cancer). Indi(v)iduals so(m)etimes co(m)(p)ensate surprisingly well for da(m)age to the articulators.

Chapter 4: Vowels and Diphthongs

1. See text, especially Figure 4-3.
2. (a) /u/, high-back
   (b) /ɔ/, low-mid-back
   (c) /ɛ/, low-mid-front
   (d) /ʊ/, high-mid-back
   (e) /i/, high-front
   (f) /ɑ/, low-back
   (g) /ʊ/, high-mid-back
   (h) /i/, high-front
   (i) /ɪ/, high-mid-front
   (j) /æ/, low-front
   (k) /ʊ/, high-mid-back
   (l) /o/, mid-back
   (m) /ɝ/, central
   (n) /ɪ/, high-mid-front
3. (a) /i/—/æ/: tongue moves down, mouth opening increases
   (b) /u/—/o/: tongue moves down, mouth opening increases
   (c) /i/—/o/: tongue moves back and down, lips round for /o/
   (d) /e͡ɪ/—/ɑ/: tongue moves back and down, mouth opening increases
   (e) /o/—/ɝ/: tongue moves forward
   (f) /i/—/æ/: tongue moves down, mouth opening increases
   (g) /u/—/ɑ/: tongue moves down, mouth opening increases, and lips go from rounded to unrounded
   (h) o—/ɛ/: tongue moves forward, lips go from rounded to unrounded
   (i) /e͡ɪ/—/ɑ/: tongue moves back and down, mouth opening increases
   (j) /o͡ʊ/—/i/: tongue moves forward and up, lips go from rounded to unrounded, and mouth opening may decrease
   (k) /i/—/ɪ/: tongue moves down, mouth opening may increase
   (l) o—/ɑ/: tongue moves down, lips go from rounded to unrounded
4. Vowels are early sounds to appear in a child's speech. Front vowels tend to predominate in an infant's early vowel usage. It has been suggested that an infant could produce a set of front vowels by holding the tongue near the front of the mouth and varying the amount of jaw opening. A closed jaw position would yield /i/ and an open jaw position would yield /æ/. (Note: The article a may be produced as either a front vowel [e] ([e͡ɪ]) or a central vowel [ə].)

4. (a) [t r $\overset{2}{\text{æ}}$ n s k r $\overset{1}{\overline{\text{ɑɪ}}}$ b]
   (b) [s $\overset{1}{\text{æ}}$ ɾ $\overset{3}{\text{ɪ}}$ s f $\overset{2}{\overline{\text{ɑɪ}}}$] (or 2-3-1 stress)
   (c) [l $\overset{1}{\text{ɛ}}$ ʤ $\overset{2}{\text{ɪ}}$ s l $\overset{2}{\overline{\text{eɪ}}}$ ʧ $\overset{3}{\text{ɚ}}$]
   (d) [f $\overset{1}{\text{ɝ}}$ n $\overset{3}{\text{ɪ}}$ ʧ $\overset{3}{\text{ɚ}}$]
   (e) [$\overset{2}{\text{ɛ}}$ r $\overset{3}{\text{ɪ}}$ z $\overset{1}{\overline{\text{oʊ}}}$ n $\overset{3}{\text{ə}}$] (sometimes 1-3-2-3)
   (f) [ʃ $\overset{3}{\text{ɪ}}$ k $\overset{1}{\text{ɔ}}$ g $\overset{2}{\text{o}}$]
   (g) [$\overset{1}{\overline{\text{oʊ}}}$ v $\overset{3}{\text{ɚ}}$ l $\overset{2}{\overline{\text{oʊ}}}$ d] (or 2-3-1)
   (h) [s k $\overset{1}{\overline{\text{ɑɪ}}}$ s k r $\overset{2}{\overline{\text{eɪ}}}$ p $\overset{3}{\text{ɚ}}$]
   (i) [t $\overset{1}{\overline{\text{aɪ}}}$ p r $\overset{2}{\overline{\text{ɑɪ}}}$ ɾ $\overset{3}{\text{ɚ}}$]
   (j) [l $\overset{2}{\text{ɪ}}$ θ $\overset{2}{\text{u}}$ $\overset{1}{\overline{\text{eɪ}}}$ n $\overset{3}{\text{ɪ}}$ $\overset{3}{\text{ə}}$]
   (k) [m $\overset{1}{\text{æ}}$ s t $\overset{3}{\text{ɚ}}$ p $\overset{2}{\text{i}}$ s] (sometimes 2-3-1)
   (l) [m $\overset{2}{\text{ɪ}}$ s $\overset{3}{\text{ɪ}}$ s $\overset{1}{\text{ɪ}}$ p $\overset{3}{\text{ɪ}}$]
5. (a) [e] has schwa [ə] offglide; checked or held terminal juncture
   (b) [$\overline{\text{ɑɪ}}$] is nasalized; rising terminal juncture
   (c) [ɛ] is produced with breathy voice; [o] is nasalized
   (d) [l] is devoiced; [i] is lengthened; checked or held juncture
   (e) numbers represent stress pattern: 1 = highest stress, 2 = less stress, 3 = least stress
   (f) [ʊ] is lowered, [ɔ] is nasalized; [ɪ] is centralized and nasalized
   (g) [$\overline{\text{oʊ}}$] is lengthened, [æ] has an [ɪ] offglide; [t] is unreleased

Chapter 10: Acoustic Phonetics

1. Assuming that the velocity of sound, *c*, is 34,000 cm/s, the quarter-length relationship $F_n = c/4$ yields a vocal tract length of 28.33 cm.
2. The fundamental period, T_0, is simply the reciprocal of the frequency value. The answers are (a) 0.002 s, or 2 ms; (b) 0.001 s, or 1 ms; and (c) 0.0002 s, or 0.2 ms.
3. The scale in (c) is not logarithmic.
4. About 20% higher, or 2400 Hz.
5. Order of increasing VOT: boat, goat, glue, par, car.
6. The circled sounds should be
   (a) s t t z ([z] is aperiodic in the sense that it has noise energy; it is periodic in the sense that it is voiced.)
   (b) θ p p
   (c) p ʃ k s t ʃ

Appendix D: Procedures to Calculate Transcription Reliability and Research Findings

1. This is not a good way for the clinician to assess her intrajudge reliability. Her score sheets are based on the child's responses on two different occasions; the child's speech may have changed between the two sampling periods.
2. This is not the best way of assessing interjudge reliability, particularly for fricatives. However, this comparison might yield a useful estimate of reliability. Any observed differences in scoring could be due to differences in the listening conditions, that is, live versus recording.
3. 88 percent
4. 73 percent (22 agreements out of 30 comparisons = 73.3 percent)
5. 84 percent (56 agreements out of 67 comparisons = 83.6 percent)

References

(see also Appendixes)

Adams, S. G. 1990. Rate and clarity of speech: An X-ray microbeam study. Ph.D. dissertation, University of Wisconsin, Madison.

Adams, S. G., Weismer, G., and Kent, R. D. 1993. Speaking rate and speech movement velocity profiles. *Journal of Speech and Hearing Research 36:* 41–54.

Armstrong, L., and Ward, I. 1926. *Handbook of English intonation.* Leipzig.

Baltaxe, C., Simmons, J., and Zee, E. 1984. Intonation patterns in normal, autistic and aphasic children. In *Proceedings of the Tenth International Congress of Phonetic Sciences,* Eds. Van den Broecke and Cohen, 713–18.

Beckman, M. E. 1986. *Stress and non-stress accent. Netherlands phonetic archives 7.* Dordrecht: Foris.

Beckman, M. E., and Edwards, J. 1990. Lengthenings and shortenings and the nature of prosodic constituency. In J. Kingston and M. E. Beckman (Eds.), *Between the grammar and physics of speech* (pp. 152–214). Cambridge, England: Cambridge University Press.

Beckman, M. E., and Edwards, J. 1991. Prosodic categories and duration control. *Journal of the Acoustical Society of America 87,* Suppl. 1: S65.

Behne, D. 1989. Acoustic effects of focus and sentence position on stress in English and French. Ph.D. dissertation, University of Wisconsin, Madison.

Benguerel, A.-P., and Cowan, H. 1974. Coarticulation of upper lip protrusion in French. *Phonetica 30:* 41–55.

Bernthal, J. E., and Bankson, N. W. 1993. *Articulation and phonological disorders.* 3rd ed. Englewood Cliffs, N.J.: Prentice-Hall.

Bloch, B., and Trager, G. 1942. *Outline of linguistic analysis.* Baltimore, MD: Waverly Press.

Bloomfield, L. [1933] 1984. *Language.* New York: Holt, Rinehart & Winston. Reprint. Chicago: University of Chicago Press.

Bonnot, J.-F. P., and Chevrie-Muller, C. 1991. Some effects of shouted and whispered conditions on temporal organization. *Journal of Phonetics, 19:* 473–83.

Boyce, S., and Espy-Wilson, C. Y. 1997. Coarticulatory stability in American English /r/. *Journal of the Acoustical Society of America 101:* 3741–53.

Bradlow, A. R. (1995). A comparative acoustic study of English and Spanish vowels. *Journal of the Acoustical Society of America, 97:* 1916–24.

Brewster, K. 1989. Assessment of prosody. In *Linguistics in clinical practice,* Ed. K. Grundy, 168–85. London: Taylor and Francis.

Bronstein, A. 1960. *The pronunciation of American English.* New York: Appleton-Century-Crofts.

Byrd, D. 1996. Influences on articulatory timing in consonant sequences. *Journal of Phonetics, 24:* 209–44.

Byrd, D., and Saltzman, E. 1998. Intragestural dynamics of multiple prosodic boundaries. *Journal of Phonetics, 26:* 173–99.

Calvert, D. 1980. *Descriptive phonetics.* New York: Thieme-Stratton.

Campbell, T. F., and Dollaghan, C. A. 1995. Phonological and speech production characteristics of children following traumatic brain injury: Principles underlying assessment and treatment. In *Phonological characteristics of special populations,* Ed. J. Bernthal and W. Bankson, New York: Thieme Medical Publishers.

Carroll, J. 1958. The assessment of phoneme cluster frequencies. *Language 34:* 267–78.

Carterette, E., and Jones, M. 1974. *Informal speech: Alphabetic and phonemic texts with statistical analyses and tables.* Berkeley: University of California Press.

Catford, J. 1968. The articulatory possibilities of man. In *Manual of Phonetics,* Ed. B. Malmberg. Amsterdam: North-Holland.

Catford, J. 1977. *Fundamental problems in phonetics.* Bloomington: Indiana University Press.

Chaney, C. 1988. Acoustic analysis of correct and misarticulated semivowels. *Journal of Speech and Hearing Research 31:* 275–87.

Chen, M. 1970. Vowel length variation as a function of the variety of the consonant environment. *Phonetica 22:* 129–59.

Chomsky, N., and Halle, M. 1968. *The sound pattern of English.* New York: Harper & Row.

Christman, S. S. 1992. Abstruse neologism formation: Parallel processing revisited. *Clinical Linguistics and Phonetics 6:* 65–76.

Clements, G. N. 1990. The role of the sonority cycle in core syllabification. In *Papers in laboratory phonology 1: Between the grammar and the physics of speech,* Eds. J. Kingston and M. Beckman. Cambridge, England: Cambridge University Press.

Cohen, A., Coller, R., and t'Hart, J. 1982. Declination: Construct or intrinsic feature of speech pitch? *Phonetica 39:* 254–73.

Costely, M., and Broen, P. 1976, November. The nature of listener disagreement in judging misarticulated speech. Paper presented at the American Speech and Hearing Association National Convention, Houston.

Crystal, D. 1982. *Profiling linguistic disability.* London: Whurr Publishers.

Cutler, A. 1992. The production and perception of word boundaries. In *Speech perception, production and linguistic structure,* Eds. Y. Tohkura, E. Vatikiotis-Bateson, and Y. Sagisaka, 419–25. Amsterdam: IOS Press.

Dalbor, J. 1980. *Spanish pronunciation: Theory and practice.* New York: Holt, Rinehart, & Winston.

Dalby, J. M. 1984. Phonetic structure of fast speech in American English. Unpublished doctoral dissertation, Indiana University.

Daniloff, R., and Moll, K. 1968. Coarticulation of lip rounding. *Journal of Speech and Hearing Research 11:* 707–21.

De Boysson-Bardies, B., Sagart, L., and Durand, C. 1984. Discernible differences in the babbling of infants to target language. *Journal of Child Language 16:* 1–17.

De Jong, K. J. 1991. The oral articulation of English stress accent. Doctoral dissertation, Ohio State University.

Delattre, P., and Freeman, D. 1968. A dialect study of American *r*'s by X-ray motion picture. *Linguistics 44:* 29–68.

Denes, P. 1955. The effect of duration on the perception of voicing. *Journal of the Acoustical Society of America 27:* 761–64.

Denes, P., and Pinson, E. 1973; 1963. *The speech chain.* Garden City, New York: Anchor Press (1973) and Bell Telephone Laboratories, Inc. (1963).

De Pijper, J. R., and Sanderman, A. A. 1994. On the perceptual strength of prosodic boundaries and its relation to suprasegmental cues. *Journal of the Acoustical Society of America, 96:* 2037–47.

Dewey, G. 1923. *Relative frequency of English speech sounds.* Cambridge, MA: Harvard University Press.

Diedrich, W., and Bangert, J. 1981. *Articulation learning.* Houston: College-Hill Press.

Dilley, L., Shattuck-Hufnagel, S., and Ostendorf, M. 1996. Glottalization of word-initial vowels as a function of prosodic structure. *Journal of Phonetics, 24:* 423–44.

DuBois, E., and Bernthal, J. 1978. A comparison of three methods for obtaining articulatory responses. *Journal of Speech and Hearing Disorders 43:* 295–305.

Duckworth, M., Allen, G., Hardcastle, W., and Ball, M. 1990. Extensions to the International Phonetic Alphabet for the transcription of atypical speech. *Clinical Linguistics and Phonetics 4:* 273–80.

Edwards, J., and Beckman, M. E. 1988. Articulatory timing and the prosodic interpretation of syllable duration. *Phonetica 45:* 156–74.

Faircloth, S., and Faircloth, M. 1973. *Phonetic science.* Englewood Cliffs, NJ: Prentice-Hall.

Fernald, A., and Mazzie, C. 1991. Prosody and focus in speech to infants and adults. *Developmental Psychology 27:* 209–21.

Flege, J. E. 1987. The production of "new" and "similar" phones in a foreign language: Evidence for the effect of equivalence classification. *Journal of Phonetics, 15:* 47–65.

Flege, J. E. 1989. Differences in inventory size affect the location but not the precision of tongue positioning in vowel production. *Language and Speech, 32:* 123–47.

Fonagy, I., and Fonagy, J. 1966. Sound pressure level and duration. *Phonetica, 15:* 14–21.

Fourgeron, C., and Keating, P. A. 1997. Articulatory strengthening at edges of prosodic domains. *Journal of the Acoustical Society of America, 101:* 3728–40.

Fowler, C. A., and Brancazio, L. 2000. Coarticulation resistance of American English consonants and its effects on transconsonantal vowel-to-vowel coarticulation. *Language and Speech, 43:* 1–41.

French, N., Carter, C., and Koenig, W. 1930. The words and sounds of telephone conversations. *Bell System Technical Journal 9:* 290–324.

French, P., and Local, J. 1986. Prosodic features and the management of interruptions. In *Intonation in Discourse,* ed. C. Johns-Lewis, 157–80. London: Croon Helm.

Fristoe, M., and Goldman, R. 1968. Comparison of traditional and condensed articulation tests examining the same number of sounds. *Journal of Speech and Hearing Research 11:* 583–89.

Fromkin, V., and Rodman, R. 1978. *An introduction to language.* 2d ed. New York: Holt, Rinehart & Winston.

Fry, D. 1955. Duration and intensity as physical correlates of linguistic stress. *Journal of the Acoustical Society of America 27:* 765–68.

Fry, D. B. 1958. Experiments in the perception of stress. *Language and Speech 1:* 126–52.

Fudge, E. C. 1969. Syllables. *Journal of Linguistics 5:* 193–320.

Gibbon, D. 1976. *Perspectives of intonation analysis. Forum linguisticum, band 9.* Bern: Herbert Lang.

Giles, S. B. 1971. A study of articulatory characteristics of /l/ allophones in English. Ph.D. dissertation, University of Iowa.

Gimson, A., 1970. *An introduction to the pronunciation of English.* 2d ed. New York: St. Martin's Press.

Gleason, H. 1961. *An introduction to descriptive linguistics.* New York: Holt, Rinehart & Winston.

Goldsmith, J. A. 1990. *Autosegmental and metrical phonology.* Oxford, England: Basil Blackwell.

Green, J. O., and Ravizza, S. M. 1995. Complexity effects on temporal characteristics of speech. *Human Communication Research, 21:* 390–421.

Gunderson, J. 1992. Perception of accelerated synthesized speech. Doctoral dissertation, University of Wisconsin, Madison.

Hargrove, P., and McGarr, N. 1993. *Prosody treatment: Working with and on prosody.* San Diego: Singular Publishing Group.

Hejna, R. 1955. *Hejna developmental articulation test.* Madison: Wisconsin College of Typing.

Hockett, C. 1958. *A course in modern linguistics.* New York: Macmillan.

Hoequist, C. E. 1983. Syllable duration in stress-, syllable-, and mora-timed languages. *Phonetica 40:* 203–37.

Hollien, H. 1980. Vocal indicators of psychological stress. In *Forensic psychology and psychiatry. Annals of the New York Academy of Sciences,* eds. F. Wright, C. Bahn, and R. W. Rieber. Vol. 347, 47–72.

Honikman, B. 1964. Articulatory settings. In D. Abercrombie (Ed.), *In honour of Daniel Jones* (pp. 73–84). London: Longmans.

Hooper, J. B. 1972. The syllable in linguistic theory. *Language 48:* 525–40.

Hubbell, A. 1950. *The pronunciation of English in New York City.* New York: Kings Crown Press.

Huber, J. E., Stathopoulos, E. T., Curione, G. M., Ash, T. A., and Johnson, K. 1999. Formants of children, women, and men: The effects of vocal intensity variation. *Journal of the Acoustical Society of America, 106:* 1532–42.

Hyman, L. 1975. *Phonology: Theory and analysis.* New York: Holt, Rinehart & Winston.

Ingram, D. 1989. *Phonological disability in children.* 2d ed. San Diego: Singular Publishing Group.

Irwin, J., Weston, A., Griffith, F., and Rocconi, C. 1976. Phoneme acquisition using the paired-stimuli technique in the public school setting. *Language, Speech and Hearing Services in Schools 7:* 220–29.

Jesperson, O. 1913. *Lehrbuch der phonetik,* 2d ed. Leipzig: B. G. Teubner.

Johns-Lewis, C., ed. 1986. *Intonation in discourse.* London: Croon Helm.

Jones, D. 1966. *The pronunciation of English,* 4th ed. Cambridge, England: Cambridge University Press.

Junqua, J.-C. 1993. The Lombard reflex and its role on human listeners and automatic speech recognizers. *Journal of the Acoustical Society of America, 93:* 510–24.

Kahn, D. 1980. Syllable-based generalizations in English phonology. Doctoral dissertation, Massachusetts Institute of Technology. New York: Garland Press.

Kantner, C., and West, R. 1941. *Phonetics.* New York: Harper & Row.

Keating, P. 1983. Comments on the jaw and syllable structure. *Journal of Phonetics 11:* 401–6.

Keating, P. A. 1990. The window model of coarticulation: Articulatory evidence. In J. Kingston and M. E. Beckman (Eds.), *Papers in laboratory phonology I. Between the grammar and physics of speech* (pp. 451–70). Cambridge, England: Cambridge University Press.

Kent, R. 1976. Anatomical and neuromuscular maturation of the speech mechanism: Evidence from acoustic studies. *Journal of Speech and Hearing Research 19:* 421–47.

Kent, R., and Moll, K. 1972. Cinefluorographic analyses of selected lingual consonants. *Journal of Speech and Hearing Research 15:* 453–73.

Kent, R. D. 1970. A cinefluorographic investigation of the component gestures in lingual articulation. Unpublished doctoral dissertation, University of Iowa, Iowa City, IA.

Kent, R. D. 1982. Contextual facilitation of correct sound production. *Language, Speech, and Hearing Services in Schools, 13:* 66–76.

Kent R. D., Mitchell, P. R., and Sancier, M. 1991. Evidence and role of rhythmic organization in early vocal development in human infants. In *The development of timing control and temporal organization in coordinated action,* eds. J. Fagard and P. Wolff, 135–49. Amsterdam: Elsevier.

Kent, R. D., and Netsell, R. 1971. Effects of stress contrasts on certain articulatory parameters. *Phonetica 24:* 23–44.

Kent, R. D., and Read, W. C. 2002. *The acoustic analysis of speech,* Albany, NY: Singular/Thomson Learning.

Kenyon, J. 1964. *American pronunciation.* 10th ed. Ann Arbor, MI: Wahr.

Kenyon, J., and Knott, T. 1953. *A pronouncing dictionary of American English.* Springfield, MA: Merriam.

Kerek, A. 1976. The phonological relevance of spelling pronunciation. *Visible Language 10:* 323–38.

Klatt, D. 1968. Structure of confusions in short-term memory between English consonants. *Journal of the Acoustical Society of America 44:* 401–7.

Klatt, D. 1976. Linguistic uses of segmental duration in English: Acoustic and perceptual evidence. *Journal of the Acoustical Society of America 59:* 1208–21.

Klatt, D. H. 1975. Vowel lengthening is syntactically determined in a connected discourse. *Journal of Phonetics, 3:* 129–40.

Ladefoged, P. 1971. *Preliminaries to linguistic phonetics.* Chicago: University of Chicago Press.

Ladefoged, P. 1975. *A course in phonetics.* New York: Harcourt Brace Jovanovich.

Ladefoged, P. 1993. *A course in phonetics.* 3rd ed. Fort Worth: Harcourt Brace Jovanovich.

Ladefoged, P., DeClerk, J., Lindau, M., and Papcun, G. 1972. An auditory-motor theory of speech production. *UCLA Working Papers in Phonetics,* No. 22, 48–75. Department of Linguistics, UCLA.

Landahl, K. H. 1980. Language-universal aspects of intonation to children's first sentences. *Journal of the Acoustical Society of America 67,* Suppl. 1: S63.

Laver, J. 1980. *The phonetic description of voice quality.* Cambridge, England: Cambridge University Press.

Lieberman, P. 1967. *Intonation, perception, and language.* Cambridge, MA: M.I.T. Press.

Lieberman, P., Katz, W., Jongman, A., Zimmerman, R., and Miller, M. 1985. Measures of the sentence intonation of read and spontaneous speech in American English. *Journal of the Acoustical Society of America 77:* 649–57.

Lieberman, P., and Tseng, C. Y. 1981. On the fall of the declination theory: Breath-group versus "declination" as the base form for intonation. *Journal of the Acoustical Society of America,* Suppl. *67:* S63.

Lienard, J. S., and Di Benedetto, M. G. 1999. Effect of vocal effort on spectral properties of vowels. *Journal of the Acoustical Society of America, 106:* 411–22.

Lindblom, B. 1990. Explaining phonetic variation: A sketch of the H&H theory. In *Speech production and speech modelling,* eds. W. J. Hardcastle and A. Marchal, 403–39. Amsterdam: Kluwer.

Lindblom, B., and Sundberg, B. 1969. A quantitative model of vowel production and the distinctive features of Swedish vowels. *Quarterly Progress and Status Report,* No. 1, 14–32. Speech Transmission Laboratory, Royal Institute of Technology, Stockholm.

Mackay, I. 1978. *Introducing practical phonetics.* Boston: Little, Brown.

Maddieson, I. 1984. *Patterns of sounds.* Cambridge, England: Cambridge University Press.

Maddieson, I., and Precoda, K. 1990. Updating UPSID. *UCLA Working Papers in Phonetics, 74:* 104–11.

Mader, J. 1954. The relative frequency of occurrence of English consonant sounds in words in the speech of children in grades one, two, and three. *Speech Monographs 21:* 294–300.

Maeda, S. 1976. *A characterization of American English intonation.* Cambridge, MA: M.I.T. Press.

Malmberg, B. 1963. *Phonetics.* New York: Dover.

Martin, J. G. 1972. Rhythmic (hierarchial) versus serial structure in speech and other behavior. *Psychological Review 79:* 487–509.

McCarthy, J. 1988. Feature geometry and dependency: A review. *Journal of Phonetics 43:* 84–108.

McDonald, E. 1964. *Articulation testing and treatment: A sensory-motor approach.* Pittsburgh: Stanwix House.

McDonald, E. 1968. *A screening deep test of articulation.* Pittsburgh: Stanwix House.

McSweeny, J. L., and Shriberg, L. D. 2001. Clinical research with the prosody-voice screening profile. *Clinical Linguistics and Phonetics, 15:* 505–28.

Mines, M., Hanson, B., and Shoup, J. 1978. Frequency of occurrence of phonemes in conversational English. *Language and Speech 21:* 221–41.

Mitchell, P. 1988. Phonetic variation and final syllable lengthening in multisyllable babbling. Doctoral dissertation, University of Wisconsin, Madison.

Moll, K. L., and Daniloff, R. G. 1971. Investigation of the timing of velar movements during speech. *Journal of the Acoustical Society of America, 50:* 678–84.

Morrison, J. A., and Shriberg, L. D. 1992. Articulation testing versus conversational speech sampling. *Journal of Speech and Hearing Research 35:* 259–73.

Moser, H. 1969. *One-syllable words.* Columbus, OH: Chas. E. Merrill.

Mowrer, D., Baker, R., and Schutz, R. 1970. *Modification of the frontal lisp: Programmed articulation control kit.* Palos Verdes Estates, Calif.: Educational Psychological Research Associates.

Mukherjee, J. 2000. Speech is silver, but silence is golden: Some remarks on the function(s) of pauses. *Anglia-Zeitschrift für Englische Philologie, 118:* 571–584.

Nearey, T. 1978. Phonetic feature systems for vowels. Ph.D. dissertation, University of Connecticut, 1977. Reproduced by Indiana University Linguistics Club.

Ogilvie, M., and Rees, N. 1969. *Communication skills: Voice and pronunciation.* New York: McGraw-Hill.

Oller, D. K. 1986. Metaphonology and infant vocalizations. In *Early precursors of speech,* eds. B. Lindblom and R. Zetterstrom, 21–35. Basingstoke: Macmillan.

Oller, D., and Eilers, R. 1975. Phonetic expectation and transcription validity. *Phonetica 31:* 288–304.

Oller, D., and Smith, B. 1977. Effect of final-syllable on vowel duration in infant babbling. *Journal of the Acoustical Society of America 62:* 994–97.

Otomo, K., and Stoel-Gammon, C. 1992. The acquisition of unrounded vowels in English. *Journal of Speech and Hearing Research 35:* 604–16.

Paynter, E., Ermey, J., Green, J., and Draper, D. 1978, November. Articulation development of English consonants in Mexican-American children. Paper presented at the American Speech and Hearing Association National Convention, San Francisco.

Perkell, J. 1969. *Physiology of speech sound production: Results and implications of a quantitative cineradiographic study.* Cambridge, MA: M.I.T. Press.

Perkell, J. 1971. Physiology of speech production: A preliminary study of two suggested revisions of the features specifying vowels. *Quarterly Progress Report,* No. 102. Cambridge, MA: M.I.T. Research Laboratory of Electronics.

Peterson, G., and Shoup, J. 1966. A physiological theory of phonetics. *Journal of Speech and Hearing Research 9:* 5–67.

Picheny, M. A., Durlach, N. I., and Braida, L. D. 1986. Speaking clearly for the hard of hearing. II.: Acoustic characteristics of clear and conversational speech. *Journal of Speech and Hearing Research 29:* 434–46.

Pickett, J. M. 1980. *The sounds of speech communication.* Baltimore: University Park Press.

Pike, K. 1943. *Phonetics.* Ann Arbor: University of Michigan Press.

Pike, K. 1947. *Phonemics.* Ann Arbor: University of Michigan Press.

Pollock, K. E. 1991. The identification of vowel errors using traditional articulation or phonological process test stimuli. *Language, Speech, and Hearing Services in Schools 22:* 39–50.

Pollock, K. E., and Keiser, N. J. 1990. An examination of vowel errors in phonologically disordered children. *Clinical Linguistics and Phonetics 4:* 161–78.

Prator, C., and Robinett, B. 1973. *A manual of English pronunciation.* 3rd ed. New York: Holt, Rinehart & Winston.

Price, P. J. 1980. Sonority and syllabicity: Acoustic correlates of perception. *Phonetica 37:* 327–43.

The Principles of the International Phonetic Association. 1949; revised to 1978. London: University College Department of Phonetics. Revised chart insert (1979) in *Journal of the International Phonetic Association 8* (1978).

Quiles, A. 1981. *Fonetica acustica de la lengua Espanola.* Madrid: Biblioteca Romanica Hispanica.

Ramig, L. 1975. Examiner bias in perceptual ratings of nasality in cleft palate speakers. Masters Thesis, University of Wisconsin–Madison.

Raphael, L., and Bell-Berti, F. 1975. Tongue musculature and the feature of tension in English vowels. *Phonetica 32:* 61–63.

Read, C., Buder, E. H., and Kent, R. D. 1990. Speech analysis systems: A survey. *Journal of Speech and Hearing Research 33:* 363–74.

Read, C., Buder, E. H., and Kent, R. D. 1992. Speech analysis systems: An evaluation. *Journal of Speech and Hearing Research 35:* 314–32.

Read, C., and Schreiber, P. A. 1982. Why short subjects are harder to find than long ones. In *Language acquisition: The state of the art,* eds. E. Wanner and L. Gleitman. Cambridge, England: Cambridge University Press.

Recasens, D. 1985. Coarticulatory patterns and degrees of coarticulatory resistance in Catalan CV sequences. *Language and Speech, 28:* 97–114.

Recasens, D., Pallares, M. D., and Fontdevila, J. 1997. A model of lingual coarticulation based on articulatory constraints. *Journal of the Acoustical Society of America, 102:* 544–61.

Renfrew, C. 1966. Persistence of the open syllable in defective articulation. *Journal of Speech and Hearing Disorders 31:* 370–73.

Roberts, A. 1965. *A statistical linguistic analysis of American English.* The Hague, Netherlands: Mouton.

Rochester, S. 1972. The significance of pauses in spontaneous speech. *Journal of Psycholinguistic Research 2:* 51–81.

Rostolland, D. 1982. Acoustic features of shouted voice. *Acustica, 51:* 80–89.

Rousey, C., and Moriarity, A. 1965. *Diagnostic implications of speech sounds.* Springfield, Ill.: Charles C. Thomas.

Russell, G. 1928. *The vowel.* Columbus: Ohio State University Press.

Sapir, E. 1921. *Language: An introduction to the study of speech.* New York: Harcourt Brace Jovanovich.

Saporta, S. 1955. Frequency of consonant clusters. *Language 31:* 25–30.

Schulman, R. 1989. Articulatory dynamics of loud and normal speech. *Journal of the Acoustical Society of America, 85:* 295–312.

Schwartz, J. L., Boe, L. J., Vallee, N., and Abry, C. 1997. Major trends in vowel system inventories. *Journal of Phonetics, 25:* 233–53.

Selkirk, E. 1982. The syllable. In *The structure of phonological representations,* Part II, eds. H. van der Hulst and N. Smith. Dordrecht: Foris Publications.

Selkirk, E. O. 1984. *Phonology and syntax: The relation between sound and structure.* Cambridge, MA: M.I.T. Press.

Shriberg, L. 1972. Articulation judgments. Some perceptual considerations. *Journal of Speech and Hearing Research, 15:* 876–82.

Shriberg, L. 1975. A response evocation program for /ɝ/. *Journal of Speech and Hearing Disorders 40:* 92–105.

Shriberg, L. 1980a. Developmental phonological disorders. In *Introduction to Communication Disorders,* eds. T. Hixon, L. Shriberg, and J. Saxman. Englewood Cliffs, NJ: Prentice-Hall.

Shriberg, L. D. 1980b. An intervention procedure for children with persistent /r/ errors. *Language, Speech, and Hearing Services in Schools 11:* 102–10.

Shriberg, L. D. 1993. Four new speech and prosody-voice measures for genetics research and other studies in developmental phonological disorders. *Journal of Speech and Hearing Research 36:* 105–40.

Shriberg, L. D., Allen, C. T., McSweeny, J. L., and Wilson, D. L. 2001. PEPPER: Programs to examine phonetic and phonologic evaluation records [Computer software]. Madison, WI: Waisman Center, University of Wisconsin.

Shriberg, L. D., Hinke, R., and Trost-Steffen, C. 1987. A procedure to select and train persons for narrow phonetic transcription by consensus. *Clinical Linguistics and Phonetics 1:* 171–89.

Shriberg, L., and Kwiatkowski, J. 1980. *Natural process analyses (NPA): A procedure for phonological analyses of continuous speech samples.* New York: John Wiley.

Shriberg, L. D., and Kwiatkowski, J. 1985. Continuous speech sampling for phonologic analyses of speech-delayed children. *Journal of Speech and Hearing Disorders 50:* 323–34.

Shriberg, L. D., and Kwiatkowski, J. 1994. Developmental phonological disorders. I.: A clinical profile. *Journal of Speech and Hearing Research, 37:* 1100–26.

Shriberg, L. D., Kwiatkowski, J., and Rassmussen, C. 1990. *Prosody-voice screening profile (PVSP).* Tucson, AZ: Communication Skill Builders.

Shriberg, L., and Swisher, W. 1972, November. Development of an articulation scoring training program (ASTP). Paper presented at the American Speech and Hearing Association National Convention, San Francisco.

Shriberg, L. D., and Widder, C. J. 1990. Speech and prosody characteristics of adults with mental retardation. *Journal of Speech and Hearing Research 33:* 627–53.

Silverman, K., and Pierrehumbert, J. B. 1990. The timing of pre-nuclear high accents in English. In *Papers in laboratory phonology I: Between the grammar and the physics of speech.* eds. J. Kingston and M. E. Beckman. Cambridge, England: Cambridge University Press.

Smit, A. B., and Bernthal, J. E. 1983. Voicing contrasts and their phonological implications in the speech of articulation-disordered children. *Journal of Speech and Hearing Research 26:* 486–500.

Smith, M. R., Cutler, A., Butterfield, S., and Nimmo-Smith, I. 1989. The perception of rhythm and word boundaries in noise-masked speech. *Journal of Speech and Hearing Research 32:* 912–20.

Sorensen, J. M., and Cooper, W. E. 1980. Syntactic coding of fundamental frequency in speech production. In *Perception and production of fluent speech,* ed. R. A. Cole, 399–440. Hillsdale, NJ: Lawrence Erlbaum.

Stetson, R. 1951. *Motor phonetics.* 2d ed. Amsterdam: North-Holland.

Stephens, I., and Daniloff, R. 1974, November. Trouble with /s/. Paper presented to the American Speech and Hearing Association National Convention, Las Vegas.

Stevens, K., and House, A. 1955. Development of a quantitative description of vowel articulation. *Journal of the Acoustical Society of America 27:* 484–93.

Stoel-Gammon, C., and Harrington, P. B. 1990. Vowel systems of normally developing and phonologically disordered children. *Clinical Linguistics and Phonetics 4:* 145–60.

Sweet, H. 1877. *A handbook of phonetics.* Oxford: Clarendon Press.

Tabain, M. 2001. Variability in fricative production and spectra: Implications for the hyper- and hypo- and quantal theories of speech production. *Language and Speech, 44:* 57–94.

Thomas, C. 1958. *An introduction to the phonetics of American English.* 2d ed. New York: The Ronald Press.

Thorsen, N. G. 1985. Intonation and text in standard Danish. *Journal of the Acoustical Society of America 77:* 1205–16.

Tiffany, W., and Carrell, J. 1977. *Phonetics: Theory and application.* 2d ed. New York: McGraw-Hill.

Trager, G., and Smith, H. 1951. *An outline of English structure. Studies in linguistics: Occasional papers,* No. 3. Norman, OK: Battenberg Press.

Traugott, E., and Pratt, M. 1980. *Linguistics for students of literature.* New York: Harcourt Brace Jovanovich.

Traunmuller, H., and Eriksson, A. 1995. The perceptual evaluation of F_0 excursions in speech as evidenced in liveliness estimations. *Journal of the Acoustical Society of America, 97:* 1905–15.

Traunmuller, H., and Eriksson, A. 2000. Acoustic effects of variation in vocal effort by men, women, and children. *Journal of the Acoustical Society of America, 107:* 3438–51.

Trim, J. 1953. Some suggestions for the phonetic notation of sounds in defective speech. *Speech 17:* 21–24.

Trost, J. E. 1981. Articulatory additions to the classic description of the speech of persons with cleft palate. *Cleft Palate Journal, 18:* 193–203.

Van den Heuvel, H., Cranen, B., and Rietveld, T. 1996. Speaker variability in the coarticulation of /a, i, u/. *Speech Communication, 18:* 113–130.

Venneman, T. 1972. On the theory of syllabic phonology. *Linguistische Berichte 18:* 1–18.

Webster's New International Dictionary. 1956. 2d ed. Springfield, MA: Merriam.

Webster's Third New International Dictionary. 1961. Springfield, MA: Merriam.

Wightman, C. W., Shuttuck-Hufnagel, S., Ostendorf, M., and Price, P. J. 1992. Segmental durations in the vicinity of prosodic phrase boundaries. *Journal of the Acoustical Society of America, 91:* 1707–17.

Winitz, H. 1969. *Articulatory acquisition and behavior.* New York: Appleton-Century-Crofts.

Wise, C. 1957. *Applied phonetics.* Englewood Cliffs, NJ: Prentice-Hall.

Wise, C. 1957. *Introduction to phonetics.* Englewood Cliffs, NJ: Prentice-Hall.

Zawadzki, P., and Kuehn, D. 1980. A cineradiographic study of static and dynamic aspects of American English /r/. *Phonetica 37:* 253–66.

Zlatin-Laufer, M. 1980. Temporal regularity in prespeech. In *Infant communication: Cry and early speech,* eds. T. Murray and A. Murray. Houston: College-Hill Press.

Index

Note: Page numbers for exercise answers are in italics